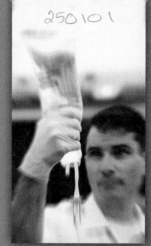

PHARMACOLOGY *for the*
PREHOSPITAL PROFESSIONAL

JEFFREY S. GUY, MD, FACS

MOSBY JEMS

ELSEVIER

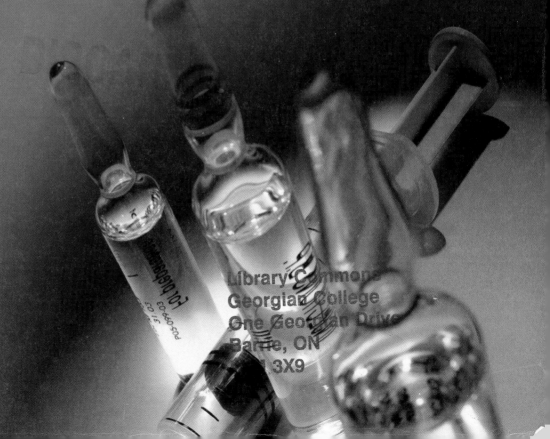

MOSBY JEMS
ELSEVIER

11830 Westline Industrial Drive
St. Louis, Missouri 63146

PHARMACOLOGY FOR THE PREHOSPITAL PROFESSIONAL

ISBN: 978-0-323-03590-3

Notice

Knowledge and best practice in this field are constantly changing. As new research and experience broaden our knowledge, changes in practice, treatment and drug therapy may become necessary or appropriate. Readers are advised to check the most current information provided (i) on procedures featured or (ii) by the manufacturer of each product to be administered, to verify the recommended dose or formula, the method and duration of administration, and contraindications. It is the responsibility of the practitioner, relying on their own experience and knowledge of the patient, to make diagnoses, to determine dosages and the best treatment for each individual patient, and to take all appropriate safety precautions. To the fullest extent of the law, neither the Publisher nor the Author assumes any liability for any injury and/or damage to persons or property arising out or related to any use of the material contained in this book.

The Publisher

Library of Congress Control Number 2007921551

Executive Editor: Linda Honeycutt
Associate Developmental Editor: Mary Jo Adams
Publishing Services Manager: Julie Eddy
Senior Project Manager: Laura Loveall
Design Manager: Margaret Reid

Printed in Canada

Last digit is the print number: 9 8 7 6 5 4 3 2 1

To my wife, Deanna, and my children
Danielle, Christian, Madeline, Spencer, and Layne
I love all of you, and I am blessed.

Contributors

Deanna L. Aftab Guy, MD
Assistant Professor of Pediatrics, Division of Pediatric
  Endocrinology
Vanderbilt University Medical Center
Nashville, Tennessee
Vanderbilt Children's Hospital
Nashville, Tennessee

Angela Allen, RN, MSN, ACNP-BC, CCRN, NREMT-B
Nurse Educator
Vanderbilt University Medical Center Burn Center
Nashville, Tennessee

Will Chapleau, EMT-P, RN, TNS
Manager, ATLS Program
American College of Surgeons
Chicago, Illinois

Gregory J. Chapman, BS, RRT, REMT-P
Program Director
Institute of Prehospital Emergency Medicine
Hudson Valley Community College
Troy, New York

Brenna Michelle Farmer, MD
Emergency Medicine Resident Physician
Vanderbilt University Department of Emergency
  Medicine
Vanderbilt University Medical Center
Nashville, Tennessee

William W. Goldsmith, D.O.
Assistant Professor of Clinical Anesthesiology
Vanderbilt University Medical Center
Nashville, Tennessee
Staff Anesthesiologist
Sacred Heart Hospital
Pensacola, Florida

Kirby R. Gross, MD, FACS
Commander
772nd Forward Surgical Team
Fort Campbell, Kentucky

Michelle M. McLean, MD, NREMT-P
Emergency Physician
Emergency Care Center
Covenant Hospital
Saginaw, Michigan

Leanna R. Miller, RN, MN, CCRN, CEN, NP
Assistant in Surgery
Vanderbilt University Medical School
Nashville, Tennessee
Educator: Trauma, Burn, Life Flight
Vanderbilt University Medical Center
Nashville, Tennessee

**Deanna Moore, RN, MSN, ACNP-BC, CCRN,
  NREMT-P, FP-C**
Acute Care Nurse Practitioner
Neurocare ICU
Vanderbilt University Hospital
Nashville, Tennessee

**Mary Jane Pavlick, RN, BA, AAS, CEN, EMT-P,
  EMS-I**
Guest Instructor
School of EMS, Cleveland Clinic Health System,
  Eastern Region
Euclid, Ohio
Human Resources Development
Hillcrest Hospital
Mayfield Heights, Ohio
Program Manager, Emergency Management
Hillcrest Hospital
Mayfield Heights, Ohio

Corey M. Slovis, MD, FACP, FACEP
Professor of Emergency Medicine
Chairman, Department of Emergency Medicine
Vanderbilt University School of Medicine
Nashville, Tennessee
Medical Director
Nashville Fire Department
Nashville, Tennessee

Steven J. White, MD, FACEP, FAAP
Assistant Professor of Emergency Medicine and
  Pediatrics
Vanderbilt University School of Medicine
Nashville, Tennessee
Emergency Department Attending Physician
Vanderbilt University Medical Center
Monroe Carrell Jr. Childrens' Hospital
Nashville, Tennessee

Stephen R. Wirth, Esq., M.S., EMT-P
Partner
Page, Wolfberg & Wirth, LLC
Mechanicsburg, Pennsylvania
Adjunct Professor
University of Pittsburgh EMS Program
Pittsburgh, Pennsylvania
Adjunct Professor
George Washington University EMS Program
Washington, DC

Douglas M. Wolfberg, JD, BS, EMT-A
Partner
Page, Wolfberg & Wirth, LLC
Mechanicsburg, Pennsylvania
Adjunct Professor
Widener University School of Law
Harrisburg, Pennsylvania
Adjunct Professor
University of Pittsburgh EMS Program
Pittsburgh, Pennsylvania
Adjunct Professor
George Washington University EMS Program
Washington, DC

Reviewers

The editors wish to acknowledge and thank the many reviewers of this book who devoted countless hours to intensive review. Their comments were invaluable in helping develop and fine tune the manuscript.

David K. Anderson, BS, EMT-P
Director, Paramedic Education Program
Northwest Regional Training Center
Vancouver, Washington

Jeffrey K. Benes, BS, NREMT-P
Owner/Consultant/Educator
Jeff Benes Company
Antioch, Illinois

Chip Boehm, RN, EMT-P/FF
EMS Educator
Portland Fire Department
Portland, Maine

Robert P. Breese, EMT-P, FP-C
Monroe Community College
Rochester, New York

Rob Brouhard, AA, EMT-P
Modesto, California

Anthony J. Brunello, RN, BS, PHRN, TNS, EMS-LI
Provena St. Mary's Hospital
Kankakee, Illinois

JoAnn Cobble, EdD, NREMT-P, RN
Dean, Division of Health Professions
Oklahoma City Community College
Oklahoma City, Oklahoma

Peter Connick, REMTP, EMT I/C
Adjunct Faculty
Cape Cod Community College
West Barnstable, Massachusetts
Captain, Chatham Fire Rescue
Chatham, Massachusetts

Ken Davis, NREMT-P, CCEMT-P, FP-C
Paramedic Coordinator
Eastern New Mexico University
Roswell, New Mexico

Daryl D. DePestel, PharmD
Clinical Assistant Professor
University of Michigan College of Pharmacology
Ann Arbor, Michigan

Dennis Edgerly, EMT-P
EMS Instructor
HealthONE EMS
Englewood, Colorado

John F. Elder, CCEMT-P, EMT-P
Director of Education
CareFlight
Fort Worth, Texas

Sloan B. Fleming, PharmD
Vanderbilt University Medical Center
Nashville, Tennessee

Fidel O. Garcia, EMT-P
EMS Education Coordinator
St. Mary's Hospital
Grand Junction, Colorado

Danna S. Hatley, PharmD
East Alabama Medical Center
Opelika, Alabama

Chad S. Kim, BA, NREMT-P, I/C
Paramedic/Firefighter Instructor/Coordinator
University of New Mexico EMSA
Eastern New Mexico University
Roswell, New Mexico
Albuquerque Fire Department
Albuquerque, New Mexico

Michael W. Lynch, AS, CCEMT-P, NREMT-P
Administrative Director
Grozer Chester Medical Center
Media, Pennsylvania

Dean Martin, AAS, EMT-P
Division Chief
Fire Marshal/Training/EMS Division
Columbia Fire Department
Columbia, Missouri

Denise Martin, MS
Oakland Community College
Auburn Hills, Michigan

Joanne McCall, RN, BAS, MA, CEN, CFN, SANE-A
Providence Park Hospital
Novi, Michigan

Christine C. McEachin, RN, BSN, CEN, Paramedic/IC
Clinical Nurse Specialist—Emergency Services
William Beaumont Hospital—Troy
Troy, Michigan

Greg Mullen, BS, MS, NREMT-P
Education Coordinator
National EMS Academy
Lafayette, Louisiana

Deborah L. Petty, EMT-P I/C
Paramedic Training Officer
St. Charles County Ambulance District
St. Peters, Missouri

Lynn Pierzchalski-Goldstein, PharmD
Clinical Coordinator Pharmacy
Penrose St. Francis Health System
Colorado Springs, Colorado

Gregg D. Ramirez, BS, EMT-P
Student Services Director
Army Medical Department, Northwest Regional
    Training Center
Vancouver, Washington

Ken Reardon, Flight Paramedic
LifeNet New York
Valhalla, New York

Judith A. Ruple, PhD, RN, NREMT-P
The Ruple Group/Education Consultants
The Villages, Flordia
Professor (Retired)
University of Toledo
Toledo, Ohio

Janet L. Schulte, BS, AS, NR-CCEMT-P
Director of Continuing Education
IHM Health Studies Center
St. Louis, Missouri

Stephen M. Setter, PharmD, CDE, CGP, DVM
Associate Professor of Pharmacotherapy
Washington State University—Spokane
Elder Services, Visiting Nurses Association
Spokane, Washington

Douglas R. Smith, MAT, EMT-P, I/C
Educational Consultant
Platinum Educational Group, LLC
Jenison, Michigan

David L. Sullivan, PhD(c), NREMT-P
St. Petersburg College EMS/CE
Pinellas Park, Flordia

Anthony Tedesco, RN, NREMT-P
St. Petersburg College
Pinellas Park, Flordia

Donna G. Tidwell, BS, RN, EMT-P
Director of EMS Personnel Licensure and Education
Tennessee Department of Health Division of EMS
Nashville, Tennessee

Preface

Finally, a textbook that makes pharmacology for prehospital providers easy and understandable! This text puts EMS pharmacology in perspective and presents information the way you learn it and use it—case-by-case and step-by-step.

This textbook uses a problem-solving approach through clinical scenarios for adult and pediatric patients. Since it is task-oriented, you are able to learn the next step—administering the drug—right along with the scenario. *You will learn the material using the same methods that you will apply the material during the care of the ill or injured!*

Chapters include scenarios to illustrate learning objectives. Each time a drug is introduced, a photograph of the medication is presented to orient you, along with an overview of the drug and the indications for use. Special boxes are also included to provide helpful tips. Detailed information about drug administration, tailored to the prehospital professional, is included for every drug introduced, including classification, action, indication, adverse effects, contraindications, dosage, and special considerations. This text contains over 90 profiles of drugs commonly used in the prehospital setting and most-commonly prescribed.

The Companion DVD includes several medical animations that will be beneficial to your training. It also includes video demonstration of critical skills. The skills are listed step-by-step in the book. An icon is next to the skill title indicating that the skill also appears in the Companion DVD.

Acknowledgments

Pharmacology for the Prehospital Professional would not have been possible without the support of all of the contributing authors. I would like to thank the following individuals:

Katherine Tomber and Linda Honeycutt from Elsevier for their endless support and technical assistance. Without either of them this project would have never have gotten off of the ground.

Missi Jarboe for always being willing to help me and my family in virtually any capacity. I value your help and your friendship.

John Howser and Anne Rayner for their assistance with the photography.

Most of all I would like to thank my wife, Deanna, for her patience, support, and love. She has been exceedingly patient while I worked on this project.

Jeffrey S. Guy, MD, FACS

Contents

PHARMACOLOGY *for the*
PREHOSPITAL PROFESSIONAL

JEFFREY S. GUY

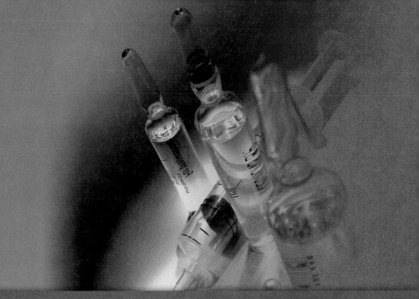

PART

I

Foundations

CHAPTER 1

Principles of Pharmacology

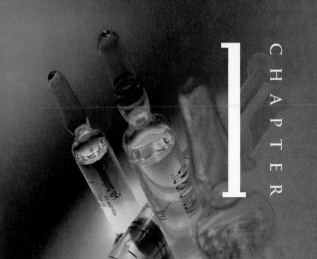

OBJECTIVES

1. Explain the difference between a drug's generic name and trade name.
2. Explain the concepts of pharmacology, pharmacokinetics, receptor interactions, and pharmacodynamics.
3. Explain the dose-response relationship.
4. Define enteral and parenteral medications and identify the routes of administration for each.
5. Explain first-pass metabolism.
6. Explain the process of drug metabolism and excretion.
7. Define passive diffusion, carrier-mediated facilitated diffusion, active transport, and passive transport.
8. Explain the difference and relationship between an agonist drug and antagonist drug.
9. Explain the role of the autonomic nervous system and alpha$_1$, alpha$_2$, beta$_1$, and beta$_2$ receptors.
10. Discuss medications used to stimulate the adrenergic receptors: epinephrine, norepinephrine (Levophed), dopamine, dobutamine, and phenylephrine (Neo-Synephrine).
11. Discuss medications used to block the adrenergic receptors: atropine sulfate and scopolamine (Transderm-Scop).

Medications that Appear in Chapter 1

Dopamine (Intropin)
Norepinephrine (Levophed)
Dobutamine (Dobutrex)
Phenylephrine (Neo-Synephrine)
Epinephrine
Propranolol (Inderal)
Labetalol (Normodyne, Trandate)
Metoprolol (Lopressor, Toprol XL)
Atenolol (Tenormin)
Atropine sulfate
Scopolamine (Transderm Scop)

Your unit is dispatched to a medical call with the report of a 42-year-old woman who has collapsed. The information you receive from the dispatcher is that her brother found her prone on the floor and that she is nonresponsive to his attempts to awaken her. The patient's brother is not aware of any preexisting medical conditions. When you arrive, you find a 42-year-old woman lying on the floor approximately 4 feet from a flight of stairs. Her family has moved her to the supine position. Some vomit has pooled next to her head, and she has some vomit on her face.

An unresponsive individual, or "man down," presents several challenges. What are the potential causes of this patient's altered level of consciousness? Cardiac arrhythmia, diabetic emergency, seizure, toxic ingestion or overdose, stroke, and traumatic brain injury are only a few of the potential causes. The treatment of each of these conditions requires unique pharmacologic interventions.

The treatment priorities for this patient are the same as for all patients: scene safety, airway, breathing, and circulation. You kneel down next to the patient and ensure that her airway is patent and free of vomitus. Her respirations are spontaneous and unlabored. Your partner checks her oxygen saturation reading and reports that it is 93%. While you place a nonrebreather oxygen mask, you also place her on the cardiac monitor and learn that she is in sinus tachycardia. She begins to have a violent tonic-clonic seizure. Your partner protects her head and closely monitors her airway.

Seizures have several causes, but your immediate priorities include ensuring airway patency and protecting the patient from harm. As the paramedic in charge you consider your options for stopping the current seizure, preventing additional seizures, preventing potential metabolic complications of seizures, and investigating the potential causes of the seizure that may require emergency treatment. What are the appropriate drugs for the treatment of seizures? What is the most rapid way of delivering those drugs? What if the routes of drug administration cannot be obtained or fail? Are additional routes of drug administration available? Is the patient taking any medications that may interact with the emergency medications? What are some of the adverse effects of the emergency medications to monitor for during and after administration? Does the patient have any allergies or conditions that contraindicate any medications? Does the patient have kidney or liver disease that may require a reduction in drug dosages?

INTRODUCTION

Pharmacology can be a challenging topic for any healthcare professional to master. Thousands of drugs are in use, all of which have specific actions, indications, dosages, and **adverse effects.** Several methods of administering drugs exist as well, depending on the drug and the patient. Providing drug therapy to patients in hectic emergency situations in which little time is available to reflect or consult a reference text is particularly challenging.

Try not to approach pharmacology as a topic that requires memorization of a multitude of facts and dosages. Instead, approach it as an opportunity to synthesize and apply all the information you have learned while studying anatomy, physiology, and the management of specific diseases. As you read this text, intermittently stop and reflect on how you will use the information to take action during an emergency. Get comfortable reciting the names and dosages of these medications. Imagine a singer who practices a song to become familiar with the lyrics. The first time you say "epinephrine 1 mg IV push" should not be at the bedside of a critical patient. When you go through this text, practice saying the names of these drugs and their dosages. Take time to study the photographs of the drugs and imagine yourself requesting a particular medication, getting it out of a box, and administering that medication to a patient. Athletes and surgeons often visualize each step of a particular event or operation before their performance. As a prehospital provider, patients' lives depend on your optimal performance. Mental rehearsal will make the topic of pharmacology more interesting and familiar.

DRUG NAMES

Many medications have complex-sounding names. You do not need to know every name of every medication you might encounter while providing emergency care. However, you must be able to recognize, document, and communicate important information about various medications that patients may be taking and you may be administering.

All drugs have at least two names: generic and trade. The **generic name** is usually an abbreviated version of the drug's chemical name. The generic name is registered with the U.S. Food and Drug Administration (FDA) and listed in a directory of medications known as the **United States Pharmacopeia-National Formulary (USP-NF).** Generic drug names are written in lower case and are also known as *nonproprietary names.*

A drug's **trade name** is created by pharmaceutical companies. When a pharmaceutical company discovers a new drug, scientists assign it a chemical name that describes its chemical structure, which is often long and difficult to remember. The manufacturer proposes a generic (nonproprietary) name to the FDA for approval. The generic name often is an abbreviated form of the chemical name. The company then creates a memorable and descriptive trade name (also known as a *proprietary* or *brand name*). Trade names always begin with a capital letter. In this text, the generic name is listed first, with the trade name in parentheses after it. The *Physician's Desk Reference* is an example of a reference that provides an exhaustive catalog of drug information. Table 1-1 shows examples of the generic and trade names of several common drugs, including their indications for use.

TABLE 1-1

Examples of Generic and Trade Names

Generic Name	Trade Name	Indication
albuterol	Ventolin	Asthma
nitroglycerin	Nitrostat	Angina
sotalol hydrochloride	Betapace	Ventricular arrhythmia
tamsulosin hydrochloride	Flomax	Benign prostatitic hypertrophy

GENERAL PRINCIPLES

Discussions about pharmacology are all too often approached as chemistry lessons. However, the information regarding any drug is relatively constant no matter which drug is being discussed.

When approaching pharmacology in general terms, consider the following questions:

▶ How does the drug get in the body?
▶ How does the drug move around the body?
▶ Which tissues is the drug able to reach?
▶ What makes the drug work?
▶ How is the drug broken down?
▶ How is the drug removed from the body?

Four major concepts address these topics: pharmacology, **pharmacokinetics,** receptor interactions, and **pharmacodynamics.** Pharmacology is the study of the biochemical and physiologic properties of medications (the suffix *-ology* means "the study of"; therefore *pharmacology* means *the study of drugs*). Some of the properties of medications include **mechanism of action,** indications, adverse effects, contraindications, and toxicity.

The pharmacology of a medication is different from its pharmacokinetics. *Kinetic* refers to movement, so pharmacokinetics refers to how a medication acts, including how it is absorbed into the bloodstream **(absorption),** how it is distributed throughout the body **(distribution),** how the body metabolizes the drug (biotransformation), and finally, how it is eliminated (elimination).

Receptors are the sites on various tissues to which drugs bind to exert their desired physiologic effects. When explaining receptors, the analogy to a lock and key is often made; the drug is the key, and the receptor is the lock. Drug/receptor interactions "unlock" the drugs to act on the target tissue.

Pharmacodynamics explains how a drug works and interacts with various receptors, other drugs, and **enzyme** systems within the body.

Absorption is the movement of a medication from the point of administration (e.g., gastrointestinal (GI) tract, skin, muscle) into the bloodstream for movement throughout the body. Two factors that affect the absorption of a drug are the dosage and the route of administration. (Absorption is discussed in greater detail later in the chapter.)

MEDICATION DOSAGE

The **dose** of a medication is the amount of medication administered, often referred to in a unit of measure such as milligram (mg) or gram (g). The **dosage** of a medication is the size, frequency, and number of doses to be administered, such as 50 mg every 4 hours. Dosage is important in determining the concentration of the drug at the site of action. Typically, the higher the dosage, the higher the concentration of the medication at the site of action. The greater the amount of drug at the site of action, the greater the physiologic effect. Typically, as the dosage of a medication increases, so does the physiologic effect manifested by the drug. This effect continues to increase with increasing doses of the medication up to a point at which increasing the medication no longer produces an increase in the desired physiologic effect. This phenomenon is referred to as a **dose-response relationship** or **dose-response curve** (Fig. 1-1).

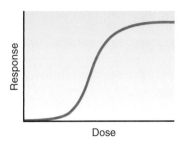

▼ **Fig. 1-1** Dose-response curve: Increasing the dose of a medication increases the physiologic effect. The physiologic effect increases to a point at which an increase in dose does not result in any further increase in the desired physiologic effect.

MEDICATION FORMS AND ROUTES

Medications come in different forms, and a single medication commonly comes in a variety of forms. The appropriate *form of medication* often is determined by the nature and urgency of the medical problem that the drug is being used to treat. To introduce the concept of the various forms of medications, consider the following patient.

> Your unit is called to a downtown office building, where a woman is having a severe asthma attack. You arrive and are escorted to a fifth-floor office by building security. There you find a 23-year-old woman bent over in a chair. She is clearly in distress, with labored breathing. Your partner takes her vital signs while you set her up with oxygen. Her blood pressure is 118/68 mm Hg, heart rate is 112 beats/min, respiratory rate is 36 breaths/min, and pulse oximeter reading is 92%.

Someone having an asthma attack needs immediate relief. Oral medications, such as a capsule or tablet, need to be swallowed, digested, absorbed, and then circulated through the body; the patient may not get relief for 30 minutes to 1 hour. Therefore, in the emergent circumstance of an asthma attack, an oral medication is inappropriate. Oral medications are appropriate for the treatment of stable, chronic conditions such as hypertension or acute, non–life-threatening conditions. Aspirin is perhaps the most commonly recognized oral medication. Everyone is aware that when taking aspirin for a headache or muscle ache, a certain amount of time must elapse before feeling any relief. This delay is because aspirin must be swallowed and travel to the stomach, where it is broken down, absorbed in the intestine, passed through the bloodstream, and delivered to the desired site of action. This delay of 20 to 60 minutes for administration of an oral medication for symptomatic relief could potentially be problematic and catastrophic for patients having an asthma attack. Asthma medications that are given orally (e.g., terbutaline [Brethine], metaproterenol [Alupent], and theophylline) are typically not used during an acute asthma attack and would be inappropriate for the patient described in the preceding scenario.

Enteral medications are drugs that are absorbed through the GI tract. Enteral medications, which are given orally or rectally, have several disadvantages. To swallow oral medications, the patient must be conscious and cooperative. Medications absorbed through the GI tract must first pass through the liver before being distributed throughout the body. At this point the drug is often partially metabolized, which reduces the amount of medication available for distribution to the body. This is called **first-pass metabolism. Enteral administration** has other disadvantages, including a variable rate of absorption, potential irritation of the mucous lining of the stomach or intestine, and patient noncompliance.

Enteral medication administration also has many advantages. It is by far the most common and safest route of drug administration. The delivery of the medication into the circulation is slow after oral administration. The slow absorption of medications into the bloodstream prevents rapid and high blood levels that often lead to adverse effects. An additional advantage of oral medications is the convenience of delivering medications without a need for sterile technique.

Parenteral medications are drugs that bypass the GI tract. **Injectable medications** are parenteral medications that can be injected directly into a muscle **(intramuscular [IM])**, a vein **(intravenous [IV])**, or the subcutaneous tissue **(subcutaneous [Sub-Q])**. Injectable medications are rapidly available and circulate throughout the body, often in minutes. The drawback of injectable medication administration is that it requires special training and, in the case of IV medications, special equipment. IV is the preferred route of administration for cardiac medications in advanced life support situations. An example of an IV medication is epinephrine. Epinephrine is a powerful drug capable of stimulating the heart to function better and faster, as well as causing relaxation of the smooth muscle that surrounds the bronchial tree. Epinephrine is typically used in the treatment of cardiac arrest, asthma attacks, and anaphylaxis. These are life-threatening emergencies that require rapid and dependable delivery of this medication. Administration of epinephrine by an IV route allows the medication to be delivered much more rapidly than if it were able to be given enterally.

To achieve a rapid therapeutic concentration of some drugs in a life-threatening emergency, a **loading dose** must be administered. Factors that determine a particular loading dose are the desired serum concentration of the drug and the volume of distribution. In emergency situations, loading doses are administered intravenously to achieve rapid 100% bioavailability of the drug. **Bioavailabilty** is the percentage of an administered drug that is available in the bloodstream to act at the target tissue. Let us illustrate this in the form of net (or take-home) pay on your paycheck. We are painfully aware that the amount on the top line of our paycheck is not the amount of money we get to take home to pay the rent and buy groceries. For the sake of this example, let us consider a paycheck with a gross amount of $1000. From that initial amount of $1000 comes federal and state income taxes, which decrease the amount of money available to take home.

Gross pay:	$1000
− Federal taxes:	$350
− State taxes:	$150
Net pay (take-home)	$500

When an enteral medication is administered (orally or rectally), not all of that medication is absorbed by the GI tract, and of the percentage that is absorbed a fraction is broken down and metabolized by the liver. The fraction of the medication that is available in the bloodstream, or bioavailable fraction, is similar to net pay.

If 1000 mg of a particular medication (medication X) is administered as a tablet (enteral administration), perhaps 35% is not absorbed by the intestine; 15% gets metabolized by the liver. That leaves only 50% (i.e., 500 mg of medication X) of the administered medication available to the bloodstream and ultimately the target tissue.

Dose administered:	1000 mg
− Amount not absorbed by the intestine	350 mg
− Amount metabolized in liver first-pass	150 mg
Bioavailable dose	500 mg

In an emergency, when a medication is given as an IV bolus, the administered dose is delivered directly into the bloodstream. IV administration of medications increases the bioavailability of the dose by removing factors such as variability in absorption from the GI tract and first-pass metabolism.

Maintenance doses maintain an average concentration of a drug at serum-steady states. In the absence of a loading dose, five half-lives must pass to achieve a steady state of the drug concentration.

A **half-life** of a medication is the time required for the concentration of a medication in the bloodstream to decrease to half of its original level. Half-life is different from the duration of action. Duration of action is the amount of time a single dose of a medication produces the desired effect. A car filled with gasoline may be able to drive 500 miles before running out of gas. When the gas gauge is on half a tank, the level of gasoline is at half of its original level. The distance the car could drive until the amount of gas in the tank was decreased to half a tank would be the equivalent of half-life. Despite having only a half a tank of gas, the car is still able to run until the there is not enough gas to power the engine, or an empty tank. The distance that the car can run using the gasoline in the tank is the duration of action. Therefore, in the car example, the half-life is 250 miles, and the duration of action is 500 miles. Although this example simplifies these concepts, it does illustrate the terms. Clearly there are differences between gasoline in an automobile and the concentration of a medication in a patient's blood. The engine of a car will run until the tank is emptied, but a medication will lose its desired biologic effect long before the serum concentrations are zero.

Let's go back to our hypothetical drug, medication X. The usual dose of medication X is 1000 mg administered intravenously every 12 hours. Medication X has a half-life of 12 hours. Without a loading dose, it takes approximately 5 doses for the level of the medication in the blood to approach a steady state of drug concentration. To illustrate the concept of loading doses and half-life, watch what happens to the serum drug levels at the end of each half-life when a medication is administered without a loading dose.

Dose Number	Amount of Drug Administered	Serum Concentration After Dose	Serum Concentration at End of Half-Life
Dose 1	1000 mg	1000 mg	1000 mg / 2 = 500 mg
Dose 2	1000 mg	500 mg + 1000 mg = 1500 mg	1500 mg / 2 = 750 mg
Dose 3	1000 mg	750 mg + 1000 mg = 1750 mg	1750 mg / 2 = 875 mg
Dose 4	1000 mg	875 mg + 1000 mg = 1875 mg	1875 mg / 2 = 938 mg
Dose 5	1000 mg	938 mg + 1000 mg = 1938 mg	1938 mg / 2 = 969 mg
Dose 6	1000 mg	969 mg + 1000 mg = 1969 mg	1969 mg / 2 = 985 mg

With the example above, you see that it takes approximately 5 doses of medication X until the serum levels at the end of a half-life begin to stabilize and approach a steady serum concentration.

Next, administer a loading dose of 2000 mg of medication X, and then start a maintenance dose of 1000 mg.

Medication X: 1000 mg every 12 hours with a loading dose of 2000 mg:

Dose Number	Amount of Drug Administered	Serum Concentration After Dose	Serum Concentration at End of Half-Life
Dose 1 (Loading)	2000 mg	2000 mg	2000 mg / 2 = 1000 mg
Dose 2	1000 mg	1000 mg + 1000 mg = 2000 mg	2000 mg / 2 = 1000 mg
Dose 3	1000 mg	1000 mg + 1000 mg = 2000 mg	2000 mg / 2 = 1000 mg
Dose 4	1000 mg	1000 mg + 1000 mg = 2000 mg	2000 mg / 2 = 1000 mg
Dose 5	1000 mg	1000 mg + 1000 mg = 2000 mg	2000 mg / 2 = 1000 mg
Dose 6	1000 mg	1000 mg + 1000 mg = 2000 mg	2000 mg / 2 = 1000 mg

This example clearly demonstrates that by administering a loading dose of 2000 mg, appropriate serum concentrations of the medication are rapidly obtained and maintained.

For a patient having an asthma attack, IV medications can provide rapid relief. However, an asthmatic patient can have several attacks a day, both at home and away from home. Starting an IV line or giving an IM injection for each asthmatic episode would be impractical. Therefore **inhaled medications** are often used to deliver medication to patients with asthma. Inhaled medications are rapidly active, easy to administer, and often convenient. Most asthmatic patients have prescribed **inhalers,** which contain medication in a fine powder that immediately acts on the lungs when administered. Inhalation is a rapid route of administration in which the medications can act directly on receptors in the lung, as well as be absorbed in the bloodstream. Albuterol (Proventil, Ventolin) is an example of an inhaled medication that is rapidly delivered to a patient having an asthma attack. Other examples include anesthetics administered to patients undergoing surgery.

Inhaled medications can also be given in liquid form. Liquid medication is **nebulized,** or made into small particles, by a delivery device and then delivered to the patient by inhalation. Nebulized medications are inhaled, but they require a device to deliver the medication called a **nebulizer.** Asthmatic patients may have a small machine at home that delivers the nebulized medication (Fig. 1-2). Ambulances and hospitals use a small nebulization chamber powered by an oxygen source.

Some medications are delivered by absorption across mucous membranes or the skin. For example, in **buccal administration,** glucose gel is administered between the cheek and gums of a diabetic patient with low blood sugar. The gel is rapidly absorbed and quickly increases the patient's serum glucose level.

Nitroglycerin is a medication available in a variety of forms and can be absorbed in several ways. One form is compressed powder, which is made into tablets. A nitroglycerin tablet can be placed under a patient's tongue, where it is rapidly absorbed though the oral mucous membranes. Alternatively, nitroglycerin is available in a form that can be sprayed under a patient's tongue for **sublingual administration.** A third method of nitroglycerin delivery is **transdermal** (across the skin) **administration.**

Gas is another form that medications can take. The drug most commonly used by prehospital providers is oxygen, which is a gaseous form of a drug. Inhaled nitrous oxide is another drug in the gaseous form that is often used in the prehospital setting.

Chapter 3 provides detailed, step-by-step explanations for delivering drugs by various routes, and Chapter 5 covers the administration of IV drugs.

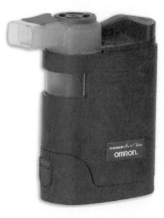

▼ **Fig. 1-2**   An example of a portable nebulizer system for home use. (Courtesy Omron Healthcare, Inc., Bannockburn, Ill.)

DRUG METABOLISM AND EXCRETION

Drug metabolism is the breakdown and change of a drug by various chemical reactions throughout the body. Medications are broken down by the liver in a series of complex chemical reactions into either an active or inactive compound. The transformation of an active drug to an inactive chemical through a series of chemical reactions is known as **biotransformation.** As previously mentioned, one disadvantage of administering a drug orally is first-pass metabolism. When a drug is absorbed by the GI tract, the drug must first go to the liver, where it is acted on by enzymes of the liver. Enzymes are proteins that act as catalysts to assist and increase the rate of breakdown of a medication; the liver is a source of plentiful enzymes and the site for the majority of drug metabolism. The kidneys and lungs are other sites of drug metabolism.

Metabolism often changes the chemical nature of a medication, making it inactive. Therefore factors that alter drug metabolism can change the effectiveness of an administered medication. Factors that increase drug metabolism break down a drug at a faster rate and perhaps render the drug less effective or completely ineffective. Therefore patients whose drug metabolism is increased will often require increased dosing for a medication to be effective.

The opposite is also true; a slowed metabolic rate results in a decrease in the breakdown of a given medication. With a slowed drug metabolism, medications can potentially reach toxic levels and have an adverse effect on a patient. A given dosage of a medication can affect individual patients differently, in part because of differences in the ways patients metabolize drugs. The following are some factors that alter drug metabolism:

- Age of the patient
- Route of drug administration
- Dosage of the medication
- Genetic predisposition of the patient
- Diet or starvation
- Preexisting disease

These specific factors are further explained in Chapter 19.

Drugs administered orally require absorption in the intestine and then proceed through the liver for first-pass metabolism. The result of first-pass metabolism is that a medication given orally requires a significantly higher dose than the same medication given by a **parenteral route.** For example, the IV dose of propranolol is 1 mg; however, the dose of the same medication given orally is 40 mg.

Drug **excretion** is the removal of a drug or metabolite from the body. The kidney typically is the organ responsible for removal of drugs and drug by-products. The liver can also excrete drugs from the body, although it does so less frequently. When the liver metabolizes medications, by-products are excreted by the liver into the bile.

PHARMACOKINETICS

Paramedics administer medications to patients to produce a desired clinical effect. That clinical effect may be to slow a heart that is beating too fast, accelerate a heart that is beating too slowly, or provide relief to a patient in pain. All medications have adverse effects, such as nausea, hypotension, and rash. The goal of drug therapy is to administer a medication to obtain the desired clinical effect while minimizing the likelihood of adverse effects.

Pharmacokinetics is the study of drug absorption, distribution, and excretion. As previously discussed, absorption is the movement of a drug from the site of administration into the bloodstream, where it can be transported throughout the body. Drug absorption determines, to a large degree, how rapidly a medication becomes available for a therapeutic effect. The more rapidly the medication is absorbed, the more quickly it will assist a patient. Absorption occurs from any site at which a medication is administered.

Absorption of most medication by any route other than the IV route (e.g., oral, rectal, IM, Sub-Q, transdermal) follows **first-order kinetics.** In first-order kinetics, a constant fraction of the medication is absorbed into the bloodstream. For example, an oral medication is absorbed from the intestine at a rate of 50% of the administered medication over a period of 20 minutes. Therefore if the patient takes 10 mg of this particular medication, 5 mg is absorbed at the end of 20 minutes, and 5 mg remains within the intestine. At the end of an additional 20 minutes (40 minutes after administration) an additional 50% (2.5 mg) is absorbed into the bloodstream. Therefore 40 minutes after administration, 7.5 mg (5 mg + 2.5 mg) has been absorbed across the intestine and is now circulating in the bloodstream, and 2.5 mg remains within the intestine waiting to be absorbed. After the third 20-minute interval, or 60 minutes after administration, an additional 50% is absorbed. Because only 2.5 mg of the medication remained, 1.25 mg is absorbed during this third 20-minute interval. This illustrates an example of first-order metabolism often called **exponential kinetics of absorption.** In this example, the rate of absorption is 50% over a 20-minute period. Some medications may have a much lower absorption rate over a much longer period, and these rates of absorption differ from medication to medication. After administration of an IV drug, a constant amount of the drug is absorbed and circulates within the bloodstream. Because the medication is administered directly into the bloodstream, absorption is not delayed; 100% of the medication is available in a brief period. This is known as **zero-order kinetics.**

Distribution of a drug refers to its transportation through the bloodstream to various tissues in the body and ultimately to the target site. Several factors determine how rapidly and to what magnitude a medication can accumulate in any given tissue. Drugs are rapidly delivered to organs such as the brain, heart, kidney, and liver because they have rich blood supplies. Drugs that are lipid or fat soluble can easily cross the membranes that separate the various body compartments, whereas drugs that are lipid insoluble take longer to cross into the various body compartments. The **volume of distribution** is the space that the drug would occupy; expressed as mg/L or such. A drug with a high volume of distribution is a drug that is fat soluble and can easily pass through membranes and into the various body compartments.

The bioavailability of a drug is the fraction of the drug that reaches circulation. The following factors may alter the bioavailability of a particular drug:

1. How rapidly the medication is broken down and absorbed in the intestinal tract
2. The dietary habits of the patient
3. The size of a tablet
4. The formulation of the medication

How a particular medication is absorbed through the intestinal tract largely depends on the physical and chemical properties of the drug. Drugs can cross the body's various membranes by several different mechanisms: **passive diffusion, carrier-mediated facilitated diffusion, active transport, passive transport,** and **endocytosis.** Passive diffusion (also known as *passive transport*) occurs when medications penetrate cells by diffusing through the cell's membrane. Factors that determine whether the medication is capable of diffusing through the cell membrane include the chemical nature of a particular drug, such as the molecular size, the chemical charge, fat or water solubility, and the concentration of the drug within the body.

Another method of transporting drugs into tissues is a process known as *carrier-mediated facilitated diffusion*. The transportation of the drug into a particular cell depends on a second molecule to carry the drug molecule into the cell. One way of visualizing carrier-mediated facilitated diffusion is to imagine a large group of people who need to be transported from one point to another by a series of buses. When a bus arrives, the people get on the bus, which takes them to their destination. Once at the destination, the people get off the bus and are free to move to their final destination. Applying this example to the transportation of medications into the cell, the administered drug accumulates at the outside of the cell membrane (the bus stop). There the medication loads (or binds) with a carrier macromolecule (bus). The carrier molecule (bus) then transports the bound medication (passengers) to its destination inside the cell. Once inside the cell, the bound medication disassociates from the carrier molecule (passengers get off the bus). Inside the cell the drug molecules go to their target site to produce the desired effect.

Carrier-mediated facilitated diffusion is a **saturable process.** As the concentration of the drug outside the cell increases, the rate of transporting the drug into the cell also increases. Eventually a point is reached at which increasing the concentration of a drug outside the cell does not result in an increase in transportation of the drug into the cell. By definition, a saturable process is one in which the external concentrations of the drug can reach a point at which increasing the concentration does not result in an increase in the rate of transportation into the cell. Returning to the bus example, assume that each bus, when full, can carry a maximum of 50 passengers. If a bus comes once an hour and only 20 people are at the bus stop, the bus will transport 20 people an hour. If 40 people are at the bus stop, the bus still has the capacity to transport 40 people in an hour. If the number of passengers at the bus stop increases to 60, the bus can load and transport only 50 passengers in an hour. Whether 70, 80, or 100 passengers are at the bus stop, that one bus can still carry only 50 passengers. This is an example of a saturable process. Applying the preceding metaphor, a saturable process is one in which the external concentrations (the number of passengers waiting for a bus) do not increase the rate of influx (the number of passengers transported by the bus in an hour).

Active transport (also a saturable process) is another method by which drug molecules are capable of crossing cell membranes. In many ways active transport and carrier-mediated facilitated diffusion are similar. Both mechanisms require a macromolecule to assist in transport. Both processes require specific binding of the drug molecule to the macromolecule, and both are capable of reaching a point of saturation. An example that illustrates active transport would be the bilge pump in a boat. A bilge pump pumps water from the bottom of a boat back into the lake or ocean. For the pump to work, it requires energy. The molecules that transport drugs by active transport also require energy.

Passive transport occurs when a drug molecule moves down a concentration gradient. This means that a drug moves from an area of high concentration to an area of low concentration. Factors that determine to what degree and how rapidly a drug may move by passive transport include the size of the drug molecule, how easily a particular drug dissolves in either water or fat, and the concentration of the drug in the various body compartments.

Endocytosis is a minor method of drug movement. In endocytosis, a cell essentially forms a sac around the drug molecule with the cell's membrane, and the cell membrane folds inward, bringing the drug into the cell.

With most medications, an amount of time elapses from when the drug is administered until the patient exhibits the desired effect. This interval can range from seconds to hours, even days in some cases. The **onset of action,** or **latent period,** is the time interval from administration to desired effect. A drug may produce its desired effect for varying periods. **Duration of action** is the period from which the drug initially exhibits its desired action to the point in time when the effect is no longer perceptible.

Duration of action is different from biologic half-life. The half-life of the particular drug is determined by the rate of transformation and excretion of a drug. A half-life is the period required to eliminate half the administered medication from the body and is not affected by the dose of the drug. In a given patient, the half-life of a medication is the same regardless of the dose of medication administered. Excretion is the process of eliminating a drug or its metabolites from the body. Some drugs are rapidly metabolized and excreted from the body, whereas others can linger for days.

The **therapeutic index (TI)** is the measurement of the relative safety of a drug. Two factors are used to determine the safety or TI of a medication. To calculate TI, the **effective dose 50 (ED50)** and the **lethal dose 50 (LD50)** must be known. The LD50 is the dose that is fatal in 50% of the laboratory animals tested. To obtain this value, researchers intentionally overdose animals to the point at which half the animals die at the administered test dose. In contrast, the ED50 is the dose that produces a therapeutic effect in 50% of laboratory animals tested. Once these two factors are determined, the TI is calculated by the following equation:

$$TI = LD50/ED50$$

This ratio provides a numeric value between 0 and 1. The closer this value is to 1, the more dangerous a drug is when administered. In contrast, the closer this number is to 0, the safer the drug.

PHARMACODYNAMICS

Simply stated, pharmacodynamics explains how drugs work. Having an understanding of how a particular drug works allows you to administer it confidently, with an awareness of its effectiveness, **side effects,** and interactions. The way a drug works at the target tissue is often called the *mechanism of action*. Drugs typically work by one of the following three mechanisms:
1. Drug/receptor interactions
2. Drug/enzyme interactions
3. Nonspecific drug interactions

DRUG/RECEPTOR INTERACTIONS

Many drugs work much like a key opening a lock. A drug, like a key, has a complex shape, and that shape determines its function. The drug binds to a receptor, as with a key in a lock. The combined drug/receptor interaction then essentially unlocks the drug to act on the target tissue. **Reversible binding** occurs when the drug is able to separate from the cell's receptor, as in removing a key from a lock. When the drug is removed from the receptor, the effect of the drug stops. With some medications, once the drug binds to the receptor, it cannot separate from the receptor; this is known as **irreversible binding.** Figure 1-3 illustrates the concepts of reversible and irreversible binding.

An **agonist** is a drug that produces the desired physiologic effect upon binding with the receptor. Agonists turn things on. In contrast, an **antagonist** is a drug that either diminishes or eradicates the physiologic effect of the agonist. That is, antagonists turn things off. **Pharmacologic antagonism** occurs when an antagonist binds to a receptor and prevents the biologic effect of an agonist. Antagonists can be either competitive or noncompetitive. **Competitive antagonists** can bind to the receptor in a reversible fashion. With increasing concentration of agonists, the competitive antagonist can be displaced by the agonists. Therefore providing additional agonists is one strategy for overcoming the effect of a competitive antagonist. A **noncompetitive antagonist** irreversibly binds to the receptor. Regardless of how much of the agonist is given, the effect of the noncompetitive antagonists on the receptor cannot be overcome.

Drugs and receptors also have some degree of chemical attraction toward one another, similar to the attraction between two magnets. This attraction between drug and receptor is known as **affinity.** Consider two magnets of opposite polarity. The stronger the attraction between two magnets, the greater the likelihood they will bind to each other if placed in

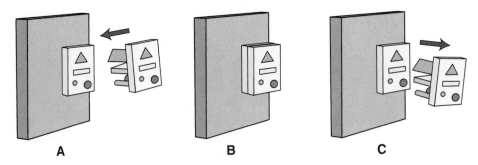

A   **B**   **C**

▼ **Fig. 1-3   A,** Drugs and their cell receptors have a very specific and complex structure. A drug binding to a specific receptor is like a key fitting into a lock. **B,** *Irreversible binding* occurs when the drug is not able to separate from the receptor, and the drug will have a prolonged effect. **C,** *Reversible binding* occurs when the drug separates from the cell receptor; this is similar to removing a key from a lock. Once the drug separates from the receptor, the effect of the drug stops.

proximity to each another. The weaker the attraction between two magnets, the closer they need to be to allow the same magnitude of attraction as two stronger magnets.

Efficacy is the ability of a drug to produce the desired biologic effect by binding to and unlocking a given receptor. For example, aspirin and morphine are two medications known to produce the effect of analgesia. Both medications are capable of producing the same desired effect—relief of pain. Which medication, aspirin or morphine, is most likely to produce the desired effect? Morphine has a greater efficacy in producing pain relief.

Potency is a term used to compare the different doses of two medications in producing the same effect. Morphine and fentanyl are both narcotics that produce analgesia. A fentanyl dose of 0.100 mg produces the same effect as 10 mg of morphine. Both drugs produce the same effect; however, a much smaller dose of fentanyl is required. In this example, fentanyl would be considered a more potent medication. The potency of a particular medication is independent of that medication's efficacy. For the purposes of selecting medications, efficacy is more important than potency.

When a patient is given two drugs that produce similar effects, the combined effects of these two drugs may be enhanced. **Summation** occurs when two medications with the same effect given together produce an effect in equal magnitude to the effects of the two drugs when given independently. In other words, the observed effect is equal to the effect of drug A plus the effect of drug B (1 + 1 = 2). In some cases, the observed effect of the two medications when given concurrently is greater than the effects of the medications when given individually. This phenomenon is known as **synergism.** With synergism, the combined effect is greater than the effect of drug A plus the effect of drug B (1 + 1 > 2).

The final enhancement of a drug's effect is known as **potentiation.** Potentiation occurs when a drug lacking an effect of its own increases the effect of a second drug.

DRUG/ENZYME INTERACTIONS

Enzymes are chemicals or compounds that control various chemical changes and reactions within the body. Drugs interact with enzymes and either increase or decrease the enzyme's mediated chemical reaction. Drugs are capable of binding or interacting with various enzymes and either accelerating or arresting their actions. An enzyme works by binding to the starting compound, known as the **substrate.** Some drugs that act on enzyme systems work by mimicking the substrate molecule, binding with the enzyme system, and essentially clogging the chemical reaction regulated by that particular enzyme. Other drugs can bind enzymes and accelerate a chemical reaction.

NONSPECIFIC DRUG INTERACTIONS

Nonspecific drug interactions occur when a drug acts on a target organ or tissue in a method that does not require binding of a drug with either a receptor or an enzyme. Nonspecific drug interactions often occur when a drug directly acts on a cell or the cell's membrane.

DRUG ACTIONS AND EFFECTS

Medications are administered to patients to achieve desired physiologic effects or actions. Unfortunately, medications often produce unwelcome physiologic side effects as well. Side effects often are considered nothing more than benign annoyances, such as headaches, nausea, and drowsiness. Side effects are often treated by reducing the dosage or eliminating the offending medication.

However, medications also can cause adverse effects, which are considered serious, undesired effects of a medication. On occasion, adverse effects are serious enough to warrant hospitalization. Examples of adverse effects include renal failure, bleeding, bone marrow suppression, and progression of heart disease. An **idiosyncratic response** is a rare and unpredicted response to a medication.

An **allergic response** typically occurs when a patient mounts an antibody response to a medication to which he or she had previously been sensitized. When the patient is reexposed to the medication, he or she responds with signs and symptoms such as rash, itching, and swelling. A patient with one drug allergy can be predisposed to manifest an allergic reaction to another medication of the same class or with similar chemical features. An **anaphylactic reaction** is an allergic reaction with life-threatening manifestations in which the patient can have swelling of the airway, inability to breathe, hypotension, and shock. This topic is further explained in Chapter 8.

Drug interaction occurs when the effects of one drug are modified by or interfere with the effects of a second drug administered concurrently. The result of a drug interaction often is that the effect of one drug is increased by the second drug.

Essentially two types of drug interactions occur: those that alter the plasma levels of the particular medication and those that alter the effects of a medication. Although essentially thousands of drug interactions are clinically relevant, most result in the prolongation of either the effect or half-life of a second medication. A large number of drugs are metabolized by the liver enzyme **cytochrome P-450.** Examples of such drugs include theophylline (Theo-24, Theolair, Uniphyl), warfarin (Coumadin), cimetidine (Tagamet), and antidepressants. Drugs are also able to interact with food and alcohol. Drug interactions with food and alcohol can occur by way of the cytochrome P-450 system, as well as through competition with the drug's binding site. Perhaps the most common drug and food interaction is with a class of drugs known as *monoamine oxidase inhibitors.* This class of drug cannot be taken with aged cheeses or many processed foods.

A large element of drug therapy is the manipulation of various physiologic functions. Depending on the disease state, the provider may need to manipulate a given patient's heart rate, blood pressure, respiratory effort, or even bowel functions. Under normal conditions, the autonomic nervous system provides minute-to-minute control of these wide-ranging functions. Therefore, in the attempt to control various disease states and reestablish a state of normal, a clinician needs to be familiar with the **autonomic nervous system.**

AUTONOMIC NERVOUS SYSTEM

The role of the autonomic nervous system is to control and integrate many major body functions. This is in contrast to the **somatic nervous system,** which controls skeletal muscles and movement. The autonomic nervous system provides involuntary control of many internal body functions. It is composed of two divisions: the **sympathetic** and **parasympathetic nervous systems** (Fig. 1-4). Both the sympathetic and parasympathetic nervous systems innervate the heart, bronchial smooth muscle, iris of the eye, salivary glands, and urinary bladder. The sympathic nervous system also innervates the vascular smooth muscle, sweat glands, and adrenal medulla.

The sympathetic nervous system readies the body to handle stress, which is commonly referred to as the **fight-or-flight response.** Most people have experienced a situation in which they felt threatened by a real or perceived risk. The physiologic changes that occur to the body when faced with that threat, such as violence or an accident, are responses to the actions of the sympathetic nervous system. Medications that exert effects on the sympathetic nervous system use **adrenergic receptors** and are called **adrenergic agonists.**

The parasympathetic nervous system is responsible for the routine housekeeping chores of the body, such as slowing the heart rate, producing acid for the stomach, and emptying the bladder and bowels. Drugs that act on the parasympathetic nervous system are referred to as **cholinergic agonists.**

ADRENERGIC RECEPTORS AND ACTIVATING DRUGS

Adrenergic receptors, which get their name from *adrenaline,* are commonly manipulated by medications. Adrenaline, more commonly known as *epinephrine,* is responsible for increasing the heart rate, increasing the contractility of the heart, increasing blood pressure, and dilating the bronchioles of the lungs. The net result of these effects is to ready the individual for the fight-or-flight response. Epinephrine regulates these effects through a series of adrenergic receptors: **alpha$_1$, alpha$_2$, beta$_1$,** and **beta$_2$.** Each receptor has unique properties, locations, and biologic effects when stimulated. A summary of these

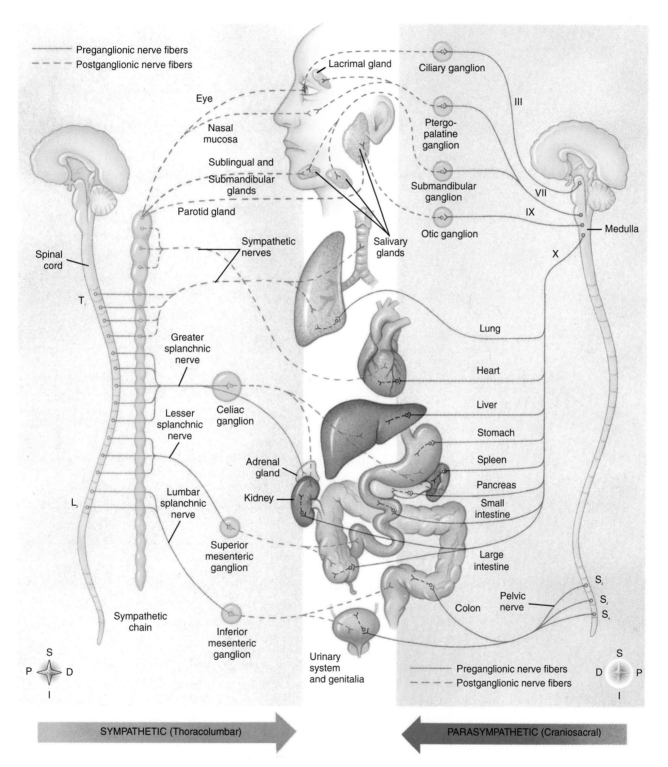

▼ **Fig. 1-4** Pathways of the sympathetic and parasympathetic nervous system. (From Thibodeau G, Patton K: *Anatomy & physiology*, ed 6, St Louis, 2007, Mosby.)

receptors is found in Table 1-2. Medications that can mimic and interact with adrenergic receptors have many effects and applications to prehospital care. Remembering the location and effects of each of these receptors can help you understand these drugs and their uses in prehospital care.

TABLE 1-2

Properties of Adrenergic Receptors

Receptor	Locations	Effects	Examples of Receptor Agonists
Alpha$_1$	Peripheral blood vessels	Vasoconstriction, elevation of systemic blood pressure	Norepinephrine, epinephrine, phenylephrine, and dopamine
Alpha$_2$	Presynaptic and postsynaptic nerve terminals	Vasodilation, anesthesia	Clonidine
Beta$_1$	Heart	Increase in heart rate and strength of cardiac contraction	Norepinephrine, epinephrine, and dobutamine
Beta$_2$	Airway, smooth muscle	Bronchodilation	Epinephrine, albuterol, and terbutaline

Alpha$_1$ receptors are primarily located on the peripheral blood vessels. Stimulation of these receptors results in vasoconstriction and elevation of systemic blood pressures. Dopamine is a drug that increases blood pressure by stimulation of the alpha$_1$ receptors on blood vessels.

Alpha$_2$ receptors are located on nerve endings and provide negative feedback to nerves in the sympathetic nervous system. The concept of negative feedback can be compared with a house thermostat. When a furnace heats a house, the temperature rises until it reaches the temperature set on the thermostat. Once the set temperature is reached, the thermostat sends a signal to the furnace to shut off and cease heating. This ability to signal a process (heating) when a goal or target (temperature) is reached is an example of negative feedback.

Beta$_1$ receptors are cardiovascular in nature. They are found on the heart and, when stimulated, increase heart rate and contractility. Increases in heart rate and contractility increase cardiac output.

Beta$_2$ receptors are located on the bronchial smooth muscle. Stimulation of beta$_2$ receptors relaxes bronchial smooth muscle and increases the diameter of the bronchial tree. Drugs that stimulate the beta$_2$ receptors are often used in respiratory emergencies.

Blood Vessels

The tone of the vascular smooth muscle is principally under the control of adrenergic receptors. Vascular smooth muscles contract and decrease the diameter of blood vessels, resulting in an increase in blood pressure or the shunting of blood from one area of the body to another. Stimulation of alpha$_1$ receptors by drugs such as dopamine results in vasoconstriction and increased blood pressure. Drugs that block the beta receptors are known as **beta blockers.** When a patient is given a beta blocker such as labetalol (Trandate, Normodyne), blood vessels relax, resulting in a decrease in systemic blood pressure.

Heart

Beta agonists are capable of mediating their effect on the heart through the action of the beta$_1$ receptor. Beta$_2$ agonists exert their effects primarily on the bronchial smooth muscles. When a cardiac beta receptor is stimulated by a beta agonist, the heart rate increases. Stimulation of beta receptors in the heart also increases cardiac output.

You can remember the distinction between beta$_1$ agonists and beta$_2$ agonists by remembering that human beings have one heart (beta$_1$) and two lungs (beta$_2$).

Eyes

The muscles of the eye responsible for pupil dilation are stimulated by alpha agonists. Drugs that act on both alpha and beta receptors can alter the pressure inside the eye, which is clinically significant in patients with glaucoma.

Respiratory Tract

Stimulation of the beta$_2$ receptors of the bronchial smooth muscles results in relaxation of these muscles and dilation of the airway. Inhaled bronchodilators commonly used by patients with asthma stimulate beta$_2$ receptors.

DRUGS THAT STIMULATE ADRENERGIC RECEPTORS

Remember that adrenergic receptors work through a receptor mechanism similar to a lock and key. These drugs must mimic the shape and structure of the native agonists of the adrenergic receptors. Drugs that mimic the actions of the sympathetic nervous system are referred to as **sympathomimetic drugs.** Epinephrine and norepinephrine are two examples of sympathomimetic drugs. Below are some of the more common sympathomimetic drugs that may be used by the prehospital provider. More detailed discussion of these agents is provided in later chapters in regard to their use in specific diseases.

In the body's natural production of sympathomimetic hormones, dopamine is the **precursor** to norepinephrine, and norepinephrine is the precursor to epinephrine. A precursor is a substance or drug that precedes another substance in the development of a substance or drug. When the body makes epinephrine, a molecule goes through a series of modifications before becoming epinephrine.

Dopamine → Norepinephrine → Epinephrine

Dopamine primarily stimulates the beta$_1$ receptors of the heart and causes the release of norepinephrine from the autonomic nervous system. As a beta$_1$ agonist, dopamine can increase heart rate and cardiac output. As the dose of dopamine is increased, it begins to stimulate alpha receptors, resulting in vasoconstriction. Therefore at higher doses dopamine acts much like an epinephrine infusion.

Norepinephrine is similar to epinephrine in its action on beta$_1$ receptors, but it has less potency on the alpha receptors and essentially no action on beta$_2$ receptors.

Dobutamine is a synthetic sympathomimetic drug that stimulates the beta$_1$ receptors. It is used to improve cardiac performance in patients with congestive heart failure, which it accomplishes with less of an increase in myocardial oxygen consumption than do other sympathomimetic agonists. This effect is caused by the drug's ability to improve cardiac output without significant increases in heart rate or systolic blood pressure.

Phenylephrine is a pure alpha agonist capable of increasing blood pressure. Because of its pure alpha activity, it is used as a vasopressor in conditions such as septic shock.

Epinephrine binds both alpha and beta receptors. The effects on the heart are mediated primarily by beta receptors. Epinephrine administration results in increases in blood pressure, heart rate, cardiac contractility, and cardiac output. Administration of epinephrine can result in cardiac arrhythmias. Alpha stimulation causes vasoconstriction and elevation of blood pressure.

DOPAMINE (INTROPIN)

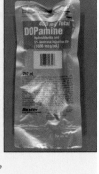

Classification: Adrenergic agonist, inotropic, vasopressor
Action: Stimulates alpha and beta adrenergic receptors. At moderate doses (2-10 mcg/kg/min), dopamine stimulates beta$_1$ receptors, resulting in inotropy and increased cardiac output while maintaining dopaminergic-induced vasodilatory effects. At high doses (>10 mcg/kg/min), alpha adrenergic agonism predominates, and increased peripheral vascular resistance and vasoconstriction result.
Indications: Hypotension and decreased cardiac output associated with cardiogenic shock and septic shock, hypotension after return of spontaneous circulation following cardiac arrest, symptomatic bradycardia unresponsive to atropine.
Adverse Effects: Tachycardia, arrhythmias, skin and soft tissue necrosis, severe hypertension from excessive vasoconstriction, angina, dyspnea, headache, nausea/vomiting.
Contraindications: Pheochromocytoma, VF, VT, or other ventricular arrhythmias, known sensitivity (including sulfites). Correct any hypovolemia with volume fluid replacement before administering dopamine.
Dosage:
- **Adult:** 2 to 20 mcg/kg/min IV, IO infusion. Starting dose 5 mcg/kg/min; may gradually increase the infusion by 5 to 10 mcg/kg/min to desired effect. Cardiac dose is usually 5 to 10 mcg/kg/min; vasopressor dose is usually 10 to 20 mcg/kg/min. Little benefit is gained beyond 20 mcg/kg/min.
- **Pediatric:** Same as adult dosing.

Special Considerations:
Half-life 2 minutes
Pregnancy class C

NOREPINEPHRINE (LEVOPHED)

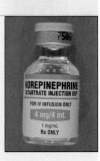

Classification: Adrenergic agonist, inotropic, vasopressor
Action: Norepinephrine is an alpha$_1$, alpha$_2$, and beta$_1$ agonist. Alpha-mediated peripheral vasoconstriction is the predominant clinical result of administration, resulting in increasing blood pressure and coronary blood flow. Beta adrenergic action produces inotropic stimulation of the heart and dilates the coronary arteries.
Indications: Cardiogenic shock, septic shock, severe hypotension.
Adverse Effects: Dizziness, anxiety, cardiac arrhythmias, dyspnea, exacerbation of asthma.
Contraindications: Patients taking MAOIs, known sensitivity. Use with caution in hypovolemia.
Dosage:
- **Adult:** Add 4 mg to 250 mL of D$_5$W or D$_5$NS, but not normal saline alone. 0.5 to 1 mcg/min as IV, IO, titrated to maintain blood pressure >80 mm Hg. Refractory shock may require doses as high as 30 mcg/min.
- **Pediatric:** 0.05 to 2 mcg/kg/min IV, IO infusion, to a maximum dose of 2 mcg/kg/min.

Special Considerations:
Do not administer in same IV line as alkaline solutions.
Half-life 1 minute
Pregnancy class C

DOBUTAMINE (DOBUTREX)

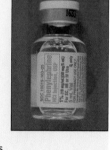

Classification: Adrenergic agent

Action: Acts primarily as an agonist at $beta_1$ adrenergic receptors with minor $beta_2$ and $alpha_1$ effects. Consequently, dobutamine increases myocardial contractility and stroke volume with minor chronotropic effects, resulting in increased cardiac output.

Indications: CHF, cardiogenic shock.

Adverse Effects: Tachycardia, PVCs, hypertension, hypotension, palpitations, arrhythmias.

Contraindications: Suspected or known poisoning/drug-induced shock, systolic blood pressure <100 mm Hg with signs of shock, idiopathic hypertrophic subaortic stenosis, known sensitivity (including sulfites). Use with caution in hypertension, recent MI, arrhythmias, hypovolemia.

Dosage:
- **Adult:** 2 to 20 mcg/kg/min IV, IO. At doses >20 mcg/kg/min, increases of heart rate of >10% may induce or exacerbate myocardial ischemia.
- **Pediatric:** Same as adult dosing.

Special Considerations:

Half-life 2 minutes

Pregnancy class C

PHENYLEPHRINE (NEO-SYNEPHRINE)

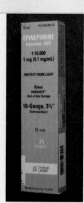

Classification: Adrenergic agonist

Action: Stimulates the alpha receptors, causing vasoconstriction, which results in increased blood pressure.

Indications: Neurogenic shock, spinal shock, cases of shock in which the patient's heart rate does not need to be increased, drug-induced hypotension.

Adverse Effects: Hypertension, VT, headache, excitability, tremor, MI, exacerbation of asthma, cardiac arrhythmias, reflex bradycardia, soft tissue necrosis.

Contraindications: Acute MI, angina, cardiac arrhythmias, severe hypertension, coronary artery disease, pheochromocytoma, narrow-angle glaucoma, cardiomyopathy, MAOI therapy, known sensitivity to phenylephrine or sulfites.

Dosage:
- **Adult:** 100 to 180 mcg/min IV, IO. Once the blood pressure has been stabilized, the dose can be reduced to 40 to 60 mcg/min.
- **Pediatric (2 to 12 years):** 5 to 20 mcg/kg IV, IO followed by 0.1 to 0.5 mcg/kg/min IV, IO (max dose: 3 mcg/kg/min IV, IO).

Special Considerations:

Pregnancy class C

EPINEPHRINE

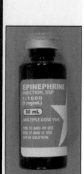

Classification: Adrenergic agent, inotropic

Action: Binds strongly with both alpha and beta receptors, producing increased blood pressure, increased heart rate, bronchodilation.

Indications: Bronchospasm, allergic and anaphylactic reactions, restoration of cardiac activity in cardiac arrest.

Adverse Effects: Anxiety, headache, cardiac arrhythmias, hypertension, nervousness, tremors, chest pain, nausea/vomiting.

Contraindications: Arrhythmias other than VF, asystole, PEA; cardiovascular disease; hypertension; cerebrovascular disease; shock secondary to causes other than anaphylactic shock; closed-angle glaucoma; diabetes; pregnant women in active labor; known sensitivity to epinephrine or sulfites.

cont'd

EPINEPHRINE—CONT'D

Dosage:

Cardiac Arrest:
- **Adult:** 1 mg (1 : 10,000 solution) IV, IO; may repeat every 3 to 5 minutes.
- **Pediatric:** 0.01 mg/kg (1 : 10,000 solution) IV, IO; repeat every 3 to 5 minutes as needed (max dose: 1 mg).

Symptomatic Bradycardia:
- **Adult:** 1 mcg/min (1 : 10,000 solution) as a continuous IV infusion; usual dosage range: 2 to 10 mcg/min IV; titrate to effect.
- **Pediatric:** 0.01 mg/kg (1 : 10,000 solution) IV, IO; may repeat every 3 to 5 minutes (max dose: 1 mg). If giving epinephrine by ET tube, administer 0.1 mg/kg.

Asthma Attacks and Certain Allergic Reactions:
- **Adult:** 0.3 to 0.5 mg (1 : 1000 solution) IM or Sub-Q; may repeat every 10 to 15 minutes (max dose: 1 mg).
- **Pediatric:** 0.01 mg/kg (1 : 1000 solution) IM or Sub-Q (max dose: 0.5 mg).

Anaphylactic Shock:
- **Adult:** 0.1 mg (1 : 10,000 solution) IV slowly over 5 minutes, or IV infusion of 1 to 4 mcg/min, titrated to effect.
- **Pediatric:** Continuous IV infusion rate of 0.1 to 1 mcg/kg/min (1 : 10,000 solution); titrate to response.

Special Considerations:

Half-life 1 minute

Pregnancy class C

DRUGS THAT BLOCK ADRENERGIC RECEPTORS

Stimulation of adrenergic receptors influences physiologic responses in different organ systems. Medications capable of binding and blocking adrenergic receptors have several therapeutic applications. Beta adrenergic receptor blockers, or beta blockers, prevent naturally occurring beta agonists from stimulating the receptor. When most beta blockers bind to the receptor, they essentially render that receptor nonfunctional. **Nonselective beta blockers** are capable of binding to both $beta_1$ and $beta_2$ receptors, whereas **selective beta blockers** bind and block either $beta_1$ or $beta_2$ receptors but not both.

Beta blockers have both negative chronotropic and inotropic effects. **Chronotropic drugs** affect the heart rate. Positive chronotropic drugs increase heart rate, and negative chronotropic drugs decrease heart rate. **Inotropic drugs** affect the magnitude of the squeeze of the heart muscle. Positive inotropic drugs make the squeeze of the heart stronger, whereas negative inotropic drugs decrease the intensity of the cardiac squeeze.

Reduction of heart rate and inotropy are useful in patients with cardiac disease. Oxygen is the fuel for the heart, and that fuel is delivered by the coronary arteries (termed *myocardial oxygen consumption*). When the heart beats fast, it burns more fuel (oxygen). With heart disease the coronary arteries narrow, decreasing the amount of oxygen that can be delivered to the heart. To conserve oxygen, beta blockers or negative chronotropic drugs are administered to patients.

Imagine driving a car, and the needle on the gas gauge is resting in that area below the large E for empty. How would you drive to the nearest gas station? Do you punch the pedal to the floor and speed to the next station? No, because that action would consume fuel at a greater rate. When trying to conserve fuel, drive with gradual accelerations and avoid excessive speed. This is similar to a concept applied to the sick heart. The consumption of fuel (oxygen) by the heart is similar to gas used in an automobile. By placing patients on drugs such as beta blockers, the rate of acceleration of the heart is limited and the amount of oxygen delivered to the heart is conserved.

The blockage of beta₂ receptors can result in bronchoconstriction in patients with asthma. Although beta-blocking drugs selective for the beta₁ receptor are advantageous in the treatment of heart disease, administration of a nonselective beta blocker to patients with asthma or chronic obstructive pulmonary disease can aggravate these pulmonary conditions. Propranolol (Inderal), a nonselective beta blocker, is capable of binding to both beta₁ and beta₂ receptors and can decrease both heart rate and cardiac output. Labetalol (Trandate, Normodyne) is another example of a nonselective beta blocker. Beta₁ selective blockers are advantageous because they provide the desired effect of reducing heart rate and consumption of oxygen by the heart without adversely affecting lung function.

Selective beta₁ blockers such as metoprolol (Lopressor, Toprol XL) and atenolol (Tenormin) are used in some prehospital settings for the treatment of hypertension. A more detailed discussion of these agents is found in Chapter 12.

PROPRANOLOL (INDERAL)

Classification: Beta adrenergic antagonist, antianginal, antihypertensive, antiarrhythmic class II

Action: Nonselective beta antagonist that binds with both the beta₁ and beta₂ receptors. Propranolol inhibits the strength of the heart's contractions, as well as heart rate. This results in a decrease in cardiac oxygen consumption.

Indications: Angina; narrow-complex tachycardias that originate from either a *reentry mechanism* (reentry SVT) or an *automatic focus* (junctional, ectopic, or multifocal tachycardia) uncontrolled by vagal maneuvers and adenosine in patients with preserved ventricular function; AF and atrial flutter in patients with preserved ventricular function; hypertension; migraine headaches.

Adverse Effects: Bradycardia, AV block, bronchospasm, hypotension.

Contraindications: Cardiogenic shock, heart failure, AV block, bradycardia, pulmonary edema, sick sinus syndrome, known sensitivity. Use with caution in chronic lung disease (asthma and COPD).

Dosage:
· **Adult:** 1 to 3 mg IV, IO at a rate of 1 mg/min; may repeat the dose 2 minutes later.
· **Pediatric:** 0.01 to 0.1 mg/kg slow IV, IO over a 10-minute period.

Special Considerations:
Monitor blood pressure and heart rate closely during administration.
Pregnancy class C

LABETALOL (NORMODYNE, TRANDATE)

Classification: Beta adrenergic antagonist, antianginal, antihypertensive

Action: Binds with both the beta₁ and beta₂ receptors and alpha₁ receptors in vascular smooth muscle. Inhibits the strength of the heart's contractions, as well as heart rate. This results in a decrease in cardiac oxygen consumption.

Indications: ACS, SVT, severe hypertension.

Adverse Effects: Usually mild and transient; hypotensive symptoms, nausea/vomiting, bronchospasm, arrhythmia, bradycardia, AV block.

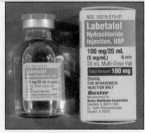

Contraindications: Hypotension, cardiogenic shock, acute pulmonary edema, heart failure, severe bradycardia, sick sinus syndrome, second- or third-degree heart block, asthma or acute bronchospasm, cocaine-induced ACS, known sensitivity. Use caution in pheochromocytoma, cerebrovascular disease or stroke, poorly controlled diabetes, with hepatic disease. Use with caution at lowest effective dose in chronic lung disease.

Dosage:
Cardiac Indications: Note: Monitor blood pressure and heart rate closely during administration.
· **Adult:** 10 mg IV, IO over a 1- to 2-minute period. May repeat every 10 minutes to a maximum dose of 150 mg or give initial bolus and then follow with infusion at 2 to 8 mg/min.
· **Pediatric:** 0.4 to 1 mg/kg/hr to a maximum dosage of 3 mg/kg/hr.

cont'd

LABETALOL (NORMODYNE, TRANDATE)—CONT'D

Severe Hypertension:

- **Adult:** Initial dose is 20 mg IV, IO slow infusion over a 2-minute period. After the initial dose, blood pressure should be checked every 5 minutes. Repeat doses can be given at 10-minute intervals. The second dose should be 40 mg IV, IO, and subsequent doses should be 80 mg IV, IO, to a maximum total dose of 300 mg. The effect on blood pressure typically will occur within 5 minutes from the time of administration. Alternatively, may be administered via IV infusion at 2 mg/min to a total maximum dose of 300 mg.
- **Pediatric:** 0.4 to 1 mg/kg/hr IV, IO infusion with a maximum dose of 3 mg/kg/hr.

Special Considerations:

Pregnancy class C

METOPROLOL (LOPRESSOR, TOPROL XL)

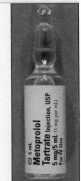

Classification: Beta adrenergic antagonist, antianginal, antihypertensive, class II antiarrhythmic

Action: Inhibits the strength of the heart's contractions, as well as heart rate. This results in a decrease in cardiac oxygen consumption. Also saturates the beta receptors and inhibits dilation of bronchial smooth muscle (beta$_2$ receptor).

Indications: ACS, hypertension, SVT, atrial flutter, AF, thyrotoxicosis.

Adverse Effects: Tiredness, dizziness, diarrhea, heart block, bradycardia, bronchospasm, drop in blood pressure.

Contraindications: Cardiogenic shock, AV block, bradycardia, known sensitivity. Use with caution in hypotension, chronic lung disease (asthma and COPD).

Dosage:

Cardiac Indications:

- **Adult:** 5 mg slow IV, IO over a 5-minute period; repeat at 5-minute intervals up to a total of three infusions totaling 15 mg IV, IO.
- **Pediatric:** Not recommended for pediatric patients; no studies available.

Special Considerations:

Blood pressure, heart rate, and ECG should be monitored carefully.

Use with caution in patients with asthma.

Pregnancy class C

ATENOLOL (TENORMIN)

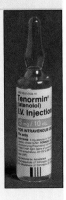

Classification: Beta adrenergic antagonist, antianginal, antihypertensive, class II antiarrhythmic

Action: Inhibits the strength of the heart's contractions and heart rate, resulting in a decrease in cardiac oxygen consumption. Also saturates the beta receptors and inhibits dilation of bronchial smooth muscle (beta$_2$ receptor).

Indications: ACS, hypertension, SVT, atrial flutter, AF.

Adverse Effects: Bradycardia, bronchospasm, hypotension.

Contraindications: Cardiogenic shock, AV block, bradycardia, known sensitivity. Use with caution in hypotension, chronic lung disease (asthma and COPD).

Dosage: ACS:

- **Adult:** 5 mg IV, IO over a 5-minute period; repeat in 5 minutes.
- **Pediatric:** Not recommended for pediatric patients.

Special Considerations:

Pregnancy class D

CHOLINERGIC RECEPTORS AND ACTIVATING DRUGS

Receptors of the parasympathetic nervous system are known as **cholinergic receptors.** The term *cholinergic* comes from the name of the principal neurotransmitter of the parasympathetic nervous system, **acetylcholine.** Acetylcholine is the neurotransmitter used by the parasympathetic nervous system to act on the various organs of the body. It can act on the heart to slow the heart rate in addition to having a negative inotropic effect. Acetylcholine is also used in the sympathetic nervous system to relay messages, not as a neurotransmitter.

Two types of cholinergic receptors are at work within the parasympathetic nervous system: **nicotinic** and **muscarinic receptors.** Nicotinic receptors are found in the central nervous system, autonomic ganglia, and striated muscle. Muscarinic receptors are found on the cardiac and smooth muscle, exocrine glands, and brain.

Several drugs bind and stimulate cholinergic receptors, although few have a role in the prehospital setting. Atropine competes with acetylcholine for the opportunity to bind muscarinic receptors, which results in an increase in heart rate. As a prehospital drug, atropine commonly is used for the treatment of bradycardia and asystole. When treating symptomatic bradycardia, the dosage guidelines must be strictly followed. In smaller doses atropine can cause further slowing of the heart. Higher doses of atropine lead to the desired acceleration of heart rate. In high enough dosages, atropine also exerts effects on the pulmonary system by causing bronchodilation and a reduction of secretions. Consequently, atropine is the drug of choice in nerve agent and organophosphate poisoning.

ATROPINE SULFATE

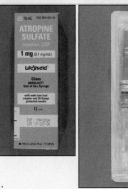

Classification: Anticholinergic (antimuscarinic)
Action: Competes reversibly with acetylcholine at the site of the muscarinic receptor. Receptors affected, in order from the most sensitive to the least sensitive, include salivary, bronchial, sweat glands, eye, heart, and GI tract.
Indications: Symptomatic bradycardia, asystole or PEA, nerve agent exposure, organophosphate poisoning.
Adverse Effects: Decreased secretions resulting in dry mouth and hot skin temperature, intense facial flushing, blurred vision or dilation of the pupils with subsequent photophobia, tachycardia, restlessness. Atropine may cause paradoxical bradycardia if the dose administered is too low or if the drug is administered too slowly.
Contraindications: Acute MI; myasthenia gravis; GI obstruction; closed-angle glaucoma; known sensitivity to atropine, belladonna alkaloids, or sulfites. Will not be effective for infranodal (type II) AV block and new third-degree block with wide QRS complex.
Dosage:
Symptomatic Bradycardia:
- **Adult:** 0.5 mg IV, IO every 3 to 5 minutes to a maximum dose of 3 mg.
- **Adolescent:** 0.02 mg/kg (minimum 0.1 mg/dose; maximum 1 mg/dose) IV, IO up to a total dose of 2 mg.
- **Pediatric:** 0.02 mg/kg (minimum 0.1 mg/dose; maximum 0.5 mg/dose) IV, IO, to a total dose of 1 mg.
Asystole/Pulseless Electrical Activity:
- 1 mg IV, IO every 3 to 5 minutes, to a maximum dose of 3 mg. May be administered via ET tube at 2 to 2.5 mg diluted in 5 to 10 mL of water or normal saline.
Nerve Agent or Organophosphate Poisoning:
- **Adult:** 2 to 4 mg IV, IM; repeat if needed every 20 to 30 minutes until symptoms dissipate. In severe cases, the initial dose can be as large as 2 to 6 mg administered IV. Repeat doses of 2 to 6 mg can be administered IV, IM every 5 to 60 minutes.
- **Pediatric:** 0.05 mg/kg IV, IM every 10 to 30 minutes as needed until symptoms dissipate.
- **Infants <15 lb:** 0.05 mg/kg IV, IM every 5 to 20 minutes as needed until symptoms dissipate.
Special Considerations:
Half-life 2.5 hours
Pregnancy class C; possibly unsafe in lactating mothers.

SCOPOLAMINE (TRANSDERM SCOP)

Classification: Neurologic antivertigo, antimuscarinic
Action: Antagonizes acetylcholine at muscarinic receptors.
Indications: Motion sickness
Adverse Effects: Dry mouth, drowsiness, dilated pupils and blurred vision, hallucinations, confusion.
Contraindications: Glaucoma, cardiac arrhythmias, coronary artery disease, known sensitivity.
Dosage:
· **Adult and children older than 12 years:** 1 disc applied to skin behind ear.
Special Considerations:
Half-life 8 hours
Pregnancy class C

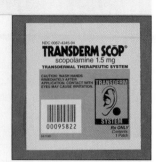

Scopolamine is another drug that competitively binds with the muscarinic receptor. Compared with atropine, scopolamine does not have as potent an effect on the heart and lungs. Scopolamine commonly is used for the treatment of motion sickness. Although dispensing a scopolamine patch would be highly unlikely for a paramedic, being dispatched to an interstate or airport for a medical call in which a patient has taken this drug is possible.

REVIEW QUESTIONS

1. Explain the difference between a drug's generic name and trade name.
2. List the properties of a medication.
3. Explain the dose-response relationship.
4. Why would an oral medication be inappropriate for an acute emergency such as an asthma attack?
5. Explain first-pass metabolism.
6. List the factors that alter drug metabolism.
7. Explain the similarities between active transport and carrier-mediated facilitated diffusion.
8. Define half-life.
9. List two factors in determining (calculating) the therapeutic index.
10. What are the roles of the agonist and antagonist in the action of a drug?
11. What is a drug interaction?
12. What are two types of drug interactions?
13. What are the physiologic effects of epinephrine?
14. What is the effect on the heart when stimulating $beta_1$ receptors?
15. What are the effects on the lungs when stimulating $beta_2$ receptors?
16. What is the effect of giving too small a dose of atropine?

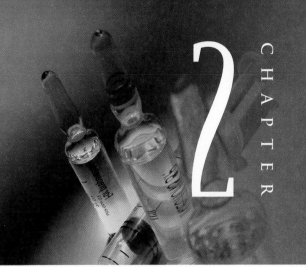

Legal Aspects and Risk Management

OBJECTIVES

1. Describe the importance of the publication *To Err Is Human: Building a Safer Health System.*
2. Define the four elements of negligence: duty to act, breach of duty to act, causation, and harm to the patient.
3. Describe the principal goal of Good Samaritan laws.
4. List the steps a provider can take to minimize the risk of a medication mistake.
5. Explain the benefits of protocols in preventing mistakes in medication administration.
6. Describe Schedule I, II, III, IV, V, and VI medications and the abuse potential for each.
7. Discuss the importance of properly storing, securing, and maintaining medications.
8. List the parts of the $A^3E^3P^3$ refusal guidelines.
9. Discuss the effect of living wills and advance directives on prehospital providers.
10. List the "dos and don'ts" of documenting medication administration.
11. Discuss the importance of properly documenting and reporting medication errors.

INTRODUCTION

The administration of medications by prehospital providers in the field can have a tremendously positive effect on patients. In terms of avoiding risk and liability, however, medication administration ideally should be performed in a more controlled environment. The administration of drugs in the field can present obstacles such as low light levels and unstable environmental conditions that test the skills of even the most competent caregiver. Nonetheless, medication administration in the field is a skill that must be mastered, and paramedics can learn to avoid mistakes that can harm patients and open the door to lawsuits.

This chapter describes the legal context of medication administration in the field and the legal basis for negligence lawsuits. The most common liability areas associated with prehospital medication administration are discussed, as well as strategies for minimizing the two key risk areas: **harm to the patient** and likelihood of a lawsuit.

Skill, knowledge, sound judgment, and strict adherence to protocols and procedures can reduce the possibility of a bad patient outcome or a lawsuit.

Your paramedic unit is dispatched to a local department store in response to a medical call. While en route, the dispatcher informs you that the patient is a 33-year-old woman with a history of diabetes. When you arrive, you find the patient sitting in a chair and holding her head in her hands. She answers all your questions, and her mental status is clear. She tells you that she is an insulin-dependent diabetic. She was rushed this morning getting her kids ready for school; she took her morning dose of insulin but failed to eat a complete breakfast. She began to run some errands and became dizzy, weak, and diaphoretic. She believes she had a hypoglycemic episode ...

... but feels a little better after having some juice. You assess the patient and measure her blood glucose level. The glucometer reads 60 mg/dL. You administer some glucose gel to the patient, and she reports feeling much better. She is more talkative. She looks at her watch and starts to gather her bundles. She reports that she is going to be late to pick up her daughter at preschool. The patient tells you that she feels fine and appreciates your concerns. You recommend that she be transported to the hospital for further evaluation. She refuses any further medical care or transport even after you have provided some initial therapy and evaluation.

What type of refusal is this? As a paramedic your job is done, right? Wrong. You tell her that she should not drive. You tell her that you would prefer she call her husband to drive her home. She responds with a prompt "no!" She does not want her husband to know about this incident. She has provided you with a partial refusal, but what are the legal obligations and potential liabilities in partially treating a patient? Are you obligated to call her husband, or would that be violating her privacy? Is not transporting her to the hospital negligent? What if she has another episode while driving the car, with or without her kids? Is the patient medically and legally competent to refuse additional care? Does the patient understand the potential risks of refusing therapy? Have you explained these concerns in a simple, nonmedical fashion so that the patient can understand? What are the protocols for patients providing consent or refusing emergency medical care?

SCOPE OF POTENTIAL LEGAL LIABILITY

On a national scale, errors in medication administration are a serious problem, even in the more controlled environment of a hospital. A medication error is a preventable occurrence caused by inappropriate use of a medication that has the potential to result in patient harm. The public first became aware of the extent of medication errors after a landmark publication by the Institute of Medicine entitled *To Err Is Human: Building a Safer Health System*.[1] This report revealed the following findings:

- Approximately 50,000 to 100,000 Americans die each year from general medical errors.
- Medical errors are the eighth leading cause of death, ranking higher than breast cancer and human immunodeficiency virus.
- Approximately 7000 people die each year from medication errors alone.

Emergency medical services (EMS) is not immune to the problem of medication errors, and in many cases the problem is made worse by the environmental conditions and other situational factors inherent in the field setting that are not present in a hospital. Little research has described the scope of the problem, but in one recent study, researchers at Western Carolina University assessed the medication calculation skills of a group of practicing paramedics, including the types of computations they found most difficult and the relationships between drug calculation skills and various demographic characteristics. The study involved a 10-item drug calculation examination administered to a group of 109 practicing paramedics who represented a cross-section of EMS system characteristics in North Carolina.[2] The researchers found that the overall performance on the drug calculation examination was poor. The mean score was 51.4%. IV flow rate and medication bolus calculation problems were answered correctly in 68.8% of the cases, followed by non–weight-based medication infusions (33.9%), weight-based medication infusions (32.5%), and percentage-based medication infusions (4.5%). Interestingly, the examination scores were higher among paramedics with college-level education but lower among paramedics with more years of experience.

The results of this study were similar to findings in other allied health professions: medication calculation skills were lacking. The paramedics in this study also reported infrequent opportunities to perform drug calculations in the clinical setting, such as during hospital skill rotations, and that medication calculations were not a routine part of EMS continuing education programs.

PRINCIPLES OF NEGLIGENCE

The same principles of negligence that can lead to liability in other areas of emergency medicine apply to medication administration. **Ordinary negligence,** or basic negligence, is defined as the failure to exercise the degree of care that another reasonable person would exercise in the same or similar situation in which harm to another person results. The average, ordinary person or professional is held to that standard when a negligence lawsuit arises. Applying this concept to medical care, actions that would be considered ordinary negligence are acts that caused harm to the patient and "deviated from good and acceptable medical standards."[3]

Negligence is defined by the following four elements, all of which must be proven in court for the plaintiff to prevail:

1. Duty to act
2. Breach of duty to act
3. Causation
4. Harm to the patient

DUTY TO ACT

Duty to act is a simple concept: Did you have a duty to provide the care to the patient? This is generally an easy element for the plaintiff to prove. Because an ambulance service or EMS organization promotes itself to the public as capable of responding to emergency requests, the service has a duty to respond to the patient and provide the level of care that reasonable paramedics are expected to provide.

However, the duty to act must be a legal duty. In other words, the defendant must have a legal obligation to respond, treat, and transport the patient before the duty to act can be breached.

> A paramedic is on his way to work the night shift at ABC Ambulance and Rescue. He hears on his scanner that a serious motor vehicle accident has occurred just a few blocks away from his location. He chooses not to respond to that call in his private vehicle and continues on his way to work.

In this case, the paramedic has no duty to act because he is not legally obligated to respond until he has officially begun work. Had he been at the station and on duty, he would have had a duty to act.

BREACH OF DUTY TO ACT

If a paramedic fails in any way to provide the level of care that the EMS agency or local protocols dictate, he or she may be guilty of **breach of duty to act.** This is the point at which the **standard of care** comes into play; that is, if an individual failed to act, was the failure to act inconsistent with local protocol or other direction to provide care? In such cases, expert witnesses are used to testify to the standard of care for EMS personnel in the community in which they serve. The key question is what would a reasonably prudent paramedic do in this same situation?

> A paramedic is at the end of her shift and is very tired—so tired that all she cares about is going home. However, right before the shift ends, a call comes in for a possible heart attack. She responds and is directed by medical command to administer 4 mg of morphine sulfate intravenously for pain. But the paramedic does not want to deal with all the paperwork that comes with administering a narcotic agent, so she decides not to give the patient the morphine and transports him to the hospital.

In this case the paramedic clearly breached her duty to act by not administering the medication to the patient as ordered by medical command. She did not provide the standard of care expected by her EMS agency and the community.

CAUSATION

Causation refers to the fact that the plaintiff must prove that the paramedic's conduct was a substantial factor in bringing about harm to the patient. This is a difficult element to prove in most EMS cases because, at the outset, the "wheels of harm" to the patient were set into motion before EMS was even activated. In other words, the paramedic responds to a patient who has already incurred harm and is merely intervening in an attempt to reduce the effect of that harm. The question the jury would have to answer is whether the paramedic's conduct was the *cause* of the harm to the patient. This is referred to as **proximate cause.** If the patient's harm can be shown to have come from other sources and not the paramedic's conduct, the causation requirement would not be met.

> A patient with severe chest pain calls 9-1-1. First responders arrive and find an unconscious patient. The automatic external defibrillator shows a shockable rhythm, and a shock is administered. The patient's pulse and respirations return. EMS then responds, and a paramedic assesses the patient. He administers a cardiac medication but gives a dose that is too high. After receiving the excessive dose, the patient has a seizure. He is later found to have incurred brain damage.

If the drug administration error in this case can be shown to have caused the seizure and subsequent brain damage, proximate causation would be proven. But in defending the paramedic or EMS agency, the defense attorney would likely argue that the patient had the seizure and incurred brain damage as a result of the heart attack and cardiac arrest itself, not the medication error.

In some cases medication errors and their effect on the patient can be isolated from the initial insult to the patient. For example, if a patient has a heart attack and is given a medication to which he is allergic, which subsequently leads to an anaphylactic reaction and death, demonstrating that conduct was a substantial factor in the harm to the patient may be relatively simple. The question would be whether the patient would have suffered an anaphylactic reaction despite the conduct of the paramedic. In this situation the answer would clearly be "no," and this element of negligence would be proven.

HARM TO THE PATIENT

A successful lawsuit based on negligence requires that there must be some harm to the patient; that is, physical or emotional injury that caused damage to the patient.

Damage can be shown in the form of the patient's own testimony, the testimony of expert witnesses, and other evidence that points to the extent of harm to the patient. The cost of this harm can be translated into medical costs for treatment, recovery, and rehabilitation; pain and suffering; and other compensatory damages. To prove negligence, the plaintiff typically must show that the harm was of the type that could have been caused by the EMS provider.

> Washington County Fire Department paramedics respond to a motor vehicle crash. On arrival, paramedics find the driver of the vehicle walking around, with no apparent injuries. His vehicle incurred minor damage when it struck a parked car. One of the paramedics approaches the patient, who refuses treatment and says he is fine. The paramedic obtains an informed refusal form, which is signed by the patient. The patient goes home and goes to sleep. The next day he wakes up with a throbbing headache and goes to the emergency department (ED). He is admitted with a cerebral aneurysm that requires surgery; he also has developed some paralysis. The patient sues the municipality, stating that the paramedics were negligent in not transporting him to the hospital.

In this case, although the patient incurred harm from the accident, that harm did not result from the acts or omissions of the paramedics. The paramedic was wise to ask the patient to sign an informed refusal.

THE IMMUNITY DEFENSE

Many states provide certain **immunities** under the law that make proving negligence against an EMS provider difficult for a plaintiff. These immunities are based on the age-old principle of the Good Samaritan, which encourages others to assist ill and injured people to the best of their ability without fear of a lawsuit if they make any mistakes.

Nearly every state has some form of **Good Samaritan legislation.** Many of these laws merely protect bystanders or individuals without medical training from getting sued for providing assistance in an emergency. Some of these laws protect physicians and nurses who render care at the scene of an emergency outside their work environment. These laws are designed to encourage off-duty health professionals to assist in an emergency without the fear of liability, which could cloud their judgment or prevent them from lending help.

Other state laws extend the immunity to EMS personnel and other emergency responders. For example, Pennsylvania's immunity statute for EMS personnel states the following:

> *No* first responder, emergency medical technician or EMT-paramedic or health professional who in good faith attempts to render or facilitate emergency medical care authorized by this act *shall be liable* for any civil damages as a result of any acts or omissions, *unless guilty of gross or willful negligence* [italics added for emphasis].[4]

Do Good Samaritan laws provide complete immunity from a negligence lawsuit? Usually they do not. The type of immunity that these laws embody is not full immunity, but rather **qualified immunity.** That is, the immunity has a qualification: the caregiver may not act in a reckless, wanton manner in total disregard to the patient. Acting in this manner would be considered **gross negligence.** Most immunity statutes provide a caregiver immunity from a negligence lawsuit unless his or her actions could be shown to constitute gross negligence.

Gross negligence is difficult to prove in many cases because actions or inactions must be found to be more than a mere mistake to be considered grossly negligent acts. As one state's supreme court described it, gross negligence is substantially more than "ordinary carelessness, inadvertence, laxity, or indifference." It is behavior that is "flagrant, grossly deviating from the ordinary standard of care."[5]

Volunteer EMS personnel often have legal protection for their conduct. The underlying philosophy is that if an individual volunteers to save a person's life or assist the person in a medical crisis, that individual should not have to worry about getting sued. Otherwise, individuals may not be willing to act as Good Samaritans and help in an emergency. In many cases these state laws require that volunteers have a minimal level of training, such as cardiopulmonary resuscitation or first aid, and that they render assistance only within the level of that certification or training.

Some states limit immunity protection to volunteer personnel and do not apply it to paid EMS personnel. Lawmakers in those states believe that healthcare providers owe a higher duty to the people they are obligated to serve as part of their profession. In other words, because responding to emergencies is part of a paramedic's responsibility as an emergency professional, paramedics should be better prepared for these situations than Good Samaritans.

> Check state laws carefully to determine whether immunity statutes apply to paid, or career, EMS personnel. If the state has no immunity statute, the standard for evaluating conduct likely will be based on ordinary negligence, which is easier to prove than gross negligence.

How does a paramedic avoid committing gross negligence? First and foremost, paramedics should function within their certification level. They should not perform skills or administer medications out of their **scope of practice** (the legally approved skills that may be performed and the medications authorized to administer) as defined by state law. For example, if you are not authorized under state law and your medical director to administer paralytic agents to combative patients who need to be intubated, you should not use that medication—even if it is available in the drug box.

Second, always act in good faith. The best way to do this is to always treat patients as though they were your own close relatives. Function in a reasonable and prudent manner with the interest of the patient in your heart and mind. Common sense often helps in this area. Ask yourself the question, "Is this the right thing to do in this situation?" If the answer is "no," reevaluate the plan of action. Failure to verify a patent vein when administering IV medication and failure to check the vial of medication to verify its concentration and expiration date are examples of not acting in good faith.

Third, do not take actions or fail to take actions that could be construed as grossly negligent. Function within your scope of practice and do what the public would expect you to do. Do not commit an action or omit an action that you had a recognized duty to do or not do, knowing or having reason to know that the act or omission could create a substantial risk of harm to the patient. Remember the first rule of medical care: do no harm. If your actions could harm the patient, do not initiate them in the first place.

MEDICATION ERRORS: MISTAKE OR NEGLIGENCE?

Mistakes occur every day in the prehospital field. It is a challenging working environment, and providers need to be vigilant and alert at all times. Even the smallest mistake can lead to serious harm to the patient. Still, a mistake does not necessarily mean negligence under the law. The successful plaintiff must prove by a preponderance of the evidence that all four elements of negligence were present; this usually is demonstrated by showing that a provider deviated from the standard of care and that his or her conduct was a substantial factor in causing the harm to the patient.

Negligence is difficult to prove, but in many cases juries are sympathetic to the plaintiff or the plaintiff's surviving family members. Many jurors view paramedics as professionals who are no different from nurses and other healthcare professionals who work in hospitals. In addition, jurors do not always decide cases on the basis of the law. This is perpetuated by the fact that, in American society, the manner in which a jury decides a negligence case is not subject to review on appeal unless clear errors occurred in trial procedures, such as evidence being admitted when the judge should have disallowed it or jury instructions that do not reflect the current state of the law. A clear basis for appeal would be tampering with the jury or juror misconduct, but even then winning an appeal on these issues is rare.

Defendants are judged by jurors who can be influenced by many factors and who make their decisions based on many sources of information. Assessment of witness credibility, opinions of the plaintiff or defense counsel, and the jurors' life experiences all weigh in on the jury's decision of liability. Other more tangible factors include the extent of harm to the patient, life expectancy of the patient, effect of the harm on the patient's activities of daily living, and other emotional issues that are part of the case. Juries are expected to follow the law and abide by the instructions read to them by the judge. However, the biases, prejudices, and persuasiveness of the attorneys greatly affect the final decision.

In all aspects of their work, prehospital care providers must avoid conducting themselves in a manner that could be construed as negligent. The following steps can be taken to minimize the risk of a medication mistake that can harm a patient and result in a lawsuit:

▷ *Be well educated.* Know drugs and everything about them, including contraindications to administration, possible side effects, and drug interactions. New medications are approved by the U.S. Food and Drug Administration at an increasingly rapid pace, and the treatment protocols for specific situations are constantly changing.

▶ *Be well rested.* Providers are more apt to make a mistake when tired and stressed. In emergency services, failure to be in the best possible physical condition can lead to serious errors. Medication administration requires providers to be sharp and at their best. Many aspects of this skill require intact thought processes and mental skill. Studies have shown that failure to be well rested can lead to mistakes in patient care, and medication errors are more likely to occur when providers are tired and unable to think clearly.

▶ *Know protocols and follow them.* In negligence cases, the standard of care is examined. The standard of care in a lawsuit is determined by that state's scope of practice and other supplemental sources, including training program curricula, textbooks, and medical expert reports and testimony. That standard is also often defined by local medical protocols, which can become direct evidence of legally authorized scope of practice and the standard of medical care for the community. Deviating from these protocols can be considered deviating from the standard of care.

▶ *Maintain knowledge and skills.* As the North Carolina study suggests, drug calculation and other medication administration skills should be practiced on a regular basis to keep the provider from getting rusty. Lack of practice leads to a greater likelihood of making mistakes.

Maintaining medication knowledge and administration skills is especially important to avoid mistakes when treating pediatric patients, who are seen less frequently than adults (thus most paramedics have less practice treating pediatric patients). The *To Err Is Human* report stated that 64% of the children in a particular study went into iatrogenic cardiac or respiratory arrest because of medical errors. Errors in pediatric drug administration can occur for a variety of reasons, including misplaced decimal points when performing calculations and rushed calculations and medication administration.

Pediatric patients require medication dosages that are not often administered in the prehospital setting. In addition, dealing with a seriously ill or injured child is an added stressor. The liability that can result from a medication error in a pediatric patient can be extensive. The emotional impact on the jury when a child is harmed by a healthcare provider and the young age of the patient generally translate to higher damage awards in pediatric cases. The court can award damages for loss of future income of the child, as well as the loss of affection for the parents. As such, the economic value of the harm to the patient or loss of life can be tremendous.

A paramedic can never be too cautious when administering medication to a pediatric patient. Always double-check procedures and have your partner or another healthcare professional check as well. Stay in close touch with online medical command if possible, and seek guidance and direction when you are unsure of yourself or if protocols require it. Be mindful that administering prehospital medications to a child is an infrequent occurrence for the prehospital provider. Therefore the likelihood of committing an error is greater.

PROTOCOLS AS A RISK MANAGEMENT TOOL

Established advanced life support (ALS) protocols are an excellent safeguard to prevent mistakes in medication administration. In some ALS systems online medical direction is extremely important, with most medication orders coming from an emergency physician in the ED. In situations in which medication orders are given over the radio or by telephone, *the paramedic must make certain that the correct medication and dosage were heard and repeated back to the physician for confirmation.* Online medical direction can give the paramedic a degree of comfort in knowing that administering a particular medication in the proper amount is not the sole decision of the field provider.

In other ALS systems medication administration is accomplished by adherence to either **standing orders** or ALS **protocols.** Standing orders serve as advance orders from medical direction that are developed ahead of time and are followed by all paramedics in that particular ALS system. They are directives to be followed in the event that certain medical conditions are determined by the paramedic. Standing orders are used routinely, and in these cases online medical direction is not necessary. The paramedic typically provides a report to medical direction either en route or on arrival in the ED to communicate the medication(s) administered, dose, route, and effect on the patient. An example of a standing order is shown in Figure 2-1—area shaded in *red*.

Protocol for Allergic Reactions

History
1. Exposure, ingestion, or contact (stings, drugs, foods, etc.)
2. Prior allergic history
3. Current medications

Symptoms
4. Itching
5. Rash
6. Swelling
7. Respiratory distress
8. Abdominal pain
9. Nausea, vomiting
10. Syncope
11. Weakness
12. Anxiety
13. Choking sensation
14. Cough

Signs
15. Vital signs: Vary (routine or shock*)
16. Skin: Rash, redness, urticaria (hives), generalized or local edema
17. HEENT: Tongue or upper airway (uvula) edema*
18. Respiratory: Wheezing, stridor, hoarseness,* cough, upper airway noise
19. Neurologic: Varies

Basic Life Support
20. Secure airway in accordance with airway protocol
21. **Administer supplemental oxygen, maintain saturation between 90% and 100%**
22. Record and monitor vital signs
23. Assist patient in self-administration of previously prescribed Sub-Q epinephrine (autoinjector)
24. Nothing by mouth

Advanced Life Support
25. Advanced airway/ventilatory management as needed
26. Initiate cardiac monitoring, record and evaluate ECG strip
27. Record and monitor O_2 saturation
28. Microstream capnography (if available), if any acute respiratory symptoms
29. If BP < 90 mm Hg systolic, **administer boluses of 0.9% NaCl at 250-500 mL to maintain systolic BP > 90 mm Hg**
   - *Contraindicated if evidence of congestive heart failure (e.g., rales)*

30. Mild Reaction (Itching/Hives)
   a) **Diphenhydramine** (Benadryl) **1 mg/kg IV** (Maximum 50 mg)
      i) May be administered IM if no IV access available
31. Moderate Reaction (Dyspnea, Wheezing, Chest tightness)
   a) **Albuterol** (Proventil) **2.5 mg/3 ml via aerosolized**
      i) May repeat Albuterol (Proventil) X 2
   b) **Diphenhydramine** (Benadryl) **1 mg/kg IV** (Maximum 50 mg)
      i) May be administered IM if no IV access available
   c) **Methylprednisolone** (Solu-Medrol) **125mg, slow IV bolus**
32. Severe Systemic Reaction (BP < 90 mm Hg, Stridor, Severe respiratory distress)
   a) **Epinephrine 1:1000 0.3 mg Sub-Q**
   b) **Albuterol** (Proventil) **2.5 mg/3 mL via aerosolized**
      i) May repeat X 2
   c) **Methylprednisolone** (Solu-Medrol) **125 mg, slow IV bolus**
   d) **Diphenhydramine** (Benadryl) **1 mg/kg IV** (Maximum 50 mg)
      i) May be administered IM if no IV access
33. Cardiopulmonary Arrest Imminent
   a) **Epinephrine 1:10,000 0.5 mg IVP** (instead of 1:1000 Sub-Q)
   b) **Albuterol** (Proventil) **2.5 mg/3 mL via aerosolized**
   c) **Diphenhydramine** (Benadryl) **1 mg/kg IV** (Maximum 50 mg)
      i) May be administered IM if no IV access available

▼ **Fig. 2-1** Example of a protocol. A protocol is a series of orders and instructions that outline the treatment required for a specific medical condition. The area shaded in *red* is an example of a standing order. Standing orders are provided in advance by medical direction to be used by providers in specific circumstances. A standing order is usually one element of a series of standing orders or instructions, referred to as a *protocol*.

In most cases protocols are orders designed to be followed in the event that online medical direction is not available for certain reasons. These reasons are spelled out as part of protocol development and can include situations such as communication systems failure and limited access to online medical direction because of system design. These protocols define what should be done for the patient in particular situations. An example of a protocol is shown in Figure 2-1.

Medication administration is a critical element of most ALS protocols because remembering the medications and doses to administer to a particular patient in a particular situation can be difficult in the often stressful field environment. Committing protocols to memory is important to help prevent administration of the wrong drug or the wrong dose of the drug.

Both standing orders and protocols are typically developed after much thought and study. In many ways they represent the standard of care for prehospital ALS in a given community or region. These procedures can be invaluable tools for the paramedic in the field and serve as a safeguard to avoiding errors in medication administration.

Most protocols are based on an either/or analysis and often are written as a flow-chart or decision tree. At a particular point in the protocol, a choice must be made. For example, a protocol for cardiac arrest or ventricular fibrillation may state that if a patient is in ventricular fibrillation, epinephrine 1 mg should be administered by IV push every 5 minutes. The first decision is to determine whether the patient is in ventricular fibrillation. If the answer is "yes," the protocol to administer the epinephrine should be followed.

An important aspect of standing orders and protocols is that they tend to be rigid and do not allow for unique patient conditions or situations. Most ALS systems require that these orders be followed exactly, except in extremely unusual situations. Because they represent the standard of care for particular patient conditions, failure to follow orders to the letter can put a paramedic at a disadvantage in court. Unfortunately, the clarity of standing orders and protocols can be quickly used against the paramedic in court if he or she did not follow them as any other reasonable and prudent paramedic would have, given the same situation. These documents are commonly entered into evidence in lawsuits through a fact witness (someone involved in the situation, such as a paramedic or emergency physician) or an expert witness hired to provide an opinion on whether the protocols were appropriate, reflected the standard of care in the community, and were properly followed.

Standing orders and protocols are important considerations in lawsuits. They work in the clinician's favor by providing direction in managing patients in difficult and stressful situations in which clarity of thinking and judgment can be skewed.

The following actions can help ensure that protocols involving medication administration work favorably for the paramedic and the patient:

▶ *Keep protocols up to date.* Protocols need to change as the standard of medical care changes. This frequently happens in EMS as treatment modalities are reevaluated by national physician groups, such as the American Heart Association's Emergency Cardiac Care Committee. When this happens, a community's ALS system needs to evaluate these changes to determine whether they should be implemented. The ALS system must provide the most current treatment modalities. Failure to keep pace with the changes in prehospital medicine can have a negative effect on patients' clinical outcomes and can work against clinicians in a negligence action. This failure can be used by the plaintiff's attorney to demonstrate what the standard of care should be in that particular case and to show that a system did not follow the appropriate standard of care. In most cases the individual paramedic is not found liable for performing treatment in accordance with outdated protocols. However, the EMS agency carries a great risk for liability in these situations.

▶ *Know the protocols.* Paramedics must know their ALS treatment protocols inside and out. Frequent review of these protocols and drills that test knowledge (such as a simulated cardiac arrest situation, or "mega code") are essential. Proper protocol use leads to positive patient outcomes and reduced risk of negligence lawsuits.

LAWS GOVERNING PREHOSPITAL PHARMACOLOGY

Numerous laws govern the use of medications and pharmacologic agents in the field. The basic laws that address the manufacturing, packaging, and labeling of medications have their roots in the early twentieth century. At that time many deaths were caused by improperly manufactured drugs, as well as the lack of education for physicians and patients about contraindications, side effects, and proper administration and use.

The federal Food, Drug, and Cosmetic Act, enacted in 1938, required detailed labeling of all medications. From this law evolved the package insert required in all medication packaging. This insert describes in detail the generic and common names of the drug, indications and contraindications for administration, directions for its use, recommended dosages, and potential side effects. This law alone eliminated scores of medication errors through proper and accurate labeling.

Narcotic agents are afforded extra scrutiny under the law because of their potential for abuse. The federal Comprehensive Drug Abuse Prevention and Control Act of 1970 classified potentially dangerous and habit-forming drugs into five different classes, or schedules, with safeguards for their prescription, use, and control.

The more dangerous drugs have a lower schedule number. **Schedule I** drugs are the most dangerous and have the highest abuse potential. Drugs in this class have no recognized medical use; examples include heroin, lysergic acid diethylamide (LSD), and methaqualone. **Schedule II** drugs are recognized as having a high potential for abuse, but they are safe and have accepted medical uses. Schedule II drugs include narcotics, stimulants, and depressant drugs. They are available only by a written prescription, and their distribution is carefully monitored by the Drug Enforcement Agency (DEA). Some medications administered in the prehospital field, such as morphine sulfate and meperidine, are Schedule II drugs, as are stimulants (e.g., amphetamines) and depressants (e.g., secobarbital). **Schedule III** drugs have less abuse potential than Schedule I and II drugs. Abuse of Schedule III drugs may lead to moderate or low physical dependence. Examples of Schedule III drugs include narcotics such as codeine, common stimulants such as benzphetamine, and depressants such as talbutal. **Schedule IV** and **Schedule V** agents are less habit forming and pose a lesser risk of harm from overdose. Examples of Schedule IV drugs include diazepam (Valium) and alprazolam (Xanax). Cough medications with codeine are an example of Schedule V drugs.

The Controlled Substances Act is enforced by the DEA. Only physicians registered with the DEA and those who have approved DEA numbers may prescribe scheduled medications. The physician's DEA number must appear on the prescription form, and serious criminal penalties can be levied for misusing this number.

In addition to the federal drug control laws, most states have enacted their own laws that address the use and misuse of medications. As with federal laws, many of these laws mandate criminal penalties for violation; so in many cases of abuse, theft, misuse, and illegal sale of scheduled drugs, both the federal and state criminal codes may have been violated.

State EMS laws also govern the use of prehospital medications. Most states have approved drug lists that outline the medications that an EMT-Intermediate or paramedic may administer in the field. Ultimately the local EMS system's medical director dictates which of those drugs may be used in the system. EMS agencies *must* maintain and use only the medications approved by the state EMS office and local medical director.

In many cases, state EMS laws mandate disciplinary sanctions against emergency personnel who misuse approved medications. Violations of the regulations that control drug administration in the prehospital setting can result in a hearing and disciplinary action, such as suspension or revocation of certification. Care must be taken at all times to follow state laws carefully and report any violations to the management of the EMS agency, the medical director, and the appropriate state or local authority.

OPERATIONAL CONSIDERATIONS

Medications used by paramedics are life-saving tools that can stabilize the heart or treat anaphylactic shock. As a comparison, consider the traditional tools commonly required for search and rescue. These tools might include Hurst Jaws of Life (Hale Products, Shelby, NC) and rams to extricate victims from motor vehicle collisions or ropes and rappelling gear for high-angle rescues. Because the lives of the victim and rescuer depend on this vital equipment, it should be meticulously stored and maintained. Because drugs are tools to the paramedic, they also must be carefully stored, secured, and maintained.

STORAGE AND SECURITY

Because of the mandate to provide proper patient care and adhere to the strict legal controls over drugs used in the prehospital setting, every EMS organization must ensure the safety and security of the medications within its control. Medications must be properly ordered, inventoried, stored, and dispensed when needed. A central storage location at the organization that is kept secure with double locking systems is often the best method for ensuring this protection.

Special care must be taken to ensure the security of narcotic agents because of the potential for theft and misuse. Narcotics should be signed in and signed out at each shift, with clear documentation of the transfer of the custody of the narcotics from one EMS crew to the next. Appropriate log books should be maintained at all times so that, in the event of lost or missing narcotics, determining who had the responsibility for protecting the drug at that time is possible (Fig. 2-2). All transfers of narcotics from one crew to the next should be witnessed so that at no time does only one person have access to the narcotic agents.

DRUG CURRENCY

All medications have varying **shelf life,** the period of time a medication can be stored and remain suitable for use. The length of a medication's shelf life depends on many factors, such as the chemical composition of the drug, its stability or volatility, and its expected period of effectiveness. Shelf life varies significantly across the spectrum of drugs used in the prehospital setting, so expiration dates must be constantly checked and rechecked. Outdated medications have no place in the prehospital setting; they will likely not have the intended beneficial effects for patients. In addition, courts look poorly on organizations and health professionals who use outdated drugs. If the use of an outdated medication can be proven in court, the plaintiff has an easier time proving a case of negligence against the EMS agency or the individual care provider.

The potential for using outdated drugs exists when the drugs are infrequently used. For this reason, daily checklists must be used to ensure that no medication carried by the EMS unit is outdated or damaged. All outdated medications should be properly disposed of according to the organization's policies. Medications also should be disposed of when they appear to have been damaged, if the seals on the packaging are broken, or if the medication may have been exposed to environmental conditions that contradict the manufacturer's instructions for storage.

ENVIRONMENTAL ISSUES

Prehospital ALS is provided in all types of weather and in a wide range of environmental conditions. In addition, the nature of emergency response necessitates that medications are portable and ready to go in a given moment. The U.S. Food and Drug Administration has strict requirements on the environmental parameters within which a medication is effective, and storage temperature ranges are established for virtually all medications.

Administering a medication that has been rendered ineffective because of exposure to excessive heat or cold does not benefit the patient and is a risk factor for liability. This is a common area in which liability is assessed against the ALS system in negligence cases. Strict adherence to medication storage and use requirements is thus absolutely essential.

Narcotic Log

Date	Patient Name	Drug Given	Amount of Drug Given	Name of Person Administering Drug	Signature of Authorizing Physician
2/10/08	S. Tombber	midazolam	1.0 mg	K. Milford, EMT-P	*(signature)*

▼ **Fig. 2-2**   Example of a log book. A medication, or narcotic, log is a record of controlled substances administered in the prehospital setting. The log allows the tracking of narcotic inventory and usage.

Where should medications be stored to ensure that they are maintained in the proper environmental conditions according to the manufacturer? Medications often are stored in sealed drug boxes in the ambulance or response vehicle. If the vehicle is parked outside rather than in an environmentally controlled garage, the vehicle itself must be appropriately connected to systems that maintain an appropriate temperature. If drugs are exposed to excessive heat or cold while in use, as in the case of a mountain rescue or other extended time situation, they should be properly discarded and replaced on return.

EXPOSURE TO BLOODBORNE PATHOGENS

Safety of self, crew members, and other responders is always a top priority. Medication administration must be conducted in a manner that is as risk free as possible. The Occupational Safety and Health Act provides clear guidelines for EMS personnel in dealing with the potential exposure to bloodborne pathogens, which can occur when administering medications by the IV route or being exposed to bodily fluids. The threat of human immunodeficiency virus (HIV), hepatitis, and other diseases spread through the blood warrants strict adherence to all safety requirements and procedures.

In recent years the federal Occupational Health and Safety Administration has intensified its interest in the safety of healthcare providers and EMS providers in particular. Recent regulatory changes require all EMS agencies to review their sharps devices and obtain the best possible devices to minimize risk of exposure. The regulations require that EMS agencies involve their personnel in the selection of safe devices.

The federal Ryan White Law provides safeguards for EMS personnel in the event of a needlestick. The law establishes a mechanism of reporting so that, if a patient tests positive for HIV, EMS personnel are advised through the medical director of the necessary precautions and other steps that should be taken.

CONSENT ISSUES AND LIMITATIONS

The United States Supreme Court has upheld the right of every patient to self-determination regarding medical care and the application of life-saving or life-sustaining measures. Put simply, every person has the right to determine whether to accept or reject any type of medical care or treatment (including any form of "laying on of hands" by healthcare providers) as long as he or she is capable of making that decision as a competent adult.

This principle of self-determination applies in the prehospital environment just as it does within a hospital. However, the likelihood of a patient not being competent to make decisions is higher in the prehospital setting because of a variety of factors, such as shock, substance abuse, and decreased level of consciousness. Prehospital professionals need to ensure that their patients give **consent** for every assessment and treatment provided. All competent adults have the right to consent to or refuse care and treatment, even in emergency situations. This includes the right to refuse parts of the care and treatment.

Patients are often leery of medication administration in the field, particularly older patients who are accustomed to traditional healthcare only and may consider an ambulance as merely a transportation system. Some patients will consent to an assessment and non-invasive treatment but will refuse invasive therapies such as parental medications. The patient may simply dislike needles or be opposed to the administration of specific medications. Remember, prehospital professionals have an obligation to inform the patient about what medication is being administered, as well as the reason for administration.

What should paramedics do when a patient refuses to consent to administration of a medication? First, ensure the patient is competent to make that refusal. Any refusal of consent to care must be carefully documented. Failure to properly assess the patient's ability to give consent and improper documentation of a refusal of consent are significant liability risks that open the door to claims of abandonment or negligence.

Refusals can be complete or partial. A **complete refusal** occurs in situations in which the patient refuses all aspects of treatment. This probably is the most common type of refusal situation. A **partial refusal** occurs when a patient agrees to some, but not all, of the treatment offered. If a patient refuses a portion of treatment, such as the administration of a specific medication, the paramedic can still provide other treatment that the patient does consent to receive. In these situations the paramedic should obtain written documentation of the refusal, even if it is just a partial refusal, when possible.

A^{3}E^{3}P^3 REFUSAL GUIDELINES

Consent and the refusal of consent must be properly handled to minimize liability. One set of guidelines, termed the **A^{3}E^{3}P^3** (*a*ssess, *a*dvise, *a*void; *e*nsure, *e*xplain, *e*xploit; *p*ersist, *p*rotocols, *p*rotect) **refusal guidelines,** helps EMS providers remember the critical considerations when faced with refusal situations.

Assess

Assess the patient's legal and mental capacity to refuse care. The patient must be a legally recognized adult (older than age 18 years) or deemed by law to be considered an adult (as with an emancipated minor or other special circumstances). However, proof that the patient is emancipated is difficult to obtain because no common form of identification exists that indicates this status. Some states, such as California, place this notation on the person's driver's license if the Division of Motor Vehicles is provided with court documentation that the minor is emancipated. Therefore always err on the side of treatment whenever doubtful of whether the patient can legally refuse treatment. Only competent adults can consent to care or refuse care. Minors are permitted by most state laws to consent to medical treatment, but they may not refuse treatment. In other words, allowing a minor to refuse care in a case in which it is clearly needed would pose significant risk of a claim for patient abandonment; minors usually are not considered legally competent to refuse treatment.

Does the patient have a mental condition that might prevent him or her from making an informed decision? Examples include permanent conditions such as Alzheimer's disease and situational conditions such as shock, alcohol or drug intoxication, and decreased level of consciousness from a head injury or other trauma.

Advise

Advise the patient of his or her medical condition and the proposed treatment. Although prehospital care providers do not make diagnoses, they are required to tell a patient what is going on regarding his or her medical condition and how the care provider proposes to help so that the refusal decision is informed. Do not be afraid to tell the patient the truth about what is happening.

Avoid

Avoid the use of confusing terminology when talking to patients; speak to them in terms they can understand. For example, rather than saying "You appear to be having a myocardial infarction with premature ventricular contractions that could cause you to go into ventricular fibrillation at any moment," explain to the patient, "You are probably having a heart attack, and you have very irregular heartbeats that could cause your heart to stop beating at any time. That is why we need to put this medication into your vein—to calm down those irregular beats."

Ensure

Ensure that the patient's decision to refuse care is the result of his or her own informed decision making and not the result of improper influence or coercion by others. Make sure the patient is not merely parroting what a family member is telling him or her to say.

Explain

Explain the alternatives to the patient if he or she refuses care and transportation. Make sure the patient knows all the options, such as calling 9-1-1 again, calling his or her physician, and going to the ED if the symptoms continue or worsen.

Exploit

Exploit uncertainty. Many patients are unsure about whether they should go to the hospital, and that uncertainty should be used to the care provider's advantage in advising the patient to obtain necessary care. For example, when a patient expresses uncertainty, he or she typically expresses it with the idea that the healthcare professional will help make the necessary decision. For example, a patient may say "I'm not sure I need to go to the hospital." The care provider could reply, "Well, if I were you, I would certainly go to the hospital, where a doctor could check me out and where all the necessary equipment is there if it is needed." A variety of creative ways can be used to make positive statements to encourage the patient to allow further care. This situation requires good communications skills.

Persist

Persist in trying to persuade the patient to obtain the necessary care. The prehospital professional may need to make several attempts to convince a patient that he or she should consent to EMS treatment and transported to the hospital. A well-documented refusal helps demonstrate this persistence in the event of a lawsuit.

Protocols

Protocols are meant to be followed. If your service or EMS system has protocols in place regarding patient refusals, be sure to adhere to them. This is especially important in regard to medication administration because of the many risks associated with deviating from the traditional treatments.

Protect

Protect yourself with adequate documentation of the refusal (Fig. 2-3). Write a thorough narrative explaining all the steps in the process, obtain the patient's signature to verify his or her understanding of the decision when possible, and try to get the names and addresses of witnesses who observed the refusal process. Describe the specifics of any partial refusal of care.

REFUSAL OF SERVICES

I hereby refuse the emergency medical services and/or transportation offered and advised by the above named service provider and its emergency personnel, _____ hospital, and the emergency medical and nursing personnel from said hospital giving directions to the service provider. I understand that my refusal may jeopardize the health of the patient, and hereby release the above named parties from any and all claims of liability in connection with my refusal.

_____
Signature of Patient or Legally Authorized Representative

_____
Signature of EMT/Field RN

_____
Witness   **Date**

▼ **Fig. 2-3** A release from liability form. (From Shade B, Collins T, Wertz E, et al: *Mosby's EMT-intermediate textbook for the 1985 National Standard Curriculum,* rev, St Louis, 2006, Mosby.)

LIVING WILLS AND ADVANCE DIRECTIVES

All states have living will statutes that allow individuals to designate in advance the level of medical intervention they want to receive in the event of a terminal illness. These legal documents provide **advance directives,** or specific orders to the caregiver, regarding what level of treatment the patient wants to receive in such a situation. Many advance directives provide limitations on treatment in the event of a cardiac arrest or coma. These directives typically allow the healthcare provider to treat the patient with palliative or comfort measures and restrict the use of resuscitative measures such as cardiopulmonary resuscitation, endotracheal **intubation,** and medication administration.

Most state laws have strict verification requirements to ensure that the directive being followed is proper. Some states require that patients wear identification tags (similar to medic alert tags that are used to identify patients with allergies or medical conditions), whereas others require a document signed by the patient's attending physician. In some states these orders are found in a red envelope on the kitchen refrigerator. Some states require that online medical direction be consulted before an advance directive can be recognized. Even if the patient has an advance directive in place, however, it can be overruled at any time by the patient. A competent patient has the right to void the directive by changing his or her mind during the course of treatment.

Restrictions on medication administration should be clearly delineated in the directive. For example, the directive could state that "no advanced cardiac life support medications" are to be administered. Or the directive could be specific to certain medications, such as stating that epinephrine and atropine should be withheld. In many situations involving terminally ill patients with cancer, morphine sulfate and other pain medications are specifically permitted to be given intravenously, but all other medications are to be withheld. Check state laws and local protocols for the correct procedures to be followed when confronted with an advance directive.

DOCUMENTATION

Clear and accurate documentation is required for quality patient care and is a necessity in a litigious society. The patient care record (PCR) is closely scrutinized in malpractice and negligence trials, so ensure that documentation is thorough and specific. If you are called to the witness stand, you will be cross-examined by the plaintiff's counsel about the quality of your documentation. If your documentation of patient care is sloppy or incomplete, this fact will reflect negatively on your credibility as a competent caregiver, even if your documentation contains no gross errors.

Following are some important dos and don'ts to consider when documenting medication administration[6]:

DOS

▶ Ensure that the documentation of medication administration is an accurate reflection of your prehospital capabilities and your scope of practice.

▶ Write legibly and in complete sentences with proper abbreviations so that all personnel can adequately read your report.

▶ Document the time, medication given, dose, method, and route of administration in the treatment section of the PCR.

▶ Document a medication refusal by the patient and state why the patient refused the medication. Document every attempt you make to persuade the patient, and ask for the patient's signature.

▶ Document why you gave the patient a particular medication.

▶ Document known medication allergies and any untoward reactions to medication you administer, as well as the treatment you provided in response.

▶ Document vital signs before and after administration of all medications.

▶ Document any changes in vital signs, especially if the patient's condition worsens.

▶ Document the name of the physician or medical director who gave the medication order and the time of the order.

DON'TS

▶ Do not scribble or write illegibly.

▶ Do not misspell words or medication names.

▶ Do not forget to check the patient's response to the medication.

▶ Do not make up abbreviations or use inappropriate acronyms in documentation. Use only approved standard abbreviations.

▶ Do not assume that other crew members will take care of your documentation. If you gave the medication, you are responsible for documenting that fact.

▶ Do not prepare your report late if you can avoid it. Document any late entries or errors if changes or entries are made after the original report is completed and submitted.

In general, always prepare your documentation as though it will be presented in a court of law. Ask yourself the question: Is my documentation for this patient the best it can be and how I would want my own care documented? Strive to answer "yes" to this question in every situation, and your reports will accurately document the care you provide, hold up in court, validate your credibility, and positively reflect your care.

SCOPE OF PRACTICE ISSUES

Critical patient care situations in the field can be stressful, especially for novice prehospital providers or the sole EMT-Intermediate or paramedic available to provide ALS treatment. Many ALS systems have worked hard to encourage basic life support (BLS) personnel participation in the ALS care of patients through "paramedic assist" courses and other programs. EMTs and first responders are quite willing to assist paramedics with specific ALS procedures.

However, EMT-Intermediates and paramedics should proceed extremely cautiously when involving BLS personnel in ALS procedures. Even when a paramedic does not have enough hands to do everything at once, assigning to BLS personnel a procedure that can be performed legally only by an advanced-level caregiver is risky. At all times, BLS and ALS personnel must function within the limitations of their respective scopes of practice, which is defined by each state's EMS act.

A good example of how scope of practice can become a problem is with establishing an IV line. Should you allow an EMT or first responder to set up the IV bag and tubing, as well as flush the line of any air? No. Allowing this level of assistance (unless BLS personnel are permitted to establish IV lines under state law) is a risk that should not be taken. Unless the EMS provider is certified to provide that level of care, allowing BLS personnel to perform any part of a procedure that requires advanced training is improper. Although properly identifying the IV solution, maintaining a sterile field when removing protective covers, hooking up the IV tubing, and flushing the line may seem like simple tasks, they do involve a level of advanced training that only EMT-Intermediates and paramedics typically receive. A paramedic who permits a basic-level EMS provider to perform an advanced skill could be considered negligent for improperly delegating the skill. In addition, the basic-level EMS provider can be in violation of his or her state's EMS act by performing a skill outside the scope of practice for the individual's level of certification.

What can the basic-level provider do to assist in this situation? In a nutshell, everything short of providing a skill considered restricted to a more advanced care provider. With the example of starting an IV, this could include getting the solutions and IV start supplies, removing them from their packages (but not exposing sterile surfaces), tearing tape, and preparing other material to be used to secure the IV site and tubing.

When administering any medication, EMT-Intermediates and paramedics must *personally* complete all the steps necessary to administer the medication properly. The following steps should be taken each time a medication is administered:

1. Ask the patient about any known allergies to medications, and check for a MedicAlert bracelet or tag.
2. Determine the patient's medical history and current medications so that drug interactions can be avoided.
3. Verify that you have the correct medication in the correct concentration. Although recent packaging procedures have significantly lowered this risk, one of the common medication errors in the field is administering the right medication in the *wrong* concentration (e.g., administering the concentrated form of the medication intended for an IV drip infusion as a direct IV bolus, or vice versa).

A common sense rule to avoid mistakes is to check the label on the medication at least four times: when selecting the medication, when preparing to draw it up, after drawing it up, and finally, while administering it.

4. Verify and repeat any order received to administer a medication. The technical quality of radio and telephone communications in the field can be unreliable.
5. Examine the packaging of the medication for discoloration and any other unusual characteristics.
6. Examine the packaging of the medication and the vial or ampule itself for the expiration date.
7. Open the medication and prepare it for administration, following proper procedures for ensuring sterility.
8. Administer the medication according to the proper procedure or protocol for the particular drug.

9. Observe the patient for any untoward reactions and any improvement or other change in condition. Report any changes to medical direction or hospital staff on arrival.

A common question that arises regarding scope of practice is whether an EMT or first responder should document on the BLS PCR interventions or assessments performed by the paramedic. This may be an issue in which EMS is provided in tiered systems; that is, when BLS and ALS are provided by separate organizations (e.g., BLS responds in a transporting ambulance and ALS responds in a nontransporting paramedic intercept or fly car unit). In some systems the practice may be to document that the ALS provider applied a cardiac monitor and what electrocardiographic rhythm was displayed on the monitor. Some EMTs also document that the paramedic started an IV, how many attempts were necessary to establish the line, what medications and solutions were administered through the IV, and other information about the ALS care provided.

As a general rule, EMS providers should document according to their scope of practice and should not attempt to document skills beyond what they are trained and certified to perform themselves. Too great a risk for inconsistent and inaccurate records is posed when a provider documents beyond his or her scope of practice. In addition, such documentation could impair the credibility of the EMS provider if he or she becomes a witness in a lawsuit. If an EMT documents a particular cardiac rhythm, for example, that provider is vulnerable to a damaging cross-examination about his or her training and qualifications, or lack thereof, to make such determinations and why he or she would document care beyond the scope of practice. An EMT who is not able to answer questions in a deposition or on the witness stand about all the documentation, including the EMT-documented ALS care, could find his or her quality of treatment and credibility called into question.

This is not to suggest that EMTs should not document any facts regarding the ALS treatment. For example, the EMT should certainly document the fact that the paramedic provided patient care in addition to the EMT's role in the care. If the paramedic intubated the patient, and the EMT handled the bag-mask ventilation, the BLS patient care report should reflect that. Other general observations on a BLS patient care report, such as "paramedic performed a patient assessment," "paramedic intubated the patient," "paramedic applied a cardiac monitor," and "IV medications administered by the paramedic" are also appropriate, as long as the EMT refrains from describing details such as the intubation technique used, tube size used, particular cardiac rhythm displayed on the monitor, and the names and dosages of specific medications administered by ALS.

In many areas the provision of EMS is a team effort between BLS and ALS providers, with both groups performing specific responsibilities and playing valuable roles in patient care. Just as EMS providers must render all patient care within their respective scope of practice, their documentation should likewise be limited to their scope of practice.

MISDIRECTION OF MEDICATIONS

A less common liability issue with respect to medication administration in EMS is "misdirection," or theft, of controlled substances. Federal and state laws place strict requirements on the purchase, storage, and use of medications, particularly controlled substances. Serious criminal penalties exist for the misappropriation of certain types of medications, such as narcotic agents, and healthcare providers who misuse medications entrusted to them are judged harshly.

The medication supply system should be closely monitored, with clearly defined purchase and security procedures in place. Common criminal activity includes stealing a medication from the storage device and replacing it with water or another substance. This gives the appearance that the caregiver is actually administering the medication, when in fact the patient is getting nothing more than a placebo. Ethically this is a particularly heinous crime because the replacement can go undetected for quite some time, and patients can be harmed by not receiving medication.

Unfortunately, because the EMS environment is a less-controlled environment than the traditional hospital setting, weaknesses often exist in the medication supply system that require close attention and monitoring. At a minimum, no person should have sole access to the medication supply system. Appropriate checks and balances should be in place. The medication supply and control system should be periodically audited by individuals who are not directly associated with it.

INCIDENT REPORTING

Every medication error must be properly documented and reported. This is essential for patient care and quality assurance to prevent the error from happening again. The ALS provider who makes a medication error and fails to properly document and report it is in violation of the law, as well as general principles of ethics.

Making these reports is a professional duty even when you know that you could be subjected to disciplinary action or other negative consequences. The failure to report errors demonstrates a lack of professionalism and can jeopardize a patient's life. Being a professional requires a high degree of self-regulation, and the prehospital care provider must adhere to all rules of conduct, particularly when a mistake is made.

National formats for reporting medication errors are available for other healthcare professions, but no national standard has been developed in EMS. Every EMS system should have its own standardized system for documenting medication errors. The system medical director should be involved in the review of any medication errors.

EMS agencies should have a policy on "unusual occurrence reporting," which defines what occurrences should be reported and the procedures for reporting them. Medication errors, such as errors in drug choice, dosage, or route of administration, are high on the list of reportable occurrences.

Incident reports should be completed promptly while the care provider's memory is fresh, providing the essential details of the incident. Once the incident report is completed, it should be submitted to the immediate supervisor. Attaching the incident report to the PCR is not advised, because anything attached to the PCR can become part of the medical record. Of course, the PCR should clearly indicate any known errors that occurred in patient care and the steps that were taken to remedy the error. However, the details of how the error occurred are best left for the separate incident report.

The incident should then be promptly investigated by appropriate management personnel and the system's medical director. Appropriate corrective action should be taken when a medication error has occurred. Corrective action can include additional continuing education for the individual and sometimes disciplinary action. Most state EMS laws may also have requirements that certain medication errors be reported to the EMS office, and a standard incident report format may be in place at that agency.

In many cases of medication errors, problems in the system may have contributed to the error. Every medication error should be reviewed from a quality assurance and risk management perspective to ensure that system problems are identified and corrected. Otherwise, the risk of a future error is not reduced, and another care provider in the system may be just as likely to make the same mistake. System-wide education may ultimately be required after the error is closely reviewed. Although medication and other treatment errors are unfortunate occurrences, these errors provide an opportunity to review the system critically and make positive changes to improve overall prehospital patient care.

Risk reduction is the key to avoiding liability in medication administration. The two primary goals should always be to eliminate or reduce the risk of harm to the patient and eliminate or reduce the risk of a successful lawsuit against the EMS organization. Improving overall patient safety is the general theme that encompasses the actions taken to reduce errors. This theme must be applied to every aspect of medication administration.

In 2001 the EMS Division of the National Highway Traffic Safety Administration sponsored a roundtable to discuss EMS patient safety and error reduction strategies. The participants discussed the types of error reduction activities occurring in other sectors of medicine, considered how errors could be reduced, and identified which patient safety activities should be pursued. The participants recognized that EMS providers need greater insight into the human factors that affect patient safety and a better reporting system when errors occur.

Accepting responsibility for the human factors that can affect your ability to function error free is the key to a professional approach to avoiding medication errors in the field. By taking this responsibility seriously, you can reduce the risk of harm to your patients and minimize the risk of liability for your EMS organization.

REVIEW QUESTIONS

1. Define ordinary negligence.
2. What is the principal goal of Good Samaritan laws?
3. If a paramedic makes an honest mistake in a medication administration, is he or she negligent?
4. Define standing orders and protocols.
5. What are the medical uses for medications categorized as Schedule I?
6. Define shelf life and explain the importance of checking a drug's expiration date.
7. What is the Ryan White Law?
8. Who decides what medications will be used by a particular EMS system?
9. What should a prehospital provider do when a patient refuses a medication or treatment?
10. Define a partial and a complete refusal.
11. In most states, can a minor refuse treatment?
12. What treatment levels are acceptable under advance directives?
13. List the "don'ts" of documenting medication administration.
14. Should an incident report be attached to a PCR?

REFERENCES

1. Institute of Medicine: *To err is human: building a safer health system,* Washington, DC, 2000, National Academies Press.
2. Hubble MW, Paschal KR, Sanders TA: Medication calculation skills of practicing paramedics, *Prehosp Emerg Care* 4(3):253-60, 2000.
3. *Hoffman v. Brandywine Hospital,* 661 A.2d 397 (Pa. Super. 1995).
4. 35 PA STAT 6931(j).
5. *Albright v. Abington Memorial Hospital,* 696 A.2d 1159 (Pa. 1997).
6. Bruce ML, Sones SS, Peck B: Medication safety. Implications for EMS, *Emerg Med Serv* 32:97, 2003.

BIBLIOGRAPHY

Page J, Wolfberg D, Wirth S: *EMS law bulletins,* www.pwwemslaw.com, Accessed February 27, 2007.
Patient safety in emergency medical services roundtable report and recommendations, Washington, DC, 2002, National Highway Traffic Safety Administration.

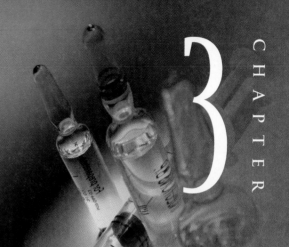

Drug Administration: Safety and Procedures

OBJECTIVES

1. Define standing orders, one-time orders, and as-needed (prn) orders.
2. Discuss the six patient rights of drug administration.
3. Explain the routes of enteral medications (oral, rectal, sublingual, and buccal) and demonstrate the proper procedure for each.
4. Explain the routes of parenteral medications (intravenous, intramuscular, subcutaneous, intraosseous, transdermal/topical, inhalation, endotracheal tube) and demonstrate the proper procedure for each.

INTRODUCTION

Administration of medication in the prehospital field can significantly improve patient outcome. To make the best use of this important patient care tool, prehospital professionals must be cognizant of rules regarding medication orders and guidelines regarding patient and provider safety. Step-by-step instructions for safe and accurate medication administration by a variety of routes are given in this chapter. Instructions for administration of intravenous drugs and intraosseous infusions are provided in Chapter 5.

You are dispatched to a medical call for a man down at a local shopping mall. Just before arriving on the scene, the dispatcher informs you that mall security has used an automated external defibrillator on the patient. At the scene, you find an elderly male approximately 70 years old who is unresponsive. You immediately reach for your defibrillator pads while your partner moves to the patient's head and begins bag-mask ventilation. The screen on the cardiac monitor displays ventricular tachycardia. You immediately defibrillate the patient, and he converts to a sinus rhythm. To prevent him from returning to ventricular tachycardia, you administer a bolus of amiodarone (Cordarone) 150 mg IV over 10 minutes. ...

MEDICATION ORDERS

A paramedic requires an order from a medical direction physician to administer a medication. **Medical direction** is the process by which physicians direct and monitor the care given in the prehospital environment within an EMS system. Medical direction can be provided either online or offline. **Online medical direction** occurs when the prehospital provider is able to consult and obtain direction and orders in real time by radio or telephone communication (Fig. 3-1). **Offline medical direction** occurs when the physician medical director is not available for real-time interactions. The majority of cases of medical direction are offline. The medical director approves a series of protocols detailing the care that the prehospital professional is to provide in a given clinical scenario.

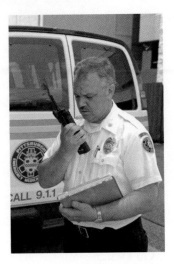

▼ **Fig. 3-1**   A paramedic online with medical direction.

Orders can take several forms: **standing orders, one-time orders,** and **as-needed (prn) orders.** All medication orders follow a standard form and include the following four elements:

1. Name of drug
2. Dose: a quantity followed by a unit of measure (e.g., 5 mg)
3. Route: oral, rectal, sublingual, buccal, endotracheal, intramuscular, subcutaneous, transdermal/topical, inhalation, intravenous, or intraosseous
4. Frequency: a one-time order, as needed, or for a duration of time

STANDING ORDERS

Standing orders are instructions for treatment that are usually specific to a particular patient presentation and may or may not require consultation with medical direction. Standing orders are most appropriate for life-threatening conditions that require immediate intervention. In such circumstances, medication standing orders are part of a larger treatment protocol, or a series of interventions and drugs used to treat an emergency condition. For example, EMS systems typically have standing orders for the treatment of life-threatening cardiac arrhythmias, which often are a component of the advanced cardiac life support (ACLS) treatment guidelines. Standing orders also exist for a variety of other conditions, such as grand mal seizures, asthma, and anaphylaxis. In the preceding scenario, the paramedic was not required to confer with medical direction before administering an ACLS drug, because most EMS systems have standing orders for such medications.

ONE-TIME ORDERS

... Your unit is called to a local park to assist a man who has injured his leg while playing baseball. At the field, you find a 28-year-old man who is reporting severe pain in his right leg. He tells you that he was running to home plate when he collided with the catcher. You remove his shoe and split the right leg of his trousers. The patient has an obvious deformity and crepitus of the lower portion of the right leg. You check the distal pulses, as well as motor and sensory function of the injured leg. No vascular or nerve injury is apparent, but the patient clearly has a closed fracture of the right tibia and fibula. Your partner brings the cot to the patient, and you begin to splint the leg and prepare the patient for transport. With any manipulation of the leg, the patient exhibits extreme pain, and you cannot adequately splint or move him without inflicting additional pain. You consult medical direction and obtain an order for 2 mg morphine to be given intravenously. The patient's pain is reduced enough to allow you to splint the injured extremity and place him on the ambulance cot for transport.

One-time orders occur when a paramedic has consulted medical direction and has received an order for immediate drug intervention for the treatment. In the preceding scenario, the paramedic was given a one-time order to administer morphine to the injured patient. This is in contrast to a standing order, in which the local protocol prescribes use of a drug without consulting medical direction. With a one-time order, the paramedic cannot repeat the order without again consulting medical direction.

AS-NEEDED ORDERS

As-needed orders are often referred to as *prn orders* (*prn* is an abbreviation for the Latin phrase *pro re nata,* which means "as the situation demands"). As-needed orders are typically given for a specific patient condition or physiologic parameter. They are commonly given for pain and abnormalities in blood pressure, heart rate, and blood sugar. As-needed orders can be obtained from medical direction to treat a condition if it develops. For example, a paramedic crew is transporting a patient with an open fracture, and the patient is in an extreme amount of pain after the initial 2 mg of IV morphine. The paramedic contacts medical direction to obtain an order for morphine. Medical direction orders morphine 4 mg IV and gives an additional order of morphine 2 mg IV as needed for pain. The second part of that order is an example of an as-needed order.

COMMUNICATION WITH MEDICAL DIRECTION

When orders are received from medical direction, communication must be concise and clear. When an order is given, the paramedic should write it down and then read the order back to medical direction. The physician serving as medical direction should then confirm that the order the paramedic read back is either correct or incorrect. If medical direction does not confirm the order, the paramedic should request confirmation before proceeding.

You are transporting a 54-year-old man who threw gasoline on a fire while burning brush. The fire flashed on the patient, and he sustained burns on approximately 25% of his total body surface area. You have started an IV and began to transport the patient. He is screaming in pain and reports the severity of pain as 10 on a scale of 0 to 10. You get on the radio to medical direction. After reporting your assessment and treatment, you request an order for morphine to treat the patient's pain.

Communication Example

Medical direction:	"Go ahead and give the patient morphine 4 mg IV."
Paramedic:	"Copy. Read back: morphine 4 mg IV push times one. Check?"
Medical direction:	(no response)
Paramedic:	"Morphine 4 mg IV push times one. Please confirm."
Medical direction:	"That's correct."
Paramedic:	"Copy."

When taking verbal orders, always read the order back and await acknowledgment that your order read back was correct. This method reduces communication errors regarding medication orders and improves patient safety.

ISSUES

PATIENT SAFETY

To ensure patient safety regarding medication administration, a checklist known as the **six patient rights of drug administration** is used that contains the elements shown in Figure 3-2.

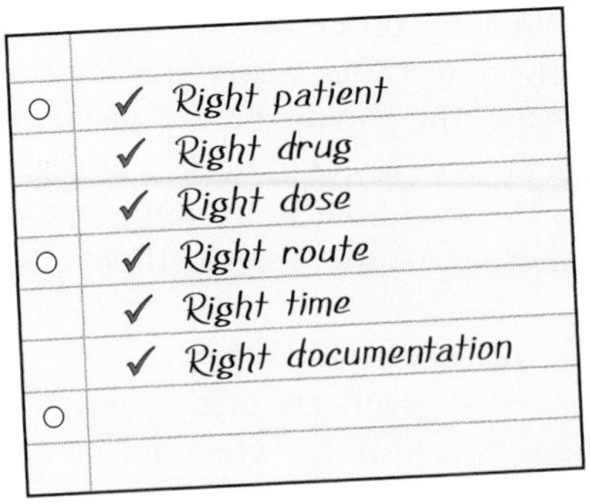

○ ✓ *Right patient*
✓ *Right drug*
✓ *Right dose*
○ ✓ *Right route*
✓ *Right time*
✓ *Right documentation*
○

▼ **Fig. 3-2** Six patient rights of drug administration. Running through this checklist before drug administration will reduce the likelihood of a medication error and improve patient safety.

Run through this checklist before administering any drug to reduce the likelihood of a medication error.

Right Patient

Is the person to whom you will administer the medication the person you think he or she is? This question is perhaps more relevant in a setting where one provider may be caring for several patients. You must ensure that the medication you will administer is meant for the correct patient. If administering or assisting with prescription medications, read the medication label and check to see whether the name on the medication bottle is the name of the patient you are treating.

Right Drug

Before administering a drug, confirm that the drug in your hand is the drug you have been ordered to give. Drugs used in ACLS and other emergency situations are commonly supplied in unassembled, preloaded syringes in color-coded boxes. However, several patient care providers often are at an emergency scene, and the individual who pulls the medications from the medication drawer and removes them from their color-coded boxes may not be the same individual who administers them. In fact, one provider can pass a rather generic-looking preloaded syringe to a second provider to administer the medication to the patient. Remember, this may all occur quickly in a tension-filled environment. Therefore the person who actually administers the medication should never assume that the medication he or she has been handed is indeed the medication ordered. When a medication has been passed to you for administration, read the label on the syringe and confirm the order with the team leader or medical direction. At a fast food restaurant, when you place your order the person taking it will recite it over a microphone, and the person back on the grill will repeat the order out loud. This is a good practice to make sure that the order is understood and that customers get what they ordered. Unfortunately, in a medical emergency the same effort is often not made to ensure that a verbal order is understood and confirmed. When receiving a verbal order in person or on the radio, read back the order and wait for confirmation that the order heard is correct. A common source for potential error is mistakenly giving a medication that either looks similar or has a similar name to the medication meant to be administered. The process of stating the order out loud double-checks the name of the medication with those giving the order, as well as other providers in the vicinity.

Right Dose

Ensure that the patient is getting the correct dose of the medication. Repeat the dose verbally before administration. If you are not directly administering the medication, listen to the dose being administered. If you question the dose, call for a "stop" or "timeout" to confirm the dosage. Patient safety is everyone's responsibility.

Right Route

Check the route of administration and whether the route is accessible. If the ordered route is oral, can the patient swallow the medication? Can the medication be crushed? Some oral medications formulated as a sustained-released medication cannot be crushed to assist in oral administration. Administering a sustained-release oral medication in a crushed form may result in overdose.

Right Time

For hospital providers, the *right time* typically refers to administering a medication at the right time of day. This usually is not a significant problem for the prehospital professional. However, the time can also refer to the time it takes to safely administer a bolus of an IV medication. Some medications, such as procainamide, have significant side effects if administered at a rate that is too rapid. When administering an IV medication as a bolus, questioning over what period the bolus should be given is in the interest of patient safety.

Right Documentation

Observe how the patient tolerated the medication. Did a change in the cardiac rhythm or vital signs occur? Document the medication given, the dose, time of administration, route, and any changes in the patient's condition.

You are back at the first scene of the man down at the shopping mall. The shift supervisor has arrived. As you are preparing to load the patient onto the cot, the patient develops a bradycardia that rapidly degenerates into asystole. The supervisor instructs you to administer epinephrine 1:10,000, 1 mg IV, in accordance with your standing order per ACLS guidelines. Another paramedic at the scene pulls epinephrine from the drug box and hands you a preloaded glass syringe. You look at the syringe and read the contents, calling out, "Epinephrine 1:10,000, 1 mg IV push." The team leader responds, "Yes, that's correct," confirming that you have the correct drug in your hands. You administer the drug as intended.

All too often, the individual running a code gives an order and is not sure that someone has heard the order or carried it out. Always acknowledge and verify medication orders.

PROVIDER SAFETY

The first rule of providing emergency care in the field is to ensure your personal safety. A fundamental concept taught to all prehospital providers is scene safety. Paramedics are taught to position emergency vehicles in areas of high visibility and physically protect the scene. When responding to a shooting or stabbing call, standard practice is for an ALS unit to delay arrival on the scene until law enforcement has determined that the scene is safe, weapons are secured, and the assailant is not in the vicinity. The practice of wearing appropriate personal protective equipment (PPE) and following universal precautions is designed to reduce the likelihood that a provider will be infected by a pathogen when exposed to infectious blood, body fluids, or respiratory droplets. The diseases these efforts are meant to prevent include those with no cure: human immunodeficiency virus (HIV), hepatitis B (HBV), and hepatitis C (HCV). Universal precautions is the practice in which the provider assumes that all blood, body fluids, and patient materials are contaminated with HIV, HBV, or HCV. When observing universal precautions, a provider dons PPE, specialized clothing or equipment to protect the provider from contamination. Gloves are a standard component of PPE. Gloves will not prevent needlesticks, but they will act as a barrier between a contaminated body fluid and an open wound on the provider's hand. Masks are another element of PPE; they should be worn when a splash of the patient's body fluids may get into the eyes, nose, or mouth of the provider. When a provider wears a mask, the mucous membranes of the eyes must be protected with goggles (Fig. 3-3). A mask is required when intubating a patient, dealing with a patient who is actively bleeding, or drawing blood. Goggles must have side shields to prevent blood from entering the eye from the side. If prescription glasses are used as eye protection, those glasses must have side shields, and a plan must be in place to decontaminate the glasses if they become contaminated.

The most obvious risk of blood contamination to a provider is being accidentally stuck by a needle, scalpel, or other sharp object. A provider should never attempt to recap or bend a needle. Immediately after using a needle or sharp, it should be placed in an approved puncture-resistant and leak-proof needle box (Fig. 3-4).

Studies of paramedics' compliance with universal precautions have revealed alarming results. Most paramedics complied with the use of gloves but properly handled sharps in only 37% of cases. The rate of appropriate use of additional protective devices such as goggles, masks, and gowns was unacceptable. Goggles were used in only 6% of the cases in which they were indicated, and gowns were never used when appropriate.[1] Figure 3-5 shows a provider wearing appropriate PPE.

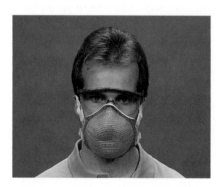

▼ **Fig. 3-3** A paramedic wearing appropriate mask and goggles. (From Stoy W, Platt T, Lejeune D: *Center for emergency medicine: Mosby's EMT-basic textbook,* ed 2 rev, St Louis, 2007, Mosby.)

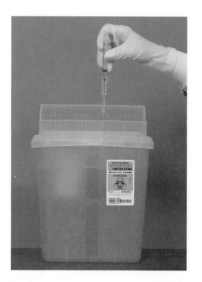

▼ **Fig. 3-4** Sharps should be discarded in an appropriate container. (From Potter PA, Perry AG: *Fundamentals of nursing,* ed 7, St Louis, 2009, Mosby.)

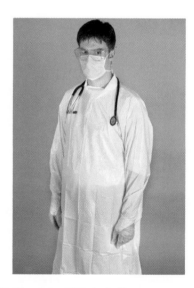

▼ **Fig. 3-5** PPE—including eyewear, mask, gown, and gloves—provides adequate body substance isolation. (From Henry M, Stapleton E: *EMT prehospital care,* ed 3 rev, St Louis, 2007, Mosby.)

ENTERAL DRUG ADMINISTRATION PROCEDURES

Chapter 1 explains that medications can be given either enterally or parenterally. Enteral medications enter the bloodstream through the gastrointestinal (GI) tract. In the prehospital care environment, enteral medications are given orally, rectally, sublingually, and buccally.

ADMINISTRATION OF ORAL MEDICATIONS

The majority of medications prescribed by physicians are taken orally in a solid form, such as a pill, tablet, or capsule, or in a liquid form. The oral route has several limitations when treating medical emergencies in the prehospital environment. Oral medications are not practical or safe to administer to patients with an altered or depressed level of consciousness. In addition, because oral medications require absorption in the GI tract, they are not rapidly available for treatment of life-threatening emergencies.

Orders for oral medications are often described as "PO," which is an abbreviation for the Latin *per os,* meaning "by mouth."

> **Assisted medication administration** occurs when a prehospital professional helps a patient take his or her own prescribed medication. Assisted medication administration often can be performed after consultation with medical direction. Before helping a patient with his or her own medication, read the label. Verify that the medication you are helping the patient administer is indeed his or her own. Read the prescription bottle to ensure that the name on the bottle is the name of the patient, and confirm that the medication and dose are the medication and dose that you intend to administer. Also, be sure the medication has not expired. If a patient has stored multiple medications in the same bottle and you cannot confirm the identification of a medication, do not help the patient take it.

ORAL MEDICATION ADMINISTRATION

Equipment Needed:
Medication, medication cup, gloves, drinking water
Procedure:
1. Observe universal precautions.
2. Verify drug order.
3. Confirm right patient, right medication, right dose, right route, and right time.
4. Confirm with the patient that he or she has no allergies to the medication, and document allergies to any other medication.
5. When possible, explain to the patient what medication you are going to administer and why.
6. Open the medication container and tap out the prescribed number of pills into a medication cup, the patient's hand, or your gloved hand.
7. *Do not crush solid medication.* Some pills and capsules are formulated as time-released medications. By crushing a tablet, the active ingredient can be absorbed into the bloodstream all at once rather than over a period of hours, which may result in an unintentional overdose. Before crushing any solid medication, consult a drug reference or medical direction.
8. Place the patient in the sitting position.
9. Ask the patient to swallow the medication with 4 to 5 oz water.
10. Record the time of drug administration in the patient care record.
11. Evaluate the patient for desired effects of the medication, as well as any adverse effects. Continued reevaluation should occur throughout transport.

ADMINISTRATION OF RECTAL MEDICATIONS

Rectal medications are not frequently used in the prehospital setting, but some indications for their use may arise. **Rectal administration** is used most commonly in situations in which oral administration would be ideal but cannot be tolerated by the patient because of nausea or vomiting. In some emergency settings the rectal route is optimal for rapidly delivering a medication to a patient who is not able to take an oral medication, such as the rectal administration of diazepam (Valium) or lorazepam (Ativan) for the treatment of pediatric seizures.

Medications formulated to be given as rectal suppositories often have a butterlike consistency. That is, the medication is a solid at room temperature, but once the suppository in placed in the rectum, the body temperature melts the medication into a liquid form, allowing more rapid absorption by the rectal mucosa.

RECTAL MEDICATION ADMINISTRATION

Equipment Needed:
Gloves, suppository or medication to be administered, lubricant (if time permits)
Procedure:
1. Observe universal precautions.
2. Verify drug order.
3. Confirm right patient, right medication, right dose, right route, and right time.
4. Confirm with the patient that he or she has no allergies to the medication, and document allergies to any other medication.
5. When possible, explain to the patient what medication you are going to administer and why.
6. Help the patient disrobe. For legal protection, ask an individual (not a family member) of the patient's same sex to be present.
7. Ask the patient to lie on one side and draw his or her knees up toward the chest.
8. Remove the suppository from its wrapper and hold it at the rectum. Gently hold pressure at the anal sphincter for a few seconds while the patient takes a slow, deep breath and gently bears down. This maneuver will relax the anal sphincter muscles and help introduce the suppository.
9. Advance the suppository into the rectum approximately 1 inch.
10. Once the suppository has been placed, keep the patient on his or her side for approximately 20 minutes if possible.
11. Record the time of drug administration in the patient care record.
12. Evaluate the patient for desired effects of the medication, as well as any adverse effects. Continued reevaluation should occur throughout transport.

Details on how to administer rectal diazepam (Valium) are provided in Chapter 15.

ADMINISTRATION OF SUBLINGUAL MEDICATIONS

Medications can be applied to mucous membranes, where the drug can be rapidly absorbed and transported by the bloodstream. For certain medications this method of drug delivery is extremely fast and effective. For example, nitroglycerin is administered to the mucous membranes beneath the tongue, or sublingually, where a rich network of blood vessels facilitates rapid absorption and distribution.

 ## ADMINISTRATION OF NITROGLYCERIN: SPRAY AND SUBLINGUAL

Equipment Needed:
Medication, PPE
Procedure:
1. Observe universal precautions.
2. Verify drug order.
3. Confirm right patient, right medication, right dose, right route, and right time.
4. Confirm with the patient that he or she has no allergies to the medication, and document allergies to any other medication.
5. When possible, explain to the patient what medication you are going to administer and why.
6. Instruct the patient to lift his or her tongue. Place one tablet under the tongue and ask the patient to close his or her mouth. Instruct the patient to not chew the tablet and to leave it under the tongue until it is completely dissolved.
7. If the patient uses nitroglycerin spray, spray once under the tongue or in the buccal membrane per protocol. Instruct the patient to close his or her mouth quickly.
8. Take the patient's blood pressure within 2 minutes of administration.
9. Record the time of drug administration in the patient care record.
10. Reassess and record vital signs.
11. Evaluate the patient for desired effects of the medication, as well as any adverse effects.

ADMINISTRATION OF BUCCAL MEDICATIONS

The **buccal area** is the mucous membrane on the inside of the check. Medication such as glucose gel for hypoglycemic patients can be administered here (termed *buccal administration*) by prehospital providers. However, this route of administration is safe only for conscious patients with an intact gag reflex.

ORAL GLUCOSE MEDICATION ADMINISTRATION

Equipment Needed:
Medication, gloves, tongue depressor or other appropriate applicator, PPE
Procedure:
1. Observe universal precautions.
2. Verify drug order.
3. Confirm right patient, right medication, right dose, right route, and right time.
4. Confirm with the patient that he or she has no allergies to the medication, and document allergies to any other medication.
5. When possible, explain to the patient what medication you are going to administer and why.
6. Place the medication between the patient's gum and cheek near the location of the molar teeth (Fig. 3-6).
7. Advise the patient not to drink any fluids while the medication is dissolving and being absorbed.
8. Record the time of drug administration in the patient care record.
9. Evaluate the patient for desired effects of the medication, as well as any adverse effects. Continued reevaluation should occur throughout transport.

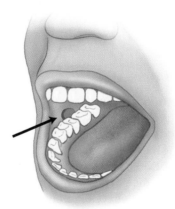

▼ **Fig. 3-6**   Oral glucose administration. Medications, such as glucose gel, can be administered in the buccal area on the inside of the check. This method of administration is only safe in conscious patients with an intact gag reflex.

PARENTERAL DRUG ADMINISTRATION PROCEDURES

The **parenteral route** is the most common route of drug administration used by paramedics. This type of route includes any route of drug administration other than absorption from the GI tract. Parenteral routes include an IV line, **IM injection**, intradermal Sub-Q injection, **intraosseous (IO) infusion, transdermal/topical administration, inhalation administration,** and **endotracheal (ET) tube** administration. Parenteral drug administration is a more effective route in the prehospital environment, because medications given intravenously produce blood levels that are reliable and available almost immediately. The limitation of parenteral drug administration is the need to have special training and equipment for drug delivery. IV and IO methods of administration are explained in Chapter 5.

EQUIPMENT

Syringes

A **syringe** is a medical instrument used for injecting fluid into or withdrawing fluid from the body. Syringes can be made of glass or plastic, but plastic syringes are used primarily in the prehospital setting. Syringes are used for a variety of purposes and come in a wide spectrum of sizes from 1 mL to 50 mL. They have three parts: the tip, barrel, and plunger (Fig. 3-7).

The **tip** of the syringe attaches the needle. With **Luer-lock syringes,** the tip is threaded, allowing a needle to be screwed into the tip. The Luer-lock allows the needle to be attached to the barrel with greater security. This type of syringe is required for use in needleless IV systems, which are increasing in popularity. With **non–Luer-lock syringes,** the needle fits tightly on the tip.

The **barrel** of the syringe contains the medication. Syringe barrels come in a variety of volumes. Volume markings are etched on the surface of most syringes, typically in milliliters. **Insulin syringes** are calibrated so that the user is able to draw up and measure the units of insulin.

The **plunger** is the inner portion of the syringe that pushes the liquid medication to the tip of the syringe and out the needle.

Needles

Needles (also called *sharps*) are a critical—and potentially dangerous—tool in drug administration. Needles have various parts and come in different sizes. A needle is composed of a hub, shaft, and bevel (see Fig. 3-7).

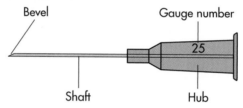

Bevel   Gauge number   25   Shaft   Hub

▼ **Fig. 3-7**   Various parts of the needle. (From Potter PA, Perry AG: *Fundamentals of nursing*, ed 7, St Louis, 2009, Mosby.)

The **hub** typically is made of plastic and, in the case of a non–Luer-lock syringe, tightly fits over the tip of a syringe. When a Luer-lock syringe is used, the needle is attached to the syringe by screwing the hub into the Luer-lock.

The **shaft** of the needle is attached to the hub.

The **bevel** is the angled surface at the end of a needle. The longer the bevel on a needle, the easier the needle will pierce the skin.

Needles also have different gauges, which are determined by their diameter. The larger the needle diameter, the smaller the gauge (e.g., a 16-gauge needle is much larger than a 25-gauge needle).

Butterfly needles are small, short needles with plastic tabs that resemble the wings of a butterfly. Attached to the needle of a butterfly needle is a small piece of clear plastic tubing with an IV connector that can be attached to a syringe or IV tubing. Butterfly needles are used to withdraw blood or establish an IV in children and adults with small or difficult-to-access veins. The needle is inserted into the vein while the wings of the butterfly are held. Access to the vein is confirmed by a small return of blood into the tubing. Many needles now contain a plastic needle cover attached to the hub of the needle by a plastic syringe. These systems allow this cover to be swung over the needle. Once in place, this plastic cover cannot be removed.

Needle safety guidelines include the following:

▸ Never resheath a needle.
▸ Never remove a plastic needle sheath with the teeth. Such maneuvers pose a serious risk of injury.
▸ Do not let needles lie around. No one ever means to get stuck with a contaminated needle. Typically, a needle is put down and someone either forgets about it or is not aware of it.

- Once a needle is used, it should immediately be discarded in an appropriate sharps container.
- Ensure that sharps containers are changed before they are full. Injuries can occur when the sharps container is full and someone tries to add one more needle.
- Never stick a needle and syringe in the cushion of a cot or bench of an ambulance. Not only is this nonsterile, it is also abusive to the equipment.

ADMINISTRATION OF INTRAMUSCULAR INJECTIONS

IM injection is a method of administering medication directly into muscle tissue, where it is absorbed in the general circulation. Several muscles of varying sizes are appropriate sites for injection. The size of the needle used for an IM injection depends on the location of the injection and the size of the muscle group. IM injections involve placing a needle deep in the muscle tissue. A needle accidentally placed into a nerve can result in permanent pain and disability. To prevent such injuries, care providers must know the proper location for placement of IM injections. Muscles used for IM injections include the deltoid, thigh, and hip.

The **deltoid muscle** is at the top of the shoulder. This muscle is an excellent choice for IM injection of emergency medications because the deltoid has a rich blood supply, allowing injected medications to be rapidly absorbed. In adults, the deltoid can tolerate an injection volume of 2 mL. The appropriate area for an IM injection of the deltoid is a triangular area on the lateral aspect (Fig. 3-8). One structure that can be damaged from an improper IM injection to the deltoid is the radial nerve.

The muscles of the thigh provide another site for IM injections. The appropriate area of injection of the thigh can be located by placing one hand on the upper thigh and one hand on the lower thigh. The area between the two hands on the anterior surface of the thigh is the correct area for an IM injection, the **vastus lateralis** (Fig. 3-9). In adults, up to 5 mL can be injected into this site. This is the preferred site for IM injections in infants until the muscle of the deltoid becomes more developed.

Injections into the hip are termed **dorsogluteal injections.** This area is the upper outer quadrant of the buttocks. This technique of IM injection should not be used in patients younger than 2 years or in patients who are very thin or emaciated. Place the patient on his or her side with the knees flexed toward the chest, and ask the patient to rotate the toes inward. Locate the posterior iliac spine, which is where the hemipelvis meets the sacrum, and then locate the greater trochanter of the femur. Imagine a line between these two points. This is the upper outer quadrant of the buttock. An IM injection in this area is a dorsogluteal IM injection (Fig. 3-10).

Because of variation in the sizes of muscles in children, a **ventrogluteal injection** is the preferred site. Place the patient on his or her side. Put your hand on the side of the

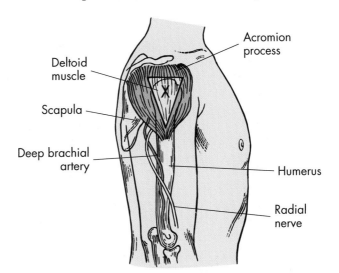

▼ **Fig. 3-8** The injection site for the deltoid muscle is roughly formed by an inverted triangle, with the acromion process as the base. The muscle may be visible in well-developed patients. (From Potter PA, Perry AG: *Fundamentals of nursing,* ed 7, St Louis, 2009, Mosby.)

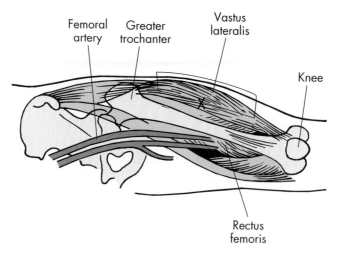

▼ **Fig. 3-9** The injection sites for the vastus lateralis muscle and the rectus femoris muscle can be defined by landmarks. One hand is placed below the greater trochanter. The other hand is placed above the knee. The space between the two hands defines the middle third of the underlying muscle. The rectus femoris is on the anterior thigh. The vastus lateralis is on the lateral side. (From Potter PA, Perry AG: *Fundamentals of nursing*, ed 7, St Louis, 2009, Mosby.)

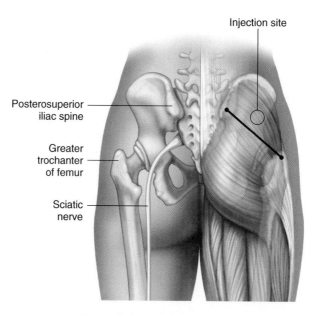

▼ **Fig. 3-10** The posterosuperior iliac spine and the greater trochanter are located by palpation. An imaginary line is drawn between the two. The injection site should be above and out from that line. (From Harkreader H, Hogan M, Thobaben M: *Fundamentals of nursing: caring and clinical judgement*, ed 3, St Louis, 2007, Saunders.)

hip with the heel of your hand resting on the greater trochanter (hip joint), the thumb toward the umbilicus, the index finger on the anterior iliac spine tubercle, and the middle finger on the posterior iliac crest. With the index finger, point to the anterior iliac spine. The area of injection is in the V formed by your hand (Fig. 3-11).

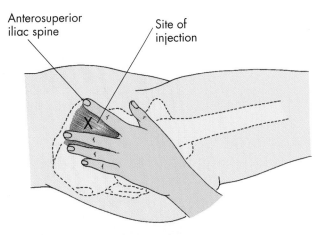

▼ **Fig. 3-11**   The injection site for the ventrogluteal muscle is defined by placing the palm of one hand on the trochanter of the femur. A V is then made with the fingers of that hand. One side runs from the greater trochanter to the anterior-superior iliac spine. The other side runs from the greater trochanter to the iliac crest. The injection is made into the center of the V. (Modified from Potter PA, Perry AG: *Fundamentals of nursing*, ed 7, St Louis, 2009, Mosby.)

INTRAMUSCULAR MEDICATION ADMINISTRATION

Equipment Needed:
21 gauge 1½ needle, syringe with desired amount of drug, alcohol wipe, gloves, sharps container, adhesive bandage, PPE

Procedure:

1. Observe universal precautions.
2. Verify drug order.
3. Confirm right patient, right medication, right dose, right route, and right time.
4. Confirm with the patient that he or she has no allergies to the medication, and document allergies to any other medication.
5. When possible, explain to the patient what medication you are going to administer and why.
6. Determine the appropriate muscle site for IM injection.
7. Identify landmarks for injection.
8. Prepare the area for injection with alcohol.
9. Insert the needle with a rapid, dartlike motion. Insert the needle at a 90-degree angle to the surface of the skin (Fig. 3-12).
10. Pull back on the syringe to ensure that the tip of the needle is not in a blood vessel.
11. Inject the medication.
12. Remove the needle.
13. Immediately dispose of the needle and syringe in an approved sharps container.
14. Apply pressure to the area.

> Massaging the area may produce pain, especially if a large volume of fluid was injected.

15. Record the time of drug administration in the patient care record.
16. Evaluate the patient for desired effects of the medication, as well as any adverse effects. Continued reevaluation should occur throughout transport.

Some medications used in IM injections are irritating to the soft tissues and can result in permanent staining of the skin. Hydroxyzine (Vistaril) is one drug that can permanently stain the skin. Such medications should be injected by the **Z-track technique** of injection, which can be used at any site and with any medication. This method allows delivery of the medication to the deep muscle tissue, preventing it from leaking back into the soft tissues and skin.

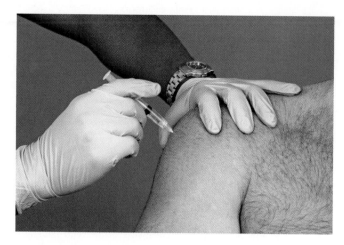

▼ **Fig. 3-12**   Appropriate site for an intramuscular injection. (From Sanders M: *Mosby's paramedic textbook,* rev ed 3, St Louis, 2005, Mosby.)

INTRAMUSCULAR MEDICATION ADMINISTRATION: Z-TRACK TECHNIQUE

Equipment Needed:
Medication, gloves, syringe, needle, alcohol prep, dressing, sharps container, PPE
Procedure:
1. Observe universal precautions.
2. Verify drug order.
3. Confirm right patient, right medication, right dose, right route, and right time.
4. Confirm with the patient that he or she has no allergies to the medication, and document allergies to any other medication.
5. When possible, explain to the patient what medication you are going to administer and why.
6. Determine appropriate muscle site for IM injection.
7. Identify landmarks for injection.
8. Prepare the area for injection with alcohol.
9. Stretch the skin to one side approximately 1 inch (Fig. 3-13, A).
10. Insert the needle with a rapid, dartlike motion at a 90-degree angle to the surface of the skin (Fig. 3-13, B).
11. Pull back on the syringe to ensure that the tip of the needle is not in a blood vessel.

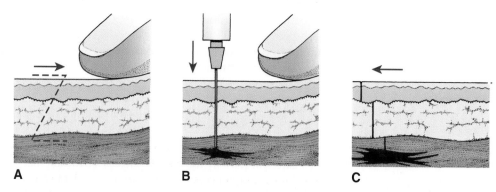

A   **B**   **C**

▼ **Fig. 3-13**   Z-track injection technique. **A,** Pull the tissue laterally. **B,** Insert the needle straight down into the muscle and inject the medication. **C,** Release the tissue as the needle is withdrawn; this allows the skin to slide over the injection track and seal the medication inside. (From Edmunds MW: *Introduction to clinical pharmacology,* ed 5, St Louis, 2006, Mosby.)

12. Inject the medication slowly, and wait approximately 5 seconds.
13. Remove the needle and let the skin slide back into place (Fig. 3-13, C).
14. Immediately dispose of the needle and syringe in an approved sharps container.
15. Apply pressure to the area. Do not massage the area.
16. Record the time of drug administration in the patient care record.
17. Evaluate the patient for desired effects of the medication, as well as any adverse effects. Continued reevaluation should occur throughout transport.

Intradermal medications are administered just below the epidermal layer of skin. The intradermal route is most often used for allergy and tuberculin testing. Local anesthetics may be administered by this route.

INTRADERMAL MEDICATION ADMINISTRATION

Equipment Needed:
Medication, gloves, syringe, needle, alcohol prep, dressing, sharps container, PPE
Procedure:
1. Observe universal precautions.
2. Verify drug order.
3. Confirm right patient, right medication, right dose, right route, and right time.
4. Confirm with the patient that he or she has no allergies to the medication, and document allergies to any other medication.
5. When possible, explain to the patient what medication you are going to administer and why.
6. Calculate the dose, and withdraw the appropriate amount of medication in a syringe (usually less than 0.5 mL).
7. Determine appropriate site for intradermal injection. Use the skin on the anterior surface of the forearm.
8. Cleanse the site with an antiseptic wipe. Begin at the desired site and cleanse outward in a circular motion.
9. Tell the patient that he or she will feel a brief discomfort during the injection.
10. Retract the skin below the site and hold taut. Insert the needle bevel up into the skin at a 10- to 15-degree angle. Pull back on the plunger to aspirate and ensure that you have not entered a vein. If no blood appears, inject the drug just below the surface of the skin until a small bump appears.
11. Remove the needle and discard into an appropriate sharps container.
12. Apply an adhesive bandage to control any bleeding.
13. Explain to the patient the need to report back for the test to be read within a specific timeframe.
14. Record the time of drug administration in the patient care record.
15. Evaluate the patient for desired effects of the medication, as well as any adverse effects.

ADMINISTRATION OF SUBCUTANEOUS INJECTIONS

The **subcutaneous (Sub-Q) space** is the tissue between the dermis of the skin and the underlying muscle. This space does not tolerate a volume of injection greater than 2 mL. The dose is usually less than 0.5 mL. The Sub-Q space does not have a rich blood supply; therefore medications injected into this space have a slow onset of action and a prolonged duration of action. Sub-Q injections are easy and quick to perform; in fact, they are performed by patients to self-administer medications, such as diabetic patients who self-administer daily insulin injections and patients with a history of allergies who commonly carry an EpiPen for rapid **Sub-Q administration** if necessary.

Small syringes and needles are used for Sub-Q injections. The sites used for Sub-Q injections in the field are the upper arms, upper back, and scapular regions (Fig. 3-14). Patients who self-administer Sub-Q injections commonly use the abdomen and anterior thigh as sites. Because the volumes of medications administered subcutaneously usually are small, the medications must be potent.

SUBCUTANEOUS MEDICATION ADMINISTRATION

Equipment Needed:

Medication, gloves, syringe, needle, alcohol prep, dressing, sharps container, PPE

Procedure:

1. Observe universal precautions.
2. Verify drug order.
3. Confirm right patient, right medication, right dose, right route, and right time.
4. Confirm with the patient that he or she has no allergies to the medication, and document allergies to any other medication.
5. When possible, explain to the patient what medication you are going to administer and why.
6. Determine appropriate muscle site for Sub-Q injection.
7. Draw the medication into the syringe.
8. Prepare the area for injection with alcohol.
9. Hold the skin at the site of the proposed Sub-Q injection flat with one hand.
10. Insert the needle at a 45-degree angle (see Fig. 3-14). When injecting in the scapular and abdominal areas, grasp a small roll of skin and insert the needle at a 90-degree angle.
11. Aspirate before injection *except* when injecting **heparin.** Aspirating back before injection of heparin leads to bruising after administration.
12. Inject the medication.
13. Remove the needle.
14. Immediately dispose of the needle and syringe in an approved sharps container.
15. Apply pressure to the area.
16. Record the time of drug administration in the patient care record.
17. Evaluate the patient for desired effects of the medication, as well as any adverse effects. Continued reevaluation should occur throughout transport.

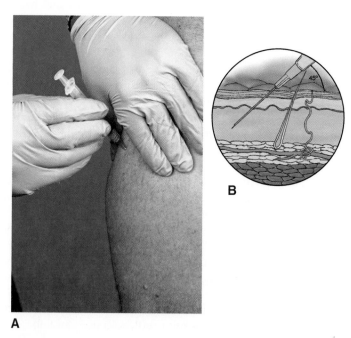

▼ **Fig. 3-14**   Technique for Sub-Q injection. **A,** Pinch the skin and inject the needle at a 45-degree angle to the skin. **B,** Cross-section view showing proper placement of the needle in the Sub-Q tissue. (**A,** From Sanders M: *Mosby's paramedic textbook,* rev ed 3, St Louis, 2005, Mosby. **B,** From Shade B, Rothenberg M, Wertz E, et al: *Mosby's EMT-Intermediate textbook,* ed 2, St Louis, 2002, Mosby.)

ADMINISTRATION OF TOPICAL MEDICATIONS

Topical medications are administered to the skin for direct treatment of a skin condition or systemic absorption through the skin and transportation through the bloodstream. The most common topical medication used by prehospital providers is nitroglycerin ointment.

Appropriate areas to apply nitroglycerin ointment are the chest, upper arm, and flank. Shaving the skin is not appropriate because it can create small nicks and irritate the skin. Ointments and creams should be applied with a tongue depressor. Nitroglycerin is now supplied with small pieces of applicator paper.

Topical patches are becoming an increasingly popular method of drug delivery for a variety of medical conditions.

TOPICAL MEDICATION ADMINISTRATION

Equipment Needed:
Medication, gloves, alcohol prep, template, adhesive dressing
Procedure:
1. Observe universal precautions.
2. Verify drug order.
3. Confirm right patient, right medication, right dose, right route, and right time.
4. Confirm with the patient that he or she has no allergies to the medication, and document allergies to any other medication.
5. When possible, explain to the patient what medication you are going to administer and why.
6. Clean the skin with an alcohol prep.
7. Apply the applicator with the nitroglycerin ointment to the skin, with the ointment side facing down (Fig. 3-15).
8. Do not rub the medication into the skin.
9. Record the time of drug administration in the patient care record.
10. Evaluate the patient for desired effects of the medication, as well as any adverse effects. Continued reevaluation should occur throughout transport.

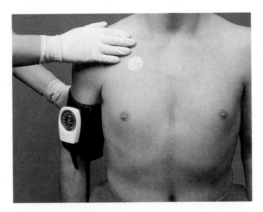

▼ **Fig. 3-15**   Patch with nitroglycerin ointment applied to the skin. (From Sanders M: *Mosby's paramedic textbook,* ed 3 rev, St Louis, 2007, Mosby.)

ADMINISTRATION OF MEDICATIONS THROUGH AN ENDOTRACHEAL TUBE

In life-threatening emergencies, such as during ACLS codes, patients often require medications immediately—even before IV or IO access has been established. If the patient is intubated, paramedics can administer several drugs through the endotracheal tube until reliable IV access is established. These include lidocaine (Xylocaine), epinephrine, atropine, naloxone (Narcan), and vasopressin.

The lungs have a large surface area with a rich blood supply. When a medication is given through an endotracheal tube, the drug is immediately delivered to the basic lung units, the alveoli, where it is rapidly absorbed by the numerous blood vessels that cover each **alveolus.**

Remember which drugs can be given through an endotracheal tube with the mnemonic NAVEL:
- **N** naloxone
- **A** atropine
- **V** vasopressin
- **E** epinephrine
- **L** lidocaine

When a medication is administered through an endotracheal tube, 2 to 2.5 times the dose of medication given intravenously is required. In addition, to help with rapid absorption, the medication should be diluted in 10 mL of normal saline or sterile water for adult patients and 5 mL of normal saline or sterile water for pediatric patients. Medication administration by this route is appropriate only until reliable IV or IO access has been established, so do not abandon attempts to secure an IV or IO.

MEDICATION ADMINISTRATION THROUGH AN ENDOTRACHEAL TUBE

Equipment Needed:
Medication, gloves, syringe, normal saline or sterile water
Procedure:
1. Observe universal precautions.
2. Verify drug order.
3. Confirm right patient, right medication, right dose, right route, and right time. Remember to double the dosage for this route of administration.
4. Confirm with the patient that he or she has no allergies to the medication, and document allergies to any other medication.
5. When possible, explain to the patient what medication you are going to administer and why.
6. Dilute the medication in 10 mL of normal saline or sterile water for adult patients and 5 mL of normal saline for pediatric patients.
7. If possible, remove the needle from the syringe.
8. If cardiopulmonary resuscitation is in progress, hold compressions.
9. Ask another EMS provider to grasp the endotracheal tube firmly, and then remove the bag-mask. Be careful not to tug or remove the endotracheal tube when disconnecting the bag-mask.
10. Administer the medication into the endotracheal tube.
11. "Push" the medication down the tube with two or three strong ventilations with the bag-mask.
12. Resume compressions if required.
13. Continue to try to obtain an IV line for additional medication if required.
14. Record the time of drug administration in the patient care record.
15. Evaluate the patient for desired effects of the medication, as well as any adverse effects. Continued reevaluation should occur throughout transport.

REVIEW QUESTIONS

1. For what conditions do standing orders usually exist?
2. Who would the paramedic contact for an as-needed order?
3. List the six patient rights of drug administration.
4. Why is the parenteral route of drug administration more effective than the enteral route in the prehospital setting?

5. What is the disadvantage of administering oral medications in a medical emergency?
6. List the precautions that should be followed when handling a needle.
7. Explain the rationale of the Z-track technique of IM injections.
8. What medications can be administered through an endotracheal tube?
9. Explain the dosage preparation for a medication for endotracheal delivery.

REFERENCES

1. Eustis TC, et al: Compliance with recommendations for universal precautions among prehospital providers, *Ann Emerg Med* 25:512, 1995.

Medication Math

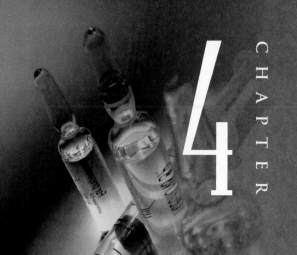

CHAPTER 4

OBJECTIVES

1. Identify the basic units of measure for weight, length, and volume.
2. Accurately convert milliliters to cubic centimeters, kilograms to pounds, and milligrams to grams (and micrograms).
3. Apply the four basic formulas (single dose, infusion of a measured amount of fluid in a set amount of time, drip infusion not based on weight, and drip infusion based on weight) to solve drug problems and determine dosages.

INTRODUCTION

Medication math can be made simple by mastering only a few basic formulas. The purpose of this chapter is to take away the mystery of medication math and replace it with confidence to learn and achieve ease in calculating drug dosages.

Anaphylaxis, as presented in the following case, is a life-threatening condition that is easily treated. However, without a grasp of the concepts of medication math, you cannot properly administer the medication epinephrine. A thorough knowledge of the concepts of pharmacology and dosing of medications is useless without the ability to make conversions of weight and volume and calculate volumes of drug to be administered based on concentration of the drug. As illustrated in the following case, to administer a simple and common medication such as epinephrine, you will need to make several calculations. To do this in a potentially life-threatening emergency requires a complete grasp of medication math principles.

Y ou and your partner are dispatched to a residence on a call for an allergic reaction. You arrive and are directed to the kitchen, where you find a 6-year-old girl who is sitting in a chair in obvious respiratory distress. The child's mother tells you she stepped on a bee while running barefoot in the backyard. The mother states that the child does not have any known allergies, but she has never been stung by a bee before. The child has stridor and a rapid respiratory rate. She is holding and rubbing a markedly swollen left foot and appears quite anxious.

Your assessment of this situation is that the child is having an anaphylactic reaction from a bee sting. You determine that epinephrine should be administered as quickly as possible, and you do not think waiting to get IV access before administering the epinephrine is prudent. You decide that the best course of action is to administer IM epinephrine (1:1000). You ask the mother how much the child weighs, and the mother replies 50 pounds. The pediatric dose for IM epinephrine is 0.01 mg/kg (1:1000). The concentration of the epinephrine (1:1000) is 1 mg/mL. How many milliliters of epinephrine (1:1000) must be administered to this child?

Several questions must be answered before determining how many milliliters to administer.

1. What is the weight of the child in kilograms?
   - ▸ The child weighs 50 pounds. To convert to kilograms, 1 kg equals 2.2 pounds.
   - ▸ $\dfrac{50\,lb}{2.2\,kg/lb} = \dfrac{50\,\cancel{lb}}{2.2\,kg/\cancel{lb}} = 22.7\,kg$
   - ▸ 22.7 kg

2. What is the weight-based dose of epinephrine (1:1000) IM?
   ▶ IM dose of epinephrine (1:1000) is 0.01 mg/kg
   ▶ $\text{Dose} = \dfrac{0.01\,\text{mg}}{\text{kg}} \times \dfrac{22.7\,\text{kg}}{1} = \dfrac{0.01\,\text{mg}}{\cancel{\text{kg}}} \times \dfrac{22.7\,\cancel{\text{kg}}}{1} = 0.01\,\text{mg} \times 22.7 = 0.23\,\text{mg}$
   ▶ Dose = 0.23 mg
3. What is the volume of epinephrine (1:1000) that needs to be administered intramuscularly by the syringe?
   ▶ Concentration of epinephrine 1 mg/mL
   ▶ $\text{Milliliters to administer} = \dfrac{\text{desired dose}}{\text{dose on hand}} \times \dfrac{\text{volume/quantity}}{1}$
   ▶ $\text{Milliliters to administer} = \dfrac{0.23\,\text{mg}}{1\,\text{mg}} \times \dfrac{1\,\text{mL}}{1}$
   ▶ $\text{Milliliters to administer} = \dfrac{0.23\,\cancel{\text{mg}}}{1\,\cancel{\text{mg}}} \times \dfrac{1\,\text{mL}}{1}$
   ▶ Milliliters to administer = 0.23 mL

You administer 0.23 mL epinephrine (1:1000) intramuscularly. Shortly after administration, the child's breathing becomes less labored and she is less anxious. You start a peripheral IV, repeat your assessment, and prepare for transport. (Drug therapy for anaphylaxis is covered in detail in Chapter 8).

SYSTEMS OF MEASUREMENT

The first system of measurement for drugs was the **apothecary system.** In that system, the weight of drugs was measured in grains. Linear measures included inches, yards, and miles. **Volume** (i.e., the measurement of fluids and liquids) was measured in minims.

The **metric system** currently is the preferred system for drug measurement and calculation. It is logical and well organized, based on a basic unit and its multiples or submultiples of 10. It is similar to the U.S. monetary system: one dollar is the basic unit of measurement, written as $1.00. It can be divided into 10 dimes (written as $0.10), which can be further divided into 10 pennies (written as $0.01). This analogy is helpful when determining drug dosages.

Just as the apothecary system has basic units of measure for weight, length, and volume, so does the metric system, as follows:
   ▶ Weight (solids or mass): gram (g)
   ▶ Length: meter (m)
   ▶ Volume (liquid or fluid): liter (L)

In addition, several prefixes are commonly used in medicine to distinguish multiples or smaller parts of these units. The four commonly used in drug calculation are **kilo, centi, milli,** and **micro.** They are defined in Table 4-1 along with calculations and examples of equivalents.

Most drugs administered in the field are measured in the following units: **gram (g), milligram (mg),** and **microgram (mcg).** Drugs present in solutions can be measured in

TABLE 4-1

Common Prefixes Used in Medication Calculation

Prefix	Calculation	Examples of Equivalents	Reverse (Also True)	Multiple or Part of a Basic Unit
kilo	1000 × basic unit	1 kg = 1000 g	1000 g = 1 kg	Multiple
centi	1/100 of a basic unit	1 cm = 1/100 m	1/100 m = 1 cm	Part
milli	1/1000 of a basic unit	1 mg = 1/1000 g	1/1000 g = 1 mg	Part
micro	1/1,000,000 of a basic unit	1 mcg = 1/1,000,000 g	1/1,000,000 g = 1 mcg	Part

milliliters (mL). At times, volumes of solutions are also reported in cubic centimeters (cc). Milliliters and cubic centimeters refer to the same volume.

CONVERSIONS

The ability to convert one unit of measure to another is vital to ensure that the intended dose of medication is administered to the patient. Failure to understand and use unit conversions may lead to overdosing the patient inadvertently or providing the patient with a less than optimal dose. Most IV medications are supplied as solutions expressed as a concentrations (e.g., milligrams per milliliter [mg/mL]). Medications are dosed as a mass (e.g., milligrams), and drug doses are often determined based on a patient's weight (e.g., pounds or kilograms) or body surface area (square meters). As mentioned in Chapter 2, lack of experience in the performance of drug calculations and conversions is a common cause of medical error, patient injury, and legal action against the prehospital professional.

MILLILITERS AND CUBIC CENTIMETERS

The milliliter is a measurement of volume (liquids or fluids in this case) and is equal to 1/1000 of a liter. The cubic centimeter is also a measurement of volume, but it is based on the centimeter, which is equal to 1/100 of a meter. Because 1 cc equals 1 mL, the terms are often used interchangeably.

For example, you may receive an order to administer 2 mL of morphine sulfate. The same order may be given as 2 cc of morphine sulfate. These two doses are considered equivalent. If a box measured 1 cm × 1 cm × 1 cm in dimension, the volume of the box would be a cubic centimeter. If the box were filled with 1 mL of water at a temperature of 4° C, the water would exactly fill the box. Therefore the *volume* is equal to the *space* that was created (Fig. 4-1).

> Remember: 1 cc = 1 mL, but 1 mL does *not* equal 1 mg. *Gram* refers to the weight of a powdered drug, not its volume or the space that it occupies.

Never take medication orders in dosages of volume. For example, you are transporting a 43-year-old man with a severe open femur fracture incurred after he fell off a roof. You call medical direction for an order for morphine, and medical direction gives the order for 3 mL (or 3 cc) of morphine sulfate. Many drugs, morphine included, come in several different concentrations. Injectable morphine comes in concentrations of 2 mg/mL, 4 mg/mL, 5 mg/mL, 8 mg/mL, and 10 mg/mL. For instance, if medical direction thought that the advanced life support (ALS) drug box was stocked with morphine sulfate with a concentration of 2 mg/mL, the intended order to give 2 mL would have resulted in 4 mg being administered. If the drug box was supplied with 4 mg/mL, the order of 2 mL would have

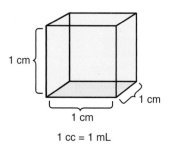

1 cm

1 cm

1 cm

1 cc = 1 mL

▼ **Fig. 4-1**   Volume is equal to the space created. The term *cc* represents cubic centimeter. A cubic centimeter is 1 cm wide, 1 cm long, and 1 cm high. One milliliter (mL) is the equivalent volume of a cubic centimeter. To avoid confusion, the term *milliliter* is preferred over cc, or cubic centimeter.

resulted in the patient getting 8 mg of morphine, or twice the intended dose. Although most drug boxes are supplied with standardized concentrations of medications, administering medications on the basis of volume alone (not concentration) is poor practice and not safe.

KILOGRAMS AND POUNDS

The next conversion commonly used to calculate drug dosages is kilograms (kg) to pounds (lb). Note that these units refer to the *patient's* weight, not the weight of the drug. Many drug dosages, particularly those administered to pediatric patients, are based on the patient's weight in kilograms to ensure safety from overdose.

The equivalent to remember is 1 kg = 2.2 lb. Therefore, to convert weight in pounds to weight in kilograms, divide the number of pounds by 2.2.

Example: If a patient weighs 154 lb, divide 154 lb by 2.2 lb/kg to determine the weight in kilograms.

$$\frac{154\,\text{lb}}{2.2\,\text{lb/kg}} = \text{weight in kilograms}$$

First, cross out "like terms" in the problem; in this case, *lb*.

$$\frac{154\,\cancel{\text{lb}}}{2.2\,\cancel{\text{lb}}/\text{kg}} = \text{weight in kilograms}$$

Now work the problem:

$$\frac{154}{2.2\,\text{kg}} = 70\,\text{kg}$$

MILLIGRAMS, MICROGRAMS, AND GRAMS

The next conversion is from milligrams to grams and, in reverse, from grams to milligrams. This process also includes converting milligrams to micrograms (mcg) and micrograms to milligrams.

Remember: *milli* means 1/1000 of a basic unit; in this case, grams. The equivalent is 1000 mg = 1 g.

To use an everyday example, when changing a dollar into coins (e.g., dimes or pennies), the *larger unit* (dollar) is changed into an equivalent sum in *smaller units* (dimes or pennies). Therefore, to get the total number of the smaller unit, multiply the number of dollars (e.g., 5 dollars) by the number of dimes or pennies *per dollar.*

Example 1:

$$\frac{5\,\text{dollars} \times 10\,\text{dimes}}{\text{dollar}} = \text{number of dimes}$$

Cross out like terms; in this case, *dollar.*

$$\frac{5\,\cancel{\text{dollars}} \times 10\,\text{dimes}}{\cancel{\text{dollar}}} = \text{number of dimes}$$

Now work the problem:

$$5 \times 10\,\text{dimes} = 50\,\text{dimes}$$

Example 2:

$$\frac{5\,\text{dollars} \times 100\,\text{pennies}}{\text{dollar}} = \text{number of pennies}$$

Cross out like terms; in this case, *dollars.*

$$\frac{5 \,\cancel{\text{dollars}} \times 100 \text{ pennies}}{\cancel{\text{dollar}}} = \text{number of pennies}$$

Now work the problem:

$$5 \times 100 \text{ pennies} = 500 \text{ pennies}$$

Note that, when converting a pocket full of change into dollar bills, *smaller units* (coins) are being changed into *larger units* (dollars). The result will be *fewer* larger units (dollars) than smaller units (coins). So, when converting between units, ask yourself, "Am I changing small units for larger units, or large units for smaller units?" This question also applies in practice; you should have an initial sense of whether the numbers and units should be increasing or decreasing in magnitude.

To convert grams to milligrams, multiply grams by 1000. Remember that every 1 g contains 1000 mg; this can be written as 1000 mg/g.

Example:

$$\frac{5 \text{ g} \times 1000 \text{ mg}}{\text{g}} = \text{number of milligrams}$$

Cross out like terms; in this case, *g.*

$$\frac{5 \,\cancel{\text{g}} \times 1000 \text{ mg}}{\cancel{\text{g}}} = \text{number of milligrams}$$

Now work the problem:

$$5 \times 1000 \text{ mg} = 5000 \text{ milligrams}$$

This can be quickly accomplished by moving the decimal point to the right the same number of spaces as there are zeros in the number. For example, because 1000 mg has 3 zeros, move the decimal point three decimal places to the right.

$$5 \text{ g} = 5\underline{000} \text{ mg}$$

The same process can be used to convert milligrams (mg) to micrograms (mcg).

milli means × 1000, or add 3 zeros
micro means × 1,000,000, or add 6 zeros

To convert milligrams (3 zeros) to micrograms (6 zeros), simply move the decimal point three more places to the right, for a total of 6 zeros.

$$5000 \text{ mg} = 5,000,\underline{000} \text{ mcg}$$

To convert milligrams to grams (smaller to larger), divide the number of grams by 1000, or simply move the decimal point three places to the *left.* This is the same as changing 100 pennies back to dollars. The 100 actually means 100 cents. Therefore move the decimal point to the left the same number of places as there are zeros in the equivalent of $1.00 (100 pennies; therefore 2 zeroes, 2 spaces):

$$100 \text{ pennies (cents)} = 1.00 \text{ dollar}$$

Following are some practice problems. Be sure to master the art of conversion before moving on so that you will understand the rest of the chapter.

Practice Problems
Convert grams to milligrams and milligrams to grams:

1. 1 g = _____ mg   3. 250 mg = _____ g

2. 1000 mg = _____ g   4. 400 mg = _____ g

5. 500 mg = _____ g   8. 10 g = _____ mg

6. 0.75 g = _____ mg   9. 2 g = _____ mg

7. 1.25 g = _____ mg   10. 2500 mg = _____ g

Convert milligrams to micrograms and micrograms to milligrams:

1. 1 mg = _____ mcg   6. 800,000 mcg = _____ mg

2. 500 mcg = _____ mg   7. 800 mg = _____ mcg

3. 250 mcg = _____ mg   8. 200 mg = _____ mcg

4. 400 mg = _____ mcg   9. 1000 mcg = _____ mg

5. 0.2 mg = _____ mcg   10. 200,000 mcg = _____ mg

Answers

Convert grams to milligrams and milligrams to grams:
1. 1 g = 1000 mg   6. 0.75 g = 750 mg
2. 1000 mg = 1 g   7. 1.25 g = 1250 mg
3. 250 mg = 0.25 g   8. 10 g = 10,000 mg
4. 400 mg = 0.4 g   9. 2 g = 2000 mg
5. 500 mg = 0.5 g   10. 2500 mg = 2.5 g

Convert milligrams to micrograms and micrograms to milligrams:
1. 1 mg = 1000 mcg   6. 800,000 mcg = 800 mg
2. 500 mcg = 0.5 mg   7. 800 mg = 800,000 mcg
3. 250 mcg = 0.25 mg   8. 200 mg = 200,000 mcg
4. 400 mg = 400,000 mcg   9. 1000 mcg = 1 mg
5. 0.2 mg = 200 mcg   10. 200,000 mcg = 200 mg

Box 4-1 summarizes basic conversions that are useful in drug calculations.

BOX 4-1

BASIC CONVERSIONS

1 g = 1000 mg
1 mg = 1000 mcg
1 L = 1000 mL or 1000 cc
1 kg = 2.2 lb
2.5 cm = 1 in
Remember: 1 mg does not equal 1 mL or 1 cc.

DRUG PREPARATIONS AND CONCENTRATIONS

Regarding drug dosage calculations, understanding that drugs are supplied in various concentrations with differing preparations is important. The same drug can come in various concentrations, and dosages must be calculated according to the particular preparation. For example, atropine sulfate, a medication commonly used to increase a slow heart rate, comes packaged in two ways in prefilled syringes: 0.5 mg/10 mL and 1 mg/10 mL. The second preparation is twice as concentrated as the first and therefore requires a dose of only half the amount. Another drug, dopamine, which is used by prehospital professionals in certain situations in the field to raise blood pressure, comes in three different concentrations: 0.8 mg/mL, 1.6 mg/mL, and 3.2 mg/mL.

FORMULAS

Formulas are used to solve drug problems or determine dosages for patients. They should be used in conjunction with the basic conversions explained previously. Four basic formulas can be used to solve all prehospital pharmacology math problems:

Formula 1
Single dose (e.g., bolus of lidocaine or IM injection of Benadryl):

$$\frac{\text{desired dose}}{\text{dose on hand}} \times \frac{\text{volume/quantity}}{1} = X$$

Formula 2
To infuse a measured amount of fluid in a set amount of time (e.g., fluid challenge):

$$\frac{\text{total volume} \times \text{drops/mL of IV set}}{\text{time in minutes}} = \text{drops/min}$$

Formula 3
Drip (infusion) not based on weight (e.g., lidocaine drip):

$$\frac{\text{dose desired}}{\text{dose on hand}} \times \frac{\text{drops/mL of IV set}}{1} = \text{drops/min}$$

Formula 4
Drip (infusion) based on weight (e.g., dopamine drip):

$$\frac{\text{dose desired}}{\text{kg}} \times \frac{\text{wt (lb)}}{2.2 \text{ lb/kg}} = \text{dose desired}$$

$$\frac{\text{dose desired}}{\cancel{\text{kg}}} \times \frac{\text{wt } \cancel{(\text{lb})}}{2.2 \ \cancel{\text{lb/kg}}}$$

$$\frac{\text{dose desired}}{\text{dose on hand}} \times \frac{\text{drops/mL of IV set}}{1} = \text{drops/min}$$

APPLICATION OF FORMULA 1

The first of the four formulas listed in the previous section is used to calculate the amount of a drug to give a patient in a single dose on the basis of the desired dose (DD), or the amount ordered by medical direction; the dose on hand (DH) or the amount of the weight of the drug (grams, milligrams, micrograms); and the volume (V) or quantity (Q), or the amount of solution in which the drug is dissolved.

> A 64-year-old woman is enjoying a round of golf when she suddenly steps in a hornets' nest and is stung multiple times. Because she is allergic to bee stings, she quickly heads back to the clubhouse and asks for help. A paramedic unit is dispatched. On arrival, the patient is in mild distress, with large hives appearing on her face and neck. Because of her age and the relatively mild signs and symptoms at this point, the paramedics avoid epinephrine and choose to administer diphenhydramine (Benadryl) 25 mg IM. Their prefilled syringe reads 50 mg/mL. How many milliliters should they administer?

Step 1: Choose the proper formula.

$$\frac{\text{desired dose}}{\text{dose on hand}} \times \frac{\text{volume (quantity)}}{1} =$$

Step 2: Fill in known values.

$$\frac{25 \text{ mg} \times 1 \text{ mL}}{50 \text{ mg}} =$$

Step 3: Cross out like terms; in this case, milligrams.

$$\frac{25\ \cancel{mg} \times 1\ mL}{50\ \cancel{mg}} = \frac{25 \times 1\ mL}{50} = \frac{25}{50}\ mL = 0.5\ mL$$

Step 4: Administer 0.5 mL of Benadryl IM to the patient.

> Remember: whenever the dosage is less than 1, always place a zero before the decimal point.

Formula 1 Practice Problems

Remember the steps: cross out like terms and multiply across.

1. Administer epinephrine (Adrenalin) 1:1000 0.3 mg Sub-Q. The prefilled syringe reads 1 mg/mL. How many milliliters should you administer?
2. Administer furosemide (Lasix) 20 mg IV. Furosemide is supplied in a concentration of 40 mg/5 mL. How many milliliters should you administer?
3. Administer atropine sulfate 0.5 mg rapid IV push. The prefilled syringe reads 1 mg/10 mL. How many milliliters should you administer?
4. Administer verapamil (Calan, Isoptin) 5 mg slow IV push. The prefilled syringe reads 5 mg/2 mL (2.5 mg/mL). How many milliliters should you administer?
5. Administer adenosine 12 mg rapid IV push. The prefilled syringe reads 6 mg/2 mL. How many milliliters should you administer?

Formula 1 Answers

1. $$\frac{DD:\ 0.3\ \cancel{mg} \times V(Q):\ 1\ mL}{DH:\ 1\ \cancel{mg}} = 0.3 \times 1\ mL = \frac{0.3 \times \cancel{1}\ mL}{\cancel{1}} = \mathbf{0.3\ mL}$$

2. $$\frac{DD:\ 20\ \cancel{mg} \times V(Q):\ 5\ mL}{DH:\ 40\ \cancel{mg}} = \frac{20 \times 5\ mL}{40} = \frac{100}{40}\ mL = \mathbf{2.5\ mL}$$

3. $$\frac{DD:\ 0.5\ \cancel{mg} \times V(Q):\ 10\ mL}{DH:\ 1\ \cancel{mg}} = \frac{0.5 \times 10\ mL}{1} = \frac{5\ mL}{1} = \mathbf{5\ mL}$$

4. $$\frac{DD:\ 5\ \cancel{mg} \times V(Q):\ 2\ mL}{DH:\ 5\ \cancel{mg}} = \frac{5 \times 2\ mL}{5} = \frac{10}{5}\ mL = \mathbf{2\ mL}$$

5. $$\frac{DD:\ 12\ \cancel{mg} \times V(Q):\ 2\ mL}{DH:\ 6\ \cancel{mg}} = \frac{12 \times 2\ mL}{6} = \frac{24}{6}\ mL = \mathbf{4\ mL}$$

APPLICATION OF FORMULA 2

Formula 2 is used to calculate the amount of a drug to give a patient when infusing a measured amount of fluid in a set amount of time, such as in fluid challenges.

> Your ALS unit is called out during a snowstorm to attend to an elderly man who has had the flu since yesterday. His daughter tells you that he has been vomiting, has had diarrhea for more than 24 hours, and has not been able to keep any fluids down. Your patient is weak and warm to the touch. He has elevated respiratory and pulse rates but a blood pressure of 88/60 mm Hg. His lung sounds are present bilaterally and clear. Medical direction tells you to administer a fluid bolus of 200 mL normal saline over a 20-minute period and then reevaluate the patient and call back. You decide to use a macrodrip infusion set that delivers 10 gtt (drops)/mL.

Step 1: Choose the proper formula.

$$\frac{\text{total volume} \times \text{gtt/mL of IV set}}{\text{time (in minutes)}} = \text{gtt/min}$$

Step 2: Fill in known values.

$$\frac{200 \text{ mL} \times 10 \text{ gtt/mL}}{20 \text{ min}} = \text{gtt/min}$$

Step 3: Cross out like terms.

$$\frac{200 \text{ mL} \times 10 \text{ gtt/mL}}{20 \text{ min}} = \text{gtt/min}$$

Step 4: Multiply across.

$$\frac{200 \times 10 \text{ gtt}}{20 \text{ min}} = \frac{2000 \text{ gtt}}{20 \text{ min}} = \frac{100 \text{ gtt}}{\text{min}}$$

Sometimes a measured amount of fluid is ordered to be given over a period of hours. To make this conversion, change hours to minutes by multiplying by 60 (for example, 5 hr × 60 min/hr = 300 min) and continue as before.

> You reassess the patient during and after the fluid challenge. His lungs remain clear, his pulse begins to drop to a normal range, his respirations are less frequent, and his blood pressure rises to 96/70 mm Hg. Medical direction tells you to continue the IV at a keep-open rate and transport the patient to the hospital.

Formula 2 Practice Problems
Remember the steps: cross out like terms and multiply across.
1. Administer 60 mL of fluid containing a medication over a 10-minute period. Use a microdrip IV infusion set that delivers 60 gtt/mL. How many drops per minute should be administered?
2. Administer 120 mL of Ringer's lactate as a fluid challenge over a 20-minute period with an IV infusion set that delivers 20 gtt/mL. How many drops per minute should be administered?
3. Administer 150 mL of normal saline over a 30-minute period with an IV infusion set that delivers 10 gtt/mL. How many drops per minute should be administered?
4. Administer 300 mL of Ringer's lactate over a 30-minute period with an IV infusion set that delivers 10 gtt/mL. How many drops per minute should be administered?
5. Administer 1000 mL of normal saline over a 5-hour period with a macrodrip IV infusion set that delivers 15 gtt/mL. How many drops per minute should be administered?

Formula 2 Answers

1. $$\frac{60 \text{ mL} \times 60 \text{ gtt/mL}}{10 \text{ min}} = \frac{60 \times 60 \text{ gtt}}{10 \text{ min}} = \frac{3600 \text{ gtt}}{10 \text{ min}} = 360 \text{ gtt/min}$$

2. $$\frac{120 \text{ mL} \times 20 \text{ gtt/mL}}{20 \text{ min}} = \frac{120 \times 20 \text{ gtt}}{20 \text{ min}} = \frac{2400 \text{ gtt}}{20 \text{ min}} = 120 \text{ gtt/min}$$

3. $$\frac{150 \text{ mL} \times 10 \text{ gtt/mL}}{30 \text{ min}} = \frac{150 \times 10 \text{ gtt}}{30 \text{ min}} = \frac{1500 \text{ gtt}}{30 \text{ min}} = 50 \text{ gtt/min}$$

$$4. \quad \frac{300 \text{ mL} \times 10 \text{ gtt/mL}}{30 \text{ min}} = \frac{3000 \text{ gtt}}{30 \text{ min}} = 100 \text{ gtt/min}$$

$$5. \quad \frac{1000 \text{ mL} \times 15 \text{ gtt/mL}}{300 \text{ min}} = \frac{15000 \text{ gtt}}{300 \text{ min}} = 50 \text{ gtt/min}$$

APPLICATION OF FORMULA 3

Formula 3 is used to calculate the amount of a drug to give a patient by drip (infusion) when the dosage is based not on weight but on dose of medication per minute.

> You are called to respond to the home of the base commander. On arrival, you find a 62-year-old male complaining of heart palpitations. You connect the cardiac monitor to find the patient with a narrow-complex supraventricular tachycardia at a rate of 178 beats/min. You have attempted to correct the arrhythmia with vagal maneuvers and adenosine to no avail. Medical direction orders you to administer an infusion of procainamide at 20 mg/min.
>
> You have a peripheral IV in place capable of delivering 60 gtt/mL. Your secondary premixed bag of procainamide reads 100 mg/mL. At how many drops per minute should you run the procainamide to administer the proper dose?

Step 1: Choose the proper formula.

$$\frac{\text{DD (in minutes)} \times \text{gtt/mL of IV set}}{\text{DH}} = \text{gtt/min}$$

Step 2: Fill in known values.

$$\frac{20 \text{ mg/min} \times 60 \text{ gtt/mL}}{100 \text{ mg/mL}} = \text{gtt/min}$$

Step 3: Cross out like terms. In this case, both mg and mL can be crossed out.

$$\frac{20 \text{ mg/min} \times 60 \text{ gtt/mL}}{100 \text{ mg/mL}} = \text{gtt/min}$$

Step 4: Multiply across for drops per minute.

$$\frac{20/\text{min} \times 60 \text{ gtt}}{100} = \frac{20/\text{min} \times 60 \text{ gtt}}{100} = \frac{1200}{100} \text{ gtt/min} = 12 \text{ gtt/min}$$

Formula 3 Practice Problems

Remember the steps: Cross out like terms and multiply across.

1. Administer an epinephrine infusion at 4 mcg/min. Add 1 mg epinephrine to a bag of 250 mL normal saline. Use a microdrip infusion set that delivers 60 gtt/mL. What is the drip rate in drops per minute?
2. Administer a procainamide infusion at 3 mg/min. Prepare the infusion by adding 1 g procainamide to a bag of 250 mL normal saline. Use a microdrip infusion set that delivers 60 gtt/mL. What is the drip rate in drops per minute?
3. Administer an epinephrine infusion at 2 mcg/min. Prepare the infusion by adding 1 mg epinephrine to a bag of 500 mL normal saline. What is the drug concentration (DH)? What is the drip rate if a microdrip infusion set that delivers 60 gtt/mL is used?

Formula 3 Answers

1. 1 mg = 1000 mcg, so the DH (drug concentration) is 1000 mcg/250 mL = 4 mcg/mL.

$$\frac{\text{DD: } 4 \text{ mcg/min} \times 60 \text{ gtt/mL}}{\text{DH: } 4 \text{ mcg/mL}} = \frac{4 \text{ meg}/\text{min} \times 60 \text{ gtt}/\text{mL}}{4 \text{ meg}/\text{mL}} = \frac{4/\text{min} \times 60 \text{ gtt}}{4}$$

$$= \frac{240}{4} \text{ gtt/min} = 60 \text{ gtt/min}$$

2. 1 g = 1000 mg, so the DH is 1000 mg/250 mL = 4 mg/mL.

$$\frac{\text{DD: } 3 \text{ mg/min} \times 60 \text{ gtt/mL}}{\text{DH: } 4 \text{ mg/mL}} = \frac{3 \text{ mg}/\text{min} \times 60 \text{ gtt}/\text{mL}}{4 \text{ mg}/\text{mL}} = \frac{3/\text{min} \times 60 \text{ gtt}}{4}$$

$$= \frac{180}{4} \text{ gtt/min} = 45 \text{ gtt/min}$$

3. 1 mg = 1000 mcg, so the DH is 1000 mcg/500 mL = 2 mcg/mL.

$$\frac{\text{DD: } 2 \text{ mcg/min} \times 60 \text{ gtt/mL}}{\text{DH: } 2 \text{ mcg/mL}} = \frac{2 \text{ meg}/\text{min} \times 60 \text{ gtt}/\text{mL}}{2 \text{ meg}/\text{mL}} = \frac{2/\text{min} \times 60 \text{ gtt}}{2}$$

$$= \frac{120}{2} \text{ gtt/min} = 60 \text{ gtt/min}$$

APPLICATION OF FORMULA 4

Formula 4 is used to calculate the amount of a drug to give a patient by drip (infusion) when the dosage is based on weight.

> ... You are transporting an elderly woman with a history of multiple cardiac events to the hospital. En route, her blood pressure begins to drop even though her cardiac rhythm shows only sinus tachycardia at a rate of 120 beats/min. You contact medical direction and are told to begin a dopamine infusion at 2 mcg/min and to titrate it until her blood pressure is approximately 90 mm Hg systolic. Prepare the infusion by adding 800 mg of dopamine to a 500-mL bag of normal saline. The patient weighs 110 pounds.

In this last formula, one more step in the process must be calculated to determine what the desired dose is on the basis of the patient's weight in kilograms. Remember that 1 kg = 2.2 pounds.

Step 1: Choose the proper formula.

$$\frac{\text{DD}}{\text{kg}} \times \frac{\text{lb}}{2.2 \text{ lb/kg}} = \frac{\text{DD}}{\text{kg}} \times \frac{\text{lb}}{2.2 \text{ lb}/\text{kg}} = \text{DD}$$

$$\frac{\text{DD}}{\text{DH}} \times \frac{\text{drops/mL of IV set}}{1} = \text{drops per minute}$$

Step 2: Determine the patient's weight in kilograms by dividing the weight in pounds by 2.2.

$$\frac{110 \text{ lb}}{2.2 \text{ lb/kg}} = \frac{110 \text{ lb}}{2.2 \text{ lb}/\text{kg}} = 50 \text{ kg}$$

Step 3: Multiply the weight in kilograms by DD/kilograms and cross out like terms to determine the DD, *with weight adjustment*. If this patient weighs 50 kg, and the DD is 2 mcg/kg per minute:

$$\frac{50 \text{ kg} \times 2 \text{ mcg}}{\text{kg/min}} = \frac{50 \text{ kg} \times 2 \text{ mcg}}{\text{kg}/\text{min}} = \frac{50 \times 2 \text{ mcg}}{\text{min}} = 100 \text{ mcg/min}$$

Step 4: Prepare the infusion and calculate the DH (drug concentration).

800 mg = 800,000 mcg to be added to 500 mL normal saline

$$\frac{800,000 \text{ mcg}}{500 \text{ mL}} = 1600 \text{ mcg/mL}$$

Step 5: Determine the drip rate with a microdrip IV infusion set that delivers 60 gtt/mL.

$$\frac{100 \text{ mcg/min} \times 60 \text{ gtt/mL}}{1600 \text{ mcg/mL}} = \text{gtt/min}$$

Step 6: Cross out like terms and multiply across.

$$\frac{100 \text{ mcg/min} \times 60 \text{ gtt/mL}}{1600 \text{ mcg/mL}} = \text{gtt/min}$$

Note: The zeros can be crossed out if only one above and one below the line are crossed out at a time, as in this example:

$$\frac{100 \text{ mcg/min} \times 60 \text{ gtt/mL}}{1600 \text{ mcg/mL}} = \text{gtt/min}$$

If the problem is rewritten by leaving out everything that has been crossed out, it becomes much simpler:

$$\frac{10/\text{min} \times 6 \text{ gtt}}{16} = 3.75 \text{ gtt/min} \quad (\text{round off to 4 gtt/min})$$

PRACTICAL APPLICATION PROBLEMS

Answers to the problems in this section are found in Appendix E.

Ventricular Fibrillation

You are assisting in the resuscitation of a 49-year-old man who is unresponsive and apneic. The cardiac monitor shows ventricular fibrillation, and the paramedic in charge has directed you to prepare and give the medications. Cardiopulmonary resuscitation (CPR) is being performed, defibrillation has been appropriately accomplished, the patient has been successfully intubated and is being bagged with 100% oxygen, and an IV has been established. ...

1. The first medication to administer is epinephrine 1:10,000 1 mg IV push. Your prefilled syringe reads epinephrine 1:10,000 1 mg/10 mL. How many milliliters should you administer?

... Five minutes later you are asked to repeat the above dose of epinephrine, but you discover that your IV has infiltrated. The paramedic directs you to administer twice the dose through the endotracheal tube. The patient has good lung sounds bilaterally with bagging. ...

2. You begin to prepare 2 mg of epinephrine 1:1000. With prefilled syringes containing 1 mg/mL each, how many milliliters of the epinephrine will you administer?

... After additional ventilating and CPR, the ventricular fibrillation continues. Another IV has been established and is patent. You are now ordered to administer amiodarone 300 mg IV. ...

3. Your prefilled syringe reads amiodarone 50 mg/mL. How many milliliters should you administer?

... CPR, artificial ventilation, and defibrillation continue, and the epinephrine has been appropriately repeated. You are now ordered to administer 150 mg of amiodarone IV. ...

4. With another prefilled syringe that reads amiodarone 50 mg/mL, how many milliliters should you administer this time?

... Attempts to resuscitate have resulted in the patient establishing a rhythm and pulse.

Pulseless Electrical Activity

You have responded to a call for help from the daughter of an 81-year-old man who has fallen. As you pull in the driveway, the dispatcher reports that the daughter called again to say that her father is now unresponsive. On arrival you assess the patient and find that he is apneic and pulseless. You begin CPR, ventilating with 100% oxygen, and apply the quick-look paddles only to see a sinus tachycardia on the monitor at 120 beats/min. You once again check for a pulse but do not find one.

Your partners continue CPR, intubate the patient, and start an IV line. You administer a dose of epinephrine and question his daughter regarding his medical history. You learn that he is a heavy drinker and was vomiting blood earlier today but refused to go to the hospital. Medical direction tells you to evaluate for hypovolemia by administering a bolus of 500 mL normal saline over the next 20 minutes. You set up your IV with a macrodrip IV infusion set that delivers 10 gtt/mL. ...

5. What is your drip rate per minute?

6. What is your drip rate per second?

... You notice that the patient's heart rate has dropped to 50 beats/min on the monitor. Medical direction now tells you to also administer a bolus of atropine 0.5 mg rapid IV push. Your prefilled syringe reads 1 mg/10 mL.

7. How many milliliters will you administer? (Show how your work fits into formula 1.)

Acute Coronary Syndromes

You are caring for a patient who reports chest pain that suggests cardiac origin. You and your partner have begun supportive care, including oxygen at 100%, vital signs, IV of normal saline to keep open, and positioning for comfort. Your protocol says to administer aspirin 320 mg. The bottle of aspirin in your drug box is labeled 160 mg/tablet.

8. How many tablets will you administer? (Hint: Use formula 1.)

Symptomatic Bradycardia

You respond to a law firm office for a 55-year-old woman with mild chest pain, dizziness, and shortness of breath that began when she returned from lunch. She is pale, cool, and moist to the touch but is oriented to person, place, time, and event. After beginning your supportive care, you find that the cardiac monitor shows a sinus bradycardia and her vital signs are as follows: blood pressure, 84/50 mm Hg; pulse, 50 beats/min; respirations, 20 breaths/min; lung sounds are clear.

You consider immediate transport, but the building's electric power is out because of a snowstorm and the elevators are not functioning. You decide to attempt to stabilize on scene.

After administering the maximum dosage of atropine without change and without response to the transcutaneous pacemaker (TCP) that you applied when the patient's heart rate did not improve with the atropine, you are advised by medical direction to initiate a dopamine infusion at 4 mcg/kg per minute. The patient weighs 110 pounds.

Your drug box contains dopamine in a prefilled syringe that reads dopamine 800 mg and bags of 500 mL normal saline. You also choose a microdrip infusion set that delivers 60 gtt/mL. ...

9. Calculate the DD by changing pounds to kilograms and then multiplying kilograms by the desired dose of 4 mcg/kg per minute.

10. Calculate the DH when you add 800 mg (800,000 mcg) to 500 mL.

11. What will the drip rate be per minute?

12. What will the drip rate be per second?

> ... The dopamine infusion is ineffective, your patient is feeling worse, and the snowstorm is getting worse. Medical direction is depending on you to "bring the emergency department to the patient." They direct you to now try administering an epinephrine infusion by adding epinephrine 1 mg to a bag of 250 mL normal saline and starting the drip at 2 mcg/min. (Hint: You can either add epinephrine 1:1000 or epinephrine 1:10,000 to the bag; both equal 1 mg, or 1000 mcg.) ...

13. What will the DH be?

14. What will the drip rate be in drops per minute?

15. What will the drip rate be in drops per second?

> ... Finally the epinephrine infusion works.

> ### Neurologic and Endocrine Emergencies
> Your patient is a severe diabetic who takes insulin on a daily basis. However, because of financial constraints, he did not take his insulin yesterday or today. He is confused and disoriented. Because you are not sure whether this is hyperglycemia or hypoglycemia and you do not have access to a glucometer, you choose to start an IV in a large vein and administer dextrose 50% 25 g (50 mL) IV push. The patient has no response, and you begin to suspect a possible drug overdose. Your next choice is naloxone (Narcan).
> Your prefilled syringe contains 0.4 mg naloxone in 2 mL normal saline. The order is for 0.4 mg naloxone. You know that if he shows no response you may need to administer as much as 10 mg naloxone depending on what drug was used. You receive an order to give 0.8 mg of naloxone.

16. How much naloxone should you administer if medical direction orders 0.8 mg?

You have now responded to an 11-year-old girl with grand mal seizures. She weighs approximately 88 pounds and has a history of seizures caused by an injury as an infant. Her mother tells you that she had to stop giving her the usual medications because of financial constraints. Medical direction tells you to administer diazepam 5 mg slow IV push or until the seizures stop. Your pre-filled syringe contains 10 mg/mL.

17. How many milliliters will you administer IV push?

Your patient is a 51-year-old man newly diagnosed with diabetes. He is exhibiting signs and symptoms of an acute diabetic emergency, and medical direction advises the administration of 50% dextrose (0.5 g dextrose/mL) IV push. Your partner has established an IV in a large vein, and you estimate his weight to be approximately 165 pounds.

18. If medical direction wants you to give 25 g of 50% dextrose IV push to this patient, how many milliliters will you give?

You have been called by the local police unit to care for a prisoner who is exhibiting signs and symptoms of drug withdrawal while at the local jail. When you discover pinpoint pupils, hypotension, respiratory depression, and nausea, you realize that you are dealing with a patient who has overdosed on a drug. You call medical direction, and they direct you to administer 2 mg of naloxone. Your vial reads 0.4 mg/mL.

19. How many mL will you administer?

On a cold winter night your unit is called to care for and transport a homeless person found in a stairwell covered only with old newspapers. He appears to be hypothermic, and an empty bottle of an alcoholic beverage is found tucked under his body. He is breathing, has a pulse, and has a readable blood pressure. However, even with your examination, he is unresponsive. His pupils are slow to respond but eventually do constrict in response to light. He appears to be malnourished for his height. No identification or other information is available to you.

You bring him immediately into your warmed ambulance and decide to give him 50% dextrose and thiamine because you suspect that he is an undernourished alcoholic. The thiamine in the drug box is packaged as 100 mg/mL.

Once you have moved him to the ambulance, you have fortunately been able to initiate an IV of normal saline to keep open. Medical direction directs you to administer 200 mg of thiamine and transport as soon as possible.

20. How many milliliters will you administer?

CHAPTER 5

Intravenous Fluids and Administration

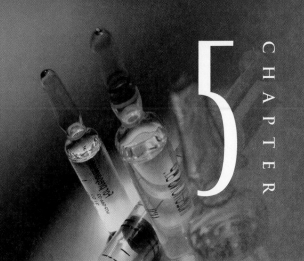

OBJECTIVES

1. Define total body water and its two main compartments (intracellular fluid and extracellular fluid).
2. Define osmosis and explain the difference between isotonic, hypotonic, and hypertonic fluids in terms in osmotic pressure.
3. Discuss colloid solutions used in intravenous therapy: albumin and hetastarch (Hespan).
4. Define hypertonic saline solutions.
5. Discuss electrolyte solutions used in intravenous therapy: calcium gluconate, sodium bicarbonate, insulin, and 5% dextrose.
6. Define drop factor, microdrip chambers, and macrodrip chambers.
7. List and discuss various appropriate sites for intravenous line insertion.
8. Demonstrate the proper procedures for the following: intravenous insertion, intravenous push, intravenous piggyback, intravenous infusion, and intraosseous infusion.
9. List the complications of intravenous infiltration, catheter shear, and phlebitis.

Medications that Appear in Chapter 5

Albumin
Hetastarch (Hespan)
Hypertonic saline (3% saline)
Calcium gluconate
Sodium bicarbonate
Insulin, regular (Humulin R, Novolin R)
Dextrose (Dextrose 50%, Dextrose 25%, Dextrose 10%)
Potassium chloride

INTRODUCTION

IV lines are started to administer IV fluids and to provide access for rapid delivery of emergency medications. Various types of IV fluids are used based on the clinical needs of the patient. Not all IV fluids are created equal, but what makes each type unique? The most obvious answer is the electrolytes and concentrations that compose the various IV fluids. The human body is essentially a bag of sea water divided into two compartments: **intracellular fluid,** which is fluid found inside the cells, and extracellular fluid. Extracellular fluid is comprised of **intravascular** and **interstitial fluid** (fluid between the cells and outside the vascular bed). A common misconception is that administered IV fluids are targeted and remain within the confines of the body's blood vessels. By altering the various concentrations of the electrolytes in the IV fluids, especially sodium, the prehospital professional can target the fluid to the body's different fluid compartments. Blood is an instrument to increase oxygen delivery to peripheral tissues. Over the past 10 years, the indications for blood transfusion have become increasingly stringent.

This chapter focuses on the different indications for IV fluid replacement and the various types of fluids used. A detailed discussion of the methods of establishing IV access is found in Chapter 3.

You are a ranger with the National Park Service. For the past 2 days, you have been involved in a search for two lost hikers. The hikers are found at the base of a canyon. You attend to the first patient, a 20-year-old man who appears weak and severely dehydrated. He tells you that he and his partner were without water for 2½ days, and the temperature was in excess of 90°F. He reports that he has not urinated in the past 24 hours and when he did, his urine was dark. On examination, the patient's skin is warm and dry. He has poor skin turgor. The mucous membranes of his mouth are dry and have an almost tacky appearance. His heart rate is 122 beats/min, blood pressure is 96/78 mm Hg, and respiratory rate is 18 breaths/min. His weight is approximately 80 kg.

The patient arrives at the hospital, and a nurse draws blood for evaluation of his serum electrolytes and renal function. The physicians agree with your assessment that the patient is significantly dehydrated. The laboratory tests results indicate some acute renal insufficiency manifested by elevated serum creatine and blood urea nitrogen levels. His serum sodium level is markedly elevated because of the dehydration. The physicians calculate that the patient's free water deficit is approximately 6 L. The physician tells you he will replace only half of that fluid in the next 24 hours. He explains that too-rapid fluid replacement causes the serum sodium level to drop too rapidly, which could potentially lead to a form of brain damage.

This patient appears to be dehydrated from a combination of excessive exposure and lack of hydration. **Dehydration** is a loss of water from the fluid space inside the cells. Dehydration can take hours to days to develop. As the cell dehydrates it begins to malfunction, leading to poor function of tissues and eventually organ failure.

Dehydration can be illustrated by imagining that a grape is a cell. The grape slowly loses fluid and dehydrates to form a raisin. With dehydration, the cells lose fluid and essentially wither.

As a general rule, conditions that quickly develop should be quickly corrected, and conditions that slowly develop should be slowly corrected. For example, after acute blood loss, such as in trauma, volume replacement occurs over a short period often measured in minutes to hours, because the blood loss occurred over a rather brief period. Fluid loss in dehydration occurs over a period of days. When such patients are evaluated at the hospital, the physician often calculates the patient's free water (or fluid) deficit. If a patient has a calculated fluid deficit of 6 L, no more than half of the calculated deficit (3 L) should be replaced in the first 24-hour period.

The above patient's condition of dehydration developed over several days; therefore his dehydration should be corrected in a slow and deliberate fashion. An initial **fluid bolus** of 1 to 2 L of isotonic crystalloid 0.9% sodium chloride (NaCl) would be appropriate, with the balance of the fluid loss replaced over a period of 24 to 48 hours. The purpose of prehospital care in this scenario is to start rehydrating the patient, which begins with choosing an IV fluid that provides rehydration to the intracellular space and expands the volume of fluid within the vascular space.

As previously mentioned, a cell that has become dehydrated is like a grape that has become a raisin. Additionally, the stranded hiker's low blood pressure and tachycardia also indicate that he has some depletion of intravascular volume. Therefore the choice of IV fluid should be one that provides some fluid resuscitation to both the intracellular space (free water) and the intravascular space. One potential choice for this setting would be isotonic crystalloids or dextrose 5% in water (D_5W).

A basic understanding of the body fluid compartments is required to understand the implications of IV fluid administration and, in this case, treat patients with dehydration.

BODY FLUID COMPARTMENTS

Most of the human body is composed of water. In adults, this amounts to approximately 45% to 65% of the body. In an average man weighing 80 kg, this equals approximately 48 L. The total amount of water in the body is known as the **total body water (TBW)** (Fig. 5-1). TBW is divided into two main compartments: intracellular fluid space and extracellular fluid space. **Intracellular fluid (ICF)** is found inside the cells, and **extracellular fluid (ECF)** is found between the cells and inside the blood vessels.[1] Two thirds of the TBW is found in the ICF, and one third is in the ECF. Of the ECF, three fourths is found in the **interstitial fluid,** and one fourth resides in the blood vessels, or the intravascular space.

> TBW: 45% to 65% of total body weight
> > ICF: two thirds of TBW
> > ECF: one third of TBW
> > > Intravascular fluid: one fourth of ECF
> > > Interstitial fluid: three fourths of ECF

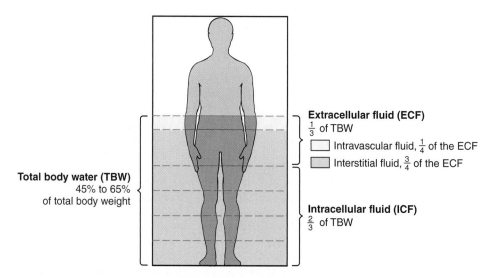

Extracellular fluid (ECF)
$\frac{1}{3}$ of TBW

☐ Intravascular fluid, $\frac{1}{4}$ of the ECF
☐ Interstitial fluid, $\frac{3}{4}$ of the ECF

Intracellular fluid (ICF)
$\frac{2}{3}$ of TBW

Total body water (TBW)
45% to 65%
of total body weight

▼ **Fig. 5-1**   Body fluid compartments. 45% to 65% of the body is composed of water. Two thirds of this fluid is inside the millions of cells making up the various tissues and organs (intracellular fluid [ICF]—*blue*). The remaining one third of the fluid is the extracellular fluid, which is found outside the cells in the blood vessels (intravascular fluid—*yellow*) and between the cells (interstitial fluid—*green*).

Interstitial fluid is the space outside the vascular space that is between the cells. For the sake of illustration, consider the blood vessels to be pipes running alongside a brick wall. The volume inside the confines of the pipes is the intravascular space. The bricks are the cells of the body, and the volume of those bricks is the intracellular volume. On a brick wall, mortar is in the narrow space between the bricks. The definition of *interstitial* is "the narrow space between things or parts." Therefore, in this example, the mortar of the wall is the interstitial space—the volume of fluid outside the bricks of cells. The mortar (interstitial fluid) and volume of the pipes (intravascular fluid) both compose the ECF (Fig. 5-2).

Water is able to move freely from one body fluid compartment to another. The compartments are separated by membranes that water can freely move across. The concentration of particles in a particular body compartment drives the movement of fluids. Particles can

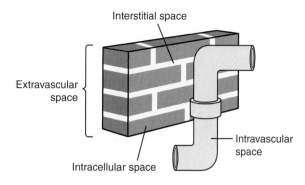

▼ **Fig. 5-2** The extravascular fluid space can be viewed to be similar to a brick wall. The bricks represent the cells, and the fluid inside the bricks is the intracellular fluid. Interstitial fluid is the fluid that resides between the cells. In this illustration, the mortar of the brick wall represents the interstitial fluid, because the mortar fills the space between the "cellular bricks." The intravascular fluid is the fluid that is within the pipes of the blood vessels.

be dissolved in salt or a body protein, but they cannot freely pass across the membranes separating the body compartments; cell membranes are quite particular regarding which types of particles they allow into the internal environment. In the body, the key particle is the electrolyte sodium. Particles that cannot freely pass across a membrane act as magnets for fluid. When particles are trapped on one side of a membrane that is permeable to water, the water will move toward the higher concentration of particles. The movement of water across such a membrane toward a higher concentration of particles is known as **osmosis** (Fig. 5-3).

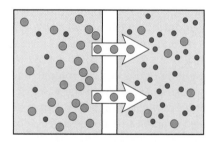

▼ **Fig. 5-3** Osmosis. The *blue* particles represent water and can move freely across the membrane in the center of the chamber. The *red* particles represent a substance that cannot move across the central membrane. The water moves across the semipermeable membrane toward the higher concentration of the trapped red particles. This is known as *osmosis*.

When "water," or D_5W, which is free of any particles, is added to one compartment, it is then freely distributed to the various body fluid compartments in proportion to their percentage of TBW. For example, if 1000 mL of water is administered as an IV bolus to a patient, it will be redistributed to the various compartments in the following way (Fig. 5-4):

1000 mL of D_5W IV
ICF (two thirds of TBW) = 666 mL
ECF (one third of TBW) = 333 mL
    Extravascular fluid (three fourths of ECF) = 250 mL
    Intravascular fluid (one fourth of ECF) = 83 mL

All this movement of water occurs within 30 minutes of administration of the IV bolus, and less than 9% of it remains in the blood vessels at the end of the 30 minutes. Because the fluid that is administered lacks any particles, the water can freely distribute itself among all the body compartments.

An IV fluid that distributes throughout several body compartments is said to have a large **volume of distribution;** this type of fluid improves a patient's intravascular and extra-

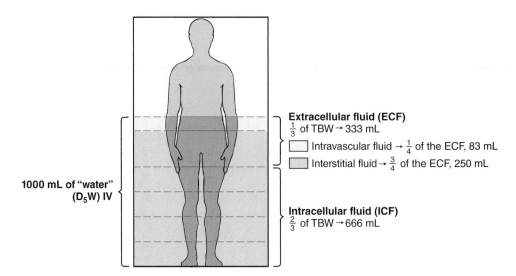

Extracellular fluid (ECF)
$\frac{1}{3}$ of TBW → 333 mL

☐ Intravascular fluid → $\frac{1}{4}$ of the ECF, 83 mL

▨ Interstitial fluid → $\frac{3}{4}$ of the ECF, 250 mL

Intracellular fluid (ICF)
$\frac{2}{3}$ of TBW → 666 mL

1000 mL of "water" (D₅W) IV

▼ **Fig. 5-4**   Administration of D₅W is free of any particles. D₅W distributes itself to the various compartments in proportion to each compartment's percentage of total body water (TBW). The extracellular fluid ([ECF]—*yellow* and *green*) is one third of the TBW. Therefore, one third of the administered D₅W (333 mL) is distributed to this space. The intravascular space *(yellow)* is only one fourth of the extracellular fluid. Only one fourth of the 333 mL remains in the intravascular space. After administering 1000 mL of D₅W, only 83 mL will remain in the intravascular space after the fluid has had an opportunity to redistribute between the various fluid spaces.

vascular volume. Chapter 1 discussed the notion that drugs must get to their intended site of action to achieve the desired effect. These same properties apply to IV fluids. If the intention of the provider is to increase the intravascular volume, the provider must choose a fluid that provides maximal expansion of the intravascular space. Attempting to improve a patient's intravascular volume by giving a fluid of which only 9 mL of every 100 mL administered remains in the vascular space is highly inefficient. A better choice of IV fluid would be one in which 25 mL of every 100 mL administered remains in the vascular space. These examples demonstrate the concept of volume of distribution. When the treatment goal is fluid resuscitation, a smaller volume of distribution is more efficient. By decreasing the distribution volume, a greater proportion of the fluid administered remains in the vascular space.

Infusion of fluids containing particles reduces the distribution volume. That is, limiting the movement of particles limits the volume of distribution, and more of the fluid remains in the vascular space. Returning to the previous example, consider a change in the type of fluid from D₅W to a fluid typically used in the prehospital setting, such as normal saline (0.9% NaCl) and Ringer's lactate solution. The salt and electrolytes in these fluids serve as particles. Their sodium concentration approximates that of the extracellular space, and the intracellular space is excluded. Such fluids are called **isotonic fluids.** Isotonic solutions have the same sodium concentration as body water.

If the patient is given 1000 mL of normal saline over a 60-minute period, the resultant increase in the intravascular volume ultimately is only 250 mL, as shown below (Fig. 5-5):

1000 mL of normal saline IV

ICF (two thirds of TBW): salt particles will not enter = 0 mL

ECF (one third of TBW) = 1000 mL

Interstitial fluid (three fourths of ECF) = 750 mL

Intravascular fluid (one fourth of ECF) = **250 mL**

Predicting the distribution of various types of IV fluids (e.g., 0.45% or 0.23% normal saline) is possible to determine the optimal fluid to administer. Table 5-1 lists the various IV fluids. For example, the patient in the preceding scenario is dehydrated and has depleted intravascular volume. Therefore the fluid this patient receives should provide

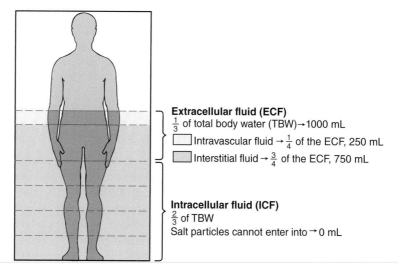

Extracellular fluid (ECF)
$\frac{1}{3}$ of total body water (TBW)→1000 mL

☐ Intravascular fluid → $\frac{1}{4}$ of the ECF, 250 mL
☐ Interstitial fluid → $\frac{3}{4}$ of the ECF, 750 mL

Intracellular fluid (ICF)
$\frac{2}{3}$ of TBW
Salt particles cannot enter into → 0 mL

▼ **Fig. 5-5** Isotonic fluids contain sodium concentrations that approximate that of the extracellular space. Isotonic fluids have sodium concentrations similar to that of body water, and this limits the distribution to the extracellular fluid compartment. The administered 1000 mL will distribute between the two compartments of the extracellular fluid (intravascular—*yellow* and interstitial—*green*) in proportion to each compartment's percentage of the extracellular fluid (intravascular—*yellow* and interstitial—*green*). After distribution, approximately 250 mL of the administered 1000 mL of isotonic fluid will remain intravascular after redistribution.

TABLE 5-1

Volume of Distribution of Various IV Fluids

1000-mL Bolus	Intracellular	Extracellular	Interstitial	Intravascular
Normal saline (0.9%) or Ringer's lactate solution (isotonic)	0 mL	1000 mL	750 mL	250 mL
½ normal saline (0.45%)	333 mL	667 mL	500 mL	167 mL
¼ normal saline (0.23%)	500 mL	500 mL	375 mL	125 mL
D₅W	666 mL	333 mL	250 mL	83 mL

some expansion of intravascular volume, as well as the fluid in the intracellular space. A good choice of IV fluid in this case is 0.45% normal saline. Following is a description of where this fluid is distributed among the vascular spaces.

Giving a patient 1000 mL of 0.45% normal saline is equivalent to giving 500 mL of normal saline and 500 mL of water. Therefore the fluids would be distributed in the amounts shown in Table 5-2. Infusion of 0.45% saline is effective in treating a dehydrated patient. This fluid replaces fluid in the vascular space but does not result in much fluid in the intracellular space. As such, this would be ineffective in treating a patient who is acutely hypovolemic from blood loss.

TABLE 5-2

Volume of Distribution of 1000 mL of 0.45% Normal Saline

	500 mL Water	500 mL Saline	Total Fluid
Intracellular fluid	333 mL	0 mL	333 mL
Extracellular fluid	167 mL	500 mL	667 mL
Interstitial fluid	125 mL	375 mL	500 mL
Intravascular fluid	42 mL	125 mL	167 mL

You are dispatched to provide assistance to a woman who is reporting severe diarrhea. After your arrival, you learn that the patient ate a buffet dinner approximately 1 hour before feeling ill. She informs you that she had abdominal cramping, followed by two bouts of emesis, followed by several episodes of severe and watery diarrhea. Your assessment of the patient reveals a 34-year-old woman who is resting on her living room couch. She reports mild abdominal discomfort. She is mildly diaphoretic. Her heart rate is 134 beats/min, blood pressure is 88/66 mm Hg, and respiratory rate is 20 breaths/min. Her mucous membranes are dry. On physical examination, she is tachycardic, lungs are clear, abdomen is soft, and only minimal tenderness is felt on deep palpation. ...

This patient has acute hypovolemia from vomiting and diarrhea. She is symptomatic, as demonstrated by tachycardia and low blood pressure. The cause of acute hypovolemia must be distinguished from hypovolemia due to acute blood loss. This patient lost fluid that is essentially composed of water and electrolytes. In contrast, acute hemorrhage is from loss of plasma and red blood cells. A blood sample from the patient with diarrhea would reveal her blood count (hemoglobin concentration and hematocrit) to be elevated. The concentration of red blood cells increases with a decrease in intravascular fluid, whereas the number of red blood cells remains unchanged. In contrast, within several hours of volume loss from acute blood loss, the blood counts (hemoglobin and hematocrit) decrease from the loss of red blood cells and intravascular fluid. Because this patient's condition developed acutely over a period of hours, the treatment needs to take place over a period of hours. The objective of treatment is volume expansion of the intravascular space. This can be accomplished by giving an infusion of an isotonic fluid, such as normal saline or Ringer's lactate, which provides reexpansion of the vascular space.

VOLUME EXPANSION

Intravascular volume is often depleted by illness and injury, and restoration of that volume is required to reestablish perfusion to vital organs and tissues. Decreased volume results in a decrease in cardiac output, and decreased cardiac output results in decreased oxygen delivery. In this case, the patient needs a fluid that maximally expands the intravascular volume. Isotonic fluids, normal saline, and Ringer's lactate allow the greatest expansion of the intravascular volume. A general rule is that for any given amount of blood loss, at least three times the amount of **crystalloid** is required to increase the intravascular volume to compensate for the loss of blood. Because of the large volume of distribution of IV fluids, the fluids shift, or leak, out of the vascular space to the interstitial and intracellular spaces. For any significant fluid or blood loss that would produce clinical symptoms of hypovolemia, the amount of required volume replacement is beyond that allowed for by most EMS protocols. From a prehospital perspective, any significant fluid resuscitation is beyond the scope of what can be accomplished in the field. Therefore hypovolemic patients must be transferred to definitive care in a timely fashion.

After a period of blood loss, the body responds by attempting to **autoresuscitate,** or shift fluid from both the intracellular space and interstitial space into intravascular space. The result is that cells can become dehydrated and malfunction, causing organ failure. Resuscitation is the administration of IV fluids to patients to replace lost fluids. Shortly after acute blood loss, the body recognizes the need to expand the intravascular volume and responds by shifting fluid from the extravascular space toward the intravascular space. In this manner the body automatically attempts to resuscitate itself (autoresuscitation).

In the case of acute blood loss, intravascular fluid replacement may need to occur in minutes to resuscitate the patient and prevent multiple organ failure. At the same time, excessive resuscitation can result in edema and pulmonary complications.

Crystalloids are IV fluids in which sodium is the primary particle that controls volume distribution. The most common types of crystalloid fluids used by prehospital providers are Ringer's lactate solution and normal saline. The movement of water through the various fluid compartments is controlled by the biologic principle of osmosis. Osmosis is the diffusion of water across a semipermeable membrane. Particles that are trapped in a particular fluid compartment act like a magnet to attract water to that compartment. In reality, the trapped particles do not attract the movement of water; the difference in concentration gradients between the two compartments does. The greater the concentration of trapped particles, the greater the movement of water. Water moves from the compartment of lower concentration to the compartment of higher concentration. As the water moves into that compartment, the concentration of the trapped particles decreases as they are diluted by the newly added water. Water continues to move down the concentration gradient until a difference in concentration between the two compartments no longer exists. In the body the particles in solution that attract water, or exert osmotic pressure, are sodium and serum proteins (e.g., albumin). Fluids that have equal osmotic pressure with the body under normal conditions are called *isotonic*. Fluids that have less osmotic pressure are hypotonic, and hypertonic fluids have greater than normal osmotic pressure. As previously mentioned, electrolytes (sodium) or large molecules, such as proteins or complex sugars, are added to IV fluids to exert osmotic pressure. Crystalloid solutions are IV fluids that use electrolytes to provide osmotic pressure. **Colloid solutions** use complex molecules such as proteins and complex sugars for osmotic pressure. Isotonic fluids contain sodium and other electrolyte concentrations that closely mimic the concentration of the ECF. In a healthy individual 1 hour after infusion of 1000 mL of isotonic fluids, only 250 mL of the infused fluid remains in the intravascular space. In critically ill or injured patients, the amount of fluid that remains in the vascular space can be less than 200 mL.[2]

A thorough understanding of hypovolemia and the various forms of volume replacement is required of all advanced prehospital providers. The causes of hypovolemia are numerous and include bleeding, burns, vomiting, diarrhea, diabetic ketoacidosis, and bowel obstruction. A healthy individual has a remarkable capacity to compensate for intravascular volume loss. Therefore, by the time a patient has symptoms of hypovolemia, the prehospital provider can assume that the magnitude of the volume loss is significant. In the case of acute blood loss, a 70-kg patient will lose greater than 30% of his or her blood volume before exhibiting hypotension.

> ... Your assessment is that the patient has acute hypovolemia as a result of food poisoning. You believe a fluid bolus is warranted because the patient has clinical signs and symptoms of hypovolemia. You insert a peripheral IV and determine that an isotonic fluid would be the best choice for this patient because you need to rehydrate both the intravascular and extravascular spaces. You start the fluid bolus of 1000 mL of Ringer's lactate to run in over a 1-hour period. You arrive at the hospital in approximately 20 minutes, and roughly 350 mL of the fluid bolus has been delivered to the patient. From a clinical standpoint, you observe a slight improvement in vital signs: heart rate of 118 beats/min, blood pressure of 102/78 mm Hg, and respiratory rate of 16 breaths/min.

In the scenario above, isotonic fluid is the fluid of choice. Isotonic fluids such as normal saline and Ringer's lactate have large volumes of distribution, and the prehospital provider needs to infuse an amount greater than the estimated fluid loss. The total volume of fluid delivered should be three to five times the amount of blood loss to increase the intravascular fluid. In this scenario, the appropriate fluid choice would be either Ringer's lactate or normal saline.

DELIVERY OF INTRAVENOUS FLUIDS

Rapid fluid losses require rapid replacement. A typical fluid bolus in an adult is 1000 mL (1 L) administered over a 15- to 60-minute period. A fluid bolus in a pediatric patient is 10 to 20 mL/kg. The key to rapid IV fluid administration for an adult is two large-bore IV catheters, either 14 or 16 gauge. The size of the catheter has a profound effect on the rate at which IV fluids can be given. The rate at which IV fluids can be administered is determined by the length and radius of the catheter. The radius of the catheter has a profound effect on determining the rate of fluid administration. Short and fat catheters typically are the most effective for rapid administration of IV fluids or medications.

Y ou are a paramedic working on the flight crew of an air medical service, and your aircraft is dispatched to an industrial accident at a saw mill. You arrive to find a 38-year-old man who has had a traumatic amputation of his right leg at the level of the mid-femur. The patient is hemorrhaging from his severed femoral artery. He is awake and alert. His airway is patent, and he is breathing spontaneously. Respiratory rate is shallow and rapid, heart rate is 138 beats/min, respiratory rate is 24 breaths/min, and blood pressure is 78/62 mm Hg. You apply direct pressure to the wound, which slows the rate of hemorrhage. Your partner applies a tourniquet, which stops the bleeding. You place a 14-gauge IV catheter in each arm. ...

This patient is in hypovolemic shock from rapid blood loss. The objective of fluid therapy in this case is to restore perfusion and oxygen delivery rapidly.

... The victim from the saw mill accident has lost approximately 45% to 50% of his circulating blood volume from the injury to his femoral artery. After your partner applies the tourniquet, you obtain a blood sample and a hemoglobin concentration. Upon arrival at the hospital, the hemoglobin level from the blood that you drew returns as normal despite the patient's profound and life-threatening blood loss.

COLLOID SOLUTIONS

Colloid solutions contain large molecules that have a preference for the vascular space. The 3 : 1 rule dictates that paramedics should administer three times the volume of crystalloid for a given loss of blood volume. However, this rule underestimates extravascular fluid shifts.

To carry a significant volume of IV fluids in an ambulance is not problematic. However, military or rural providers are limited by what they can carry. Colloids and hypertonic fluids provide an advantage for these providers by providing greater volume expansion with less fluid administered. Albumin is an IV fluid that can expand the intravascular volume by 80% of the infused volume (compared with 25% for Ringer's lactate and normal saline). Another fluid, hetastarch (Hespan), can increase the intravascular volume to 100% of the infused volume.[3] After 36 hours, approximately 33% of the infused volume of hetastarch remains in the intravascular space.

The role of albumin and other colloids in the resuscitation of critically ill and injured patients has been the source of great debate for decades, with no current consensus. Nevertheless, prehospital providers may be exposed to patients who are being treated with albumin and other colloid-containing solutions.

The idea that albumin is limited to the intravascular space is a widely held misconception. Under normal conditions, 30% to 40% of albumin is in the intravascular space and 50% to 60% is in the interstitial space. The intravascular half-life of albumin is 16 hours, and 2 hours after infusion, 90% of albumin remains in the intravascular space. Albumin, as a colloid, is capable of recruiting extravascular water into the intravascular space; each gram of albumin is capable of "pulling" 18 mL of water.[4]

ALBUMIN

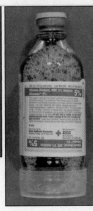
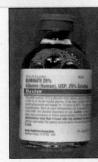

Classification: Volume expander, colloid
Action: Increases oncotic pressure in intravascular space.
Indications: Expand intravascular volume.
Adverse Effects: Allergic reaction in some patients; an excessive volume of fluid can result in CHF and pulmonary edema in susceptible patients.
Contraindications: Severe anemia or cardiac failure in the presence of normal or increased intravascular volume, solution appears turbid or after 4 hours since opening the container, known sensitivity.
Dosage: Two preparations: 500 mL of a 5% solution and 100 mL of a 25% solution.
  · **Adult:**
    · **5% albumin:** 500 to 1000 mL IV, IO.
    · **25% albumin:** 50 to 200 mL IV, IO.
  · **Pediatric:**
    · **5% albumin:** 12 to 20 mL/kg IV; the initial dose may be repeated in 15 to 30 minutes if the clinical response is inadequate.
    · **25% albumin:** 2.5 to 5 mL/kg IV, IO.
    · Alternatively, one may administer based on grams of albumin at 0.5 to 1 g/kg/dose IV, IO. May repeat as needed (max dose: 6 g/kg/day).
Special Considerations:
Patients with a history of CHF, cardiac disease, hypertension, and pulmonary edema should be given 5% albumin, or the 25% albumin should be diluted. Because 25% of albumin increases intravascular volume greater than the volume administered, slowly administer 25% albumin in normovolemic patients to prevent complications such as pulmonary edema.
Pregnancy class C

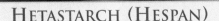

HETASTARCH (HESPAN)

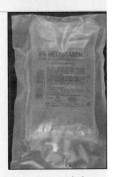

Classification: Volume expander, colloid
Action: Causes water to move from interstitial spaces, thereby increasing the oncotic pressure within the intravascular space.
Indications: Hypovolemia when volume must be increased only in the intravascular compartment.
Adverse Effects: Anaphylactic reactions, CHF, pulmonary edema, cardiac arrhythmias, cardiac arrest, severe hypotension, pruritus, edema, platelet dysfunction, bleeding complications, dilution of the serum proteins responsible for the formation of blood clots, nausea/vomiting.
Contraindications: Bleeding disorders, intracranial bleeding, CHF, pulmonary edema, renal failure, thrombocytopenia or other coagulopathy (e.g., hemophilia), known sensitivity to hetastarch or corn.
Dosage: Note: The dosage of hetastarch required is determined by the clinical situation and the severity of the hypovolemia.
  · **Adult:** 500 to 1000 mL IV, IO; more than 1500 mL of hetastarch typically is not administered because of concerns that larger doses can interfere with platelet function and promote bleeding.
  · **Pediatric:** 10 mL/kg per dose IV; the total daily dosage should not exceed 20 mL/kg.
Special Considerations:
Pregnancy class C

HYPERTONIC SALINE SOLUTIONS

Hypertonic saline solutions have a concentration greater than the isotonic concentration of 0.9%. (Recall that isotonic solutions have the same sodium concentration as body water.) Typical hypertonic solutions are 3%, 5%, or 7% saline, roughly three to five times higher sodium concentration than standard normal saline. The higher concentration of sodium pulls more volume into the vascular space. Some solutions use particles other than sodium to make the fluid hypertonic. The net effect is that intravascular volume is increased by a greater volume than the total volume infused. Such a notion is attractive to military and rural providers, who are limited in the amount of supplies they can carry.

Critics of hypertonic fluid resuscitation have argued that pulling or mobilizing fluids from the interstitial and intracellular spaces results in the dysfunction of cells and tissues. However, research has shown that during periods of stress and shock, cells actually become fat and swell with additional water. The administration of hypertonic saline results in normalization of cellular water and volume. Although hypertonic fluids were previously believed to reduce cell volume below normal, animal research has demonstrated that administration of 7.5% hypertonic solution rapidly restores both blood pressure and cardiac output in the treatment of hemorrhagic shock. However, these improvements were short lived; after 30 minutes, both blood pressure and cardiac output were similar to those animals treated with standard normal saline. Research remains active in this area, with the goal of identifying a fluid capable of rapid volume expansion limited to the vascular space and sustained improvement in blood pressure and cardiac output.[5,6]

HYPERTONIC SALINE (3% SALINE)

Classification: Volume expander, electrolyte solution
Action: The hypertonic nature of this fluid pulls extravascular fluid into the vascular space. Hypertonic saline may therefore be used as a volume expander in cases of hypovolemia or to reduce the edema of the swollen brain. Three percent saline has an electrolyte concentration of 514 mEq/L sodium.
Indications: Reduction of increased intracranial pressure resulting from traumatic brain injury, hypovolemic shock.
Adverse Effects: Increased rate of bleeding, alteration of blood clotting ability, osmotic demyelination syndrome.
Contraindications: Pulmonary congestion, pulmonary edema, known sensitivity. Hypertonic saline should not be administered by the IO route.
Dosage: Note: Hypertonic saline is available in several concentrations from 3% to 5%.
· **Adult:** 250-mL bag of hypertonic saline infused IV slowly over a 1-hour period.
· **Pediatric:** 6.5 to 10 mL/kg infused slowly IV over a 2-hour period.
Special Considerations:
Hypertonic saline can cause damage to the vein in which it is administered.
Pregnancy class C

ELECTROLYTES

Your paramedic unit is dispatched to a long-term care facility for a medical call. The dispatcher reports that the patient, who has a medical history of renal failure requiring hemodialysis, is reporting nausea, vomiting, and diarrhea. You arrive to find a 78-year-old man lying in his bed. He appears weak and pale and tells you that he has felt ill all afternoon. He has had several episodes of vomiting and one episode of diarrhea. He underwent dialysis 2 days ago. His blood pressure is 146/92 mm Hg, heart rate is 94 beats/min, respiratory rate is 20 breaths/min, and oxygen saturation is 93%. His lungs are clear, and his heartbeat is regular. A dialysis fistula is noted in his left forearm. You place the patient on oxygen, start an IV of normal saline, and place the patient on the cardiac monitor, at which time you note that the patient has peaked T waves.

This case presents one of the few situations in which a prehospital professional may need to treat an electrolyte disorder without the benefit of laboratory tests. Prehospital providers do not have the luxury of laboratory blood tests. In contrast, hospital providers such as nurses and physicians typically treat various electrolyte disorders identified by laboratory blood tests. The paramedic, however, treats electrolyte disorders that have clinical manifestations. With the exception of **hyperkalemia** (elevated levels of potassium), the majority of electrolyte disorders are not immediately life-threatening and often can wait for treatment until confirmation by laboratory tests at a hospital. Hyperkalemia may occur in the presence of renal failure and presents with gastrointestinal symptoms of nausea, abdominal pain, and/or diarrhea. Other causes of hyperkalemia include burns, crush injuries, diabetic ketoacidosis, and severe infections. Patients with hyperkalemia can have cardiovascular signs of initially peaked T waves, widening of the QRS complex, and depression of the ST segment. If left untreated, hyperkalemia can progress to heart block and cardiac arrest.

In the preceding scenario, the paramedic should suspect hyperkalemia because the patient has a history of renal failure and has gone several days without hemodialysis. He has gastrointestinal symptoms of nausea, vomiting, and diarrhea, as well as peaked T waves on electrocardiography. The treatment objectives for this patient are to protect his heart from the effects of hyperkalemia and "hide" the potassium inside the cells. Protection of the potentially life-threatening cardiac complications from hyperkalemia can be achieved by administering 1 g 10% calcium gluconate. Calcium can also be administered as calcium chloride. Administration of calcium does nothing to alter the serum level of potassium. To "hide the potassium," the potassium must be shifted from the extracellular space into the intracellular space. This can be achieved by administration of sodium bicarbonate, 50% dextrose, and insulin.

Sodium bicarbonate rapidly shifts the potassium into the cells within minutes of administration, and the effect lasts up to 12 hours. Sodium bicarbonate works by pushing potassium into the cell in exchange for a hydrogen ion. One to two **ampules** (50 to 100 mEq) are usually required in adults. Insulin (10 U regular insulin) allows additional potassium to be hidden inside the cells. Dextrose (2.5 g) is given with the insulin to prevent hypoglycemia.

CALCIUM GLUCONATE

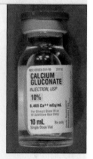

Classification: Electrolyte solution
Action: Counteracts the toxicity of hyperkalemia by stabilizing the membranes of the cardiac cells, reducing the likelihood of fibrillation.
Indications: Hyperkalemia, hypocalcemia, hypermagnesemia.
Adverse Effects: Soft tissue necrosis, hypotension, bradycardia (if administered too rapidly).
Contraindications: VF, digitalis toxicity, hypercalcemia.
Dosage: Supplied as 10% solution; therefore each milliliter contains 100 mg of calcium gluconate.
· **Adult:** 500 to 1000 mg IV, IO administered slowly at a rate of approximately 1 to 1.5 mL/min; maximum dose 3 g IV, IO.
· **Pediatric:** 60 to 100 mg/kg IV, IO slowly over a 5- to 10-minute period; maximum dose 3 g IV, IO.
Special Considerations:
Do not administer by IM or Sub-Q routes, which causes significant tissue necrosis.
Pregnancy class C

SODIUM BICARBONATE

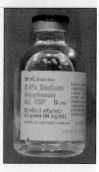

Classification: Electrolyte replacement
Action: Counteracts existing acidosis.
Indications: Acidosis, drug intoxications (e.g., barbiturates, salicylates, methyl alcohol).
Adverse Effects: Metabolic alkalosis, hypernatremia, injection site reaction, sodium and fluid retention, peripheral edema.
Contraindications: Metabolic alkalosis.
Dosage:
Metabolic Acidosis during Cardiac Arrest:
- **Adult:** 1 mEq/kg slow IV, IO; may repeat at 0.5 mEq/kg in 10 minutes.
- **Pediatric:** Same as adult dosing.
Metabolic Acidosis Not Associated with Cardiac Arrest:
- **Adult:** Dosage should be individualized.
- **Pediatric:** Dosage should be individualized.
Special Considerations:
Do not administer into an IV, IO line in which another medication is being given.
Because of the high concentration of sodium within each ampule of sodium bicarbonate, use with caution in patients with CHF and renal disease.
Pregnancy class C

INSULIN, REGULAR (HUMULIN R, NOVOLIN R)

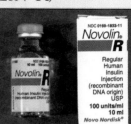

Classification: Hormone
Action: Binds to a receptor on the membrane of cells and facilitates the transport of glucose into cells.
Indications: Hyperglycemia, insulin-dependent diabetes mellitus, hyperkalemia.
Adverse Effects: Hypoglycemia, tachycardia, palpitations, diaphoresis, anxiety, confusion, blurred vision, weakness, depression, seizures, coma, insulin shock, hypokalemia.
Contraindications: Hypoglycemia, known sensitivity.
Dosage:
Diabetic Ketoacidosis:
- **Adult:** 0.1 U/kg IV, IO, or Sub-Q. Because of poor perfusion of the peripheral tissues, Sub-Q administration is much less effective than the IV, IO route. IV, IO insulin has a very short half-life; therefore IV, IO insulin without an infusion is not that effective. The rate for an insulin infusion is 0.05 to 0.1 U/kg/hr IV, IO. When dosing insulin, use a U-100 insulin syringe to measure and deliver the insulin. The time from administration to action, as well as the duration of action, varies greatly among different individuals, as well as at different times in the same individual.
Hyperkalemia:
- **Adult:** 10 U IV, IO of regular insulin (Insulin R), coadministered with 50 mL of $D_{50}W$ over 5 minutes.
- **Pediatric:** 0.1 U/kg Insulin R IV, IO.
Special Considerations:
Only regular insulin can be given IV, IO.
Pregnancy class B

DEXTROSE (DEXTROSE 50%, DEXTROSE 25%, DEXTROSE 10%)

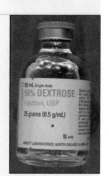

Classification: Antihypoglycemic
Action: Increases blood glucose concentrations.
Indications: Hypoglycemia
Adverse Effects: Hyperglycemia, warmth, burning from IV infusion. Concentrated solutions may cause pain and thrombosis of the peripheral veins.
Contraindications: Intracranial and intraspinal hemorrhage, delirium tremens, solution is not clear, seals are not intact.
Dosage:
Hyperkalemia:
- **Adult:** 25 g of dextrose 50% IV, IO.
- **Pediatric:** 0.5 to 1 g/kg IV, IO.
Hypoglycemia:
- **Adult:** 10 to 25 g of dextrose 50% IV (20 to 50 mL of dextrose solution).
- **Pediatric:**
  - **Older than 2 years:** 2 mL/kg of dextrose 50%.
  - **Younger than 2 years:** 2 to 4 mL/kg of dextrose 10%.
Special Considerations:
Pregnancy class C

Hypokalemia, or low serum concentration of potassium, is a condition that is nearly impossible to diagnose without the benefit of a laboratory blood test. Hypokalemia is typically a result of chronic medical conditions such as reduced dietary intake of potassium, chronic diuretic therapy, diarrhea, short bowel syndrome, vomiting, and burns. Because paramedics lack the benefit of laboratory tests, they must rely on symptoms. Unfortunately, the symptoms of hypokalemia are nonspecific. The clinical manifestations of hypokalemia include muscle weakness (which in its most severe form can lead to paralysis), abdominal distension, and constipation. On an electrocardiogram, the T waves tend to flatten and progress to atrioventricular block and cardiac arrest.

Administration of IV potassium in the prehospital setting is an unlikely occurrence. However, in the hospital setting potassium infusions and supplementation commonly occur. Therefore the paramedic in the transport of patients between various facilities may likely encounter patients who have potassium as a supplement to their IV fluids or who are receiving a potassium infusion.

Potassium replacement in chronic conditions and nonemergent conditions is provided with oral supplements. A medical condition needing oral potassium replacement is often not a medical emergency and does not require intervention by a paramedic. IV administration of potassium can potentially be dangerous because too-vigorous replacement leads to hyperkalemia. IV potassium should always be diluted and slowly administered to reduce the likelihood of pain from inflammation of the vein **(phlebitis).** Potassium should be administered only to patients with adequate renal function and good urine output. Several forms of potassium can be administered intravenously: potassium chloride, potassium acetate, and potassium phosphate. Potassium chloride is the most commonly used form of potassium administered. Potassium should not be administered to patients who are dehydrated. IV fluids with supplemental potassium should not contain more than 40 mEq/L of potassium, and the rate of administration should not exceed 20 mEq/hr.

POTASSIUM CHLORIDE

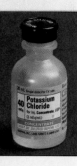
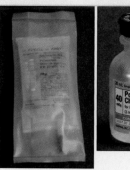

Classification: Electrolyte replacement
Action: Replaces potassium. Slight alterations in extracellular potassium levels can cause serious alterations in both cardiac and nervous function.
Indications: Hypokalemia
Adverse Effects: Hyperkalemia; AV block; cardiac arrest; GI bleeding, obstruction, or perforation; tissue necrosis if the infusion infiltrates into the soft tissues.
Contraindications: Use with caution in patients with cardiac arrhythmias, renal failure, muscle cramps, severe tissue trauma.
Dosage:
  · **Adult:** Dosage must be individualized according to patient serum potassium concentration.
  · **Pediatric:** Dosage must be individualized according to patient serum potassium concentration.
Special Considerations:
Pregnancy class C

Other common electrolyte disorders include disorders of calcium, magnesium, and phosphorus (Table 5-3). Disorders of these electrolytes are usually caused by chronic medical conditions and produce vague and non–life-threatening clinical symptoms. Therefore prehospital care providers rarely treat any of these conditions in the absence of laboratory blood tests.

TABLE 5-3

Common Electrolyte Problems

Electrolyte Disorder	Causes	Signs and Symptoms
Hypocalcemia	Sepsis, inadequate vitamin D, pancreatitis, parathyroid disease	Irritability, hyperactive deep tendon reflexes, twitching of the face or spasms of the hand, tetany, convulsions, paresthesia, abdominal cramps, muscle cramps, neural excitability
Hypercalcemia	Cancer with metastases and parathyroid disease, overactivity	Weakness, irritability, dehydration, headache, hypertension, renal stone
Hypomagnesemia	Malnutrition, cirrhosis, pancreatitis, diarrhea	Weakness, confusion, irritability, tremors, nausea, hypotension, seizures, and arrhythmias
Hypermagnesemia	Chronic renal failure	Reduced neuromuscular irritability, loss of deep tendon reflexes, sedation, confusion
Hypophosphatemia	Long-term IV nutrition, sustained vomiting or diarrhea, alcoholism, parathyroid disease	Weakness, tremors, eventually numbness of the face and fingers, irritability to seizures
Hyperphosphatemia	Chronic renal failure, treatment of acute leukemia and lymphoma	Hypocalcemia

INTRAVENOUS THERAPY: EQUIPMENT AND ADMINISTRATION

Starting IV lines is a skill that requires a great deal of practice and patience. Starting an IV in a hospital is much different from starting an IV in the field or in the back of an ambulance. The paramedic is often starting IVs in conditions of inclement weather, poor lighting, and unstable movement of the ambulance.

EQUIPMENT

Equipment needed to start an IV includes catheters, tubing sets, and bags of IV solutions. Do not omit the appropriate personal protective equipment required to protect yourself from blood and body fluids—eye protection and gloves.

Catheters

Like needles, IV catheters are composed of a hub and catheter shaft. Catheters used for IV infusions have a plastic catheter that fits over a needle. The advantage of over-the-needle catheters is that, once the metal needle has been removed from the vein, the possibility of puncturing the wall of the vein with prolonged insertion or movement is lessened.

Administration Sets

IV administration sets, or setups, include a bag of IV fluids, **drip chamber, roller clamp,** and administration port (Fig. 5-6). The drip chamber is the compartment immediately below the IV bag where the IV fluid drips at a predetermined volume. When the IV fluid drips at a uniform rate, the healthcare provider can control the volume and rate of administration with a reasonable degree of accuracy. Drip chambers allow the provider to count the number of drops over a period and calculate the rate of fluid or drug administration. **Drop factor** is the number of drops into the chamber required to administer 1 mL of fluid. Drip chambers come in two forms: microdrip and macrodrip.

Microdrip chambers administer 60 gtt/mL. The number of drops counted per minute equals the rate of infusion in milliliters per hour. Therefore, if 30 drops occur per minute, the infusion rate is 30 mL/hr. These chambers are useful when administering IV medications such as adrenergic agents and cardiac antiarrhythmics. Microdrip chambers are also useful when administering IV fluids to children or other patients who are likely to be sensitive to large amounts of IV fluids.

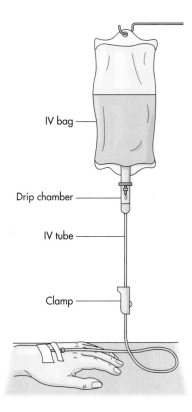

▼ **Fig. 5-6**   Intravenous administration setup. (From Elkin MK: *Nursing interventions and clinical skills,* ed 4, St Louis, 2008, Mosby.)

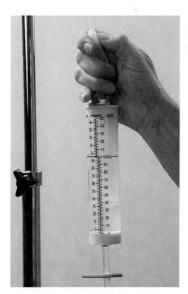

▼ **Fig. 5-7**   The volume-control chamber provides an additional level of safety to avoid inadvertent infusion of fluids to a pediatric patient or other volume-sensitive patient. (From Potter PA, Perry AG: *Fundamentals of nursing,* ed 7, St Louis, 2009, Mosby.)

Macrodrip chambers come in a variety of sizes, with drip factors of 10, 12, 15, and 20 gtt/mL. Most EMS agencies carry only one type of macrodrip chamber.

Volume-control chambers are also used to control the amount of fluids delivered (Fig. 5-7). In small children, inadvertent administration of a large volume of fluids can result in significant complications. A volume chamber can be inserted between the drip chamber and the IV bag. A roller clamp between the IV bag and volume chamber controls the amount of fluid in the chamber. The advantage of the volume chamber is that the provider can set the maximal amount of fluid to be infused by filling the chamber from the IV. Once the volume chamber empties, the patient cannot receive any more fluid.

Y-tubing is used in patients who require volume expansion and possibly transfusion of blood products. Y-tubing is also known as a blood solution set. When caring for a trauma patient, start an IV with Y-tubing and hang a bag of normal saline. With Y-tubing primed with normal saline, a transfusion of blood can be started as soon as blood is available or the patient arrives at the hospital.

During a violent spring thunderstorm, your unit is dispatched to a structure fire. The house was struck by lightning. When the fire department arrived on the scene, the house was fully engulfed. The owner of the house, a 66-year-old man, ran back in the house to get the keys for his truck, sustaining deep and partial-thickness burns to both arms and the anterior part of his chest. You and your partner remove the burned clothing, stop the burning process, start two IVs, and obtain orders to administer morphine 6 mg IV push. You estimate the patient has burns on 25% of his body surface area. Once at the hospital, the emergency department physician determines that this patient will need to be transported to the regional burn center by ambulance because of the inclement weather. You and the physician calculate the patient's fluid needs during transport and run the IV fluid rate at 450 mL/hr. When you started the IV, you used an IV set with a drip factor of 10 gtt/mL. You must determine the drops per minute required to deliver the appropriate amount of IV fluids.

$$\frac{\text{Drop factor of IV set (gtt/mL)}}{60\,\text{min/hr}} \times \text{total hourly volume to be infused} = \text{gtt/min}$$

$$\frac{10\,\text{gtt/mL}}{60\,\text{min/hr}} \times 450\,\text{mL/hr} = \text{gtt/min}$$

$$75 = \text{gtt/min}$$

You need a drip rate of 75 gtt/min into the chamber to deliver an IV flow rate of 450 mL/hr.

IV fluids infused without an **infusion pump** use the force of gravity. In the absence of a pump, many factors can alter the rate of infusion, so the fluid must frequently be verified as flowing at the intended rate. Factors affecting the drip rate include the height of the IV bag, position of the extremity with the IV, and coiling of the IV tubing. Determination of fluid rates is explained in Chapter 4.

The indication for starting an IV line often determines the rate of fluid administration. When an IV is started on medical calls, it often serves as a vehicle to allow rapid administration of medications as the patient's condition dictates. Under these conditions the fluid rate is often referred to as **TKO** (to keep open) or **KVO** (keep vein open). The KVO rate can typically be achieved with a microdrip set running at 30 to 50 gtt/min, which translates to a rate of 30 to 50 mL/hr. Failure to infuse some fluids slowly can result in the IV line clotting, which means the vein will not be available in the event of an emergency. When caring for small children, be mindful that fluid amounts that would seem small and insignificant in an adult are much more significant in a child. For example, in a 22-pound (10-kg) child, an infusion rate of 50 mL/hr would exceed the child's hourly maintenance rate (Box 5-1).

BOX 5-1

PEDIATRIC MAINTENANCE FLUIDS

To determine the appropriate rate of maintenance fluid, the provider must know or estimate the child's weight in kilograms. Remember that 1 kg equals approximately 2.2 pounds.
- For the first 10 kg of weight, the IV fluid rate is 4 mL/hr per kilogram.
  - A 5-kg child has an IV rate of 20 mL/hr (4 mL/hr per kilogram × 5 kg)
  - A 10-kg child has an IV rate of 40 mL/hr (4 mL/hr per kilogram × 10 kg)
- For the second 10 kg of weight (i.e., 10 to 20 kg of body weight), add 2 mL/kg for each additional kilogram.
  - For a 12-kg child, start with a rate of 40 mL/hr for the first 10 kg of body weight and then add 4 mL/hr for the remaining 2 kg. The IV rate then is 44 mL/hr.
    - 10 kg × 4 mL/kg per hour = 40 mL/hr
    - 2 kg × 2 mL/kg per hour = 4 mL/hr
    - Total maintenance rate: 44 mL/hr
- To calculate the IV maintenance rate for children heavier than 20 kg, add an additional 1 mL/hr per kilogram.
  - A 25-kg child will have a maintenance rate as follows:
    - First 10 kg = 40 mL/hr
    - Second 10 kg = 20 mL/hr
    - Remaining 5 kg = 1 mL/kg per hour × 5 kg = 5 mL/hr
- Therefore the total maintenance rate is 65 mL/hr.

When caring for patients who have undergone trauma, IVs are started for rapid administration of fluids or blood to expand the intravascular volume. Considerable debate exists about what constitutes the appropriate rate and magnitude of IV fluid administration in the prehospital setting. Some conditions require the paramedic to administer fluids rapidly. Running fluids wide open means opening the roller clamp all the way to allow for maximal fluid delivery with the aid of gravity. To increase the rate of fluid delivery, the paramedic can place the IV bag in a pressure bag or have someone manually squeeze the bag of fluids. Both methods increase the rate of fluid delivery.

The size of the IV catheter is the principal determinant of the maximal rate of fluid administration that can be achieved. An increase in the radius of the catheter results in a profound increase in IV flow rate. For example, water will flow through a pipe with a 5-inch diameter 2.5 times faster than through a 4-inch diameter pipe of equal length.

The rate that fluid can flow through a tube is defined by the laws of physics with the following formula:

$$\frac{(\text{Change in pressure}) \times \text{Radius}^4}{\text{Length of the catheter}}$$

Based on this formula, increasing the change in pressure by increasing the height of the bag, adding a pressure bag, or manually squeezing the bag increases the rate of fluid delivery. Increasing the length of tubing by adding tubing extension sets actually *decreases* the IV fluid rate.

In helicopters and mobile intensive care units, prehospital providers may encounter a variety of electric infusion pumps (Fig. 5-8). Numerous pumps are available with a variety of features. A well-calibrated pump offers several advantages over microdrip and macrodrip sets. The pump can easily regulate the rate of fluid administration by letting the paramedic directly enter the fluid rate into a keypad rather than count drips per minute and convert that rate to a volume per hour. Many pumps allow the provider to enter the patient's weight and desired dose of a medication, and the pump automatically calculates and sets the rate of delivery. Pumps also allow the user to set a volume to be delivered, and the pump will stop the infusion after delivering the set volume.

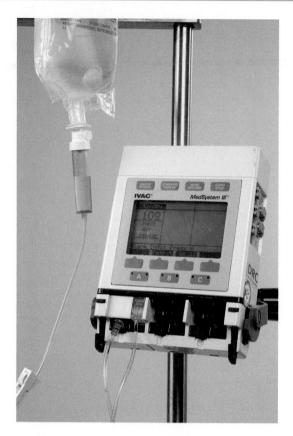

▼ **Fig. 5-8**   Intravenous infusion pump. (From Aehlert B, ed: *Paramedic practice today: above and beyond,* St Louis, 2009, Mosby.)

SITE SELECTION AND PREPARATION

IVs are most commonly inserted in the veins of the hands and arms. In cases of trauma or shock, the provider should place the IV in a larger vein of the antecubital fossa. In less critical cases, starting an IV in the most distal aspect of the extremity preserves the more proximal veins for later IV access. When possible, avoid starting an IV in the dominant hand or in an injured extremity. Avoid IVs in the lower extremities of adults because of potential complications with infections. In children, insertion of an IV into the dorsal aspect of the foot or the scalp is common.

Depending on local protocols, alcohol or povidone iodine (Betadine) is most commonly used to prepare a site for the placement of an IV catheter. Start preparing the area by cleansing the proposed site of the IV. Start and continue in a circular motion with an increasing radius. Allow the site to dry.

PROCEDURES

Following are step-by-step procedures for IV assembly, IV assembly with Volutrol, peripheral IV access, withdrawing medication from a vial, assembly of a preloaded syringe, withdrawing medication from an ampule, IV drug administration, IV infusion (piggyback): preparing medication for infusion and attaching infusion solution to primary IV line, and intraosseous infusion (tibial and sternal).

 ## IV ASSEMBLY

Equipment Needed:
IV solution, IV tubing
Procedure:
1. Observe universal precautions.
2. When possible, explain to the patient what procedure you are going to perform and why.

3. Select the appropriate IV fluid.
4. Remove cover from both IV part of IV bag of fluids and the spike on the IV tubing drip chamber.
5. Insert the spike of the tubing drip chamber into the IV tubing part of the bag of IV fluids.
6. Open the roller clamp on the IV tubing to flush the IV fluid through the tubing.
7. Once tubing has been flushed, close the roller clamp or set fluid infusion rate as prescribed.

IV ASSEMBLY WITH VOLUTROL

Equipment Needed:
IV solution, IV tubing with Volutrol
Procedure:
1. Observe universal precautions.
2. Confirm with the patient that he or she has no allergies to the medication, and document allergies to any other medication.
3. When possible, explain to the patient what procedure you are going to perform and why.
4. Select the appropriate IV fluid and spike the bag in the same way you would for a regular IV.
5. Connect and hang the drip set. Close the flow clamp at the bottom of the volume-control changer.
6. Open the flow clamp above the chamber. Fill the chamber with the appropriate amount of IV solution. Close the clamp. Open the bottom flow clamp and fill the drip chamber and tubing.
7. Cannulate the vein, connect the IV tubing, and set the drip rate by using the flow regulation clamp below the volume chamber.
8. Monitor the fluid in the chamber at all times.
9. When the volume regulation chamber is almost empty, reassess the patient's condition and lung fields to determine whether the procedure should be continued as a premeasured infusion or in a TKO format.
10. Document the medication, dose, route, needle size, and time in the patient care record.
11. Evaluate the patient for desired effects of the medication, as well as any adverse effects. Continued reevaluation should occur throughout transport.

PERIPHERAL IV ACCESS

Equipment Needed:
Alcohol or Betadine prep, tourniquet, IV catheter, IV tubing, IV solution, adhesive tape or dressing to secure IV line, sharps, PPE
Procedure:
1. Observe universal precautions.
2. Confirm with the patient that he or she has no allergies to the medication, and document allergies to any other medication.
3. When possible, explain to the patient what procedure you are going to perform and why.
4. Position the patient to stabilize the extremity where the IV is to be inserted with pillows or a cot that is easily accessible.
5. Ensure that all IV tubing and equipment are assembled and flushed and that all materials required for securing and dressing the catheter are immediately available.
6. Determine the location for IV catheter placement.
7. Apply the tourniquet several inches proximal to the proposed IV site.
8. Prepare the area.
9. Hold the needle in your dominant hand at a 30-degree angle, with the needle bevel up. Insert the needle through the skin approximately ½ to 1 inch distal to the site

where it will enter the vein. As you slowly advance the needle through the skin, reduce the angle to approximately 15 degrees while advancing through the soft tissues and into the vein.

10. Once the needle has entered into the vein, blood will flow back into the hub of the needle. Holding the needle still, slowly advance the catheter over the needle and into the vein.

11. Discard the needle immediately into an appropriate sharps container.

12. While securing the catheter with one hand, release the tourniquet and connect the hub of the catheter to the preassembled IV tubing set.

13. Open the clamp on the IV tubing and observe the flow in the drip chamber.

14. Secure the IV catheter in place with tape or adhesive dressings. Anchoring an IV in the elderly or burn and trauma patients can be difficult because adhesive tapes and dressings do not always adhere. In these cases, consider securing the catheter in place with a roller gauze.

> In conditions in which adhesive dressings or tapes will not adequately secure an IV line, secure the line with roller gauze.

15. Document the medication, dose, route, needle size, and time in the patient care record.

16. Evaluate the patient for desired effects of the medication, as well as any adverse effects. Continued reevaluation should occur throughout transport.

Once an IV line has been established, prehospital care providers can deliver medications directly into the circulatory system. IV medications can be delivered by three methods:

1. IV push
2. IV piggyback
3. IV infusion

IV Push

IV push involves using a syringe connected to the **injection port** of an IV line so that the provider can rapidly administer medications or slowly empty the syringe over a period of several minutes, depending on the particular medication. Injection ports are areas placed along the IV tubing where the provider can inject the contents of a syringe into the IV line.

Many of the medications used in the prehospital environment are supplied in preloaded syringes. To use a **preloaded syringe,** the paramedic must assemble the syringe by removing the yellow caps on the ends of the two pieces and then screwing the two pieces together. Prefilled tubes of medication are also available to emergency providers to deliver medications rapidly. **Prefilled tubes** are glass syringes or tubes that are rapidly screwed in a plastic or metal tubex. This type of medication delivery is becoming rare as disposable preloaded syringes become more prevalent. Medications not supplied in preloaded syringes are provided in **vials** or ampules. To administer the medication contained within the ampule or vial, the provider must transfer the medication into a syringe. Vials are often glass bottles with a sealed opening, rubber diaphragm, and aluminum rim and cover. Ampules are small glass containers that typically contain a single dose of a medication.

WITHDRAWING MEDICATION FROM A VIAL

Equipment Needed:
Alcohol prep, vial of medication, syringe, needle for syringe, sharps

Procedure:
1. Observe universal precautions.
2. Verify drug order.
3. Confirm right patient, right medication, right dose, right route, and right time.
4. Confirm with the patient that he or she has no allergies to the medication, and document allergies to any other medication.
5. When possible, explain to the patient what medication you are going to administer and why.
6. Peel back the aluminum lid of the vial to expose the rubber diaphragm.
7. Wipe the rubber diaphragm with an alcohol wipe.
8. Fill the syringe with the volume of air equal to the amount of medication desired to be removed from the vial.
9. With the bevel of the needle facing you, insert the needle into the vial and inject the air from the syringe.
10. Load the medication from the vial into the syringe.
11. When withdrawing a medication from a vial for use by the IM or Sub-Q routes, place a new needle on the syringe before administering the medication.

 ## ASSEMBLY OF A PRELOADED SYRINGE

Equipment Needed:
Medication in preloaded syringe, sharps
Procedure:
1. Observe universal precautions.
2. Verify drug order.
3. Confirm right patient, right medication, right dose, right route, and right time.
4. Confirm with the patient that he or she has no allergies to the medication, and document allergies to any other medication.
5. Calculate the volume of medication to be administered.
6. Remove the protective cap from the barrel and cartridge.
7. Screw the cartridge into the barrel.
8. Push in the plunger to expel the air.

 ## WITHDRAWING MEDICATION FROM AN AMPULE

Equipment Needed:
Ampule of medication, two pieces of 4 × 4 gauze, syringe, filtered needle for drawing the medication into the syringe, needle for injection, sharps
Procedure:
1. Observe universal precautions.
2. Verify drug order.
3. Confirm right patient, right medication, right dose, right route, and right time.
4. Confirm with the patient that he or she has no allergies to the medication, and document allergies to any other medication.
5. When possible, explain to the patient what medication you are going to administer and why.
6. Shift all the medication into the lower portion of the ampule by tapping the top half of the ampule.
7. Hold the ampule between your hands by wrapping it with two pieces of gauze. In one hand, hold the top of the ampule in a piece of gauze; with the other hand, hold the lower portion of the glass ampule. Break the top off the ampule by bending it away from you.
8. With a filtered needle to prevent any glass shards from being drawn up, draw the medication up into the syringe. Discard this needle and switch to a different needle if using a needle to administer medication.

Whether you are using preloaded syringes or medication from a vial or ampule, you are now ready to administer the medication as an IV push.

IV DRUG ADMINISTRATION

Equipment Needed:

Alcohol prep, medication loaded in a syringe, needle for the syringe, sharps, PPE

Procedure:

1. Observe universal precautions.
2. Verify drug order.
3. Confirm right patient, right medication, right dose, right route, and right time.
4. Confirm with the patient that he or she has no allergies to the medication, and document allergies to any other medication.
5. When possible, explain to the patient what procedure you are going to perform and why.
6. Locate the medication port of the IV line and wipe it clean with alcohol.
7. Clamp or pinch the IV tubing above the site of the medication port.
8. Insert the needle of the syringe through the diaphragm of the medication port. If using a needleless system, first unscrew needle.

> Be careful not to insert the needle through the back wall of the tubing. A short needle can help avoid this problem. Needleless systems in which the syringe is screwed to the port also work well.

9. Gently pull back on the plunger of the syringe until you see a small flow of blood in the IV tubing. This maneuver ensures that the catheter is in the vein and prevents infiltration of the medication into the soft tissues.
10. Inject the medication into the IV line at the rate appropriate for the particular medication.
11. Once all the medication has been injected, remove the needle from the medication port, unclamp the IV tubing, and dispose the needle and syringe into the appropriate container.
12. Document the medication, dose, route, needle size, and time in the patient care record.
13. Evaluate the patient for desired effects of the medication, as well as any adverse effects. Continued reevaluation should occur throughout transport.

IV Piggyback

IV piggyback infusions are secondary infusions attached to the primary infusion line. Rather than directly injecting the medication into the line as an IV push, the medication is added to a smaller bag of IV fluid and slowly infused through the medication port of the main IV line. Many IV medications are administered over a projected period of 30 minutes to hours. To administer medications intravenously over such a long period by a syringe would be highly inconvenient and impractical. Such medications are given by injecting the medication into a smaller bag of IV fluids (100 or 250 mL). The smaller IV bag containing the medication is then connected by an injector port into the main IV line. This technique of slow IV medication administration is known as *IV piggyback*.

IV INFUSION (PIGGYBACK)

I. PREPARING MEDICATION FOR INFUSION

Equipment Needed:

Alcohol prep, medication, syringe, needle, small bag of compatible IV fluids (100 or 250 mL), IV tubing, medication label, sharps

Procedure:
1. Observe universal precautions.
2. Verify drug order.
3. Confirm right patient, right medication, right dose, right route, and right time.
4. Confirm with the patient that he or she has no allergies to the medication, and document allergies to any other medication.
5. When possible, explain to the patient what procedure you are going to perform and why.
6. To prepare the medication for piggyback infusion, draw it into a syringe by the techniques previously explained.
7. Wipe the injection port of the smaller bag of IV fluids being used for the piggyback infusion with alcohol.
8. Inject the medication into the IV bag.
9. Mix the solution by shaking the IV bag.
10. Label the bag with a medication label. Document the name and amount of the medication added.
11. Document the medication, dose, route, needle size, and time in the patient care record.
12. Evaluate the patient for desired effects of the medication, as well as any adverse effects. Continued reevaluation should occur throughout transport.

II. ATTACHING INFUSION SOLUTION TO PRIMARY IV LINE

Equipment Needed:
Alcohol prep, medication, syringe, needle, small bag of compatible IV fluids, IV tubing, medication label, sharps

Procedure:
1. Observe universal precautions.
2. Verify drug order.
3. Confirm right patient, right medication, right dose, right route, and right time.
4. Confirm with the patient that he or she has no allergies to the medication, and document allergies to any other medication.
5. When possible, explain to the patient what procedure you are going to perform and why.
6. Wipe clean the medication port of the IV line with alcohol.
7. Clamp the IV tubing of the primary line above the site of the medication port.
8. Place the needle of the line containing the piggyback medication through the diaphragm of the medication port.
9. Infuse the medication into the primary IV line at the rate appropriate for the particular medication.
10. Hang the smaller IV bag containing the medication given by piggyback infusion at a level higher than the bag used for the primary IV infusion.
11. Once the infusion of the medication is complete, remove the piggyback infusion and unclamp the tubing of the primary IV line.
12. Document the medication, dose, route, needle size, and time in the patient care record.
13. Evaluate the patient for desired effects of the medication, as well as any adverse effects. Continued reevaluation should occur throughout transport.

Intraosseous Infusions

When providing care in the emergent prehospital environment, starting and maintaining vascular access is essential. **Intraosseous (IO) infusion** involves placement of a needle set into the highly vascular **intramedullary space** of the bone and infusion of fluids or medications into this space (Fig. 5-9). In cases of hypovolemic shock, veins often collapse, making access with IV catheters difficult or impossible. However, even in such cases, the intramedullary cavity of the bone remains open. Fluids, blood, and medications administered through an IO line can be delivered to the central circulation by this route as rapidly

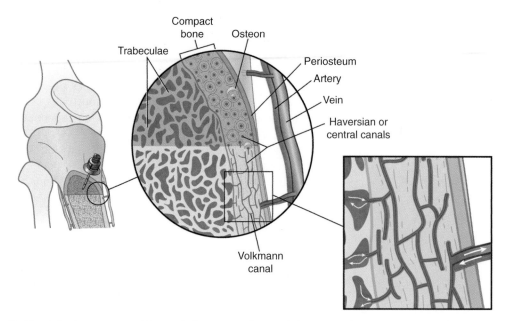

▼ **Fig. 5-9**   Bone composition and placement of an IO infusion needle set. (Courtesy Vidacare Corporation, San Antonio, Texas.)

as though administered through peripheral or central venous catheters. The use of IO infusions has been well established in the pediatric literature and, since 2005, has become increasingly popular in the adult population, as well. Use of IO infusions is of great interest to military and civilian EMS because of the ease and reliability of starting such access in suboptimal and hostile conditions.

The most common site for placement of an IO line is the proximal tibia. This site is ideal because of its flat nature and lack of extensive overlying muscle and soft tissue. Other sites, such as the distal tibia and proximal humerus, are also well studied. To locate the proximal tibia site, palpate the proximal tibia immediately below the knee and feel for a marked bump in the bone. This prominent portion of the tibia is called the **tibial tuberosity.** The optimal location for IO needle placement is medial to the tibial tuberosity on the anteromedial portion of the bone. If possible, avoid placing an IO needle in an extremity with a suspected injury.

Several different types of devices are used to gain access to the intramedullary cavity, including the Jamshidi intraosseous needle (Manan Medical, Northbrook, Ill.) and other commercial devices for use in adults and children. These devices vary in their application and techniques. Some devices use manual application, whereas others use spring-loaded devices and even electrical drills. The EZ-IO device (Vidacare Corporation, San Antonio, Tex.) is shown in Figure 5-10. The Jamshidi needle set, which was originally used as a bone marrow aspiration, is the most widely used IO device. The depth of the needle set can be controlled by the end user. The needle set has a stylet that is locked in place with a plastic cap (Fig. 5-11).

In adults, the **sternum** is occasionally used as an IO infusion site because it is thin and flat, contains a high proportion of red marrow, is easy to penetrate and less likely to be fractured in certain situations, and is close to the central circulation.[7] The recommended insertion site is in the manubrium, 1.6 cm below the sternal notch. Use of a specifically designed device is critical for sternal applications.

 ## IO INFUSION—TIBIAL APPROACH

Equipment Needed:
Alcohol or chlorhexidine prep, IO needle set, 10-mL syringe, IV tubing, bag of IV compatible fluids, several rolls of gauze, tape, sharps, PPE

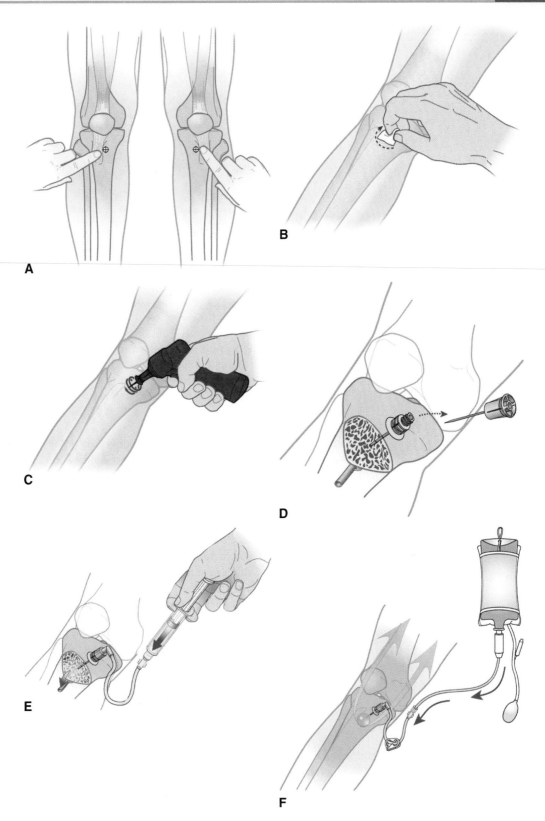

▼ **Fig. 5-10** The EZ-IO device. **A,** Identify the tibial tuberosity. **B,** Prepare the site in sterile fashion. **C,** Insert the IO needle with the EZ-IO device. **D,** Remove the inner stylus from the needle. **E,** Attach tubing and flush with sterile normal saline. **F,** Attach to IV tubing setup. (Courtesy Vidacare Corporation, San Antonio, Tex.)

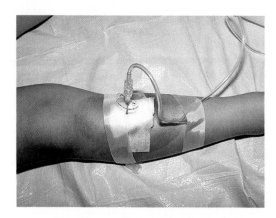

▼ **Fig. 5-11**   The IO needle can be further secured by placing two Kerlix rolls (Kendall, Mansfield, Mass.) on either side of the needle. (From Aehlert B: *Mosby's comprehensive pediatric emergency care*, rev, St Louis, 2007, Mosby.)

Procedure:
1. Observe universal precautions.
2. Verify drug order.
3. Confirm right patient, right medication, right dose, right route, and right time.
4. Confirm with the patient that he or she has no allergies to the medication, and document allergies to any other medication.
5. When possible, explain to the patient what procedure you are going to perform and why.
6. Identify the site of insertion.
7. Prepare the insertion site with either alcohol or chlorhexidine.
8. Make sure that the angle of needle set insertion is 90 degrees to the bone.
9. Advance the needle set with a back-and-forth screwing motion. Entrance into the intramedullary cavity will be apparent by a gentle give and a marked decrease in resistance to needle advancement. Avoid excessive insertion pressure.
10. Unlock and remove the stylet. Dispose the stylet as a sharp.
11. Confirm proper placement of the catheter by aspirating marrow back into a syringe that is attached to the catheter or verifying that fluids infuse freely and without any noted swelling (which would indicate infiltration) and that the catheter stands in place without any support.
12. Attach the preassembled administration set to the IO catheter.
13. Secure the IO line in place with bulky dressings. This can easily be done by placing two roller gauze dressings on either side of the IO needle and then wrapping the entire area.
14. Document the medication, dose, route, needle size, and time in the patient care record.
15. Evaluate the patient for desired effects of the medication, as well as any adverse effects. Continued reevaluation should occur throughout transport.

 ## IO INFUSION—STERNAL APPROACH FOR FAST1 IO

Equipment Needed:
Alcohol or Betadine prep, IO needle, 10-mL syringe, IV tubing, bag of IV compatible fluids, several rolls of gauze, tape, sharps, PPE

Procedure:
1. Observe universal precautions.
2. Verify drug order.
3. Confirm right patient, right medication, right dose, right route, and right time.
4. Confirm with the patient that he or she has no allergies to the medication, and document allergies to any other medication.

5. When possible, explain to the patient what procedure you are going to perform and why.
6. Locate the patient's manubrium and prepare the site with aseptic solution.
7. Use the index finger to align the target patch with the patient's sternal notch. Place the target patch.
8. Place the introducer into the target zone on the patch, perpendicular to the skin. Firmly push on the introducer to insert the infusion tube into the correct site and to the right penetration depth. Pull the introducer straight back, exposing the infusion tube and a two-part support sleeve, which falls away.
9. Verify correct placement by observing marrow entering the infusion tube.
10. Connect the IV solution and tubing to the infusion tube on the patch, and adjust the flow rate.
11. Place the protective dome over the site by pressing firmly over the target patch to engage the Velcro fastening.
12. Document the medication, dose, route, needle size, and time in the patient care record.
13. Evaluate the patient for desired effects of the medication, as well as any adverse effects. Continued reevaluation should occur throughout transport.

COMPLICATIONS OF INTRAVENOUS THERAPY

Every medication and therapy has potential complications, and the same is true for IV therapy. Complications of IV therapy include **infiltration, catheter shear,** phlebitis, infection, and infected phlebitis.

The most troublesome IV complication for the patient is infiltration. Infiltration occurs when the tip of the catheter dislodges from the lumen of the vein; the fluid or medication is then delivered to soft tissues around the vein. Infiltration of medications into the soft tissues can result in tissue destruction and necrosis at the site of infiltration.

Infiltration of an IV can be suspected when the fluid no longer freely drips. Other signs of an IV infiltration include pain and swelling at the IV site. Often the only treatment required for an IV infiltration is discontinuation of the IV and starting a new IV either proximal to the infiltration or in another uninjured extremity. Infiltration of a large amount of fluids in areas such as the hand and foot can cause pressure damage to the underlying and adjacent structures. Infiltration in these areas should be treated by elevation of the affected area and serial examinations to evaluate vascular, motor, and sensory function.

If medication infiltration is suspected, clearly communicate that information to the receiving hospital and document the communication. Also document findings about the site, the time of the incident, and any treatment rendered. Many medications and electrolytes that can cause vasoconstriction require injection of medications into the infiltrated site, intensive monitoring, and even surgical debridement and reconstruction.

Catheter shear is a complication that occurs when a segment of the catheter breaks off and is either retained in the vein or, even worse, embolizes through the venous system. This complication can occur when a provider attempts to pull a catheter back over a needle. This typically occurs when blood return appears while starting an IV. While attempting to advance the catheter into the vein over the needle, the provider either encounters resistance or loses the blood return and tries to salvage the IV by pulling the catheter back over the needle. After advancing the catheter, the catheter follows the course of the vein, which is at an angle from the needle. When the provider pulls the catheter back over the straight needle, the tip of the needle can cut the catheter into two pieces, and the severed piece of the IV catheter can remain at the site of the attempted IV start. The severed IV catheter can also float away in the vein to a site more proximal in the limb or even the heart and lungs. Sheared catheters can require retrieval by surgery or angiography. If shearing of an IV catheter is suspected, notify medical direction and document the communication.

Less-immediate complications of IVs include phlebitis, infection, and infected phlebitis. None of these infectious complications will become apparent to the paramedic who starts the IV line in the prehospital setting. However, exercising strict sterile technique can reduce the incidence of these complications. IV lines started in the field are often started in less than optimal conditions. For this reason, many hospitals have policies about prompt removal of field lines.

Phlebitis is an inflammation of the vein that can manifest as pain, redness, and edema. Many different conditions can irritate the vein and cause the inflammation of phlebitis, including concentrated fluids, certain electrolyte solutions, various medications, and simply the presence of the catheter in the lumen of the vein. When phlebitis causes the blood inside of the lumen to clot, the condition is known as **thrombophlebitis.** When a patient has thrombophlebitis, he or she can often feel the thrombosed vessel along the length of the thrombosis, and palpation of the vein elicits tenderness. On occasion, the thrombophlebitis can become infected. **Suppurative thrombophlebitis** occurs when the clot of thrombophlebitis becomes infected. Suppurative thrombophlebitis is a potentially fatal condition. The treatment for this type of thrombophlebitis is excision of the infected vein (Fig. 5-12).

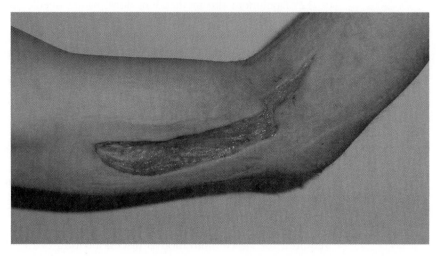

▼ **Fig. 5-12** Excision of an infected vein after suppurative thrombophlebitis.

REVIEW QUESTIONS

1. Define ICF space. What portion of the TBW is ICF?
2. What types of fluid compose the ECF space?
3. Define osmosis.
4. If you give a patient a 1000-mL bolus of D_5W, how much of that volume will remain within the vascular space?
5. After giving a patient a 1000-mL bolus of 0.9% normal saline, how much of the volume will remain in the vascular space?
6. What are the differences among crystalloid solutions, colloid solutions, and isotonic fluids?
7. What are some of the causes of hyperkalemia?
8. What is a typical fluid bolus in a pediatric patient?
9. What is the drop factor?
10. When using a microdrip chamber, how many drops compose 1 mL?
11. With a microdrip chamber attached to an IV, what is the rate of IV fluids in milliliters per hour if you count 60 gtt/min?
12. When administering IV fluids without an infusion pump, what factors can alter the rate of IV fluid delivery?
13. What determines the maximal rate of IV fluid administration?
14. What occurs when an IV infiltrates?
15. What are the signs that indicate an IV is infiltrating?
16. How can you prevent IV catheter shear?

REFERENCES

1. Mange K, et al: Language guiding therapy: the case of dehydration versus volume depletion, *Ann Intern Med* 127:848, 1997.
2. Hauser CJ, Shoemaker WC, Turpin I: Oxygen transport responses to colloids and crystalloids in critically ill surgical patients, *Surg Gynecol Obstet* 150:811, 1980.
3. Lamke LO, Liljedahl SO: Plasma volume changes after infusion of various plasma expanders, *Resuscitation* 5:93, 1976.
4. Granger DN, et al: Physiological basis for the clinical use of albumin solutions, *Surg Gynecol Obstet* 146:97, 1978.
5. Velasco IT, Pontieri V, Rocha e Silva M: Hypertonic NaCl and severe hemorrhagic shock, *Am J Physiol* 239:H664, 1980.
6. Nakayama S, et al: Small volume resuscitation with hypertonic saline resuscitation (2400 mOsm/L) during hemorrhagic shock, *Circ Shock* 13:149, 1984.
7. Aehlert B: *ACLS study guide,* ed 3, St. Louis, 2007, Mosby.

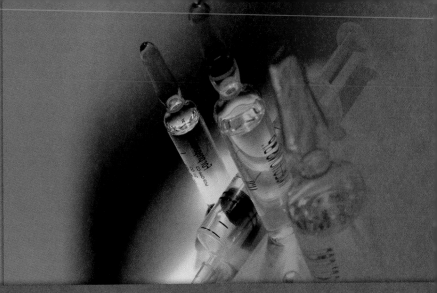

PART

II

Problem-Oriented
Pharmacology

Acute Coronary Syndromes

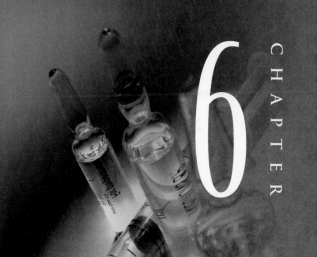

CHAPTER 6

OBJECTIVES

1. Define acute coronary syndromes, angina, unstable angina pectoris (UA), non-ST-segment elevation myocardial infarction (NSTEMI), and ST-segment elevation myocardial infarction (STEMI).
2. Discuss out-of-hospital morbidity and mortality issues.
3. List the signs and symptoms of chest pain that indicate ischemia.
4. List risk factors for acute myocardial ischemia.
5. Discuss the medications used to treat stable angina pectoris.
6. Discuss the medications used to treat UA and NSTEMI.
7. List the benefits of beta blockers on the ischemic heart and discuss the beta-blocking medications metoprolol (Lopressor), atenolol (Tenormin), esmolol (Brevibloc), propranolol (Inderal), and labetalol (Trandate).
8. List the benefits of antiplatelet agents on the ischemic heart and discuss the antiplatelet medication clopidogrel (Plavix).
9. Discuss anticoagulant medications including unfractionated heparin (heparin) and low-molecular-weight heparin (LMWH).
10. Discuss the role of angiotensin-converting enzyme (ACE) inhibitors and 3-hydroxy-3-methylglutaryl (HMG) coenzyme A reductase inhibitors.
11. Describe the two methods of reperfusion therapy: percutaneous coronary intervention (PCI) and fibrinolytics.

Medications that Appear in Chapter 6

Oxygen
Aspirin, ASA
Nitroglycerin (Nitrolingual, NitroQuick, Nitro-Dur)
Morphine sulfate
Metoprolol (Lopressor, Toprol XL)
Atenolol (Tenormin)
Esmolol (Brevibloc)
Propranolol (Inderal)
Labetalol (Normodyne, Trandate)
Clopidogrel (Plavix)
Heparin (unfractionated heparin)
Abciximab (ReoPro)
Eptifibatide (Integrilin)
Tirofiban (Aggrastat)
Angiotensin-Converting Enzyme (ACE) Inhibitors: Captopril (Capoten), Enalapril (Vasotec), Lisinopril (Prinivil, Zestril), Ramipril (Altace)
HMG Coenzyme A Statins: Atorvastatin (Lipitor), Fluvastatin (Lescol), Lovastatin (Mevacor), Pravastatin (Pravachol), Rosuvastatin (Crestor), Simvastatin (Zocor)
Fibrinolytics: Tissue Plasminogen Activator (tPA), Streptokinase (Streptase, Kabikinase), Reteplase (Retavase), Tenecteplase (TNKase)

INTRODUCTION

Acute coronary syndrome (ACS) is the leading cause of death in adults in the United States, accounting for approximately 1 million deaths annually.[1] ACS encompasses a spectrum of conditions that occur when the heart muscle is deprived of oxygen. This deprivation of oxygen is called *ischemia*. Ischemia of the heart can occur as a brief and temporary condition referred to as *stable angina pectoris* or can progress to cause death to a portion of the cardiac muscle, which is referred to as an *acute myocardial infarction*.

Morbidity and mortality for ACS in the prehospital environment is due to arrhythmias, most of which occur within the first 4 hours after symptom onset. In-hospital deaths are often caused by low cardiac output such as that seen in acute congestive heart failure and cardiogenic shock. Additional causes of in-hospital deaths include recurrent acute myocardial infarction and cardiac wall rupture. The severity of the damage is directly related to the size of the infarction. Therefore the goal of prehospital therapy is directed at limiting the size of the infarct and preserving left ventricular function.

Great strides have been made in diagnosing and treating ischemic heart disease, and developments in EMS over the past decade have allowed prehospital professionals across the country to intervene quickly and efficiently to manage these critical patients. This chapter highlights the current pharmacologic treatments for ACS. Chapters 9, 10, and 12 address the treatment of patients with cardiac arrhythmias, congestive heart failure, and hypertensive emergencies.

OVERVIEW OF ACUTE CORONARY SYNDROMES

ACS defines a progression of cardiac disease that results from ischemia. Coronary artery disease begins with early plaque formation within an artery. Plaque formation is an inflammatory response caused by deposition of lipoproteins that carry cholesterol. Rupture of these plaques can cause obstruction of the artery by thrombus formation and can interfere with blood delivery to the heart muscle. There is a spectrum of pathophysiologic and clinical progression of ACS. Ischemia occurs when the heart is deprived of oxygen. This is a reversible process, and permanent damage does not occur unless there is prolonged oxygen deprivation. Stable angina pectoris occurs when the oxygen demand of the heart exceeds the oxygen supplied to the heart. The pain associated with stable angina pectoris may be relieved with rest or oxygen supplementation. Unstable angina pectoris (UA) typically occurs when a partially occluding thrombus produces symptoms of ischemia, including chest pain. This chest pain may occur at rest or with little provocation. The pain of UA is also longer in duration and may not be relieved by rest or medication. This very serious condition requires immediate attention and may actually cause a non-ST-segment elevation myocardial infarction (NSTEMI). The definition of an NSTEMI is the acute process in which ischemia affects the myocardium with no elevation of the ST segment on the electrocardiogram (ECG). The difference between NSTEMI and UA is that with the NSTEMI, cardiac enzymes will be elevated, indicating necrosis of the cardiac tissue. ST-segment elevation myocardial infarction, or STEMI, is actual infarction of the cardiac tissue secondary to oxygen deprivation. Cell death occurs and there is permanent, irreversible damage to cardiac muscle cells. A STEMI will have elevation of the ST segments on ECG.

OVERVIEW OF STABLE ANGINA PECTORIS

You are dispatched to the home of a man with a chief complaint of chest pain. You arrive to find a 55-year-old obese man sitting in a chair. He states the he was shoveling snow and felt pressure in his chest. He continued shoveling, but the pain would not go away, so he went inside the house and sat down. After approximately 10 minutes, just before your arrival, the pain subsided. The patient denies previous episodes of chest pain and states that he has no medical history of coronary artery disease. He denies diabetes, smoking history, and hypercholesterolemia. He does state that his father died of a heart attack at the age of 62 years, and his mother has coronary artery disease. ...

Angina means "tightening," not pain. Classic angina pectoris may be described by a patient as squeezing, pressure, burning, heaviness, or bandlike pain. It typically is felt in the center of the chest or on the left side of the rib cage. The sensation may radiate to the jaw or to the right or left arm. Stable angina pectoris is described as periodic chest discomfort that occurs when oxygen demand exceeds the oxygen supply of cardiac muscle. This discomfort is typically predictable and reproducible. The attacks may become more frequent over time. Physical activity, psychologic stress, anemia, arrhythmias, and certain environmental conditions can precipitate an attack of angina. Rest, supplemental oxygen, or the administration of nitroglycerin will typically resolve stable anginal pain. The pain is usually short in duration—usually 2 to 5 minutes. It almost always lasts less than 20 minutes. The pathophysiology of this condition is caused by a reduction in the diameter of the coronary arteries that supply blood to the heart. This narrowing occurs because of the long-term deposition of atherosclerotic plaque. When the heart muscle is stressed by exertion, an increased need for oxygen occurs. However, because of the decreased diameter of these vessels, delivery of oxygenated blood cannot be increased to accommodate the heart's demands. This results in ischemia and chest pain, pressure, or discomfort. When the patient rests, the heart's oxygen demand is once again met and the ischemia and pain subside. The patient in the previous scenario represents the classic presentation of stable angina pectoris.

> ... You recommend to the patient that he should allow you to transport him to the emergency department for further evaluation, but he refuses. He tells you that he often gets this type of pain in his chest when he overexerts himself. ...

Management

Chest pain that is relieved with rest is an indication that the patient should be evaluated for cardiac damage and coronary artery disease in the emergency department. The patient in the previous scenario should be transported to the emergency department even though he is feeling better at the time of evaluation. The clinical presentation of cardiac ischemia can mislead even the most seasoned prehospital professionals. The consequences of failed or delayed treatment could be catastrophic. For these reasons, the evaluation and treatment of the symptom of chest pain should follow standardized protocols.

After completing the primary assessment of a patient reporting chest pain, oxygen should be administered. Based on the patient's presentation, oxygen supplementation may be in the form of a nasal cannula or nonrebreather mask. The patient should be placed on a cardiac monitor and IV access should be obtained. A 12-lead ECG should also be completed.

> ... Your attempts to convince the patient to go to the emergency department appear to have failed. The patient argues that he only has heartburn and is too busy to spend the rest of his day in the emergency department. He removes the blood pressure cuff and stands up. As he stands up, he appears weak and puts his right hand on his chest. His color is poor, and he is diaphoretic. You rapidly help him sit back down in the chair. You place an oxygen mask on him while your partner sets up to start an IV line. You administer a 325-mg nonenteric coated aspirin and instruct him to chew it, then swallow. ...

Oxygen is a naturally occurring gas that exists in the atmosphere at an approximately 21% concentration. It is odorless, tasteless, and colorless. Oxygen is an important drug used in the management of a large number of medical emergencies. A detailed description of oxygen is covered in Chapter 14. Oxygen is used in ACS and is indicated in the treatment of all patients with chest pain. When a patient has angina pectoris, oxygen demand exceeds the body's ability to deliver adequate oxygen to the heart muscle. By providing these patients with supplemental oxygen, the red blood cells become loaded with oxygen for delivery to the heart muscle. The goal is to increase the supply of oxygen to the heart muscle to meet the demand.

Oxygen has an immediate onset of action, and its duration is less than 2 minutes. Individuals who are new to medicine may not consider oxygen a drug, but in fact oxygen has a clear, beneficial physiologic effect when given at the appropriate dose; when given in excess it can have negative effects.

Aspirin is an antiplatelet medication that prohibits platelets from adhering to each other. It can also be used for analgesic, antiinflammatory, and antipyretic effects. In acute myocardial infarction, reducing clot formation in the coronary arteries is of paramount concern. Aspirin prevents the clot from growing larger by inhibiting the platelets from adhering to one another and preventing clots from forming. In cases of stable angina, such as in the previous scenario, aspirin helps prevent clots from forming and the condition from progressing to an acute myocardial infarction. Prehospital providers do not administer aspirin for its pain-relieving attribute but rather for its antiplatelet properties. Reduction of pain in chest pain is accomplished more commonly with morphine sulfate. This is discussed in greater detail in the next section.

OXYGEN

Classification: Elemental gas
Action: Facilitates cellular energy metabolism.
Indications: Hypoxia, ischemic chest pain, respiratory distress, suspected carbon monoxide poisoning, traumatic injuries, shock.
Adverse Effects: High concentrations can cause decreased level of consciousness and respiratory depression in patients with chronic carbon dioxide retention or chronic lung disease.
Contraindications: Known paraquat poisoning.
Dosage:
Low-Concentration Oxygen:
· A dose of 1 to 4 L/min by a nasal cannula is appropriate.
High-Concentration Oxygen:
· A dose of 10 to 15 L/min via nonrebreather mask is appropriate.
Special Considerations:
Pregnancy class A

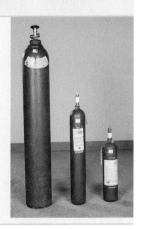

ASPIRIN, ASA

Classification: Antiplatelet, nonnarcotic analgesic, antipyretic
Action: Prevents the formation of a chemical known as thromboxane A_2, which causes platelets to clump together, or aggregate, and form plugs that cause obstruction or constriction of small coronary arteries.
Indications: Fever, inflammation, angina, acute MI, and patients complaining of pain, pressure, squeezing, or crushing in the chest that may be cardiac in origin.
Adverse Effects: Anaphylaxis, angioedema, bronchospasm, bleeding, stomach irritation, nausea/vomiting.
Contraindications: GI bleeding, active ulcer disease, hemorrhagic stroke, bleeding disorders, children with chickenpox or flulike symptoms, known sensitivity.
Dosage: Note: "Baby aspirin" 81 mg, standard adult aspirin dose 325 mg.

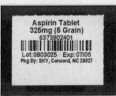

Aspirin Tablet
325mg (5 Grain)
6373902401
Lot:0803025 Exp:07/05
Pkg By: SKY, Concord, NC 28027

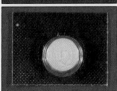

cont'd

ASPIRIN, ASA—CONT'D

Myocardial Infarction:
- **Adult:** 160 to 325 mg PO (alternatively, four 81-mg baby aspirin are often given), 300-mg rectal suppository.
- **Pediatric:** 3 to 5 mg/kg/day to 5 to 10 mg/kg/day given as a single dose.

Pain or Fever:
- **Adult:** 325 to 650 mg PO (1 to 2 adult tablets) every 4 to 6 hours.
- **Pediatric:** 60 to 90 mg/kg/day in divided doses every 4 to 6 hours.

Special Considerations:
Pregnancy class C except the last 3 months of pregnancy, when aspirin is considered pregnancy class D.

... After starting the patient on oxygen and administering 325 mg of a nonenteric coated aspirin, the patient agrees to be transported to the local emergency department. Your partner is able to start the IV line without difficulty, and you place the patient on the ECG and pulse oximeter monitors. You transport him in a position of comfort. During transport the patient's pain subsides. A week later you see the patient's wife and ask her about her husband's condition. She tells you that he had a cardiac catheterization and has undergone angioplasty of several vessels. She expresses her gratitude for insisting that her husband go to the hospital and saving his life.

OVERVIEW OF UNSTABLE ANGINA PECTORIS AND NON-ST-SEGMENT ELEVATION MYOCARDIAL INFARCTION

You are called to assist a 68-year-old woman with chest pain. You arrive to find the patient sitting at her kitchen table with her hand on her chest. She states the pain has been there on and off for 2 weeks. It usually starts while she is resting and lasts approximately 25 minutes. She describes the pain as "an elephant sitting on my chest." She feels like she cannot catch her breath. Her history is significant for hypertension: smoking, high cholesterol, and a positive family history for myocardial infarction. Her heart rate is 96 beats/min, blood pressure is 146/98 mm Hg, and respirations are 22 breaths/min. ...

This patient is displaying symptoms of UA. UA is defined as chest pain or discomfort that occurs with minimal exertion or at rest. It may not follow a pattern. It can also be defined as new-onset angina or a significant change in previously stable angina. Patients may experience chest discomfort with minimal exertion or even while at rest. The episode may also be longer in duration. The patient's description of chest pain at rest that lasts more than 20 minutes is typical for UA/NSTEMI. NSTEMI is an acute myocardial infarction without the characteristic ST-segment elevation seen in acute myocardial infarction.

The characteristics are classic with UA/NSTEMI:
- Symptoms of angina at rest
- New-onset exertional angina
- Recent acceleration of angina
- Variant angina
- Post–myocardial infarction angina (more than 24 hours)

The patient in this scenario is displaying symptoms of UA or NSTEMI. Additional terms for this condition include rest angina, crescendo angina, and preinfarction angina. UA/NSTEMI differs from stable angina by both the pathophysiology and the duration of the pain. UA/NSTEMI may not follow a pattern. In particular, woman may present atypically. Their chief complaint may be weakness, shortness of breath, or fatigue. Variant or Prinzmetal's angina is a form of UA caused by coronary artery spasm at rest. Little atherosclerotic disease is typically noted in these patients. The pain of variant angina is often severe and occurs between midnight and the early hours of the morning. This form of angina can also display characteristics of a STEMI.

The pathophysiology of UA and NSTEMI is the same as that of STEMI. The atherosclerotic changes of coronary artery disease form plaques. These plaques may rupture and a platelet-rich thrombus can form. This can occlude or partially occlude an artery. Arterial occlusion causes decreased blood flow to a portion of the cardiac muscle. Ischemia occurs, and this can lead to infarction.

Management

Every complaint of chest pain or pressure should be treated emergently. All forms of ischemia present similarly and therefore must be treated aggressively. Patients with this condition can display all the characteristics of an acute myocardial infarction and thus should be treated and transported immediately.

Initial management is similar to that of a patient with stable angina pectoris. A thorough history and physical assessment should be performed. The patient should receive supplemental oxygen, IV access, a 12-lead ECG, and aspirin. He or she should be monitored with an ECG and pulse oximeter monitor. In addition, the American Heart Association (AHA) has developed an algorithm for UA/NSTEMI (Fig. 6-1).

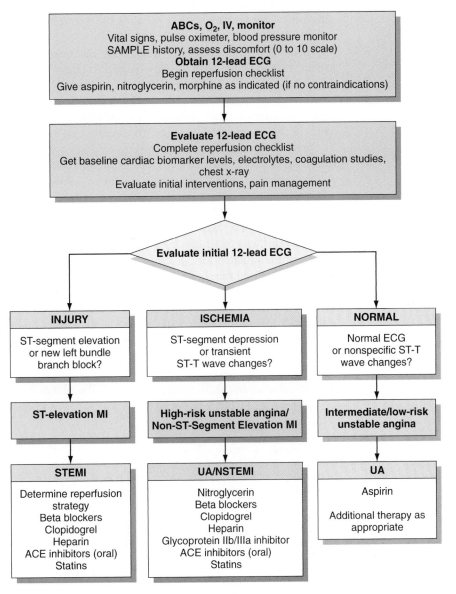

▼ **Fig. 6-1**   Ischemic chest discomfort algorithm. (Modified from Aehlert B: *ACLS study guide*, ed 3, St Louis, 2007, Mosby.)

Medications that are indicated for UA/NSTEMI include nitroglycerin, beta blockers, antiplatelet medications (clopidogrel), anticoagulant medications (heparin, enoxaparin), glycoprotein IIb/IIIa inhibitors, angiotensin-converting enzyme (ACE) inhibitors, and statins. Many of these medications are not initiated in the prehospital environment but are part of the emergency department and definitive treatment.

> ... You place the patient on oxygen 4 L/min by nasal cannula. While your partner is starting an IV, you place her on the cardiac monitor, as well as the pulse oximeter. Her heart rate is 104 beats/min and her blood pressure is 188/98 mm Hg. Her pulse oximeter reads 98% on 4 L/min via nasal cannula. You administer one 325-mg tablet of nonenteric coated aspirin and instruct her to chew the aspirin before swallowing it. Because she has been having pain for 20 minutes, you are appropriately worried that the patient has myocardial ischemia, and you prepare to administer nitroglycerin. ...

Nitroglycerin is a commonly used medication in the treatment of UA/NSTEMI. It is typically administered by the sublingual (SL) route, which allows for rapid absorption. Once in the body, the nitroglycerin is converted to nitric oxide, which is a potent vasodilator. The dilation of the venous system reduces the amount of blood returning to the heart with each heartbeat. This reduces the workload on the heart and decreases tension on the walls of the heart. These changes result in a significant reduction in the amount of oxygen consumed by the heart, which helps balance oxygen supply and demand, a classic problem in cardiac ischemia and infarction.

Although nitroglycerin causes both venous and arterial dilation, the veins dilate more than the arteries. This produces an increase in the diameter of the coronary vessels, and the heart muscle subsequently receives more oxygen-enriched blood flow. These properties make nitroglycerin a desirable choice for a UA/NSTEMI/STEMI. SL nitroglycerin has long been considered the gold standard of drugs used in the treatment of angina. Nitroglycerin has many benefits. It is easy to administer, effective, and safe. Nitroglycerin also reduces blood pressure. Therefore, vital signs must be monitored and blood pressure evaluated after each administration of an SL nitroglycerin tablet or a dose of nitroglycerin spray. An additional discussion of nitroglycerin and its various forms is included in Chapter 12.

Morphine sulfate is a medication that is often used for pain control. It is an opioid agonist and has benefit in treating refractory pain in ACS. In addition to treating pain, it has some vasodilating properties that reduce preload, thus decreasing stroke volume and blood flow to the coronary arteries. Morphine sulfate has not been studied extensively and is still indicated as a Class I recommendation for STEMI. It is a Class IIa recommendation for UA and NSTEMI. Fentanyl and hydromorphone (Dilaudid) are narcotics that are also being used for pain management in ACS.

NITROGLYCERIN (NITROLINGUAL, NITROQUICK, NITRO-DUR)

Classification: Antianginal agent
Action: Relaxes vascular smooth muscle, thereby dilating peripheral arteries and veins. This causes pooling of venous blood and decreased venous return to the heart, which decreases preload. Nitroglycerin also reduces left ventricular systolic wall tension, which decreases afterload.
Indications: Angina, ongoing ischemic chest discomfort, hypertension, myocardial ischemia associated with cocaine intoxication.
Adverse Effects: Headache, hypotension, bradycardia, lightheadedness, flushing, cardiovascular collapse, methemoglobinemia.

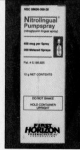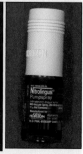

cont'd

NITROGLYCERIN (NITROLINGUAL, NITROQUICK, NITRO-DUR)—CONT'D

Contraindications: Hypotension, severe bradycardia or tachycardia, increased ICP, intracranial bleeding, patients taking any medications for erectile dysfunction (such as sildenafil [Viagra], tadalafil [Cialis], or vardenafil [Levitra]), known sensitivity to nitrates. Use with caution in anemia, closed-angle glaucoma, hypotension, postural hypotension, uncorrected hypovolemia.

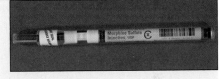

Dosage:
- **Adult:**
  - **Sublingual tablets:** 1 tablet (0.3-0.4 mg) at 5-minute intervals to a maximum of 3 doses.
  - **Translingual spray:** 1 (0.4 mg) spray at 5-minute intervals to a maximum of 3 sprays.
  - **Ointment:** 2% topical (Nitro-Bid ointment): Apply 1 to 2 inches of paste over the chest wall, cover with transparent wrap, and secure with tape.
  - **IV:**
    - **Bolus:** 12.5 to 25 mcg
    - **Infusion:** 5 mcg/min; may increase rate by 5 to 10 mcg/min every 5 to 10 minutes as needed. End points of dose titration for nitroglycerin include a drop in the blood pressure of 10%, relief of chest pain, and return of ST segment to normal on a 12-lead ECG.
  - **Pediatric IV infusion:** The initial pediatric infusion is 0.25 to 0.5 mcg/kg/min IV, IO titrated by 0.5 to 1 mcg/kg/min. Usual required dose is 1 to 3 mcg/kg/min to a maximum dose of 5 mcg/kg/min.

Special Considerations:
Administration of nitroglycerin to a patient with right ventricular MI can result in hypotension. Pregnancy class C

MORPHINE SULFATE

Classification: Opiate agonist, Schedule C-II

Action: Binds with opioid receptors. Morphine is capable of inducing hypotension by depression of the vasomotor centers of the brain, as well as release of the chemical histamine. In the management of angina, morphine reduces stimulation of the sympathic nervous system caused by pain and anxiety. Reduction of sympathetic stimulation reduces heart rate, cardiac work, and myocardial oxygen consumption.

Indications: Moderate to severe pain, including chest pain associated with ACS, CHF, pulmonary edema.

Adverse Effects: Respiratory depression, hypotension, nausea/vomiting, dizziness, lightheadedness, sedation, diaphoresis, euphoria, dysphoria, worsening of bradycardia and heart block in some patients with acute inferior wall MI, seizures, cardiac arrest, anaphylactoid reactions.

Contraindications: Respiratory depression, shock, known sensitivity. Use with caution in hypotension, acute bronchial asthma, respiratory insufficiency, head trauma.

Dosage:

Pain:
- **Adult:** 2.5 to 15 mg IV, IO, IM, or Sub-Q administered slowly over a period of several minutes. The dose is the same whether administered IV, IO, IM, or Sub-Q.
- **Pediatric:**
  - **6 months to 12 years:** 0.05 to 0.2 mg/kg IV, IO, IM, or Sub-Q.
  - **Younger than 6 months:** 0.03 to 0.05 mg/kg IV, IO, IM, or Sub-Q.

Chest Pain Associated with Acute Coronary Syndromes, Congestive Heart Failure, and Pulmonary Edema:
Administer small doses and reevaluate the patient. Large doses may lead to respiratory depression and worsen the patient's hypoxia.
- **Adult:** 2 to 4 mg slow IV, IO over a 1- to 5-minute period with increments of 2 to 8 mg repeated every 5 to 15 minutes until patient relieved of chest pain.
- **Pediatric:** 0.1 to 0.2 mg/kg/dose IV, IO.

cont'd

MORPHINE SULFATE—CONT'D

Special Considerations:
Monitor vital signs and pulse oximetry closely. Be prepared to support patient's airway and ventilations.
Overdose should be treated with naloxone.
Pregnancy class C

Beta Blockers. Beta blockers help the ischemic heart by reducing chronotropic and inotropic activity. These two actions reduce the consumption of oxygen by the heart. Beta blockers should be administered to all patients (lacking a contraindication) with UA/NSTEMI. Beta blockers administered within the first few hours following ischemia have demonstrated decreased myocardial damage and decreased long-term complications.[2] Beta blockers should be administered as soon as possible. The choice of beta blocker is not as important as ensuring that at-risk patients receive beta blockade. When administering IV beta blockers to patients, frequently reevaluate the patient's heart rate, blood pressure, and ECG monitor. In addition, frequently auscultate the patient's lungs to evaluate for the development of rales, bronchospasms, or signs of bronchospasm. Beta blockers should be avoided in patients with current cocaine abuse. Cocaine is a sympathetic stimulant. With beta blockade, unopposed alpha-receptor stimulation can lead to life-threatening hypertension.

Beta blockers should be administered for STEMI patients unless the following contraindications occur:

- Signs of heart failure
- Evidence of low output state
- Cardiogenic shock or increased risk for cardiogenic shock
- PR interval greater than 0.24 second
- Second- or third-degree heart block
- Active asthma or reactive airway disease

Patients who have atrial fibrillation or sinus tachycardia should have left ventricular function rapidly evaluated before administration of IV beta blockers.

Information about specific beta blockers metoprolol (Lopressor), atenolol (Tenormin), esmolol (Brevibloc), propranolol (Inderal), and labetalol (Trandate) follows.

METOPROLOL (LOPRESSOR, TOPROL XL)

Classification: Beta adrenergic antagonist, antianginal, antihypertensive, class II antiarrhythmic
Action: Inhibits the strength of the heart's contractions, as well as heart rate. This results in a decrease in cardiac oxygen consumption. Also saturates the beta receptors and inhibits dilation of bronchial smooth muscle (beta$_2$ receptor).
Indications: ACS, hypertension, SVT, atrial flutter, AF, thyrotoxicosis.
Adverse Effects: Tiredness, dizziness, diarrhea, heart block, bradycardia, bronchospasm, drop in blood pressure.
Contraindications: Cardiogenic shock, AV block, bradycardia, known sensitivity. Use with caution in hypotension, chronic lung disease (asthma and COPD).
Dosage:
Cardiac Indications:
- **Adult:** 5 mg slow IV, IO over a 5-minute period; repeat at 5-minute intervals up to a total of three infusions totaling 15 mg IV, IO.
- **Pediatric:** Not recommended for pediatric patients; no studies available.

Special Considerations:
Blood pressure, heart rate, and ECG should be monitored carefully.
Use with caution in patients with asthma.
Pregnancy class C

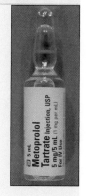

ATENOLOL (TENORMIN)

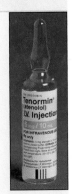

Classification: Beta adrenergic antagonist, antianginal, antihypertensive, class II antiarrhythmic

Action: Inhibits the strength of the heart's contractions and heart rate, resulting in a decrease in cardiac oxygen consumption. Also saturates the beta receptors and inhibits dilation of bronchial smooth muscle (beta$_2$ receptor).

Indications: ACS, hypertension, SVT, atrial flutter, AF.

Adverse Effects: Bradycardia, bronchospasm, hypotension.

Contraindications: Cardiogenic shock, AV block, bradycardia, known sensitivity. Use with caution in hypotension, chronic lung disease (asthma and COPD).

Dosage: ACS:
- **Adult:** 5 mg IV, IO over a 5-minute period; repeat in 5 minutes.
- **Pediatric:** Not recommended for pediatric patients.

Special Considerations:
Pregnancy class D

ESMOLOL (BREVIBLOC)

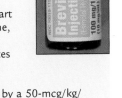

Classification: Beta adrenergic antagonist, class II antiarrhythmic

Action: Inhibits the strength of the heart's contractions, as well as heart rate, resulting in a decrease in cardiac oxygen consumption.

Indications: ACS, MI, acute hypertension, supraventricular tachyarrhythmias, thyrotoxicosis.

Adverse Effects: Hypotension, sinus bradycardia, AV block, cardiac arrest, nausea/vomiting, hypoglycemia, injection site reaction.

Contraindications: Acute bronchospasm, COPD, second- or third-degree heart block, bradycardia, cardiogenic shock, pulmonary edema, sick sinus syndrome, known sensitivity. Use with caution in patients with pheochromocytoma, Prinzmetal's angina, cerebrovascular disease, stroke, poorly controlled diabetes mellitus, hyperthyroidism, thyrotoxicosis, renal disease.

Dosage:
- **Adult:** 500 mcg/kg (0.5 mg/kg) IV, IO over a 1-minute period, followed by a 50-mcg/kg/min (0.05 mg/kg) infusion over a 4-minute period (maximum total: 200 mcg/kg). If patient response is inadequate, administer a second bolus 500 mcg/kg (0.5 mg/kg) over a 1-minute period, and then increase infusion to 100 mcg/kg/min. Maximum infusion rate: 300 mcg/kg/min.
- **Pediatric:** 500 mcg/kg (0.5 mg/kg) IV, IO over a 1-minute period, followed by an infusion at 25 to 200 mcg/kg/min.

Special Considerations:
Half-life 5 to 9 minutes

Any adverse effects caused by administration of esmolol are brief because of the drug's short half-life.

Resolution of effects usually within 10 to 20 minutes.

Pregnancy class C

PROPRANOLOL (INDERAL)

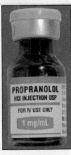

Classification: Beta adrenergic antagonist, antianginal, antihypertensive, antiarrhythmic class II

Action: Nonselective beta antagonist that binds with both the beta$_1$ and beta$_2$ receptors. Propranolol inhibits the strength of the heart's contractions, as well as heart rate. This results in a decrease in cardiac oxygen consumption.

Indications: Angina; narrow-complex tachycardias that originate from either a *reentry mechanism* (reentry SVT) or an *automatic focus* (junctional, ectopic, or multifocal tachycardia) uncontrolled by vagal maneuvers and adenosine in patients with preserved ventricular function; AF and atrial flutter in patients with preserved ventricular function; hypertension; migraine headaches.

Adverse Effects: Bradycardia, AV block, bronchospasm, hypotension.

Contraindications: Cardiogenic shock, heart failure, AV block, bradycardia, pulmonary edema, sick sinus syndrome, known sensitivity. Use with caution in chronic lung disease (asthma and COPD).

cont'd

PROPRANOLOL (INDERAL)—CONT'D

Dosage:
- **Adult:** 1 to 3 mg IV, IO at a rate of 1 mg/min; may repeat the dose 2 minutes later.
- **Pediatric:** 0.01 to 0.1 mg/kg slow IV, IO over a 10-minute period.

Special Considerations:
Monitor blood pressure and heart rate closely during administration.
Pregnancy class C

LABETALOL (NORMODYNE, TRANDATE)

Classification: Beta adrenergic antagonist, antianginal, antihypertensive

Action: Binds with both the beta$_1$ and beta$_2$ receptors and alpha$_1$ receptors in vascular smooth muscle. Inhibits the strength of the heart's contractions, as well as heart rate. This results in a decrease in cardiac oxygen consumption.

Indications: ACS, SVT, severe hypertension.

Adverse Effects: Usually mild and transient; hypotensive symptoms, nausea/vomiting, bronchospasm, arrhythmia, bradycardia, AV block.

Contraindications: Hypotension, cardiogenic shock, acute pulmonary edema, heart failure, severe bradycardia, sick sinus syndrome, second- or third-degree heart block, asthma or acute bronchospasm, cocaine-induced ACS, known sensitivity. Use caution in pheochromocytoma, cerebrovascular disease or stroke, poorly controlled diabetes, with hepatic disease. Use with caution at lowest effective dose in chronic lung disease.

Dosage:

Cardiac Indications: Note: Monitor blood pressure and heart rate closely during administration.
- **Adult:** 10 mg IV, IO over a 1- to 2-minute period. May repeat every 10 minutes to a maximum dose of 150 mg or give initial bolus and then follow with infusion at 2 to 8 mg/min.
- **Pediatric:** 0.4 to 1 mg/kg/hr to a maximum dosage of 3 mg/kg/hr.

Severe Hypertension:
- **Adult:** Initial dose is 20 mg IV, IO slow infusion over a 2-minute period. After the initial dose, blood pressure should be checked every 5 minutes. Repeat doses can be given at 10-minute intervals. The second dose should be 40 mg IV, IO, and subsequent doses should be 80 mg IV, IO, to a maximum total dose of 300 mg. The effect on blood pressure typically will occur within 5 minutes from the time of administration. Alternatively, may be administered via IV infusion at 2 mg/min to a total maximum dose of 300 mg.
- **Pediatric:** 0.4 to 1 mg/kg/hr IV, IO infusion with a maximum dose of 3 mg/kg/hr.

Special Considerations:
Pregnancy class C

... You have administered nitroglycerin SL tablets 0.4 mg three times. The patient states there is a reduction in her pain from an 8 of 10 to a 4 of 10. You arrive at the hospital. Immediately the emergency team prepares the patient for a 12-lead ECG. Oxygen is connected and vital signs are assessed. The patient is asked questions for medical allergies and conditions. The physician orders metoprolol 5-mg IV push and a nitroglycerin drip at 10 mg/min. The patient's heart rate is reduced to 62 beats/min and blood pressure is now 124/84 mm Hg. ...

Antiplatelets. The development of platelet plugs within the coronary arteries resulting in decreased blood flow to the oxygen-hungry cardiac muscle is the underlying mechanism for ACS. As discussed earlier, aspirin is rapid and effective in reducing aggregation. Clopidogrel (Plavix) is a medication that is categorized as an antiplatelet and anticoagulant medication. Clopidogrel inhibits a specific site on the platelet, rendering it incapable of binding to other platelets. This medication alters the platelet for the remainder of its life span. This makes clopidogrel a powerful anticoagulant. It is often used in conjunction with aspirin, as well as other anticoagulants, in the treatment of UA/NSTEMI. Clopidogrel 75 mg should be added to aspirin in patients with STEMI regardless of whether they undergo reperfusion with fibrinolytic therapy or do not receive reperfusion therapy. If coronary artery bypass graft (CABG) surgery is planned, the drug should be withheld for at least 5 days, or preferably 7 days. In patients younger than 75 years of age who receive fibrinolytic therapy or who do not receive reperfusion therapy, it is reasonable to administer an oral loading dose of clopidogrel 300 mg.

CLOPIDOGREL (PLAVIX)

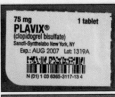

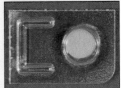

Classification: Antiplatelet
Action: Blocks platelet aggregation by antagonizing the GP IIb/IIIa receptors.
Indications: ACS, chronic coronary and vascular disease, ischemic stroke.
Adverse Effects: Nausea, abdominal pain, and hemorrhage.
Contraindications: History of intracranial hemorrhage, GI bleed or trauma, known sensitivity.
Dosage:
Unstable Angina Pectoris or Non–Q-Wave Acute Myocardial Infarction:
· **Adult:** Single loading dose of 300 mg PO followed by a daily dose of 75 mg PO.
· **Pediatric:** Not recommended for pediatric patients.
Special Considerations:
Pregnancy class B

... The 12-lead ECG demonstrates T-wave inversion in the lateral leads. There is no ST-segment elevation. The patient is still having pain and rates it a 4 of 10. Because of this continued pain, the emergency physician provides the patient with clopidogrel 300 mg PO. He is contacting a nearby cardiac center for transfer of this patient for further evaluation. ...

Anticoagulants. Unfractionated heparin and low-molecular-weight heparin (LMWH) are anticoagulants that inhibit thrombin. Heparin acts at multiple sites in the normal coagulation system. Heparin prevents fibrin formation and inhibits the activation of platelets. LMWH works by inhibiting two proteins in the clotting cascade. It also inhibits the formation of clots. Compared with unfractionated heparin, which requires a loading dose, IV access, and laboratory monitoring, LMWH has greater bioavailability and is administered daily or twice daily by Sub-Q injection. The only detriment to LMWH is that there is no way to completely reverse its anticoagulant effects. Both medications are considered "blood thinners," but they do not dissolve existing clots. They are both used in ACS. They are typically initiated in the emergency department; however, prehospital providers may transport patients who are receiving these medications.

HEPARIN (UNFRACTIONATED HEPARIN)

Classification: Anticoagulant
Action: Acts on antithrombin III to reduce the ability of the blood to form clots, thus preventing clot deposition in the coronary arteries.
Indications: ACS, acute pulmonary embolism, deep venous thrombosis.
Adverse Effects: Bleeding, thrombocytopenia, allergic reactions.
Contraindications: Predisposition to bleeding, aortic aneurysm, peptic ulceration; known sensitivity or history of heparin-induced thrombocytopenia, severe thrombocytopenia, sulfite sensitivity.
Dosage:
Cardiac Indications:
· **Adult:** 60 U/kg IV (max 4000 units), followed by 12 U/kg/hr (max 1000 units). Once in the hospital, additional dosing is determined based on laboratory blood tests.
· **Pediatric:** 75 U/kg followed by 20 U/kg/hr.
Pulmonary Embolism and Deep Vein Thrombosis:
· **Adult:** 80 U/kg IV, followed by 18 U/kg/hr.
· **Pediatric:** 75 U/kg IV followed by 20 U/kg/hr.
Special Considerations:
Half-life approximately 90 minutes
Pregnancy class C

Glycoprotein IIb/IIIa Inhibitors. Glycoprotein IIb/IIIa inhibitors are medications that are used in patients with UA/NSTEMI/STEMI. They are often used in conjunction with heparin or aspirin to prevent clotting before and during invasive heart procedures. The mechanism of action of these medications is that they inhibit platelet aggregation by inhibiting the integrin glycoprotein IIb/IIIa receptor, as well as the final common pathway of platelet aggregation. These medications are very potent platelet inhibitors.

There are three medications in this class:

- Abciximab (ReoPro)
- Eptifibatide (Integrilin)
- Tirofiban (Aggrastat)

The use of this class has shown definite reduction in death, myocardial infarction, and the need for revascularization. These medications are used in the emergency department and extensively by cardiology. Currently they are not used in the prehospital environment. However, they remain an important treatment modality for UA/NSTEMI/STEMI, so prehospital professionals may transport patients receiving glycoprotein IIb/IIIa inhibitors.

ABCIXIMAB (REOPRO)

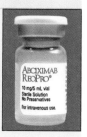

Classification: GP IIb/IIIa inhibitor
Action: Prevents the aggregation of platelets by inhibiting the integrin GP IIb/IIIa receptor.
Indications: UA/NSTEMI patients undergoing planned or emergent percutaneous coronary intervention.
Adverse Effects: Bleeding from the GI tract, internal bleeding, intracranial hemorrhage, hypotension, stroke, anaphylactic shock.
Contraindications: Bleeding from any source, severe uncontrolled hypertension, surgery or trauma within the previous 6 weeks, stroke within the previous 30 days, renal failure, thrombocytopenia, intracranial mass.
Dosage:
UA/NSTEMI with Planned PCI within 24 Hours:
- 0.25 mg/kg IV, IO (10 to 60 minutes before procedure), then 0.125 mcg/kg/min IV, IO infusion for 12 to 24 hours.

Percutaneous Coronary Intervention Only:
- 0.25 mg/kg IV, IO, then 10 mcg/min IV, IO infusion.

Special Considerations:
Pregnancy class C

EPTIFIBATIDE (INTEGRILIN)

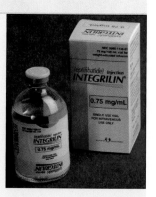

Classification: GP IIb/IIIa inhibitor
Action: Prevents the aggregation of platelets by binding to the GP IIb/IIIa receptor.
Indications: UA/NSTEMI—to manage medically and for those undergoing percutaneous coronary intervention.
Adverse Effects: Bleeding from the GI tract, internal bleeding, intracranial hemorrhage, hypotension, stroke, anaphylactic shock.
Contraindications: Bleeding from any source, severe uncontrolled hypertension, surgery or trauma within the previous 6 weeks, stroke within the previous 30 days, renal failure, thrombocytopenia.
Dosage:
- **Adult:** Loading dose: 180 mcg/kg IV, IO (max dose: 22.6 mg) over 1 to 2 minutes, then 2 mcg/kg/min IV, IO infusion (max dose: 15 mg/hr).
- **Pediatric:** No current dosing recommendations exist for pediatric patients.

Special Considerations:
Half-life approximately 90 to 120 minutes
Pregnancy class B

TIROFIBAN (AGGRASTAT)

Classification: GP IIb/IIIa inhibitor
Action: Prevents the aggregation of platelets by binding to the GP IIb/IIIa receptor.
Indications: UA/NSTEMI—to manage medically and for those undergoing percutaneous coronary intervention.
Adverse Effects: Bleeding from the GI tract, internal bleeding, intracranial hemorrhage, hypotension, stroke, anaphylactic shock.
Contraindications: Bleeding from any source, severe uncontrolled hypertension, surgery or trauma within the previous 6 weeks, stroke within the previous 30 days, renal failure, thrombocytopenia.
Dosage: 0.4 mcg/kg/min IV, IO for 30 minutes, then 0.1 mcg/kg/min IV, IO infusion for 48 to 96 hours.
Special Considerations:
Half-life approximately 2 hours
Pregnancy class B

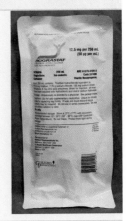

Angiotensin-Converting Enzyme Inhibitors. ACE inhibitors are often used to treat patients with congestive heart failure and postinfarction and are usually administered orally. Although these medications are not initiated in all prehospital systems, they are an integral treatment modality for UA/NSTEMI/STEMI treatment. In addition, patients may already be taking a medication from this class. It is currently believed that this class of medications reduces morbidity and mortality in severe ACS. The reduction of future exacerbations of NSTEMI/STEMI has been linked to reduction in plaque rupture and shear force within the artery.

The body produces a hormone called *angiotensin I*, which is inactive. It is converted to the active form, angiotensin II, by the action of the ACE. Angiotensin II causes significant vasoconstriction and aldosterone secretion. Aldosterone causes retention of salt and water at the kidney with increased excretion of potassium. Both of these actions increase blood volume and blood pressure. Using an ACE inhibitor prevents the conversion of angiotensin I to angiotensin II. This causes a drop in blood pressure and reduces the stress on myocardial tissue.

The medications in this class include the following:

▶ Captopril
▶ Enalapril
▶ Lisinopril
▶ Ramipril

There has been no documented study to suggest one ACE inhibitor delivers better outcomes.

ANGIOTENSIN-CONVERTING ENZYME (ACE) INHIBITORS: CAPTOPRIL (CAPOTEN), ENALAPRIL (VASOTEC), LISINOPRIL (PRINIVIL, ZESTRIL), RAMIPRIL (ALTACE)

Classification: ACE inhibitors
Action: Blocks the enzyme responsible for the production of angiotensin II, resulting in a decrease in blood pressure.
Indications: Congestive heart failure, hypertension, post-myocardial infarction.
Adverse Effects: Headache, dizziness, fatigue, depression, chest pain, hypotension, palpitations, cough, dyspnea, upper respiratory infection, nausea/vomiting, rash, pruritus, angioedema, renal failure.

cont'd

ANGIOTENSIN-CONVERTING ENZYME (ACE) INHIBITORS: CAPTOPRIL (CAPOTEN), ENALAPRIL (VASOTEC), LISINOPRIL (PRINIVIL, ZESTRIL), RAMIPRIL (ALTACE)—CONT'D

Contraindications: Angioedema related to previous treatment with an ACE inhibitor, known sensitivity. Use with caution in aortic stenosis, bilateral renal artery stenosis, hypertrophic obstructive cardiomyopathy, pericardial tamponade, elevated serum potassium levels, acute kidney failure.
Dosage:
  · **Adult:** Medication is administered orally. Dosage is individualized.
  · **Pediatric:** Medication is administered orally. Dosage is individualized.
Special Considerations:
Pregnancy class D

HMG Coenzyme A Reductase Inhibitors (Statins). HMG coenzyme A reductase inhibitors have been shown to reduce the incidence of morbidity when administered within a few days after the onset of ACS. They have also been shown to reduce the incidence of reinfarction, recurrent angina, rehospitalization, and stroke when initiated within a few days after onset of ACS.[3] Although these medications are not typically initiated in the prehospital environment, they are part of the AHA algorithm for UA/NSTEMI. These medications are often referred to as the *statins*.

HMG COENZYME A STATINS: ATORVASTATIN (LIPITOR), FLUVASTATIN (LESCOL), LOVASTATIN (MEVACOR), PRAVASTATIN (PRAVACHOL), ROSUVASTATIN (CRESTOR), SIMVASTATIN (ZOCOR)

Classification: HMG coenzyme A statins
Action: Reduces the level of circulating total cholesterol, LDL cholestrol, and serum triglycerides; reduces the incidence of reinfarction, recurrent angina, rehospitalization, and stroke when initiated within a few days after onset of ACS.
Indications: Acute coronary syndromes/acute myocardial infarction prophylaxis, hypercholesterolemia, hyperlipoproteinemia, hypertriglyceridemia, stroke prophylaxis.
Adverse Effects: Constipation, flatulence, dyspepsia, abdominal pain, infection, headache, flu-like symptoms, back pain, allergic reaction, asthenia, diarrhea, sinusitis, pharyngitis, rash, arthralgia, nausea/vomiting, myopathy, myasthenia, renal failure, rhabdomyolysis, chest pain, bronchitis, rhinitis, insomnia.
Contraindications: Active hepatic disease, pregnancy, breast-feeding, rhabdomyolysis.
Dosage:
  · **Adult:** Medication is administered orally. Dosage is individualized.
  · **Pediatric:** Safe use has not been established.
Special Considerations:
Pregnancy class X

... The patient is started on heparin with a 4200-U bolus dose followed by an 840-U/kg bolus. A nitroglycerin drip is started at 5 mcg/min. The patient is prepared for transport. During transport the patient develops increased pain. Per medical control, you adjust the nitroglycerin drip to 15 mcg/min. A repeat blood pressure is 130/88 mm Hg. You arrive at the receiving facility and the staff immediately obtains a 12-lead ECG that demonstrates no acute change. The cardiologist arrives and schedules the patient for percutaneous coronary intervention (PCI) immediately. He requests abciximab 0.25 mg IV and an infusion of 0.125 mg/kg/hr to be administered. In addition, he requests an initial IV dose of enalapril 1.25 mg IV and atorvastatin 5 mg PO. The patient is prepared for PCI and transferred to the cardiac catheterization laboratory.

OVERVIEW OF ST-SEGMENT MYOCARDIAL INFARCTION

You receive a call for a 61-year-old man with a chief complaint of chest pain. On arrival, you find an obese man sitting in a chair. He is dyspneic and diaphoretic. He states that his chest pain has been present for 45 minutes and is "like a ton of bricks on my chest." The patient describes the pain as radiating to his jaw and left arm. He has a history of hypertension, diabetes, smoking, and a positive family history of heart disease. He denies a history of congestive heart failure, chronic obstructive pulmonary disease, asthma, or emphysema. His last cardiac workup was 3 years ago. His pulse is 96 beats/min, blood pressure is 138/98 mm Hg, and respiratory rate is 24 breaths/min. Your 12-lead ECG demonstrates elevations in leads I, aV_L, V_5, and V_6. ...

This patient has a significant number of risk factors for ACS and infarction. He has chest pain that is pressure-like and lasts longer than 30 minutes. Radiation to the jaw and left arm are also common symptoms significant of anginal pain. He has shortness of breath and diaphoresis. Chest pain itself is a poor predictor of the prehospital diagnosis of acute myocardial infarction; however, diaphoresis in a patient with chest pain is definitely suggestive of ACS and infarction. ST-segment elevation in leads I, aV_L, V_5, and V_6 are specific for a lateral wall STEMI. This patient should be aggressively treated and prepared for transport.

The pathophysiology of STEMI is usually the complete blockage of an artery by a ruptured plaque and thrombus formation. Occasionally, the decreased blood flow can occur secondary to vasospasm. This can be caused by cocaine abuse. Thrombus or vasospasm actually causes blood flow to the heart to stop or diminish considerably. Decreased oxygen delivery causes ischemia. If not reversed, infarction will occur and result in cell death. After heart cells are damaged, they are unable to respond to electrical stimulus, which alters the conduction and contraction of cardiac muscle.

... You place the patient on oxygen 4 L/min by nasal cannula. Your partner places the patient on a cardiac monitor and gets ready to start an IV line while you prepare to administer several medications. You give the patient four 81-mg baby aspirins. You tell him to chew and then swallow the aspirins. You ask the patient whether he is taking any medications for erectile dysfunction or impotence, and the patient denies use of these medications. You administer one SL nitroglycerin 0.4 mg, then reassess the patient, including a complete set of vital signs. The patient reports that he has no reduction in his chest pain. Repeat vitals show heart rate of 92 beats/min, blood pressure 142/96 mm Hg, and respiratory rate of 18 breaths/min. Pulse oximeter reading is 95% on 4 L/min oxygen. Because the patient is still having chest pain after 5 minutes, you administer a second dose of nitroglycerin 0.4 mg SL. You take his blood pressure again, and it is 140/96 mm Hg. You then administer morphine sulfate 2 mg slow IV push. On reassessment of the patient, he reports significant improvement in his chest pain. ...

Management

Initial care for this patient is the same as for patients with UA. Appropriate prehospital care would include starting the patient on oxygen; initiating an IV; placing the patient on a cardiac monitor; and administering aspirin, nitroglycerin, and morphine sulfate. Additional medications that are used in STEMI treatment include those medications discussed in the section on UA/NSTEMI. This includes the antiplatelet medications, anticoagulant medications, ACE inhibitors, beta blockers, glycoprotein IIb/IIIa inhibitors, and HMG coenzyme A reductase inhibitors (statins). Reperfusion therapy is also indicated.

Reperfusion Therapy. Reperfusion therapy is the gold standard for the treatment of STEMI. The two methods for reperfusion are pharmacologic reperfusion (fibrinolytics) and PCI. Fibrinolytic treatment is indicated in those patients who have onset of symptoms of less than 12 hours, ST-segment elevation greater than 1 mm in two or more contiguous leads (or bundle branch block obscuring ST-segment analysis), and a history suggesting STEMI (Box 6-1). PCI is preferred if the patient comes to a facility where PCI is available and if it can be accomplished within 90 minutes of the onset of symptoms. It is also preferred if there is increased bleeding risk. Patients with STEMI who come to a hospital with PCI capability should be treated with primary PCI within 90 minutes of first medical contact as a systems goal. Patients with STEMI who come to a hospital without PCI capability and who cannot be transferred to a PCI center and undergo PCI within 90 minutes should be treated with fibrionlytic therapy within 30 minutes. Bottom-line faster reperfusion is endorsed.[4]

BOX 6-1

REPERFUSION THERAPY: FIBRINOLYTICS OR PERCUTANEOUS CORONARY INTERVENTION?

Fibrinolysis is generally preferred if
- Patient presents ≤3 hours from symptom onset.
- Invasive strategy is not an option (catheterization laboratory occupied/not available, vascular access difficulties, lack of access to skilled PCI facility).
- Invasive strategy would be delayed (prolonged transport, medical contact-to-balloon or door-balloon >90 minutes, [door-to-balloon] minus [door-to-needle] is >1 hour).
- No contraindications to fibrinolysis.

An invasive strategy is generally preferred if
- Patient presents >3 hours from symptom onset.
- Diagnosis of STEMI is in doubt.
- Skilled PCI facility available with surgical backup (medical contact-to-balloon or door-balloon <90 minutes, [door-to-balloon] minus [door-to-needle] is <1 hour).
- Contraindications to fibrinolysis, including increased risk of bleeding and intracranial hemorrhage.
- High risk from STEMI (such as congestive heart failure [CHF]).

If presentation <3 hours and no delay for PCI, then no preference for either strategy.

From Antman EM, et al: 2005 American Heart Association Guidelines for cardiopulmonary resuscitation and emergency cardiovascular care, part 8. Circulation 112(suppl IV):IV-95, 2005. Available online: www.acc.org/clinical/guidelines/stemi/index.pdf.

FIBRINOLYTICS: TISSUE PLASMINOGEN ACTIVATOR (tPA), STREPTOKINASE (STREPTASE, KABIKINASE), RETEPLASE (RETAVASE), TENECTEPLASE (TNKASE)

Classification: Thrombolytic agent
Action: Dissolves thrombi plugs in the coronary arteries and reestablishes blood flow.
Indications: ST-segment elevation (≥1 mm in two or more contiguous leads), new or presumed-new left bundle branch block.
Adverse Effects: Bleeding, intracranial hemorrhage, stroke, cardiac arrhythmias, hypotension, bruising.
Contraindications: ST-segment depression, cardiogenic shock, recent (within 10 days) major surgery, cerebrovascular disease, recent (within 10 days) GI bleeding, recent trauma, hypertension (systolic blood pressure ≥180 mm Hg or diastolic blood pressure ≥110 mm Hg), high likelihood of left heart thrombus, acute pericarditis, subacute bacterial endocarditis, severe renal or liver failure with bleeding complications, significant liver dysfunction, diabetic hemorrhagic retinopathy, septic thrombophlebitis, advanced age (older than 75 years), patients taking warfarin (Coumadin).
Dosage: Dosing per medical direction.
Special Considerations:
Pregnancy class C

... You arrive at the emergency department. The physician orders a 12-lead ECG. The ST-segment elevation has worsened. The patient is started on a nitroglycerin drip at 10 mcg/min. Heparin is initiated with a bolus of 7200 U and a drip of 1080 U/hr. The patient is given clopidogrel 300 mg PO. Atorvastatin 10 mg PO is given, as well as enalapril 1.25 mg IV. Abciximab is ordered from the pharmacy. The PCI team is in place and the patient is taken to the catheterization laboratory for intervention. On your next call, you stop back to check on your patient. He received a drug-eluting stent in the circumflex artery. He has been placed on atorvastatin and captopril. He will be discharged home in the morning.

ACS represents a spectrum of diseases. The most benign form of ACS is stable angina. This is chest pain that generally occurs with exertion, is relieved by rest, and lasts less than 5 minutes. This may progress to UA, which is pain that follows no pattern. Chest pressure may occur at rest, during sleep, or during activity. This pain typically lasts less than 20 minutes. NSTEMI is very similar to UA in its presentation. The difference is that with NSTEMI there is alteration in cardiac enzymes that reflect myocardial damage. To the prehospital professional, these two conditions will be indistinguishable. STEMI occurs when there is a significant decrease in coronary blood flow. This is often caused by a rupture of the atherosclerotic plaque. A thrombus rich in platelets obstructs blood flow and oxygen delivery to the myocardial cell. This can lead to cell death and loss of cardiac muscle function.

The primary goal of treatment is to minimize the damage to the myocardial cells. This can be accomplished by a variety of medications.

- Oxygen is used to help increase the supply of oxygen to the ischemic cells.
- Nitroglycerin is a vasodilating medication that increases blood flow to the coronary arteries.
- Morphine sulfate, fentanyl, and hydromorphone are narcotic pain medications that reduce the sympathetic response to pain.
- Aspirin is an antiplatelet medication that reduces platelet clumping and formation of thrombus.
- Clopidogrel is an antiplatelet medication that also inhibits the clumping of platelets and affects the platelet for its entire life.
- Heparin and LMWH affect the clotting cascade and inhibit further clotting at the site of thrombus.
- Glycoprotein IIb/IIIa inhibitors also prevent the terminal step in platelet aggregation.
- Beta blockers reduce the heart rate and blood pressure, lowering the sheer stress on the myocardial muscle cells.
- ACE inhibitors reduce volume and blood pressure.
- Fibrinolytics are the only medications that actually will break an existing thrombus.
- PCI is the mechanical opening of the blocked artery by either balloon or stent placement.

ACS is a major cause of morbidity and mortality in this country and around the world. Research and development continue to advance the science of the treatment for ACS. With the common goal of reperfusion to minimize cardiac damage as the gold standard, prehospital professionals will continue to be at the forefront of this fascinating change in treating this disease process.

REVIEW QUESTIONS

1. List risk factors for acute myocardial ischemia.
2. Why is oxygen administration critical to a patient with stable angina pectoris?
3. Before administering nitroglycerin to a male patient, you should ask whether the patient is taking medications for what condition?

4. Name two benefits of administering morphine to a patient with chest pain.
5. What is the effect of beta blockers on the ischemic heart?
6. Name three contraindications for the use of beta blockers.
7. Explain the role of antiplatelets know as glycoprotein IIb/IIIa receptor antagonists.
8. What are the contraindications for fibrinolytic drug administrations?

REFERENCES

1. Rosen P, Barker FJ, Braen R: *Rosen's emergency medicine concepts and clinical practice*, ed 6, St Louis, 2006, Mosby.
2. About.com: Health Topics A-Z: *Heart attack and acute coronary syndrome* (website): http://adam.about.com/reports/000012_8.htm. Accessed April 9, 2008.
3. 2005 American Heart Association, Inc: 2005 American Heart Association guidelines for cardiopulmonary resuscitation and emergency cardiovascular care. Part 8: Stabilization of the patient with acute coronary syndromes, *Circulation* 112:IV89–IV110, 2005.
4. Antman EM, et al: 2007 Focused update of the ACC/AHA 2004 guidelines for the management of patients with ST-elevation myocardial infarction: A report of the American College of Cardiology/American Heart Association task force on practice guidelines developed in collaboration with the Canadian Cardiovascular Society endorsed by the American Academy of Family Physicians, *J Am Coll Cardiol* Published online: 10 Dec 2007; doi:10.1016/j.jacc.2007.10.001.

BIBLIOGRAPHY

Bertrand ME, et al: Management of acute coronary syndromes in patients presenting without persistent ST elevation: the task force on the management of acute coronary syndromes of the European Society of Cardiology, *Eur Heart J* 23:1809, 2002.
Braunwald E, et al: *Unstable angina: diagnosis and management.* Clinical Practice Guideline Number 10 (amended) AHCPR Publication No. 94-0602, Agency for Health Care Policy and Research and the National Heart, Lung, and Blood Institute, Public Health Service, US Department of Health and Human Services, Rockville, Md, May 1994.
Gibler WB, et al: Practical implementation of the guidelines for unstable angina/non-ST-segment elevation myocardial infarction in the emergency department, *Ann Emerg Med* 46:185, 2005.
Lange RA, Hills LD: Cardiovascular complications of cocaine use, *N Engl J Med* 345:351, 2001.
Meier MA, et al: The new definition of myocardial infarction: diagnostic and prognostic implications in patients with acute coronary syndromes, *Arch Intern Med* 162:1585, 2002.
Pollack CV Jr, et al: 2004 American College of Cardiology/American Heart Association guidelines for the management of patients with ST elevation myocardial infarction: implications for emergency department practice, *Ann Emerg Med* 45:363, 2005.
Sabatine MS, et al: Addition of clopidogrel to aspirin and fibrinolytic therapy for myocardial infarction with ST-segment elevation, *N Engl J Med* 352:1179, 2005.
www.mdconsult.com

Analgesia and Sedation

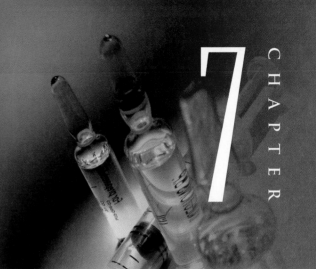

OBJECTIVES

1. Discuss why, despite the frequency of patient reports of pain, it often is not treated in the field.
2. Discuss the narcotics (opiates) that the prehospital provider may encounter: morphine sulfate, fentanyl citrate (Sublimaze), meperidine (Demerol), butorphanol (Stadol), and nalbuphine (Nubain).
3. Discuss the effects of nonsteroidal antiinflammatory drugs such as ketorolac (Toradol).
4. List the benefits of nitrous oxide and demonstrate the proper procedure for administering the drug.
5. Discuss various roles of ketamine (Ketalar), etomidate (Amidate), and propofol (Diprivan) in prehospital care.
6. Explain the benefit of the ability of benzodiazepines to induce anterograde amnesia.
7. Discuss the role of sedatives (benzodiazepines) in pain management, including the following drugs: diazepam (Valium), midazolam (Versed), lorazepam (Ativan), flumazenil (Romazicon), and naloxone (Narcan).
8. Explain why antiemetics may be necessary in the treatment of pain.
9. Discuss the effects of the following antiemetics: promethazine (Phenergan), ondansetron (Zofran), and dolasetron (Anzemet).

Medications that Appear in Chapter 7

Morphine sulfate
Fentanyl citrate (Sublimaze)
Meperidine (Demerol)
Butorphanol (Stadol)
Nalbuphine (Nubain)
Aspirin, ASA
Ibuprofen
Ketorolac (Toradol)
Nitrous oxide
Ketamine (Ketalar)
Etomidate (Amidate)
Propofol (Diprivan)
Diazepam (Valium)
Midazolam (Versed)
Lorazepam (Ativan)
Flumazenil (Romazicon)
Naloxone (Narcan)
Promethazine (Phenergan)
Dolasetron (Anzemet)

INTRODUCTION

Pain is a common complaint in the prehospital field. Paramedics often encounter reports of headaches, chest pain, pain from trauma such as fractures, and abdominal discomfort. Innumerable medical conditions can present as pain. A variety of agents and treatments are available to reduce a patient's discomfort and even allow a more thorough patient assessment. These include **narcotics (opiates)**, nonsteroidal antiinflammatory drugs, **sedatives (benzodiazepines)**, antiemetics, and miscellaneous pain medications.

> Your unit is dispatched to a local park. On arrival, you find a 34-year-old man lying on a paved running path. The patient's distraught wife explains that her husband fell while rollerblading. The patient is experiencing extreme pain in his left leg. You perform an assessment. The patient has a heart rate of 130 beats/min, blood pressure of 160/102 mm Hg, respiratory rate of 18 breaths/min, and an oxygen saturation level of 97%. The patient has gross deformity of the left thigh, indicating a closed femur fracture. He has good motor and sensory function, as well as pulses distal to the fracture.

OVERVIEW OF ANALGESIA AND SEDATION

Despite the frequency of patient reports of pain, it is often not treated in the prehospital setting. Several reasons explain this fact, with the principal one being the concern that administration of **analgesics** (compounds that relieve pain), especially narcotics, can cause respiratory depression and hypotension. Providers are also concerned that analgesics may mask the progression of symptoms.

Another argument against the liberal use of analgesics in the field is that administration of these agents can complicate assessment of the patient after arrival at the hospital. For example, in a patient with a head injury or another neurologic condition, the administration of analgesics or sedatives (calming, quieting drugs) can mask the progression of the condition. In the case of abdominal pain, narcotics have historically been withheld until a diagnosis or a decision for surgery has been made. However, this philosophy originated in an era when the principal method for determining that a patient needed surgery was physical examination of the abdomen. The near-universal use of computer tomographic scanning for the evaluation of abdominal pain makes analgesia less of a concern. Narcotics in excessive doses can reduce the patient's ability to protect the airway and decrease respirations. Fear of these complications results in a lower rate of authorization for narcotics administration. Unfortunately, the result is that patients endure pain that can be easily treated. Apnea and loss of an airway are potentially catastrophic complications. Therefore the provider must closely monitor the patient's oxygen saturation, ventilations, and airway. If any of these becomes compromised, the paramedic needs to be prepared and equipped to intervene to support oxygenation and ventilation.

A patient's discomfort can be composed of several elements. The most obvious is pain, which can be treated with analgesics. A second element of a patient's distress is often anxiety, which is best treated with sedative drugs. Sedatives result in a generalized and nonspecific depression of the central nervous system (CNS). Narcotic drugs such as opiates produce both analgesia and some degree of sedation as a secondary effect.

MANAGEMENT

NARCOTICS (OPIATES)

Narcotics are the class of drugs typically used to treat moderate and severe pain. They are also known as *opiates* because they either derive from or contain chemical structures similar to opium. Opiates that a prehospital provider may encounter include morphine sulfate, fentanyl citrate (Sublimaze), meperidine (Demerol), butorphanol (Stadol), and nalbuphine (Nubain).

Opiates bind with **opiate receptors** in the CNS, resulting in a reduction of the pain sensation. However, opiates do not address the underlying mechanism producing the pain. If the muffler fell off your car, you would be disturbed by the loud noise your car now makes. One solution would be to increase the volume of the car's radio. The result is that you can no longer hear the rumble of your car, so it no longer disturbs you. However, as with the use of opiates, the underlying problem still exists.

The patient in the preceding scenario is reporting severe pain from a fracture of his femur. The administration of a narcotic to this patient will decrease his pain sensation but will do nothing to treat the fracture. Despite subjective improvement after administration of an opiate, the patient still requires specific therapy for the underlying problem, in this case the fractured femur. The fact that narcotics can mask the principal problem by altering the patient's perception of pain is one argument for conservative use of prehospital analgesics.

Another example is a patient with abdominal pain from possible appendicitis. The provider may not know that the patient's appendix perforated if the pain is masked by excessive narcotics. Although this is certainly a valid concern, the judicious use of narcotics—versus withholding all analgesia—provides patients with some degree of relief and allows the examiner to obtain a reliable physical examination. "Judicious" is a subjective term and impossible to quantify. A safe practice is to administer small doses with frequent reevaluation between each dose. The administration of several small doses is better practice than administering one large dose.

The patient in the preceding scenario exhibits many of the typical signs of a patient with severe pain: agitation and restlessness, tachycardia, and hypertension. Although the tachycardia could be caused by blood loss associated with the femur fracture, the concomitant presentation of pain and hypertension supports the fact that the patient's elevated heart rate is most likely caused by severe discomfort. Tachycardia from hypovolemia is usually associated with a normal or depressed blood pressure.

Excessive administration of narcotics can result in respiratory depression, so prehospital providers should give supplemental oxygen and be equipped and skilled to intervene and support a patient's airway in the event of respiratory depression or arrest.

Administration of some narcotics, such as morphine sulfate, can result in hypotension, particularly in hypovolemic patients. For example, some trauma patients can lose 25% of their blood volume without any depression of their blood pressure. Patients can often tolerate such blood loss because they are able to compensate for this decrease of their circulatory volume. However, administration of a narcotic to such a patient can result in vasodilation and subsequent hypotension. Therefore paramedics need to ensure that patients have adequate intravascular blood volume before administering narcotics. This may require administration of several hundred milliliters of an intravascular fluid bolus before administration of narcotics.

Morphine induces the release of **histamine,** which causes vasodilation, which in turn produces hypotension. Fentanyl citrate (Sublimaze), although rarely used in the prehospital setting, does not result in the release of histamine and therefore is less associated with hypotension after IV administration. For this reason, if a patient who is hypovolemic requires narcotic administration, consider the use of fentanyl instead of morphine.

Meperidine (Demerol) is a synthetic narcotic commonly used to treat moderate to severe pain. Meperidine can decrease cardiac output in higher dosage ranges. It is broken down or metabolized by the liver, and its metabolites can cause confusion, hallucinations, and seizures. However, in a **single dose** it is unlikely that these toxic metabolites will become clinically significant.

The patient has a femur fracture and is reporting severe pain. His heart rate is elevated at 130 beats/min. You consider that the heart rate could be elevated as a result of blood loss from the fracture. However, given the elevated blood pressure and the patient's agitation from pain, you consult with medical direction. You present the patient's case, mentioning the patient's reported ...

... pain, hypertension, and tachycardia. Given the thigh deformity from the fracture, you are concerned that the patient may have had substantial blood loss. Medical direction approves the administration of fentanyl 50 mcg IV push. After administering the fentanyl, you repeat a set of vitals and patient assessment. After 5 minutes, the patient reports that his pain has not changed, and his blood pressure is 182/108 mm Hg, heart rate is 136 beats/min, and oxygen saturation is 98%. Medical control approves a second 50-mcg IV dose. After the second dose, the patient reports that his pain improves from 8 of 10 to 4 of 10. His repeat blood pressure is 138/88 mm Hg and heart rate is 110 beats/min. The pulse oximeter displays a saturation of 95%.

MORPHINE SULFATE

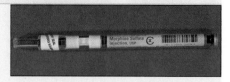

Classification: Opiate agonist, Schedule C-II
Action: Binds with opioid receptors. Morphine is capable of inducing hypotension by depression of the vasomotor centers of the brain, as well as release of the chemical histamine. In the management of angina, morphine reduces stimulation of the sympathic nervous system caused by pain and anxiety. Reduction of sympathetic stimulation reduces heart rate, cardiac work, and myocardial oxygen consumption.
Indications: Moderate to severe pain, including chest pain associated with ACS, CHF, pulmonary edema.
Adverse Effects: Respiratory depression, hypotension, nausea/vomiting, dizziness, lightheadedness, sedation, diaphoresis, euphoria, dysphoria, worsening of bradycardia and heart block in some patients with acute inferior wall MI, seizures, cardiac arrest, anaphylactoid reactions.
Contraindications: Respiratory depression, shock, known sensitivity. Use with caution in hypotension, acute bronchial asthma, respiratory insufficiency, head trauma.
Dosage:
Pain:
- **Adult:** 2.5 to 15 mg IV, IO, IM, or Sub-Q administered slowly over a period of several minutes. The dose is the same whether administered IV, IO, IM, or Sub-Q.
- **Pediatric:**
  - **6 months to 12 years:** 0.05 to 0.2 mg/kg IV, IO, IM, or Sub-Q.
  - **Younger than 6 months:** 0.03 to 0.05 mg/kg IV, IO, IM, or Sub-Q.

Chest Pain Associated with Acute Coronary Syndromes, Congestive Heart Failure, and Pulmonary Edema:
Administer small doses and reevaluate the patient. Large doses may lead to respiratory depression and worsen the patient's hypoxia.
- **Adult:** 2 to 4 mg slow IV, IO over a 1- to 5-minute period with increments of 2 to 8 mg repeated every 5 to 15 minutes until patient relieved of chest pain.
- **Pediatric:** 0.1 to 0.2 mg/kg/dose IV, IO.

Special Considerations:
Monitor vital signs and pulse oximetry closely. Be prepared to support patient's airway and ventilations.
Overdose should be treated with naloxone.
Pregnancy class C

FENTANYL CITRATE (SUBLIMAZE)

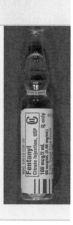

Classification: Narcotic analgesic; Schedule C-II
Action: Binds to opiate receptors, producing analgesia and euphoria.
Indications: Pain
Adverse Effects: Respiratory depression, apnea, hypotension, nausea/vomiting, dizziness, sedation, euphoria, sinus bradycardia, sinus tachycardia, palpitations, hypertension, diaphoresis, syncope, pain at injection site.
Contraindications: Known sensitivity. Use with caution in traumatic brain injury, respiratory depression.
Dosage: Note: Dosage should be individualized.
- **Adult:** 50 to 100 mcg/dose (0.05 to 0.1 mg) IM or slow IV, IO (administered over 1 to 2 minutes).
- **Pediatric:** 1 to 2 mcg/kg IM or slow IV, IO (administered over 1 to 2 minutes).
Special Considerations:
Pregnancy class B

MEPERIDINE (DEMEROL)

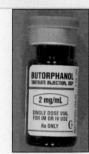

Classification: Narcotic analgesic, Schedule C-II
Action: Binds to opiate receptors, producing analgesia and euphoria.
Indications: Moderate to severe pain.
Adverse Effects: Respiratory depression, nausea/vomiting, sinus bradycardia, sinus tachycardia, palpitations, hypertension, hypotension, orthostatic hypotension, diaphoresis, syncope, shock, cardiac arrest.
Contraindications: Patients who have taken an MAOI in the past 2 weeks, patients who are using other CNS depressants or alcohol, known sensitivity. Use with caution in patients with chronic respiratory conditions (asthma or COPD), pregnant or nursing women, atrial flutter.
Dosage: If given IV, IO, administer slowly.
  · **Adult:** 50 to 150 mg IV, IO, IM, or Sub-Q. Elderly: 50 mg IV, IO, IM, or Sub-Q.
  · **Pediatric:** 1 to 2 mg/kg IV, IO, IM, or Sub-Q.
Special Considerations:
In adults, half-life approximately 4 hours, but its active metabolites may last 30 hours. Pregnancy class C; class D near term.

BUTORPHANOL (STADOL)

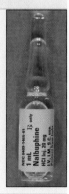

Classification: Opioid agonist-antagonist; Schedule C-IV controlled substance
Action: Produces analgesia by binding to the opioid receptor.
Indications: Moderate to severe pain.
Adverse Effects: Drowsiness, dizziness, confusion, respiratory depression, nausea/vomiting, bradycardia, hypotension.
Contraindications: Patients with active substance abuse, sensitivity to opiate agonists. Use with caution in kidney, liver, or pulmonary problems.
Dosage:
  · **Adult:** 0.5 to 2 mg IV, IO every 3 to 4 hours.
  · **Pediatric:** Not recommended for pediatric patients.
Special Considerations:
Pregnancy class C

NALBUPHINE (NUBAIN)

Classification: Synthetic opioid agonist-antagonist
Action: Produces analgesia by binding to the opioid receptor.
Indications: Moderate to severe pain.
Adverse Effects: Drowsiness, diaphoresis, headache, nausea/vomiting, dry mouth, respiratory depression, hypotension, bradycardia.
Contraindications: Known sensitivity.
Dosage:
  · **Adult:** 10 mg IV, IO, IM, or Sub-Q.
  · **Pediatric:** Not recommended for pediatric patients.
Special Considerations:
Pregnancy class B

NONSTEROIDAL ANTIINFLAMMATORY DRUGS

> On a hot Saturday afternoon, a 42-year-old man mows the lawn and then proceeds to enjoy the remainder of his day watching a baseball game on television and drinking cool iced tea. You are called to his home because he has a rapid onset of severe left flank pain. He describes the pain as rapid in onset, 10 on a 0 to 10 scale, located on his left side, and radiating down to his left testicle. He passed some bloody urine before your arrival. He denies any chest pain or shortness of breath. He has no significant medical history. His vital signs are heart rate, 122 beats/min; blood pressure, 132/88 mm Hg; respiratory rate, 16 breaths/min; and pulse oximetry reading, 97%.

The patient in this scenario presents with the classic signs and symptoms of **nephrolithiasis,** or kidney stones. Patients with nephrolithiasis typically have flank pain with radiation to the groin and, occasionally, hematuria. A nonsteroidal antiinflammatory drug (NSAID) would be an appropriate drug choice for this patient. NSAIDs work by inhibiting the body's pathways for producing an inflammatory response. They provide pain relief and decrease the inflammation partly responsible for generation of the pain.

The most commonly used NSAIDs are aspirin and ibuprofen. Ketorolac (Toradol) is another powerful analgesic that belongs to this drug class. It is currently the only NSAID that can be delivered IV, IO, or IM. A dose of 60 mg ketorolac IM is equivalent to 800 mg ibuprofen.[1] Ketorolac can provide pain relief at the level traditionally provided by narcotics.[1,2] Additionally, ketorolac holds advantages over narcotics in the treatment of renal colic from kidney stones. NSAIDs block the production of prostaglandins, which subsequently blocks the spasms and peristalsis of the ureter. Conversely, narcotics increase the ureteral spasm and may actually increase the patient's discomfort.

NSAIDS lack the most common and dreaded adverse effect of the narcotic agents: respiratory depression. However, NSAIDs still possess some serious complications, including gastric ulcers, prolongation of bleeding time, and decreased kidney function.

ASPIRIN, ASA

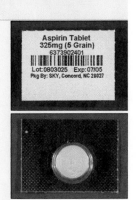

Classification: Antiplatelet, nonnarcotic analgesic, antipyretic
Action: Prevents the formation of a chemical known as thromboxane A_2, which causes platelets to clump together, or aggregate, and form plugs that cause obstruction or constriction of small coronary arteries.
Indications: Fever, inflammation, angina, acute MI, and patients complaining of pain, pressure, squeezing, or crushing in the chest that may be cardiac in origin.
Adverse Effects: Anaphylaxis, angioedema, bronchospasm, bleeding, stomach irritation, nausea/vomiting.
Contraindications: GI bleeding, active ulcer disease, hemorrhagic stroke, bleeding disorders, children with chickenpox or flulike symptoms, known sensitivity.
Dosage: Note: "Baby aspirin" 81 mg, standard adult aspirin dose 325 mg.
Myocardial Infarction:
- **Adult:** 160 to 325 mg PO (alternatively, four 81-mg baby aspirin are often given), 300-mg rectal suppository.
- **Pediatric:** 3 to 5 mg/kg/day to 5 to 10 mg/kg/day given as a single dose.
Pain or Fever:
- **Adult:** 325 to 650 mg PO (1 to 2 adult tablets) every 4 to 6 hours.
- **Pediatric:** 60 to 90 mg/kg/day in divided doses every 4 to 6 hours.
Special Considerations:
Pregnancy class C except the last 3 months of pregnancy, when aspirin is considered pregnancy class D.

IBUPROFEN

Classification: NSAID

Action: Inhibits prostaglandin synthesis by inhibiting cyclooxygenase (COX) isoenzymes, resulting in analgesic, antipyretic, and antiinflammatory effects.

Indications: Mild to moderate pain, fever, osteoarthritis, rheumatoid arthritis.

Adverse Effects: Anorexia, nausea/vomiting, epigastric/abdominal pain, dyspepsia, constipation, diarrhea, gastritis, melena, flatulence, headache, dizziness.

Contraindications: Sensitivity to NSAID or salicylate. Use with caution in asthma, hepatic disease, renal disease, congestive heart failure, hypertension, cardiac disease, cardiomyopathy, cardiac arrhythmias, significant coronary artery disease, peripheral vascular disease, cerebrovascular disease, fluid retention, or edema.

Dosage:

Mild to Moderate Pain:
- **Adult:** 400 mg PO every 4 hours as needed, not to exceed 1200 mg per day.
- **Pediatric: 6 months to 12 yrs:** 5 to 10 mg/kg PO every 6 to 8 hours as needed, not to exceed 40 mg/kg/day.

Fever:
- **Adult:** 200 to 400 mg PO every 4 to 6 hours as needed, not to exceed 1200 mg per day.
- **Pediatric: 6 months to 12 years:** 5 mg/kg PO if baseline temperature is less than 102.5° F, or 10 mg/kg PO if baseline temperature is greater than 102.5° F (max dose: 40 mg/kg/day).

Osteoarthritis or Rheumatoid Arthritis:
- **Adult:** 400 to 800 mg PO 3 to 4 times per day, not to exceed 3200 mg/day.
- **Pediatric: 1 to 12 years:** 30 to 40 mg/kg/day PO in 3 to 4 divided doses, not to exceed 50 mg/kg/day.

Special Considerations:
Pregnancy class B

KETOROLAC (TORADOL)

Classification: NSAID

Action: Inhibits the production of prostaglandins in inflamed tissue, which decreases the responsiveness of pain receptors.

Indications: Moderately severe acute pain.

Adverse Effects: Headache, drowsiness, dizziness, abdominal pain, dyspepsia, nausea/vomiting, diarrhea.

Contraindications: Patients with a history of peptic ulcer disease or GI bleed, patients with renal insufficiency, hypovolemic patients, pregnancy (third trimester), nursing mothers, allergy to aspirin or other NSAIDs, stroke or suspected stroke or head trauma, need for major surgery in the immediate or near future (i.e., within 7 days).

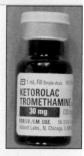

Dosage: Note: The following dosage regimen applies to single-dose administration only. IV, IO administration should occur over a period of at least 15 seconds.
- **Adult:**
  - **Younger than 65 years:** 30 mg IV, IO or 60 mg IM.
  - **Older than 65 years:** 15 mg IV, IO or 30 mg IM.
- **Pediatric:** 0.5 mg/kg IV, IO to a maximum dose of 15 mg, or 1 mg/kg IM to a maximum dose of 30 mg.

Special Considerations:
Pregnancy class C; class D in third trimester

OTHER PAIN MEDICATIONS

The need to induce or maintain an altered level of consciousness may require a variety of medications that are neither narcotic analgesics nor benzodiazepine sedatives. Nitrous oxide is an inhaled agent capable of providing some relief associated with fractures. Ketamine is a drug that provides anesthesia, allowing for the performance of invasive procedures. Ketamine is used by air medical services, combat medics, and prehospital providers in Europe. Etomidate is used in rapid sequence and pharmacologically assisted intubations. Propofol is a sedative agent administered to intubated patients being transported from one hospital to another.

Inhaled nitrous oxide is a long-standing and safe method of providing rapid analgesia for procedure-related pain. Nitrous oxide, commonly known as *laughing gas,* is routinely used to provide analgesia for dental and surgical procedures. Patient-administered, inhaled nitrous oxide is safe and easy to administer. The agent is delivered by a demand-valve face mask as a 50:50 mixture with oxygen[3] (Fig. 7-1).

Once the patient has received an adequate amount of nitrous oxide, the mask simply falls away from the face, preventing the patient from inhaling any additional anesthetic.

Nitrous oxide can provide mild analgesia and sedation. Inhaled nitrous oxide has a rapid onset of action, typically within 30 to 60 seconds. The patient's ability to protect and maintain an airway is preserved.[4,5] No adverse cardiovascular effects have been reported after patient-administered nitrous oxide.[6] Nitrous oxide has been effectively used in the prehospital setting for analgesia.[7,8]

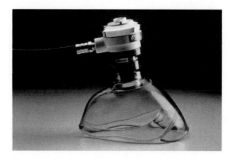

▼ **Fig. 7-1** Face mask for a nitrous oxide system. The nitrous oxide is patient administered, not paramedic administered. When the patient begins to near oversedation, the mask falls away from the patient's face and the patient begins to breathe room air. (From Roberts J, Hedges J: *Clinical procedures in emergency medicine,* ed 4, Philadelphia, 2004, WB Saunders.)

NITROUS OXIDE ADMINISTRATION

Equipment Needed:
Nitrous oxide and oxygen cylinders, blender, mask with demand valve, gas scavenger circuit

Procedure:
1. Tell the patient (not the provider) to hold the mask tightly against the face.
2. Instruct the patient not to talk or remove the mask between breaths.
3. Instruct the patient to breathe normally.

Providers assisting with nitrous oxide administration must choose their words carefully and control the environment because patients who receive this medication can be open to suggestion after nitrous oxide administration. Keep the environment quiet and avoid any unnecessary conversation.

4. Monitor the patient's vital signs and pulse oximetry.
5. Continuously assess the patient for lightheadedness, restlessness, and nausea.[9-10]

NITROUS OXIDE

Classification: Inorganic gas, inhaled anesthetic
Action: Exact mechanism is not known.
Indications: Mild to severe pain.
Adverse Effects: Delirium, hypoxia, respiratory depression, nausea/vomiting.
Contraindications: Use with caution in head trauma, increased ICP, pneumothorax, bowel obstruction, patients with COPD who require a hypoxic respiratory drive.
Dosage: Inhaled: 20% to 50% concentration mixed with oxygen.
Special Considerations:
Ensure the safety of healthcare professionals. Use only with a scavenger gas system to ensure that unused gas is collected, or scavenged, and that providers are not exposed to significant levels of the agent.
Pregnancy class not noted

You are a member of a flight crew that is responding to the scene of a burned child. You are told by dispatch that the patient is a 3-year-old child whose clothes caught on fire when she came too close to a fire used to burn trash. When you arrive, you find a child who is essentially being controlled with physical restraint by several adults. She is in extreme pain and is violently thrashing about. You perform your primary assessment. The child's airway is patent, and she is screaming in pain. You cannot obtain a blood pressure. She has good distal pulses. You determine that she has approximately 40% total body surface area burns that are deep, full-thickness burns. You consider placing an IV, but this seems impractical given the child's violent movements and the severity of pain. Nevertheless, you need to obtain access for fluid resuscitation and pain control, as well as to maintain the child's airway. ...

Ketamine is a drug that is not often used by the average prehospital provider in the United States. However, it is extremely effective when used by advanced providers in air medical services and providers in the military. Ketamine is a derivative of phencyclidine and is often referred to as a *dissociative anesthetic*. Dissociative anesthetics cause a state in which the patient feels "dissociated" from their environment. Ketamine has been used for decades with a proven record of safety. Ketamine is unique among the anesthetic drugs in that the patient can maintain spontaneous ventilation and airway patency.[11]

Many analgesics and sedatives are relatively contraindicated in hypovolemic patients because many agents cause vasodilation and subsequent hypotension. In contrast, ketamine stimulates the cardiovascular system by increasing heart rate and mean arterial blood pressure.

Etomidate (Amidate) is a hypnotic drug that induces a rapid and brief state of deep sleep or unconsciousness. It is most commonly used as an induction agent for rapid-sequence orotracheal intubation. After a bolus of etomidate, the patient is typically ready for intubation within 1 minute, and the duration of the hypnotic state lasts only 3 to 5 minutes. Despite causing unconsciousness, etomidate provides little analgesia.[12] After a dose of etomidate, the patient becomes unconscious and stops most movement.

Just because a patient is not moving when experiencing a painful procedure does not mean the patient is not feeling pain. This is a common misconception.

Administration of etomidate typically does not cause depression of the cardiovascular system.

Propofol (Diprivan) is a drug with few applications in the initial prehospital care of ill or injured patients. However, propofol is commonly used when transporting critically ill patients over long distances. Propofol is used by air ambulance services, interhospital critical care transport services, and military medicine units. For example, a provider may use propofol to keep an intubated patient sedated. A bolus of propofol can be used to induce an almost immediate state of unconsciousness; an infusion is required to maintain that state. Patients are able to wake from unconsciousness rapidly with only minimal confusion. Because propofol is metabolized by both the liver and kidney, the duration of action after a single dose is usually only 2 to 3 minutes. Propofol does not provide the patient any pain relief. Therefore if a patient needs a chest tube, for example, he or she will require analgesics in the form of narcotics.

KETAMINE (KETALAR)

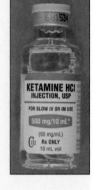

Classification: General anesthetic
Action: Produces a state of anesthesia while maintaining airway reflexes, heart rate, and blood pressure.
Indications: Pain and as anesthesia for procedures of short duration.
Adverse Effects: Emergence phenomena, hypertension and sinus tachycardia, hypotension and sinus bradycardia, other cardiac arrhythmias (rare), respiratory depression, apnea, laryngospasms and other forms of airway obstruction (rare), tonic and clonic movements, vomiting.
Contraindications: Patients in whom a significant elevation in blood pressure would be hazardous (hypertension, stroke, head trauma, increased intracranial mass or bleeding, MI). Use with caution in patients with increased ICP or increased intraocular pressure (glaucoma) and patients with hypovolemia, dehydration, or cardiac disease (especially angina and CHF).
Dosage: Administer slowly over a period of 60 seconds.
IV, IO:

- **Adult:** 1 to 4.5 mg/kg IV, IO. 1 to 2 mg/kg produces anesthesia usually within 30 seconds that typically lasts 5 to 10 minutes.
- **Pediatric:** 0.5 to 2 mg IV, IO over a 1-minute period.

IM:

- **Adult:** 6.5 to 13 mg/kg IM. 10 mg/kg IM is capable of producing anesthesia within 3 to 4 minutes with an effect typically lasting 12 to 25 minutes. In adults, concomitant administration of 5 to 15 mg of diazepam reduces the incidence of emergence phenomena.
- **Pediatric:** 3 to 7 mg IM.

Special Considerations:
Pregnancy class C

ETOMIDATE (AMIDATE)

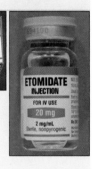

Classification: Hypnotic, anesthesia induction agent
Action: Although the exact mechanism is unknown, etomidate appears to have GABA-like effects.
Indications: Induction for rapid sequence intubation and pharmacologic-assisted intubation, induction of anesthesia.
Adverse Effects: Hypotension, respiratory depression, pain at the site of injection, temporary involuntary muscle movements, frequent nausea/vomiting on emergence, adrenal insufficiency, hyperventilation, hypoventilation, apnea of short duration, hiccups, laryngospasm, snoring, tachypnea, hypertension, cardiac arrhythmias.
Contraindications: Known sensitivity. Use in pregnancy only if the potential benefits justify the potential risk to the fetus. Do not use during labor and avoid in nursing mothers.
Dosage:

- **Adult:** 0.2 to 0.6 mg/kg slow IV, IO (over 30 to 60 seconds). A typical adult intubating dose of etomidate is 20 mg slow IV. Consider less (e.g., 10 mg) in the elderly or patients with cardiac conditions.
- **Pediatric:**
  - **Older than 10 years:** Same as adult dosing.
  - **Younger than 10 years:** Safety has not been established.

Special Considerations:
Etomidate is used to prepare a patient for orotracheal intubation. Both personnel and equipment must be present to manage the patient's airway before administration.
Pregnancy class C

PROPOFOL (DIPRIVAN)

Classification: Anesthetic

Action: Produces rapid and brief state of general anesthesia.

Indications: Anesthesia induction.

Adverse Effects: Apnea, cardiac arrhythmias, asystole, hypotension, hypertension, pain at injection site.

Contraindications: Hypovolemia, known sensitivity (including soybean oil, eggs).

Dosage: A general induction dose used to produce a state of unconsciousness rapidly is 1.5 to 3 mg/kg IV, IO.

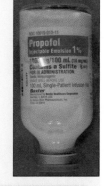

Patient Group	Dosage	Rate of Administration (10 mg/mL)
Healthy adults younger than 55 years	2 to 2.5 mg/kg IV, IO	40 mg every 10 seconds
Elderly or debilitated patients	1 to 1.5 mg/kg IV, IO	20 mg every 10 seconds
Cardiac patients	0.5 to 1.5 mg/kg IV, IO	20 mg every 10 seconds
Patients with head injuries	1 to 2 mg/kg IV, IO	20 mg every 10 seconds
Pediatric (3 to 16 years)	2.5 to 3.5 mg/kg IV, IO	20 mg every 10 seconds

After the induction bolus, the patient must be given intermittent boluses or a maintenance infusion. For an average adult, an intermittent dose is 20 to 50 mg as needed. Alternatively, a propofol infusion may be ordered. Maintenance of anesthesia with a propofol infusion can be achieved by following the following protocols:

· **Adult patients:** 25 to 75 mcg/kg/min IV, IO.
· **Elderly, debilitated, or head-injured patients:** Use approximately 80% of the normal adult dose.
· **Pediatric:** 125 to 300 mcg/kg/min IV, IO.

Special Considerations:

Propofol should be administered only by personnel trained and equipped to manage the patient's airway and provide mechanical ventilation. In elderly and debilitated patients, avoid rapid administration to prevent hypotension, apnea, airway obstruction, and/or oxygen desaturation. Continue to monitor the patient's oxygenation and vital signs and try to limit use of propofol to patients who are intubated. Propofol should not be administered through the same IV catheter as blood or plasma. Pain can occur at the site of injection, which can be minimized by use of larger veins, slower rates of administration, and administration of 1 mL 1% lidocaine before propofol administration.

Propofol is listed as a pregnancy class B; however, propofol should be avoided in pregnant women because it crosses the placenta and can cause neonatal depression.

... The child is badly burned and needs IV fluid resuscitation. Additionally, the child cannot be safely placed in the helicopter in such an agitated state. You estimate that the patient weighs approximately 15 kg. The plan is to administer IM ketamine. Once the child is sedated with the ketamine, then you will start an IV line and continue with analgesia and sedation with IV morphine and midazolam (Versed). Because the patient weighs 15 kg, you administer 45 mg IM (3 mg/kg). Within a few minutes the child begins to calm down and has an almost faraway stare. You place her on the helicopter cot without any objection. You start a peripheral IV in her left arm and some IV fluids. To prevent emergence phenomena and provide some additional sedation, you administer midazolam 1 mg IV. Approximately 15 minutes after administration of the ketamine, the child begins to report severe pain, which you treat with morphine sulfate 2 mg IV push. The remainder of the transport to the hospital goes well. You have to administer 1 mg of morphine immediately before arrival at the hospital.

SEDATIVES (BENZODIAZEPINES)

> You are dispatched to assist a despondent woman. Police are on the scene and have informed dispatch that the patient is hysterical after being informed of the death of a relative. You arrive to find an approximately 35-year-old woman who is crying and cannot be consoled. She has no medical or psychiatric history. Her vital signs are all within normal limits. You obtain additional history and learn that she was recently informed of her brother's death in an airplane crash. You try to control the scene by asking law enforcement to clear the scene of any bystanders. You try talking to her calmly, but your efforts fail. She then starts pounding the wall with her fists to the point at which her hands begin to bleed. Individuals on the scene are concerned that the woman is going to hurt herself and perhaps someone else. Law enforcement begins to talk about physically restraining her, but you are concerned that physical restraints will only frustrate her and make matters worse. You elect to chemically restrain her with an IV sedative. ...

This case represents a patient who is likely to benefit from the administration of a sedative. The most commonly used class of medications that provide sedation are benzodiazepines. Benzodiazepines are also used to reduce anxiety (anxiolytics), relax muscles, and treat seizures. They cause a generalized depression of the CNS. Benzodiazepines have the added benefit of inducing a state of **anterograde amnesia,** or amnesia regarding events occurring after the trauma or disease that caused the condition. Patients who receive a benzodiazepine before an unpleasant procedure or situation are often unable to recall the objectionable event at a later time.

Commonly used benzodiazepine drugs include diazepam (Valium), lorazepam (Ativan), and midazolam (Versed).

In the preceding case, diazepam could be administered as a sedative. After IV administration, diazepam has a rapid onset of CNS effects. It is considered to have a long duration of action, with clinical effects lasting several hours and a half-life ranging from 20 to 70 hours. Diazepam can be quite irritating at the site of injection and can cause inflammation of the vein, or phlebitis. For this reason, diazepam should be injected into larger veins and administered slowly.

Midazolam is a short-acting benzodiazepine with peak sedation occurring in 30 to 60 minutes and a half-life of approximately 2.5 hours. Onset of action is seen in 3 to 5 minutes after IV administration. In the preceding case, midazolam could also be used to provide sedation. When compared with diazepam, patients will have a briefer period of sedation (30 to 60 minutes) after administration of midazolam. Its rapid onset of action and brief duration of action make midazolam an effective medication for use in the prehospital setting.

Lorazepam is used by prehospital providers as a sedative and to reduce anxiety. Like diazepam, lorazepam has a duration of action measured in hours and a half-life of 10 to 20 hours. Studies have shown that lorazepam takes approximately 30 minutes until CNS depression occurs as measured by electroencephalography. This delay in clinical effect, coupled with a prolonged duration of action, limits the prehospital usefulness of this drug.[13]

DIAZEPAM (VALIUM)

Classification: Benzodiazepine; Schedule C-IV
Action: Binds to the benzodiazepine receptor and enhances the effects of GABA. Benzodiazepines act at the level of the limbic, thalamic, and hypothalamic regions of the CNS and can produce any level of CNS depression required (including sedation, skeletal muscle relaxation, and anticonvulsant activity).

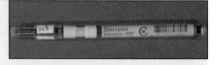

Indications: Anxiety, skeletal muscle relaxation, alcohol withdrawal, seizures.

cont'd

DIAZEPAM (VALIUM)—CONT'D

Adverse Effects: Respiratory depression, drowsiness, fatigue, headache, pain at the injection site, confusion, nausea, hypotension, oversedation.

Contraindications: Children younger than 6 months, acute-angle glaucoma, CNS depression, alcohol intoxication, known sensitivity.

Dosage:

Anxiety:

- **Adult:**
  - **Moderate:** 2 to 5 mg slow IV, IM.
  - **Severe:** 5 to 10 mg slow IV, IM (administer no faster than 5 mg/min).
  - **Low:** Low dosages are often required for elderly or debilitated patients.
- **Pediatric:** 0.04 to 0.3 mg/kg/dose IV, IM every 4 hours to a maximum dose of 0.6 mg/kg.

Delirium Tremens from Acute Alcohol Withdrawal:

- **Adult:** 10 mg IV

Seizure:

- **Adult:** 5 to 10 mg slow IV, IO every 10 to 15 minutes; maximum total dose 30 mg.
- **Pediatric:**
  - **IV, IO:**
    - **5 years and older:** 1 mg over a 3-minute period every 2 to 5 minutes to a maximum total dose of 10 mg.
    - **Older than 30 days to younger than 5 years:** 0.2 to 0.5 mg over a 3-minute period; may repeat every 2 to 5 minutes to a maximum total dose of 5 mg.
    - **Neonate:** 0.1 to 0.3 mg/kg/dose given over a 3- to 5-minute period; may repeat every 15 to 30 minutes to a maximum total dose of 2 mg. (Not a first-line agent due to sodium benzoic acid in the injection.)
  - **Rectal administration:** If vascular access is not obtained, diazepam may be administered rectally to children.
    - **12 years and older:** 0.2 mg/kg.
    - **6 to 11 years:** 0.3 mg/kg.
    - **2 to 5 years:** 0.5 mg/kg.
    - **Younger than 2 years:** Not recommended.

Special Considerations:

Make sure that IV, IO lines are well secured. Extravasation of diazepam causes tissue necrosis.

Diazepam is insoluble in water and must be dissolved in propylene glycol. This produces a viscous solution; give slowly to prevent pain on injection.

Pregnancy class D

MIDAZOLAM (VERSED)

Classification: Benzodiazepine, Schedule C-IV

Action: Binds to the benzodiazepine receptor and enhances the effects of the brain chemical (neurotransmitter) GABA. Benzodiazepines act at the level of the limbic, thalamic, and hypothalamic regions of the CNS to produce short-acting CNS depression (including sedation, skeletal muscle relaxation, and anticonvulsant activity).

Indications: Sedation, anxiety, skeletal muscle relaxation.

Adverse Effects: Respiratory depression, respiratory arrest, hypotension, nausea/vomiting, headache, hiccups, cardiac arrest.

Contraindications: Acute-angle glaucoma, pregnant women, known sensitivity.

Dosage:

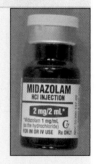

Sedation:

Note: The dose of midazolam needs to be individualized. Every dose should be administered slowly over a period of 2 minutes. Allow 2 minutes to evaluate the clinical effect of the dose given.

- **Adult:**
  - **Healthy and younger than 60 years:** *Some patients require as little as 1 mg IV, IO. No more than 2.5 mg should be given over a 2-minute interval.* If additional sedation is required, continue to administer small increments over 2-minute periods (max dose: 5 mg). If the patient also has received a narcotic, he or she will typically require 30% less midazolam than the same patient not given the narcotic.

cont'd

MIDAZOLAM (VERSED)—CONT'D

- **60 years and older and debilitated or chronically ill patients:** This group of patients has a higher risk of hypoventilation, airway obstruction, and apnea. The peak clinical effect can take longer in these patients; therefore dose increments should be smaller, and the rate of injection should be slower. *Some patients require a dose as small as 1 mg IV, IO, and no more than 1.5 mg should be given over a 2-minute period.* If additional sedation is required, additional midazolam should be given at a rate of no more than 1 mg over a 2-minute period (max dose: 3.5 mg). If the patient also has received a narcotic, he or she will typically require 50% less midazolam than the same patient not given the narcotic.
- **Continuous infusion:** Continuous infusions can be required for prolonged transport of intubated, critically ill, and injured patients. After an initial bolus dose, the adult patient will require a maintenance infusion dose of 0.02 to 0.1 mg/kg/hr (1-7 mg/hr).
- **Pediatric (weight-based):** Pediatric patients typically require higher doses of midazolam than do adults on the basis of weight (in mg/kg). Younger pediatric patients (younger than 6 years) require higher doses (in mg/kg) than older pediatric patients. Midazolam takes approximately 3 minutes to reach peak effect; therefore wait at least 2 minutes to determine effectiveness of drug and need for additional dosing.
  - **12 to 16 years:** Same as adult dosing. Some patients in this age group require a higher dose than that used in adults, but rarely does a patient require more than 10 mg.
  - **6 to 12 years:** 0.025 to 0.05 mg/kg IV, IO up to a total dose of 0.4 mg/kg. Exceeding 10 mg as total dose usually is not necessary.
  - **6 months to 5 years:** 0.05 to 0.1 mg/kg IV, IO up to a total dose of 0.6 mg/kg. Exceeding 6 mg as total dose usually is not necessary.
  - **Younger than 6 months:** Dosing recommendations for this age group is unclear. Because this age group is especially vulnerable to airway obstruction and hypoventilation, use small increments with frequent clinical evaluation. Dose: 0.05 to 0.1 mg/kg IV, IO.

Special Considerations:
Patients receiving midazolam require frequent monitoring of vital signs and pulse oximetry. Be prepared to support patient's airway and ventilation.
Pregnancy class D

LORAZEPAM (ATIVAN)

Classification: Benzodiazepine; Schedule C-IV
Action: Binds to the benzodiazepine receptor and enhances the effects of the brain chemical GABA, an inhibitory transmitter, and may result in a state of sedation, hypnosis, skeletal muscle relaxation, anticonvulsant activity, coma.
Indications: Preprocedure sedation induction, anxiety, status epilepticus.
Adverse Effects: Headache, drowsiness, ataxia, dizziness, amnesia, depression, dysarthria, euphoria, syncope, fatigue, tremor, vertigo, respiratory depression, paradoxical CNS stimulation.
Contraindications: Known sensitivity to lorazepam, benzodiazepines, polyethylene glycol, propylene glycol, or benzyl alcohol; COPD; sleep apnea (except while being mechanically ventilated); shock; coma; acute closed-angle glaucoma.

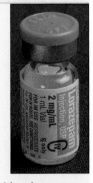

Dosage: Note: IV, IO lorazepam needs to be administered slowly.
Analgesia and Sedation:
- **Adult:** 2 mg or 0.44 mg/kg IV, IO, whichever is smaller. This dosage will provide adequate sedation in most patients and should not be exceeded in patients older than 50 years.
- **Pediatric:** 0.05 mg/kg IV, IO. Each dose should not exceed 2 mg IV, IO.

Seizures:
- **Adult:** 4 mg IV, IO given over 2 to 5 minutes; may repeat in 10 to 15 minutes (max total dose: 8 mg in a 12-hour period).
- **Pediatric:**
  - **Adolescents:** 0.07 mg/kg slow IV, IO given over 2 to 5 minutes (max single dose: 4 mg). May repeat in 10 to 15 minutes (max dose: 8 mg in a 12-hour period).
  - **Children and infants:** 0.1 mg/kg slow IV, IO given over 2 to 5 minutes (max single dose: 4 mg). May repeat at half the original dose in 10 to 15 minutes if seizure activity resumes.
  - **Neonates:** 0.05 mg/kg slow IV, IO given over 2 to 5 minutes. May repeat in 10 to 15 minutes.

Special Considerations:
Be prepared to support the patient's airway and ventilation.
Pregnancy class D

... You administer 2 mg of midazolam slowly by IV to the patient over a 2-minute period. Two to 3 minutes after your initial dose you determine that the patient is still agitated. You decide to give her a second dose of 2 mg of midazolam. She calms down and slowly appears to be falling asleep. You monitor her vital signs; her pulse oximetry reading is 94%. Three minutes later her pulse oximetry reading decreases to 87%. You apply a jaw thrust, insert a nasopharyngeal airway, and use a bag-mask to get her oxygen saturation up to 97%. You retake her vital signs. Her blood pressure has declined from 114/74 to 68/48 mm Hg. ...

The preceding scenario is that of an inadvertent iatrogenic (caused by the medical treatment itself) benzodiazepine overdose. Airway maintenance, assisted ventilations, and IV fluid bolus are necessary in this case. In addition, the benzodiazepine antagonist, flumazenil (Romazicon), is needed for the treatment of benzodiazepine overdose. Flumazenil works by competing with the same receptor used by the benzodiazepines.

Flumazenil does not reverse the excessive sedation or other ill effects of narcotics and other nonbenzodiazepine drugs, and it will not reverse the respiratory depression caused by benzodiazepines.[14] Therefore, in this case, the prehospital provider must continue to provide airway and ventilatory support after administration of flumazenil.

... You administer 0.2 mg flumazenil over a period of 15 seconds and start a bolus of Ringer's lactate. After 1 minute, the patient is still minimally responsive and requires airway and ventilatory assistance. You repeat the dose of 0.2 mg of flumazenil, again over a 15-second period. The patient begins to become more responsive, and her blood pressure begins to improve. You recheck her vital signs. Her blood pressure has improved to 104/76 mm Hg. She is breathing spontaneously, but her respirations remain shallow. You are aware that flumazenil does not reverse the hypoventilation associated with benzodiazepines; therefore you continue to monitor both her airway and vital signs closely for the duration of the transport.

FLUMAZENIL (ROMAZICON)

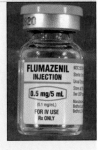

Classification: Benzodiazepine receptor antagonist, antidote
Action: Competes with benzodiazepines for binding at the benzodiazepine receptor, reverses the sedative effects of benzodiazepines.
Indication: Benzodiazepine oversedation
Adverse Effects: Resedation, seizures, dizziness, pain at injection site, nausea/vomiting, diaphoresis, headache, visual impairment.
Contraindications: Cyclic antidepressant overdose; life-threatening conditions that require treatment with benzodiazepines, such as status epilepticus and intracranial hypertension; known sensitivity to flumazenil or benzodiazepines. Use with caution where there is the possibility of unrecognized benzodiazepine dependence and in patients who have a history of substance abuse or who are known substance abusers.
Dosage:
  · **Adult:** Initial dose is 0.2 mg IV, IO over a 15-second period. If the desired effect is not observed after 45 seconds, administer a second 0.2-mg dose, again over a 15-second period. Doses can be repeated a total of four times until a total dose of 1 mg has been administered.
  · **Pediatric:** Children older than 1 year, 0.01 mg/kg IV, IO given over a 15-second period. May repeat in 45 seconds and then every minute to a maximum cumulative dose of 0.05 mg/kg or 1 mg, whichever is the lower dose.
Special Considerations:
Monitor for signs of hypoventilation and hypoxia for approximately 2 hours.
If the half-life of the benzodiazepine is longer than flumazenil, an additional dose may be needed.
May precipitate withdrawal symptoms in patients dependent on benzodiazepines.
Flumazenil has not been shown to benefit patients who have overdosed on multiple drugs.
Pregnancy class C

Naloxone (Narcan) is a **narcotic antagonist** that reverses the effects of opiate narcotics in the event of adverse effects such as CNS and respiratory depression. Naloxone is effective in reversing opiate-induced respiratory depression. However, the effects of this narcotic reversal are relatively short lived, lasting approximately 20 minutes.[15] A second dose of naloxone may be required 20 minutes after the initial dose to prevent the patient from again experiencing opiate-induced respiratory depression.

NALOXONE (NARCAN)

Classification: Opioid antagonist
Action: Binds the opioid receptor and blocks the effect of narcotics.
Indications: Narcotic overdoses, reversal of narcotics used for procedure-related anesthesia.
Adverse Effects: Nausea/vomiting, restlessness, diaphoresis, tachycardia, hypertension, tremulousness, seizures, cardiac arrest, narcotic withdrawal. Patients who have gone from a state of somnolence from a narcotic overdose to wide awake may become combative.
Contraindications: Known sensitivity to naloxone, nalmefene, or naltrexone. Use with caution in patients with supraventricular arrhythmias or other cardiac disease, head trauma, brain tumor.
Dosage:
- **Adult:** 0.4 to 2 mg IV, IO, ET, IM, or Sub-Q. Alternatively, administer 2 mg intranasally. Higher doses (10-20 mg) may be required for overdoses of synthetic narcotics. A repeat dose of one third to two thirds the original dose is often necessary.
- **Pediatric:**
  - **5 years or older or weight >20 kg:** 2 mg IV, IO, ET, IM, or Sub-Q.
  - **Younger than 5 years or weight <20 kg:** 0.1 mg/kg IV, IO, ET, IM, or Sub-Q; may repeat every 2 to 3 minutes.

Special Considerations:
Pregnancy class C

ANTIEMETICS

Y|ou are called to the home of a 36-year-old man who reports several hours of excruciating abdominal pain. The patient tells you that he has had the pain for several hours. It is localized to the lower midline portion of the abdomen, and he is unable to stand or walk because of the severity of the pain. Your assessment reveals an otherwise healthy man who is lying in the fetal position in pain. His abdomen is rigid and extremely tender to any type of touch or manipulation. The patient is having dry heaves, which are aggravating his severe discomfort. You consult medical direction and obtain authorization to administer morphine 4 mg IV, as well as an antiemetic. Once inside the ambulance, you administer 12.5 mg of promethazine slow IV push. The patient has significant improvement in his nausea, his dry heaves stop, and his pain is significantly decreased.

Antiemetics are a class of drugs used to treat nausea and vomiting, which are common adverse effects of the administration of narcotics analgesics. In emergency departments and hospitals, narcotics and antiemetics are often administered simultaneously to prevent the patient from experiencing the discomfort of nausea and vomiting. These agents can also be used to treat nausea and vomiting caused by conditions unrelated to the administration of narcotics. Common antiemetics are promethazine and dolasetron.

Promethazine (Phenergan) is often used to prevent or control nausea and vomiting. It is also used as an adjunct for the control of pain. This class of drugs is typically used for prevention of chemotherapy-associated nausea and nausea that fails to respond to treatment with promethazine. Dolasetron (Anzemet) is a **5-HT$_3$ receptor antagonist** used to prevent nausea and vomiting.

PROMETHAZINE (PHENERGAN)

Classification: Antiemetic, antihistamine
Action: Decreases nausea and vomiting by antagonizing H_1 receptors.
Indications: Nausea/vomiting
Adverse Effects: Paradoxic excitation in children and elderly patients.
Contraindications: Altered level of consciousness, jaundice, bone marrow suppression, known sensitivity. Use with caution in seizure disorder.
Dosage:
- **Adult:** 12.5 to 25 mg IV, IO or IM.
- **Pediatric:**
  - **2 years and older:** 0.25 to 1 mg/kg IV, IO, IM (maximum rate of IV, IO administration is 25 mg/min).

Special Considerations:
Pregnancy class C

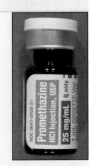

DOLASETRON (ANZEMET)

Classification: Antiemetic
Action: Prevents/reduces nausea/vomiting by binding and blocking a receptor for the brain chemical serotonin.
Indications: Prevent and treat nausea/vomiting.
Adverse Effects: Headache, fatigue, diarrhea, dizziness, abdominal pain, hypotension, hypertension, ECG changes (prolonged PR and QT intervals, widened QRS), bradycardia, tachycardia, syncope.
Contraindications: Known sensitivity. Use with caution in hypokalemia, hypomagnesemia, cardiac arrhythmias.
Dosage:
- **Adult:** 12.5 mg IV, IO.
- **Pediatric: 2 to 16 years:** 0.35 mg/kg IV, IO (max dose: 12.5 mg).

Special Considerations:
Pregnancy class B

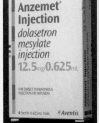
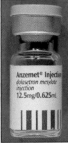

REVIEW QUESTIONS

1. Analgesics are used to treat what condition?
2. Discuss why, despite the frequency of patient reports of pain, it is often not treated in the field.
3. How does morphine produce hypotension?
4. Which narcotic is less likely to produce hypotension in a hypovolemic patient?
5. Explain the risks of administering narcotics to a patient with abdominal pain.
6. What NSAID analgesic can be administered parenterally?
7. List the advantages of nitrous oxide administration in pain management.
8. What class of medications is used to produce sedation?
9. Define antegrade amnesia and identify the class of medications that can produce this effect.
10. Explain why antiemetics may be necessary in the treatment of pain.

REFERENCES

1. Turturro MA, et al: Intramuscular ketorolac versus oral ibuprofen in acute musculoskeletal pain, *Ann Emerg Med* 26:117, 1995.
2. Cordell WH, et al: Comparison of intravenous ketorolac, meperidine, and both (balanced analgesia) for renal colic, *Ann Emerg Med* 28:151, 1996.
3. Annequin D, et al: Fixed 50% nitrous oxide mixture for painful procedures: a French survey, *Pediatrics* 105:850, 2000.
4. Burton JH, et al: Effectiveness of 50% nitrous oxide/50% oxygen during laceration repair in children, *Acad Emerg Med* 5:112, 1998.

5. Wattenmaker I, Kasser JR, McGravey A: Self-administered nitrous oxide for fracture reduction in children in an emergency room setting, *J Orthop Trauma* 4:35, 1990.
6. Eisele JH: Cardiovascular effects of nitrous oxide. In Eger II EI, editor: *Nitrous oxide,* New York, 1985, Elsevier, pp 125-156.
7. White LJ, et al: Prehospital use of analgesia for suspected extremity fractures, *Prehosp Emerg Care* 4:205, 2000.
8. Borland ML, Jacobs I, Rogers IR: Options in prehospital analgesia, *Emerg Med* 14:77, 2002.
9. Paris PM, Yealy DM: Pain management. In Marx J, Hockberger R, Walls R: *Rosen's emergency medicine: concepts and clinical practice,* ed 6, Philadelphia, 2005, Mosby.
10. Munson ES: Transfer of nitrous oxide into body air cavities, *Br J Anaesth* 46:202, 1974.
11. Roberts FW: A new intramuscular anesthetic for small children: a report of clinical trials of CI-581, *Anesthesia* 22:23, 1967.
12. Van Hamme MJ, Ghoneim NM, Amber JJ: Pharmacokinetics of etomidate, a new intravenous anesthetic, *Anesthesiology* 49:274, 1978.
13. Greenblatt DJ, Ehrenberg BL, Gunderman: Pharmacokinetic and electroencephalographic study of intravenous diazepam, midazolam, and placebo, *Clin Pharmacol Ther* 45:356, 1989.
14. Abramowicz M: Flumazenil, *Med Lett* 34:66, 1992.
15. Anderson R, Dobloug I, Refstad S: Postanesthetic use of naloxone hydrochloride after moderate doses of fentanyl, *Acta Anaesth Scand* 20:255, 1976.

Anaphylaxis

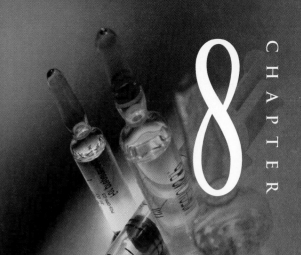

OBJECTIVES

1. List the symptoms of anaphylactic shock.
2. Discuss the role of the immune system in fighting antigens.
3. Define an allergic response.
4. Describe the body's response to a foreign substance.
5. Identify the most common cause of death from anaphylaxis.
6. Discuss medications used to treat anaphylaxis: epinephrine, epinephrine autoinjectors (EpiPen and EpiPen Jr), albuterol (Proventil, Ventolin), diphenhydramine hydrochloride (Benadryl), hydrocortisone (Solu-Cortef), and methylprednisolone (Solu-Medrol).
7. Demonstrate the proper procedure for using an EpiPen.

Medications that Appear in Chapter 8

Epinephrine
Epinephrine autoinjectors (EpiPen, EpiPen Jr)
Albuterol (Proventil, Ventolin)
Diphenhydramine hydrochloride (Benadryl)
Hydrocortisone sodium succinate (Cortef, Solu-Cortef)
Methylprednisolone sodium succinate (Solu-Medrol)

INTRODUCTION

Anaphylaxis and allergic reactions are included in a wider group of conditions called **hypersensitivity reactions.** Anaphylaxis, an exaggerated hypersensitivity reaction to a previously encountered **antigen,** is a potentially life-threatening series of events that affects multiple body systems. **Anaphylactic shock** is a serious and rapid allergic reaction that can be severe enough to result in death. The symptoms of anaphylactic shock include shortness of breath, syncope, itching, swelling of the throat, and a sudden drop in blood pressure. Anaphylactic shock causes hundreds of deaths each year in the United States. The **allergic responses** most often are stimulated by drugs such as penicillin or insect bites and stings. For prehospital providers to give optimal care to the patient experiencing anaphylaxis, they must understand the mechanism and the pharmacologic treatment necessary to prevent and resolve this life-threatening condition.

You respond to a call for a man in respiratory distress. The address is a local football field. It is a warm, sunny day. As you walk on the field, you notice bees swarming around garbage cans and discarded beverage cans. You find the patient, a 32-year-old man, sitting against a concession stand in the shade. He is wheezing audibly and is in obvious distress. His skin is warm and flushed. His wife tells you a bee stung him, and he is allergic to stings. She states that he is supposed to carry a medication pack for this type of situation, but he never got the prescription filled. ...

OVERVIEW OF ANAPHYLAXIS

IMMUNE RESPONSE

The body's normal defense against intruding antigens (substances that invade the body and induce the formation of **antibodies**) or infection is the immune system. The immune system can be considered the body's "smart bombs." Imagine a solider on a battlefield who marks a target with a special laser. A smart bomb or missile can focus on that target and selectively destroy it. In the same way the immune system selectively identifies targets for destruction. When functioning normally, the body produces antibodies, which are protective protein substances that bind to antigens and neutralize or remove them. The antibodies essentially allow special killer cells to identify and destroy those identified targets.

ALLERGIC RESPONSE

An allergic response is brought about by a hypersensitivity to a particular antigen out of proportion to its hazard to the body. The allergic response, not the antigen, is the real threat. Human beings can be hypersensitive or allergic to a variety of things: animals, vegetables, and minerals (Box 8-1). In fact, people can be sensitive to almost anything, including medications, foods, and even dust. Materials that can induce a hypersensitivity or allergic reaction are known as **allergens.**

> Foreign materials that initiate a normal immune response are antigens; antigens that produce an exaggerated allergic reaction are allergens.

Individuals with allergies to an agent should avoid contact with the allergen and be medically prepared to treat inadvertent exposure. In many individuals, an accidental exposure to an allergen may cause a rapidly developing, life-threatening condition; these individuals need to carry medication to be administered in case of exposure.

BOX 8-1

COMMON ALLERGENS

Foods	Drugs
Milk	Antibiotics (e.g., cephalosporins, tetracyclines, penicillin, streptomycin,
Egg whites	neomycin, bacitracin)
Shellfish	Aspirin
Beans	
Nuts	**Insect Bites and Stings**
Citrus fruits	Honeybees
Bananas	Yellow jackets
Fish	Wasps
Chocolate	Hornets
Chamomile tea	Fire ants
Grains	
Sulfites	

MECHANISMS OF AN ANAPHYLACTIC REACTION

When a hypersensitive person is exposed to an allergen, cells within the body release the chemicals **histamine, serotonin, bradykinin,** and **slow-reacting substance of anaphylaxis.** The chief chemical among these is histamine. The release of histamine causes vasodilation, increased capillary permeability, and smooth muscle spasm. These effects cause the signs and symptoms of an allergic reaction, and the magnitude of this response determines whether the patient has an allergic reaction or anaphylaxis. Allergic responses can be minor, affecting only one body system, or severe, affecting multiple organ systems and even causing shock from respiratory and circulatory complications. The typical allergic response involves skin rashes, hives (urticaria), itching, redness, and edema (Fig. 8-1). The patient can feel warm and flushed, exhibit edema of the lips and eyelids, and have watery eyes.

When confronted with a patient having a mild allergic response, determining whether the patient will progress to anaphylactic shock is not possible. However, always assume the potential for the development of shock and closely monitor the patient so that quick action can arrest or reverse anaphylaxis. Patients in anaphylaxis are having a serious medical event and require immediate intervention.

> The most common cause of death from an allergic reaction is obstruction of the airway.

Although rash and hives are the most common manifestations of an allergic reaction, more severe complications can arise quickly and without warning. The signs and symptoms of a more serious anaphylactic reaction are best understood by reviewing the body's responses to invading foreign substances, including the following (Fig. 8-2):

- After a foreign invader or material has been targeted, various cells attack the invader, releasing various chemicals—principally histamine.
- What distinguishes a normal immune response from an anaphylactic reaction is the magnitude of the chemical release.
- Histamine causes vasodilation, increased capillary permeability, and smooth muscle spasm.
- Vasodilation results in a drop in the systemic blood pressure and a decrease in peripheral tissue perfusion and oxygen delivery.
- Spasm of smooth muscle produces diarrhea, vomiting, and laryngospasm.
- Increased capillary permeability results in edema of the airway. The most common cause of death from an allergic reaction is obstruction of the airway.

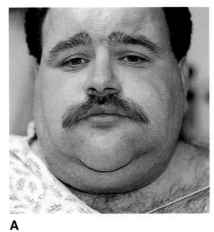 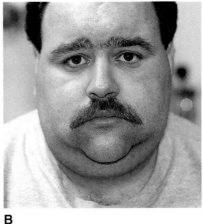

A   **B**

▼ **Fig. 8-1**   Patient with anaphylaxis. **A,** Patient has hives and swelling of the face and lips. **B,** After treatment with epinephrine and antihistamines. (From Henry M, Stapleton E: *EMT prehospital care,* ed 3 rev, St Louis, 2007, Mosby.)

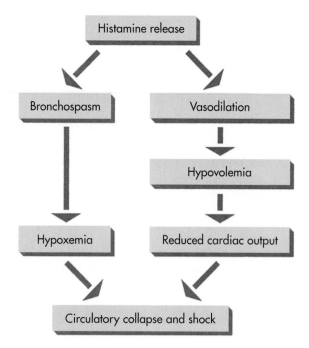

▼ **Fig. 8-2**   Pathophysiology of anaphylactic shock. (From Sanders M: *Mosby's paramedic textbook,* ed 3 rev, St Louis, 2007, Mosby.)

The faster the onset of symptoms of an allergic reaction, the more serious the threat to life.

Most patients begin to show symptoms within minutes to an hour after exposure. The faster the onset of symptoms, the more serious the threat to life. As the condition progresses, laryngoedema can cause varying degrees of airway obstruction along with tightness in the chest, shortness of breath, and lightheadedness. Continuing development of anaphylaxis can be accompanied by a decrease in the level of consciousness, respiratory distress, and circulatory collapse. When a patient having an allergic reaction reports hoarseness or describes a "full feeling," the provider should assume the patient is progressing toward life-threatening anaphylaxis.

The patient's history often confirms the diagnosis of allergic response and anaphylaxis. While monitoring the airway and respiratory status, a history of allergies and any recent exposure should be obtained. In the event that the material the patient has been exposed to is still present, decontamination or removal of the substance from the patient should be accomplished immediately.

Management

With the knowledge that most deaths caused by allergy are the result of airway obstruction, rapid and thorough assessment of the airway and breathing is of utmost importance. Patients with airway or ventilatory deficits should be assisted as their history is obtained. If the patient's airway is rapidly collapsing, **intubation** must be considered. Rapidly developing edema can make intubation impossible after the airway obstructs.

The first-line medication for anaphylaxis is epinephrine 1:10,000 IV push. Epinephrine is a catecholamine that stimulates alpha-adrenergic and beta-adrenergic receptors. This increases the rate and force of heart contractions, increasing cardiac output, and relaxes bronchial smooth muscle. By relaxing smooth muscle, lung capacity is enhanced. Edema in the bronchioles is reduced by constriction of the arterioles of the bronchioles. Epinephrine also causes peripheral vasoconstriction, which raises the arterial blood pressure.

Epinephrine should be administered as quickly as possible; waiting to start an IV line to administer epinephrine often is not prudent. Therefore, in the treatment of an allergic reaction and anaphylaxis, consider epinephrine administration by an alternative route. Epinephrine 1:10,000 can be given through the endotracheal tube, or epinephrine 1:1000 can be given as a Sub-Q or IM injection. The IM route is preferred because the epinephrine is more rapidly absorbed by that route than by the Sub-Q route.

What is the difference between epinephrine 1:1000 and 1:10,000?
The two forms of epinephrine refer to the concentration, or potency, of the solution. Epinephrine 1:10,000 is 10 times more diluted than the epinephrine 1:1000 solution.

Why is one preparation used for intravenous use and another for subcutaneous and intramuscular use?
For IV administration, the more diluted preparation of epinephrine is used: 1:10,000. When the medication is injected using Sub-Q or IM methods, it is not being delivered directly to the circulatory system. For Sub-Q and IM injection, use the more concentrated, or more potent, 1:1000 preparation.

Once patients have a significant allergic reaction, they often are prescribed an epinephrine autoinjector (EpiPen or EpiPen Jr), which is an epinephrine self-injection system. This system allows patients to inject themselves, even through clothing, with an amount of epinephrine that should decrease their symptoms in time to seek medical attention. In many EMS systems, basic and intermediate providers are trained and permitted to help patients self-administer epinephrine with these devices.

 ## USE OF THE EPIPEN

Equipment needed:
EpiPen, sharps, PPE
Procedure:
1. Unscrew the cap from the carrying case and remove the EpiPen.
2. The black tip of the EpiPen is where the needle comes out. Hold the EpiPen with the black tip pointing downward.
3. With the other hand, remove the gray safety release on the other end of the EpiPen.
4. Hold the black tip near the outer portion of the thigh. The autoinjector is designed to work through clothing. Do not inject into any area other than the outer thigh.
5. With a swinging motion of your arm, jab the EpiPen into the outer portion of the thigh so that the EpiPen clicks and the unit is perpendicular to the thigh.
6. Hold the autoinjector in place for 10 seconds. The color in the window of the autoinjector will change from clear to red, indicating completion of the injection.
7. Remove the autoinjector and massage the area for 10 seconds.

The next concern in treating anaphylaxis is maintaining circulatory integrity. Infusions of crystalloids, normal saline, or Ringer's lactate solution should be given to maintain sufficient volume in the vascular space to promote adequate perfusion. This usually means an initial bolus of 1 to 2 L of fluids in patients with hypotension.

EPINEPHRINE

Classification: Adrenergic agent, inotropic
Action: Binds strongly with both alpha and beta receptors, producing increased blood pressure, increased heart rate, bronchodilation.
Indications: Bronchospasm, allergic and anaphylactic reactions, restoration of cardiac activity in cardiac arrest.
Adverse Effects: Anxiety, headache, cardiac arrhythmias, hypertension, nervousness, tremors, chest pain, nausea/vomiting.
Contraindications: Arrhythmias other than VF, asystole, PEA; cardiovascular disease; hypertension; cerebrovascular disease; shock secondary to causes other than anaphylactic shock; closed-angle glaucoma; diabetes; pregnant women in active labor; known sensitivity to epinephrine or sulfites.

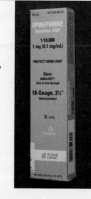
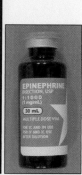

Dosage:
Cardiac Arrest:
- **Adult:** 1 mg (1:10,000 solution) IV, IO; may repeat every 3 to 5 minutes.
- **Pediatric:** 0.01 mg/kg (1:10,000 solution) IV, IO; repeat every 3 to 5 minutes as needed (max dose: 1 mg).

Symptomatic Bradycardia:
- **Adult:** 1 mcg/min (1:10,000 solution) as a continuous IV infusion; usual dosage range: 2 to 10 mcg/min IV; titrate to effect.
- **Pediatric:** 0.01 mg/kg (1:10,000 solution) IV, IO; may repeat every 3 to 5 minutes (max dose: 1 mg). If giving epinephrine by ET tube, administer 0.1 mg/kg.

Asthma Attacks and Certain Allergic Reactions:
- **Adult:** 0.3 to 0.5 mg (1:1000 solution) IM or Sub-Q; may repeat every 10 to 15 minutes (max dose: 1 mg).
- **Pediatric:** 0.01 mg/kg (1:1000 solution) IM or Sub-Q (max dose: 0.5 mg).

Anaphylactic Shock:
- **Adult:** 0.1 mg (1:10,000 solution) IV slowly over 5 minutes, or IV infusion of 1 to 4 mcg/min, titrated to effect.
- **Pediatric:** Continuous IV infusion rate of 0.1 to 1 mcg/kg/min (1:10,000 solution); titrate to response.

Special Considerations:
Half-life 1 minute
Pregnancy class C

EPINEPHRINE AUTOINJECTORS (EPIPEN, EPIPEN JR)

Classification: Adrenergic agonist, inotropic
Action: Binds strongly with both alpha and beta receptors, producing increased blood pressure, increased heart rate, bronchodilation.
Indications: Anaphylactic shock, certain allergic reactions, asthma attacks.
Adverse Effects: Headaches, nervousness, tremors, arrhythmias, hypertension, chest pain, nausea/vomiting.
Contraindications: Arrhythmias other than VF, asystole, PEA; cardiovascular disease; hypertension; cerebrovascular disease; shock secondary to causes other than anaphylactic shock; closed-angle glaucoma; diabetes; pregnant women in active labor; known sensitivity to epinephrine or sulfites.

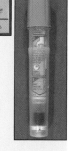

Dosage:
- **Adult:** An EpiPen contains 0.3 mg epinephrine to be administered IM into the anterolateral thigh area.
- **Pediatric:** For children weighing <30 kg, an EpiPen Jr delivers 0.15 mg IM.

Special Considerations:
Half-life 1 minute
Pregnancy class C

... After placing the patient on 100% oxygen by a nonrebreather mask, you obtain IV access. Vital signs are respiratory rate of 30 breaths/min and shallow, pulse of 120 beats/min, and blood pressure of 90/60 mm Hg. The patient's continued distress causes you to suspect he is progressing to anaphylaxis, so you prepare to administer 0.3 to 0.5 mg of 1:10,000 epinephrine IV push. You also rapidly infuse 500 mL crystalloids for his hypotension. You follow the epinephrine with 50 mg of diphenhydramine IV push over a 2- to 3-minute period. With his continuing respiratory distress, you choose to administer 2.5 mg albuterol by **nebulizer.** The patient begins to improve, and you load him into the ambulance. While transporting, you contact medical direction and communicate the patient report. As you continue to monitor the patient, you prepare to repeat dosages of the medications already delivered because your protocol allows at least one repeat dose of the epinephrine and albuterol after 5 minutes if needed.

Second-line medications can include antihistamines, corticosteroids, and bronchodilators. Antihistamines should be administered to all patients who have had an anaphylactic reaction. Diphenhydramine is the most commonly used antihistamine. It controls the histamine release and, in turn, the allergic response to the antigen. Methylprednisolone and hydrocortisone frequently are used to reduce edema and limit the recurrence of symptoms. Steroids are not helpful in the acute treatment of anaphylaxis, but they do prevent some of the later reactions of an allergic response.

For continuing respiratory distress, nebulizer treatments of bronchodilators such as albuterol frequently are used. Many prehospital protocols do not include the use of steroids, but most use epinephrine, crystalloid infusions, diphenhydramine, and albuterol or other bronchodilating medications. The use of steroids is more prevalent in protocols for extended transport times, such as prolonged interhospital ground transport and air medical services.

Albuterol (Proventil, Ventolin) is a direct-acting beta-adrenergic bronchodilator. By stimulating $beta_2$ receptors, albuterol causes bronchodilation. In the case of the bee sting victim having an anaphylactic reaction, albuterol relaxes the bronchial smooth muscle that has been thrown into spasm by the release of histamine.

Diphenhydramine hydrochloride (Benadryl) is also used to treat anaphylactic reactions because it competes with histamine for H_1 receptor sites and has significant anticholinergic properties. Diphenhydramine blocks the effects of histamine, including vasodilation, increased gastrointestinal tract secretions, increased heart rate, and hypotension.

Hydrocortisone (Solu-Cortef) is a corticosteroid that has antiinflammatory properties. It is used in the treatment of allergic reactions, anaphylaxis, asthma, and chronic obstructive pulmonary disease. Although hydrocortisone generally is not helpful in the acute treatment of anaphylaxis, it does help prevent some of the later complications of laryngoedema and urticaria. As a prehospital drug, hydrocortisone generally is used only during extended transports as a single dose.

Methylprednisolone (Solu-Medrol) is a corticosteroid that decreases the body's inflammatory response and suppresses the immune system. It is used to treat severe anaphylaxis, asthma, and chronic obstructive pulmonary disease.

ALBUTEROL (PROVENTIL, VENTOLIN)

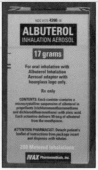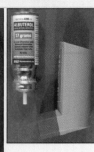

Classification: Bronchodilator, beta agonist
Action: Binds and stimulates beta$_2$ receptors, resulting in relaxation of bronchial smooth muscle.
Indications: Asthma, bronchitis with bronchospasm, and COPD.
Adverse Effects: Hyperglycemia, hypokalemia, palpitations, sinus tachycardia, anxiety, tremor, nausea/vomiting, throat irritation, dry mouth, hypertension, dyspepsia, insomnia, headache, epistaxis, paradoxical bronchospasm.
Contraindications: Angioedema, sensitivity to albuterol or levalbuterol. Use with caution in lactating patients, cardiovascular disorders, cardiac arrhythmias.
Dosage:
Acute Bronchospasm:
- **Adult:**
  - **MDI:** 4 to 8 puffs every 1 to 4 hours may be required.
  - **Nebulizer:** 2.5 to 5 mg every 20 minutes for a maximum of three doses. After the initial three doses, escalate the dose or start a continuous nebulization at 10 to 15 mg/hr.
- **Pediatric:**
  - **MDI:**
    - **4 years and older:** 2 inhalations every 4 to 6 hours; however, in some patients, 1 inhalation every 4 hours is sufficient. More frequent administration or more inhalations are not recommended.
    - **Younger than 4 years:** Administer by nebulization.
  - **Nebulizer:**
    - **Older than 12 years:** The dose for a continuous nebulization is 0.5 mg/kg/hr.
    - **Younger than 12 years:** 0.15 mg/kg every 20 minutes for a maximum of three doses. Alternatively, continuous nebulization at 0.5 mg/kg/hr can be delivered to children younger than 12 years.

Asthma in Pregnancy:
- **MDI:** Two inhalations every 4 hours. In acute exacerbation, start with 2 to 4 puffs every 20 minutes.
- **Nebulizer:** 2.5 mg (0.5 mL) by 0.5% nebulization solution. Place 0.5 mL of the albuterol solution in 2.5 mL of sterile normal saline. Flow is regulated to deliver the therapy over a 5- to 20-minute period. In refractory cases, some physicians order 10 mg nebulized over a 60-minute period.

Special Considerations:
Pregnancy class C

DIPHENHYDRAMINE HYDROCHLORIDE (BENADRYL)

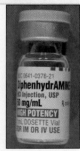

Classification: Antihistamine
Action: Binds and blocks H$_1$ histamine receptors.
Indications: Anaphylactic reactions
Adverse Effects: Drowsiness, dizziness, headache, excitable state (children), wheezing, thickening of bronchial secretions, chest tightness, palpitations, hypotension, blurred vision, dry mouth, nausea/vomiting, diarrhea.
Contraindications: Acute asthma, which thickens secretions; patients with cardiac histories; known sensitivity.
Dosage:
- **Adult:** 25 to 50 mg IV, IO, IM.
- **Pediatric: 2 to 12 years:** 1 to 1.25 mg/kg IV, IO, IM.
Special Considerations:
Pregnancy class B

HYDROCORTISONE SODIUM SUCCINATE (CORTEF, SOLU-CORTEF)

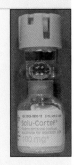

Classification: Corticosteroid
Action: Reduces inflammation by multiple mechanisms. As a steroid, it replaces the steroids that are lacking in adrenal insufficiency.
Indications: Adrenal insufficiency, allergic reactions, anaphylaxis, asthma, COPD.
Adverse Effects: Leukocytosis, hyperglycemia, increased infection, decreased wound healing, increased rate of death from sepsis.
Contraindications: Cushing's syndrome, known sensitivity to benzyl alcohol. Use with caution in diabetes, hypertension, CHF, known systemic fungal infection, renal disease, idiopathic thrombocytopenia, psychosis, seizure disorder, GI disease, glaucoma, known sensitivity.
Dosage:
Anaphylactic Shock:
 · **Adult:** 100 to 500 mg IV, IO, or IM.
 · **Pediatric:** 2 to 4 mg/kg/day IV, IO, or IM (max: 500 mg).
Adrenal Insufficiency:
 · **Adult:** 100 to 500 mg IV, IO, or IM.
 · **Pediatric:** 1 to 2 mg/kg IV, IO, or IM.
Asthma and Chronic Obstructive Pulmonary Disease:
 · **Adult:** 100 to 500 mg IV, IO, IM.
 · **Pediatric:** 1 mg/kg IV, IO. The dose may be reduced for infants and children, but it is governed more by the severity of the condition and response of the patient than by age or body weight. Dose should not be less than 25 mg daily.
Special Considerations:
Pregnancy class C

METHYLPREDNISOLONE SODIUM SUCCINATE (SOLU-MEDROL)

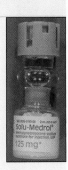

Classification: Corticosteroid
Action: Reduces inflammation by multiple mechanisms.
Indications: Anaphylaxis, asthma, COPD.
Adverse Effects: Depression, euphoria, headache, restlessness, hypertension, bradycardia, nausea/vomiting, swelling, diarrhea, weakness, fluid retention, paresthesias.
Contraindications: Cushing's syndrome, fungal infection, measles, varicella, known sensitivity (including sulfites). Use with caution in active infections, renal disease, penetrating spinal cord injury, hypertension, seizures, CHF.
Dosage:
Asthma and Chronic Obstructive Pulmonary Disease:
 · **Adult:** 40 to 80 mg IV.
 · **Pediatric:** 1 mg/kg (up to 60 mg) IV, IO per day in two divided doses.
Anaphylactic Shock:
 · **Adult:** 1 to 2 mg/kg/dose, then 0.5 to 1 mg/kg every 6 hours.
 · **Pediatric:** Same as adult dosing.
Blunt Spinal Cord Injury:
 · **Adult:** 30 mg/kg IV, IO over a period of 1 hour, then as an infusion to run for the remaining 23 hours at a dose of 5.4 mg/kg/hr.
 · **Pediatric:** Same as adult dosing.
Special Considerations:
May mask signs and symptoms of infection.
Pregnancy class C

REVIEW QUESTIONS

1. List the symptoms of anaphylactic shock.
2. Explain why the allergic response and not the antigen is the greater threat in a hypersensitivity reaction.
3. What is the principal chemical released by the body that produces many of the symptoms of anaphylaxis?
4. What is the most common cause of death from anaphylaxis?
5. What is the suspected diagnosis of a patient reporting difficulty breathing and swelling of the lips who remembers a reaction to seafood several years ago?
6. What is the first line of drug therapy for the patient in anaphylaxis?
7. What are the effects of epinephrine on smooth muscle and blood vessels?
8. What is the handheld form of epinephrine prescribed to patients for home use?

BIBLIOGRAPHY

Kasper D, et al: *Harrison's principles of internal medicine,* ed 16, New York, 2005, McGraw-Hill.

Kemp SF, Lockey RF: Anaphylaxis: a review of causes and mechanisms, *J Allergy Clin Immunol* 110:341, 2002.

McCance K, Huether S: *Pathophysiology, the biologic basis for disease in adults and children,* ed 5, St Louis, 2005, Mosby.

Pons P, Cason D: *Paramedic field care—a complaint based approach,* St Louis, 1997, Mosby.

Stewart AG, Ewan PW: The incidence, etiology, and management of anaphylaxis presenting to an accident and emergency department, *Q J Med* 89:859, 1996.

Tintinalli JE, Kelen GD, Stapcyzynski JS: *Emergency medicine: a comprehensive study guide,* ed 6, New York, 2004, McGraw-Hill.

Winberry SL, Lieberman PL: Histamine and antihistamines in anaphylaxis, *Clin Allergy Immunol* 17:287, 2002.

Cardiac Arrhythmias

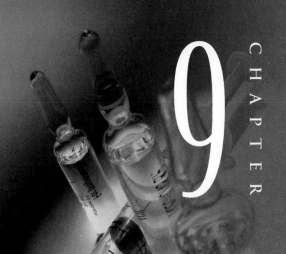

OBJECTIVES

1. Define electrical therapy.
2. Explain why electrical therapy is the preferred initial therapy over drug administration for cardiac arrest and some arrhythmias.
3. Discuss medications used to treat symptomatic bradycardia: atropine sulfate, epinephrine, and dopamine.
4. Discuss adenosine (Adenocard) and its role in the treatment of supraventricular tachycardia.
5. List and discuss three classes of antiarrhythmic agents.
6. Discuss the beta blocker atenolol (Tenormin), anticoagulant warfarin (Coumadin), and calcium channel blockers diltiazem (Cardizem) and verapamil (Isoptin).
7. Explain the benefit of beta blockers in the treatment of arrhythmias.
8. Discuss the following ventricular antiarrhythmic agents: amiodarone (Cordarone), lidocaine (Xylocaine), procainamide (Pronestyl), and magnesium sulfate.
9. Discuss medications used to treat pulseless electrical activity and asystole: epinephrine and vasopressin.

Medications that Appear in Chapter 9

Atropine sulfate
Epinephrine
Dopamine (Intropin)
Adenosine (Adenocard)
Diltiazem (Cardizem)
Verapamil (Isoptin)
Propranolol (Inderal)
Metoprolol (Lopressor, Toprol XL)
Atenolol (Tenormin)
Esmolol (Brevibloc)
Amiodarone (Cordarone)
Lidocaine (Xylocaine)
Procainamide (Pronestyl)
Magnesium sulfate
Vasopressin

INTRODUCTION

Cardiac **arrhythmias,** the loss or abnormality of cardiac rhythms, are commonly encountered in the prehospital setting. A particular arrhythmia can be longstanding, such as chronic **atrial fibrillation,** or it can be the reason that 9-1-1 was called, such as a cardiac arrest caused by **ventricular fibrillation.** Prehospital professionals must be familiar with the most commonly used antiarrhythmic agents and be proficient in administration of

Y ou receive a 9-1-1 call for a patient who had a syncopal episode. You arrive to find a 72-year-old man who is awake and talking. He reports to you that he feels dizzy, and he denies any chest pain or shortness of breath. You take a pulse while your partner places the patient on the cardiac monitor/defibrillator. The pulse feels slow, and when the patient is on the monitor you note that his rhythm is a sinus bradycardia at a rate of 48 beats/min. ...

medications used to provide advanced cardiac life support. In this chapter, we will discuss therapies to manage various cardiac arrhythmias.

BASIC ELECTROPHYSIOLOGY

The heart is a complex muscular organ composed of four smaller pumps. Each pump is made up of millions of cardiac muscle cells, and each cell is capable of contracting independently. For the heart to pump blood effectively, the muscle cells and the four chambers of the heart must work in a coordinated fashion. The muscle cells composing the four chambers must contract at precise moments. This complex process is coordinated by the heart's electrical system. Under normal conditions, an electrical impulse originates in the sinoatrial (SA) node and travels through the heart's electrical system in a predictable fashion. As each impulse moves through the heart, it signals each portion of the heart to contract in the required organized fashion. These electrical impulses coordinating cardiac contraction give the heart its rhythm. When electrical impulses controlling cardiac contraction are too slow, too fast, or irregular, the heart chambers do not contract in an organized fashion, the amount of blood pumped by the heart (cardiac output) drops, and the blood pressure falls.

OVERVIEW OF ARRHYTHMIAS

In the previous case, the patient's heart is in sinus bradycardia (Fig. 9-1). Cardiac output (CO) is determined by the patient's heart rate (HR) multiplied by the amount of blood pumped with each heartbeat (stroke volume [SV]).

$$CO = HR \times SV$$

The decrease in the heart rate causes a drop in cardiac output, producing reduced blood flow in the brain, which then causes the patient to experience dizziness and syncope.

A cardiac rhythm that is a common cause for out-of-hospital cardiac arrest is ventricular fibrillation (VF) (Fig. 9-2). VF has been described as a "bag of worms," referring to a situation in which all the cardiac cells are trying to contract independently and are not cooperating or communicating with one another. The aim of **electrical therapy** is to reset the heart and cause all the cardiac cells to pause and restart in an organized fashion. This allows a stable rhythm to be reestablished.

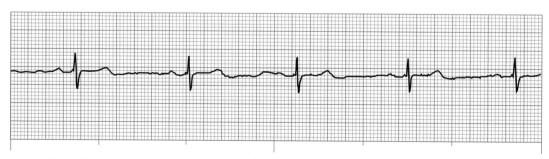

▼ **Fig. 9-1** Sinus bradycardia. (From Aehlert B: *ECGs made easy,* ed 3, St Louis, 2006, Mosby.)

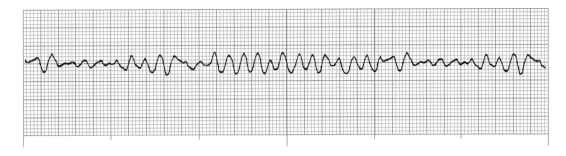

▼ **Fig. 9-2**   Ventricular fibrillation. (From Aehlert B: *ECGs made easy,* ed 3, St Louis, 2006, Mosby.)

Cardiac arrest is usually caused by the sudden onset of a cardiac arrhythmia. The typical prehospital patient in nontraumatic cardiac arrest is found to have VF when initially placed on a cardiac monitor. In the prehospital setting, VF is thought to occur from chronic myocardial ischemia resulting in electrical instability of the heart. In the hospital, a cardiac arrest typically follows an acute myocardial infarction (AMI). The initial management of the victim of a cardiac arrest varies depending on the equipment that is immediately available. Electrical defibrillation, not drug therapy, is without debate the single best method of treatment for the patient with VF. The likelihood that a patient will survive an arrest from VF will significantly diminish the longer this rhythm is not converted using electrical therapy. When defibrillation is applied within 1 minute of the development of VF, the survival rate is greater than 70%. This rate of successful defibrillation drops by 10% for each minute defibrillation is delayed.[1]

MANAGEMENT

BRADYCARDIA

A heart rate of less than 60 beats/min is the definition of bradycardia. Many individuals will have a heart rate of less than 60 beats/min and be physiologically normal. For instance, a well-conditioned athlete such as a marathon runner will have a heart rate of less than 60 beats/min and be symptom free. Other patients may require a high resting heart rate to maintain an adequate cardiac output. Such individuals may be accustomed to having a resting heart rate of 90 beats/min, and a decrease of their heart rate to 70 beats/min may be inappropriately slow for them and may produce symptoms. The initial treatment of these symptomatic patients is the same as in any emergency: ensure a patent airway, provide supplemental oxygen, monitor the cardiac rhythm, evaluate oxygen saturation and blood pressure, and place an IV line. The decreased heart rate will decrease cardiac output and may produce symptoms of decreased mental status, syncope, hypotension, chest pain, congestive heart failure, dyspnea, seizures, or shock.

The treatment of symptomatic bradycardia is both drug and electrical therapy. Electrical therapy for bradycardia is transcutaneous pacing. When confronted with a symptomatic patient with bradycardia, prepare for transcutaneous pacing. Immediately start external pacing for patients with type II second-degree heart blocks and patients with third-degree heart blocks. It usually takes time to apply a transcutaneous pacemaker, so drug therapy may be required while preparing the patient and equipment. The initial medication used for treatment of symptomatic bradycardia is atropine 0.5 mg IV. Atropine is used to treat sinus bradycardia because it inhibits the effects of the vagus nerve. The vagus nerve, when stimulated, causes slowing of the heart rate, much like applying the brakes when driving a vehicle. Therefore a drug that inhibits the vagus nerve will increase the heart rate, as if you took your foot off the brake pedal in the vehicle. Atropine may be repeated to a total dose of 3 mg. If atropine is not effective in the treatment of the bradycardia, start transcutaneous pacing as soon as possible. Infusions of epinephrine (2 to 10 mcg/min) or dopamine (2 to 10 mcg/kg/min) may be used while waiting to establish transcutaneous pacing or if pacing is ineffective. Both epinephrine and dopamine are beta-adrenergic drugs, meaning that they bind and stimulate the beta$_1$ receptors of the heart. These properties make these drugs chronotropic, which results in an increase in heart rate.

ATROPINE SULFATE

Classification: Anticholinergic (antimuscarinic)
Action: Competes reversibly with acetylcholine at the site of the muscarinic receptor. Receptors affected, in order from the most sensitive to the least sensitive, include salivary, bronchial, sweat glands, eye, heart, and GI tract.
Indications: Symptomatic bradycardia, asystole or PEA, nerve agent exposure, organophosphate poisoning.
Adverse Effects: Decreased secretions resulting in dry mouth and hot skin temperature, intense facial flushing, blurred vision or dilation of the pupils with subsequent photophobia, tachycardia, restlessness. Atropine may cause paradoxical bradycardia if the dose administered is too low or if the drug is administered too slowly.
Contraindications: Acute MI; myasthenia gravis; GI obstruction; closed-angle glaucoma; known sensitivity to atropine, belladonna alkaloids, or sulfites. Will not be effective for infranodal (type II) AV block and new third-degree block with wide QRS complex.
Dosage:
Symptomatic Bradycardia:

- **Adult:** 0.5 mg IV, IO every 3 to 5 minutes to a maximum dose of 3 mg.
- **Adolescent:** 0.02 mg/kg (minimum 0.1 mg/dose; maximum 1 mg/dose) IV, IO up to a total dose of 2 mg.
- **Pediatric:** 0.02 mg/kg (minimum 0.1 mg/dose; maximum 0.5 mg/dose) IV, IO, to a total dose of 1 mg.

Asystole/Pulseless Electrical Activity:

- 1 mg IV, IO every 3 to 5 minutes, to a maximum dose of 3 mg. May be administered via ET tube at 2 to 2.5 mg diluted in 5 to 10 mL of water or normal saline.

Nerve Agent or Organophosphate Poisoning:

- **Adult:** 2 to 4 mg IV, IM; repeat if needed every 20 to 30 minutes until symptoms dissipate. In severe cases, the initial dose can be as large as 2 to 6 mg administered IV. Repeat doses of 2 to 6 mg can be administered IV, IM every 5 to 60 minutes.
- **Pediatric:** 0.05 mg/kg IV, IM every 10 to 30 minutes as needed until symptoms dissipate.
- **Infants <15 lb:** 0.05 mg/kg IV, IM every 5 to 20 minutes as needed until symptoms dissipate.

Special Considerations:
Half-life 2.5 hours
Pregnancy class C; possibly unsafe in lactating mothers.

EPINEPHRINE

Classification: Adrenergic agent, inotropic
Action: Binds strongly with both alpha and beta receptors, producing increased blood pressure, increased heart rate, bronchodilation.
Indications: Bronchospasm, allergic and anaphylactic reactions, restoration of cardiac activity in cardiac arrest.
Adverse Effects: Anxiety, headache, cardiac arrhythmias, hypertension, nervousness, tremors, chest pain, nausea/vomiting.
Contraindications: Arrhythmias other than VF, asystole, PEA; cardiovascular disease; hypertension; cerebrovascular disease; shock secondary to causes other than anaphylactic shock; closed-angle glaucoma; diabetes; pregnant women in active labor; known sensitivity to epinephrine or sulfites.
Dosage:
Cardiac Arrest:

- **Adult:** 1 mg (1 : 10,000 solution) IV, IO; may repeat every 3 to 5 minutes.
- **Pediatric:** 0.01 mg/kg (1 : 10,000 solution) IV, IO; repeat every 3 to 5 minutes as needed (max dose: 1 mg).

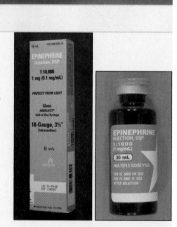

cont'd

EPINEPHRINE—CONT'D

Symptomatic Bradycardia:
- **Adult:** 1 mcg/min (1:10,000 solution) as a continuous IV infusion; usual dosage range: 2 to 10 mcg/min IV; titrate to effect.
- **Pediatric:** 0.01 mg/kg (1:10,000 solution) IV, IO; may repeat every 3 to 5 minutes (max dose: 1 mg). If giving epinephrine by ET tube, administer 0.1 mg/kg.

Asthma Attacks and Certain Allergic Reactions:
- **Adult:** 0.3 to 0.5 mg (1:1000 solution) IM or Sub-Q; may repeat every 10 to 15 minutes (max dose: 1 mg).
- **Pediatric:** 0.01 mg/kg (1:1000 solution) IM or Sub-Q (max dose: 0.5 mg).

Anaphylactic Shock:
- **Adult:** 0.1 mg (1:10,000 solution) IV slowly over 5 minutes, or IV infusion of 1 to 4 mcg/min, titrated to effect.
- **Pediatric:** Continuous IV infusion rate of 0.1 to 1 mcg/kg/min (1:10,000 solution); titrate to response.

Special Considerations:
Half-life 1 minute
Pregnancy class C

DOPAMINE (INTROPIN)

Classification: Adrenergic agonist, inotropic, vasopressor
Action: Stimulates alpha and beta adrenergic receptors. At moderate doses (2-10 mcg/kg/min), dopamine stimulates beta$_1$ receptors, resulting in inotropy and increased cardiac output while maintaining dopaminergic-induced vasodilatory effects. At high doses (>10 mcg/kg/min), alpha adrenergic agonism predominates, and increased peripheral vascular resistance and vasoconstriction result.
Indications: Hypotension and decreased cardiac output associated with cardiogenic shock and septic shock, hypotension after return of spontaneous circulation following cardiac arrest, symptomatic bradycardia unresponsive to atropine.
Adverse Effects: Tachycardia, arrhythmias, skin and soft tissue necrosis, severe hypertension from excessive vasoconstriction, angina, dyspnea, headache, nausea/vomiting.
Contraindications: Pheochromocytoma, VF, VT, or other ventricular arrhythmias, known sensitivity (including sulfites). Correct any hypovolemia with volume fluid replacement before administering dopamine.
Dosage:
- **Adult:** 2 to 20 mcg/kg/min IV, IO infusion. Starting dose 5 mcg/kg/min; may gradually increase the infusion by 5 to 10 mcg/kg/min to desired effect. Cardiac dose is usually 5 to 10 mcg/kg/min; vasopressor dose is usually 10 to 20 mcg/kg/min. Little benefit is gained beyond 20 mcg/kg/min.
- **Pediatric:** Same as adult dosing.

Special Considerations:
Half-life 2 minutes
Pregnancy class C

... Because the patient is feeling dizzy with a slow heart rate, you determine that the patient is experiencing symptomatic bradycardia. You place the patient on the cardiac monitor and oxygen while you start an IV line. You feel a weak radial pulse while your partner measures a blood pressure of 92/74 mm Hg. You administer atropine 0.5 mg IV and watch the heart rate on the monitor increase to 88 beats/min. Your partner repeats the blood pressure reading; it has increased to 122/81 mm Hg. The patient reports feeling better.

TACHYCARDIA

> You receive a 9-1-1 call for a patient with palpitations. Your patient is a 25-year-old woman with no medical problems except that she feels as though her heart is racing. Her ABCs are intact. You take her pulse, which is 180 beats/min. You attach the cardiac monitor, which shows supraventricular tachycardia (SVT) as the rhythm (Fig. 9-3). As you establish the IV line, you try to break the SVT by performing some vagal maneuvers. You perform the Valsalva maneuver on the patient. She remains in SVT, so you try carotid massage, which returns her to a normal sinus rhythm.

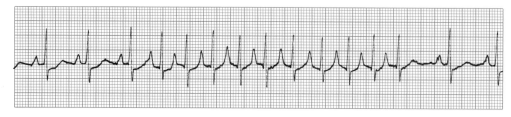

▼ **Fig. 9-3** Supraventricular tachycardia. (From Aehlert B: *ECGs made easy,* ed 3, St Louis, 2006, Mosby.)

In young patients with symptomatic SVT, vagal maneuvers and carotid massage can be used to return the patient to normal sinus rhythm. Carotid massage should never be attempted in older persons who have a high likelihood of carotid stenosis because of plaque formation. The only vagal maneuver that should be performed in older patients is a Valsalva maneuver. Remember, synchronized cardioversion is indicated if your patient is unstable, such as having altered mental status, hypotension, or chest pain. The following scenario takes a different approach to treating SVT and includes pharmacologic management.

> You respond to a call for an individual with palpitations. Your patient is a 65-year-old man with many medical problems, including heart disease. His mental status is normal and he has no abnormal vital signs, except for a pulse rate of 180 beats/min. He is in SVT according to your interpretation of the cardiac monitor. While you establish an IV line, you instruct him through the Valsalva maneuver. His rhythm continues to be SVT. You decide not to use carotid massage because of his age and medical problems. The IV line is established and you decide to administer adenosine 6 mg IV push.

When drug therapy is required, adenosine is the drug of choice for stable patients in SVT. Adenosine (Adenocard) works by altering the movement of potassium in the action potential of the heart, which slows the conduction of the action potential through the SA node. This creates a short period of asystole or ventricular escape beats and is usually seen for a few seconds after adenosine has been given. Short, self-limited episodes of ventricular tachycardia (VT) are not uncommon. Adenosine's only use is as an antiarrhythmic for SVT. Adenosine has no effect on ventricular arrhythmias.

Adenosine has an ultrashort half-life of 5 to 20 seconds and works only when the majority of the administered dose reaches the heart quickly. Consequently, it is given by rapid IV push and immediately followed by a flush solution. The 2005 American Heart Association Emergency Cardiovascular Care Guidelines recommendation is 6 mg IV, followed immediately by a normal saline bolus of 20 mL, and then the extremity should be elevated. If the SVT does not resolve within 1 to 2 minutes, the dose should be increased to 12 mg and repeated up to two times.

ADENOSINE (ADENOCARD)

Classification: Antiarrhythmic
Action: Slows the conduction of electrical impulses at the AV node.
Indications: Stable reentry SVT. Does not convert AF, atrial flutter, or VT.
Adverse Effects: Common adverse reactions are generally mild and short-lived: sense of impending doom, complaints of flushing, chest pressure, throat tightness, numbness. Patients will have a brief episode of asystole after administration.
Contraindications: Sick sinus syndrome, second- or third-degree heart block, poison-/drug-induced tachycardia.
Dosage: Note: Adenosine should be delivered only by rapid IV bolus with a peripheral IV or directly into a vein, in a location as close to the heart as possible, preferably in the antecubital fossa. Administration of adenosine must be immediately followed by a saline flush, and then the extremity should be elevated.

- **Adult:** Initial dose 6 mg rapid IV, IO (over a 1- to 3-second period) immediately followed by a 20-mL rapid saline flush. If the first dose does not eliminate the rhythm in 1 to 2 minutes, 12 mg rapid IV, IO, repeat a second time if required.
- **Pediatric:**
  - **Children >50 kg**: Same as adult dosing.
  - **Children <50 kg**: Initial dose 0.1 mg/kg IV, IO (max dose: 6 mg) immediately followed by a ≥5-mL rapid saline flush; may repeat at 0.2 mg/kg (max dose: 12 mg).

Special Considerations:
Use with caution in patients with preexisting bronchospasm and those with a history of AF.
Elderly patients with no history of PSVT should be carefully evaluated for dehydration and rapid sinus tachycardia requiring volume fluid replacement rather than simply treated with adenosine.
Pregnancy class C

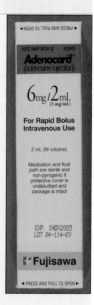

ANTIARRHYTHMIC DRUGS
Calcium Channel Blockers

A 70-year-old man calls 9-1-1 because of palpitations. He has a long history of atrial fibrillation with a rapid ventricular rate and usually takes the beta blocker atenolol (Tenormin) for rate control, as well as warfarin (Coumadin) for anticoagulation. He has been noncompliant with his atenolol and started feeling as though his heart was racing this morning.

Calcium channel blockers are class IV antiarrhythmics that bind to calcium channels. They block the influx of calcium into cardiac cells and arterial smooth muscle cells. This slows conduction velocity of the cardiac action potential and prolongs the period of repolarization. The overall effect is that the rapid electrical impulses traveling down from the atria to the ventricles through the atrioventricular (AV) node are slowed, and the ventricular rate is slowed. In the case presented previously, the administration of a calcium channel blocker will decrease the ventricular rate, but the rhythm will remain an atrial fibrillation. Calcium channel blockers also cause peripheral arterioles to dilate. Some calcium channel blockers have more of an ability to result in arteriole dilation than others. Why is this important to the prehospital provider? If you are administering a calcium channel blocker to treat a rapid heart rate like that in atrial fibrillation with a rapid ventricular rate, be mindful that the medication used to treat the heart rate may have the undesirable effect of dropping the blood pressure. Therefore, following administration for treatment of the heart rate, be sure to observe the patient closely and monitor the blood pressure frequently.

The actions of calcium channel blockers provide many clinical applications in both the acute setting and for long-term therapy. Calcium channel blockers are useful for controlling and/or converting certain supraventricular arrhythmias—stable, narrow-complex reentry SVT, and automatic focus (junctional, ectopic, and multifocal) tachycardias not converted or controlled by adenosine or vagal maneuvers. Calcium channel blockers do not convert atrial fibrillation or atrial flutter into a sinus rhythm; they only slow the ventricular rate by slowing conduction through the AV node. Because of their arterial dilatory effects, calcium channel blockers are used to treat hypertension. Because they also block vasospasm, calcium channel blockers can be used to decrease anginal episodes and even decrease the incidence of migraine headaches. Various calcium channel blockers have different proportions of vasodilator, antihypertensive, and antiarrhythmic effects.

Diltiazem (Cardizem) can be used for acute ventricular rate control and the management of hypertension. Advanced life support drug boxes that carry calcium channel blockers invariably use diltiazem. Verapamil (Isoptin) is no longer routinely used for acutely treating arrhythmias and is more likely to be prescribed for blood pressure control or continued rate control in chronic atrial fibrillation.[2,3]

DILTIAZEM (CARDIZEM)

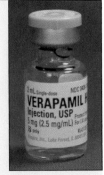

Classification: Calcium channel blocker, class IV antiarrhythmic
Action: Blocks calcium from moving into the heart muscle cell, which prolongs the conduction of electrical impulses through the AV node.
Indications: Ventricular rate control in rapid AF.
Adverse Effects: Flushing; headache; bradycardia; hypotension; heart block; myocardial depression; severe AV block; and, at high doses, cardiac arrest.
Contraindications: Hypotension, heart block, heart failure.
Dosage:
- **Adult:** Optimum dose is 0.25 mg/kg IV, IO over a 2-minute period to control rapid AF; 20 mg is a reasonable dose for the average adult patient. A second, higher dose of 0.35 mg/kg IV, IO (25 mg is a typical second dose) may be administered over a 2-minute period if rate control is not obtained with the lower dose. For continued reduction in heart rate, a continuous infusion can be started at a dose range of 5 to 15 mg/hr.
- **Pediatric:** Not recommended for pediatric patients.

Special Considerations:
Use with extreme caution in patients who are taking beta blockers because these two drug classes potentiate each other's effects and toxicities.
Patients with a history of heart failure and heart block are at a higher risk for toxicity.
Pregnancy class C

VERAPAMIL (ISOPTIN)

Classification: Calcium channel blocker; class IV antiarrhythmic
Action: Blocks calcium from moving into the heart muscle cell, which prolongs the conduction of electrical impulses through the AV node. Also dilates arteries.
Indications: Atrial fibrillation, hypertension, PSVT, PSVT prophylaxis.
Adverse Effects: Sinus bradycardia; first-, second-, or third-degree AV block; congestive heart failure; reflex sinus tachycardia; transient asystole; AV block; hypotension.
Contraindications: Second- or third-degree AV block (except in patients with a functioning artificial pacemaker); hypotension (systolic pressure <90 mm Hg) or cardiogenic shock; sick sinus syndrome (except in patients with a functioning artificial pacemaker); Wolff-Parkinson-White syndrome; Lown-Ganong-Levine syndrome; severe left ventricular dysfunction; known sensitivity to verapamil or any component of the formulation; atrial flutter or fibrillation and an accessory bypass tract (WPW, Lown-Ganong-Levine syndrome); in infants <1 yr.

cont'd

VERAPAMIL (ISOPTIN)—CONT'D

Dosage:
- **Adult:** 2.5 to 5 mg IV, IO over 2 minutes (3 minutes in elderly patients). May repeat at 5 to 10 mg every 15 to 30 minutes to a maximum dose of 30 mg.
- **Pediatric:**
  - **Children 1 to 16 years:** 0.1 mg/kg IV, IO (maximum 5 mg/dose) over 2 minutes. May repeat in 30 minutes to a maximum dose of 10 mg.
  - **Infants <1 year:** Not recommended.

Special Considerations:
Pregnancy class C

Beta Blockers

> A patient you previously saw with atrial fibrillation calls 9-1-1 on another occasion. He is again in atrial fibrillation with a rapid ventricular rate. This time, however, he also has anginal chest pain. Medical direction asks you to administer a beta blocker rather than a calcium channel blocker.

As discussed in Chapters 1 and 6, **beta blockers** exert their pharmacologic effects on both beta$_1$ and beta$_2$ receptors. Beta$_1$ receptors are located in the heart and act as the main mediator of rate and contractility. Beta blockers are negative inotropic drugs that decrease the force and velocity of myocardial contractility, thus lowering blood pressure and oxygen consumption. The negative chronotropic effects of beta blockers result in a lower heart rate, automaticity, and conduction. Thus beta blockers can dramatically decrease cardiac output. Beta$_2$ blockers prevent vasoconstriction and contribute to lowering of blood pressure.[2]

For these reasons, beta blockers are highly effective drugs for people with angina and hypertension. Research has shown that beta blockers decrease mortality rate during and after AMIs.[4,5]

Beta blockers also decrease infarct size, reduce the risk of recurrent ischemia, and decrease the incidence of sudden death from arrhythmias. Because of their ability to decrease both heart rate and myocardial contractility, beta blockers are useful in the treatment of dissecting aortic aneurysms.[2,6-8]

Beta blockers can also be used as antiarrhythmics, especially in high catecholamine or epinephrine states such as alcohol withdrawal, panic attacks, and hyperthyroidism. Beta blockers are useful for controlling heart rate in SVTs, decrease AV nodal conduction, and depress ventricular automaticity. They may be effective in the rate control of atrial fibrillation, SVT, and sinus tachycardia. They can be used to suppress premature ventricular contractions (PVCs), especially in anginal patients, because of their antiarrhythmic effects combined with oxygen-sparing properties.

Numerous beta blockers are available. The most common are propranolol, metoprolol, atenolol, and the short-acting esmolol. These agents are discussed in detail in Chapter 6.

PROPRANOLOL (INDERAL)

Classification: Beta adrenergic antagonist, antianginal, antihypertensive, antiarrhythmic class II

Action: Nonselective beta antagonist that binds with both the $beta_1$ and $beta_2$ receptors. Propranolol inhibits the strength of the heart's contractions, as well as heart rate. This results in a decrease in cardiac oxygen consumption.

Indications: Angina; narrow-complex tachycardias that originate from either a *reentry mechanism* (reentry SVT) or an *automatic focus* (junctional, ectopic, or multifocal tachycardia) uncontrolled by vagal maneuvers and adenosine in patients with preserved ventricular function; AF and atrial flutter in patients with preserved ventricular function; hypertension; migraine headaches.

Adverse Effects: Bradycardia, AV block, bronchospasm, hypotension.

Contraindications: Cardiogenic shock, heart failure, AV block, bradycardia, pulmonary edema, sick sinus syndrome, known sensitivity. Use with caution in chronic lung disease (asthma and COPD).

Dosage:
- **Adult:** 1 to 3 mg IV, IO at a rate of 1 mg/min; may repeat the dose 2 minutes later.
- **Pediatric:** 0.01 to 0.1 mg/kg slow IV, IO over a 10-minute period.

Special Considerations:
Monitor blood pressure and heart rate closely during administration.
Pregnancy class C

METOPROLOL (LOPRESSOR, TOPROL XL)

Classification: Beta adrenergic antagonist, antianginal, antihypertensive, class II antiarrhythmic

Action: Inhibits the strength of the heart's contractions, as well as heart rate. This results in a decrease in cardiac oxygen consumption. Also saturates the beta receptors and inhibits dilation of bronchial smooth muscle ($beta_2$ receptor).

Indications: ACS, hypertension, SVT, atrial flutter, AF, thyrotoxicosis.

Adverse Effects: Tiredness, dizziness, diarrhea, heart block, bradycardia, bronchospasm, drop in blood pressure.

Contraindications: Cardiogenic shock, AV block, bradycardia, known sensitivity. Use with caution in hypotension, chronic lung disease (asthma and COPD).

Dosage:
Cardiac Indications:
- **Adult:** 5 mg slow IV, IO over a 5-minute period; repeat at 5-minute intervals up to a total of three infusions totaling 15 mg IV, IO.
- **Pediatric:** Not recommended for pediatric patients; no studies available.

Special Considerations:
Blood pressure, heart rate, and ECG should be monitored carefully.
Use with caution in patients with asthma.
Pregnancy class C

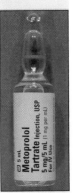

ATENOLOL (TENORMIN)

Classification: Beta adrenergic antagonist, antianginal, antihypertensive, class II antiarrhythmic

Action: Inhibits the strength of the heart's contractions and heart rate, resulting in a decrease in cardiac oxygen consumption. Also saturates the beta receptors and inhibits dilation of bronchial smooth muscle ($beta_2$ receptor).

Indications: ACS, hypertension, SVT, atrial flutter, AF.

Adverse Effects: Bradycardia, bronchospasm, hypotension.

Contraindications: Cardiogenic shock, AV block, bradycardia, known sensitivity. Use with caution in hypotension, chronic lung disease (asthma and COPD).

Dosage: ACS:
- **Adult:** 5 mg IV, IO over a 5-minute period; repeat in 5 minutes.
- **Pediatric:** Not recommended for pediatric patients.

Special Considerations:
Pregnancy class D

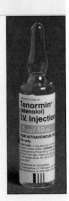

ESMOLOL (BREVIBLOC)

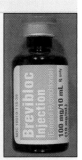

Classification: Beta adrenergic antagonist, class II antiarrhythmic
Action: Inhibits the strength of the heart's contractions, as well as heart rate, resulting in a decrease in cardiac oxygen consumption.
Indications: ACS, MI, acute hypertension, supraventricular tachyarrhythmias, thyrotoxicosis.
Adverse Effects: Hypotension, sinus bradycardia, AV block, cardiac arrest, nausea/vomiting, hypoglycemia, injection site reaction.
Contraindications: Acute bronchospasm, COPD, second- or third-degree heart block, bradycardia, cardiogenic shock, pulmonary edema, sick sinus syndrome, known sensitivity. Use with caution in patients with pheochromocytoma, Prinzmetal's angina, cerebrovascular disease, stroke, poorly controlled diabetes mellitus, hyperthyroidism, thyrotoxicosis, renal disease.
Dosage:
  · **Adult:** 500 mcg/kg (0.5 mg/kg) IV, IO over a 1-minute period, followed by a 50-mcg/kg/min (0.05 mg/kg) infusion over a 4-minute period (maximum total: 200 mcg/kg). If patient response is inadequate, administer a second bolus 500 mcg/kg (0.5 mg/kg) over a 1-minute period, and then increase infusion to 100 mcg/kg/min. Maximum infusion rate: 300 mcg/kg/min.
  · **Pediatric:** 500 mcg/kg (0.5 mg/kg) IV, IO over a 1-minute period, followed by an infusion at 25 to 200 mcg/kg/min.
Special Considerations:
Half-life 5 to 9 minutes
Any adverse effects caused by administration of esmolol are brief because of the drug's short half-life.
Resolution of effects usually within 10 to 20 minutes.
Pregnancy class C

Ventricular Antiarrhythmic Drugs

> **Y**ou receive a 9-1-1 call for a patient who is unresponsive. When you arrive, you determine the patient is apneic and pulseless. You begin CPR, establish an airway, and ventilate the patient. Once the patient is connected to your cardiac monitor/defibrillator, you see VF on the monitor. He is successfully shocked into a sinus rhythm with a pulse but has multiple PVCs, some of which occur in couplets and triplets.
>   What antiarrhythmic is best in this situation? Are there other therapeutic options?

A number of drugs can be used to treat patients with ventricular arrhythmias. Antiarrhythmic medications are divided into the following four classes based on their mechanisms of action:
1. Class I: Sodium channel blockers. These agents are further divided into subclasses according to their effect on the sodium channel.
   1A: Agents that block the fast sodium channels and depress depolarization.
   1B: Sodium channel blockers that shorten the action potential duration.
   1C: Sodium channel blockers that depress depolarization and conductivity. This subclass of agents is the most potent sodium channel blocker.
2. Class II: Beta blockers.
3. Class III: Potassium channel blocking agents.
4. Class IV: Calcium channel blocking agents.

In the previous scenario, amiodarone would be the drug of choice. Although it is classified as a class III agent, amiodarone is the only commonly used antiarrhythmic drug that has actions from every class of antiarrhythmics. That is, it has some sodium-blocking effects, some beta-blocking effects, and some calcium-blocking effects in addition to predominant effects on the potassium channels.[2,3] Amiodarone is used to treat arrhythmias that originate both above and below the AV node. It is widely accepted as the drug of choice in cardiac arrest from VF and **pulseless ventricular tachycardia.**[9]

Amiodarone can also be used to convert acute atrial fibrillation (Fig. 9-4) or **atrial flutter** (Fig. 9-5) pharmacologically.[2,3,6] Amiodarone increases the duration of the action potential, as well as the refractory period of the atria, AV node, and ventricular tissues. Because amiodarone exerts its effect in both atrial and ventricular tissue, the drug is capable of treating both atrial and ventricular arrhythmias.

When a drug increases the duration of the action potential or the refractory period, what does that mean? To explain this you need to imagine that you are standing on a bridge that passes over an interstate highway. Below you is a constant stream of automobiles speeding down the highway. In the heart, the specialized tissue that conducts electrical impulses or action potential from the SA node through the ventricles, past the SA node and down into the ventricles is similar to the interstate highway in this example. What determines how many cars rush underneath your bridge in a matter of 1 minute? The velocity of the cars and the distance between those cars are the principal elements that determine the number of cars that can pass underneath the bridge. The speed, or velocity, of the cars rushing down the highway can be likened to the action potential duration. The faster the action potential duration, the faster the action potential will move down the conduction system. Various medications and shifts of electrolytes can affect the duration of the action potential, and therefore, how rapid that particular impulse moves down the system. Let us go back to watching the traffic on the interstate. Between each car on the highway is a certain amount of space. If the cars are all traveling at 55 miles per hour, the greater the space between the cars, at a given speed, the fewer cars can pass under the bridge. In the heart, each electrical action potential has a period known as the *refractory period.* This refractory period is similar to the space between the cars. The greater the refractory period, the fewer action potentials will travel down the through the heart in 1 minute.

Amiodarone is a class III antiarrhythmic drug that increases the action potential duration and refractory period. It has been shown to decrease short-term mortality rates in patients with congestive heart failure after a myocardial infarction.[10] In cases of chronic heart failure, amiodarone reduces the risk of developing atrial fibrillation and can convert patients who are in atrial fibrillation to a **sinus rhythm.**[7]

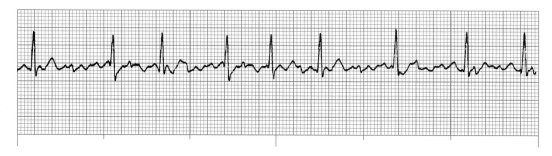

▼ **Fig. 9-4**   Atrial fibrillation. (From Aehlert B: *ECGs made easy,* ed 3, St Louis, 2006, Mosby.)

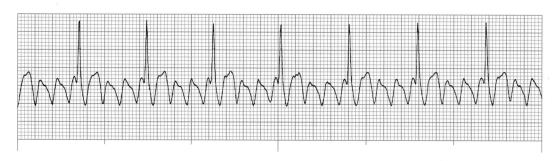

▼ **Fig. 9-5**   Atrial flutter. (From Aehlert B: *ECGs made easy,* ed 3, St Louis, 2006, Mosby.)

Because of amiodarone's irritating effects to veins and soft tissues, be careful not to allow amiodarone infusions to infiltrate into the soft tissue. It should always be administered by a secure, large-bore IV line.

Amiodarone is superior to lidocaine because it significantly improves the likelihood of converting VF and pulseless VT to a perfusing rhythm.[11,12]

Lidocaine is a class 1B antiarrhythmic because it blocks the sodium channel and it decreases the amount of time required for repolarization. These effects also make lidocaine an excellent short-acting anesthetic.

Based on multiple studies, it appears that lidocaine converts only approximately 11% to 12% of cases of VT. Research has shown that in cases of VF, amiodarone helped successfully convert significantly more patients in VF than did lidocaine.[11,12] It is for these reasons that amiodarone is the drug of choice in the treatment of life-threatening ventricular arrhythmias.

Procainamide (Pronestyl) is a class IA antiarrhythmic that works by binding to fast sodium channels and slows almost all phases of the action potential. It slows depolarization, repolarization, and impulse conduction. Procainamide can prolong the PR and QT intervals and at higher dosing can cause the QRS complex to widen. Because it decreases nodal conductivity, it can be used for both atrial and ventricular arrhythmias. It has often been used as the second-line agent of choice for atrial fibrillation, atrial flutter, and SVT in addition to its role as an effective ventricular antiarrhythmic.[2] Procainamide is usually the drug of choice when amiodarone is not effective. However, because it cannot be given rapidly and can take 20 to 40 minutes to work, most out-of-hospital providers do not use procainamide.

AMIODARONE (CORDARONE)

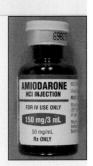

Classification: Antiarrhythmic, class III
Action: Acts directly on the myocardium to delay repolarization and increase the duration of the action potential.
Indications: Ventricular arrhythmias; second-line agent for atrial arrhythmias.
Adverse Effects: Burning at the IV site, hypotension, bradycardia.
Contraindications: Sick sinus syndrome, second- and third-degree heart block, cardiogenic shock, when episodes of bradycardia have caused syncope, sensitivity to benzyl alcohol and iodine.
Dosage:
Ventricular Fibrillation and Pulseless Ventricular Tachycardia:
- **Adult:** 300 mg IV, IO. May be followed by one dose of 150 mg in 3 to 5 minutes.
- **Pediatric:** 5 mg/kg (max dose: 300 mg); may repeat 5 mg/kg IV, IO up to 15 mg/kg.
Relatively Stable Patients with Arrhythmias such as Premature Ventricular Contractions or Wide-Complex Tachycardias with a Strong Pulse:
- **Adult:** 150 mg in 100 mL D₅W IV, IO over a 10-minute period; may repeat in 10 minutes up to a maximum dose of 2.2 g over 24 hours.
- **Pediatric:** 5 mg/kg very slow IV, IO (over 20 to 60 minutes); may repeat in 5-mg/kg doses up to 15 mg/kg (max dose: 300 mg).
Special Considerations:
Pregnancy class D

LIDOCAINE (XYLOCAINE)

Classification: Antiarrhythmic, class IB
Action: Blocks sodium channels, increasing the recovery period after repolarization; suppresses automaticity in the His-Purkinje system and depolarization in the ventricles.
Indications: Ventricular arrhythmias, when amiodarone is not available: cardiac arrest from VF/VT, stable monomorphic VT with preserved ventricular function, stable polymorphic VT with normal baseline QT interval and preserved left ventricular function (when ischemia and electrolyte imbalance are treated), stable polymorphic VT with baseline QT prolongation suggestive of torsades de pointes.
Adverse Effects: Toxicity (signs may include anxiety, apprehension, euphoria, nervousness, disorientation, dizziness, blurred vision, facial paresthesias, tremors, hearing disturbances, slurred speech, seizures, sinus bradycardia), seizures without warning, cardiac arrhythmias, hypotension, cardiac arrest, pain at injection site.
Contraindications: AV block; bleeding; thrombocytopenia; known sensitivity to lidocaine, sulfite, or paraben. Use with caution in bradycardia, hypovolemia, cardiogenic shock, Adams-Stokes syndrome, Wolff-Parkinson-White syndrome.
Dosage:
Pulseless Ventricular Tachycardia and Ventricular Fibrillation:
- **Adult IV, IO:** 1 to 1.5 mg/kg IV, IO; may repeat at half the original dose (0.5-0.75 mg/kg) every 5 to 10 minutes to a maximum dose of 3 mg/kg. If a maintenance infusion is warranted, the rate is 1 to 4 mg/min.
- **Adult ET tube:** 2 to 10 mg/kg ET tube, diluted in 10 mL normal saline or sterile distilled water.
- **Pediatric IV, IO:** 1 mg/kg IV, IO (maximum: 100 mg). If a maintenance infusion is warranted, the rate is 20 to 50 mcg/kg/min.
- **Pediatric ET tube:** 2 to 3 mg/kg ET tube, followed by a 5-mL flush of normal saline.
Perfusing Ventricular Rhythms:
- **Adult:** 0.5 to 0.75 mg/kg IV, IO (up to 1-1.5 mg/kg may be used). Repeat 0.5 to 0.75 mg/kg every 5 to 10 minutes to a maximum total dose of 3 mg/kg. A maintenance infusion of 1 to 4 mg/min (30-50 mcg/kg/min) is acceptable.
- **Pediatric:** 1 mg/kg IV, IO. May repeat every 5 to 10 minutes to a maximum dose of 3 mg/kg. Maintenance infusion rate is 20 to 50 mcg/kg/min.
Special Considerations:
Half-life approximately 90 minutes
Pregnancy class B

PROCAINAMIDE (PRONESTYL)

Classification: Antiarrhythmic, class IA
Action: Blocks influx of sodium through membrane pores, consequently suppresses atrial and ventricular arrhythmias by slowing conduction in myocardial tissue.
Indications: Alternative to amiodarone for stable monomorphic VT with normal QT interval and preserved ventricular function, reentry SVT if uncontrolled by adenosine and vagal maneuvers if blood pressure stable, AF with rapid rate in Wolff-Parkinson-White syndrome.
Adverse Effects: Asystole, VF, flushing, hypotension, PR prolongation, QRS widening, QT prolongation.
Contraindications: AV block, QT prolongation, torsades de pointes. Use with caution in hypotension, heart failure.
Dosage:

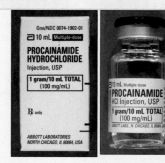

- **Adult:** 20 mg/min slow IV, IO (max total dose: 17 mg/kg until one of the following occurs: arrhythmia resolves, hypotension, QRS widens by >50% of original width).
- **Maintenance:** Infusion (after resuscitation from cardiac arrest): mix 1 g in 250 mL solution (4 mg/mL), infuse at 1 to 4 mg/min.
- **Pediatric:** 15 mg/kg slow IV, IO over 30 to 60 minutes.
Special Considerations:
Pregnancy class C

You are dispatched to a local apartment building for a 72-year-old man who suddenly collapsed. When you arrive you find an unresponsive elderly man in a chair. You rapidly get him to the floor while your partner prepares the defibrillator. The daughter is telling you that her father has never had any problems with his heart but does have a history of alcoholism, as well as some problems with his liver. The ECG monitor shows an unusual type of VT. That is, the tachycardia is not monomorphic, with every QRS complex looking the same. Instead it is polymorphic, with many different-shaped complexes that appear to rotate by 180 degrees over time, almost like it is twisting. You recognize this as **torsades de pointes** (Fig. 9-6). ...

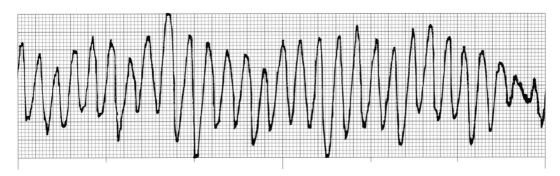

▼ **Fig. 9-6**   Torsades de pointes. (From Aehlert B: *ECGs made easy*, ed 3, St Louis, 2006, Mosby.)

Torsades de pointes is French for the phrase "twisting of points." This rhythm is often confused with VT. It is easier to detect the twisting of points on a printed strip.

Magnesium sulfate is an electrolyte and an extremely effective antiarrhythmic. Magnesium can be used to treat patients with torsades de pointes (such as in the previous scenario) successfully and decrease PVCs caused by a prolonged QT interval.[13] The exact mechanism of how magnesium prevents torsades is not defined, but it may block the sodium channels. Alcoholics typically have poor diets that cause several nutritional and electrolyte abnormalities that can result in arrhythmias. Therefore magnesium should always be considered in alcoholics and malnourished patients.

MAGNESIUM SULFATE

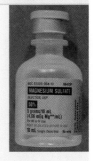

Classification: Electrolyte, tocolytic, mineral

Action: Required for normal physiologic functioning. Magnesium is a cofactor in neurochemical transmission and muscular excitability. Magnesium sulfate controls seizures by blocking peripheral neuromuscular transmission. Magnesium is also a peripheral vasodilator and an inhibitor of platelet function.

Indications: Torsades de pointes, cardiac arrhythmias associated with hypomagnesemia, eclampsia and seizure prophylaxis in preeclampsia, status asthmaticus.

Adverse Effects: Magnesium toxicity (signs include flushing, diaphoresis, hypotension, muscle paralysis, weakness, hypothermia, and cardiac, CNS, or respiratory depression).

Contraindications: AV block, GI obstruction. Use with caution in renal impairment.

Dosage:

Pulseless Ventricular Fibrillation/Ventricular Tachycardia with Torsades de Pointes or Hypomagnesemia:

· **Adult:** 1 to 2 g in 10 mL D_5W IV, IO administered over 5 to 10 minutes.
· **Pediatric:** 25 to 50 mg/kg IV, IO over 10 to 20 minutes; may administer faster for torsades de pointes (max single dose: 2 g).

cont'd

MAGNESIUM SULFATE—CONT'D

Torsades de Pointes with a Pulse or Cardiac Arrhythmias with Hypomagnesemia:
- **Adult:** 1 to 2 g in 50 to 100 mL D$_5$W IV, IO administered over 5 to 60 minutes. Follow with 0.5 to 1 g/hr IV, IO titrated to control torsades de pointes.
- **Pediatric:** 25 to 50 mg/kg IV, IO over 10 to 20 minutes (max single dose: 2 g).

Eclampsia and Seizure Prophylaxis in Preeclampsia:
- **Adult:** 4 to 6 g IV, IO over 20 to 30 minutes, followed by an infusion of 1 to 2 g/hr.

Status Asthmaticus:
- **Adult:** 1.2 to 2 g slow IV, IO (over 20 minutes).
- **Pediatric:** 25 to 50 mg/kg (diluted in D$_5$W) slow IV, IO (over 10 to 20 minutes).

Special Considerations:
Pregnancy class A

... Because the patient has been converted back into a sinus rhythm with a pulse and he is having PVCs, it would be prudent to administer an antiarrhythmic drug. You administer amiodarone 150 mg IV over a 10-minute period.

Cardiopulmonary Arrest

There are four arrhythmias associated with cardiac arrest: pulseless electrical activity (PEA), asystole, VT, and VF. Although some of the medications used to treat all four rhythms are the same, there are variations.

Pulseless Electrical Activity and Asystole. PEA and asystole are the most dreaded cardiac arrhythmias. PEA is characterized by detectable electrical activity on the monitor but no mechanical cardiac activity as detected by the presence of a pulse or audible heart tones. In asystole, the patient has neither electrical nor mechanical cardiac activity. Only two medications, epinephrine and vasopressin, are indicated in the treatment of either of these arrhythmias. Both drugs have very strong inotropic and chronotropic effects on the heart. In an arrest situation, 1 mg IV, IO of epinephrine can be administered every 3 to 5 minutes. In cases in which you are treating an overdose of a beta blocker or calcium channel blocker, high doses up to 0.2 mg/kg may be used. In emergency situations in which the prehospital professional cannot rapidly obtain either IV or IO access, epinephrine can be administered down the endotracheal tube at a dose of 2 to 2.5 mg. Another medication that is used in the treatment of PEA and asystole is vasopressin. Vasopressin is a vasoconstrictor that, unlike epinephrine, does not use the adrenergic receptors. Why is it important that vasopressin does not use adrenergic receptors? In the case of asystole, epinephrine is stimulating the adrenergic receptors, trying to reestablish a rhythm. If epinephrine is binding and stimulating all of the adrenergic receptors on the heart, the addition of a second drug, working by the same mechanism on the same receptor, is not likely to be successful. Put more simply, if plan A doesn't work, don't stick with plan A. So what's plan B? Give a second drug, vasopressin, that is a powerful inotropic and chronotropic drug but stimulates the heart via a different receptor mechanism. In cases of cardiac arrest, a single dose of 40 units IV or IO can be administered. No evidence exists to indicate that either vasopressin or epinephrine is superior in the treatment of cardiac arrest.

VASOPRESSIN

Classification: Nonadrenergic vasoconstrictor
Action: Vasopressin causes vasoconstriction independent of adrenergic receptors or neural innervation.
Indications: Adult shock-refractory VF or pulseless VT, asystole, PEA, vasodilatory shock.
Adverse Effects: Cardiac ischemia, angina.
Contraindications: Responsive patients with cardiac disease.
Dosage:
  · **Adult:** 40 U IV, IO may replace either the first or second dose of epinephrine.
  · May be given ET but the optimal dose is not known.
Special Considerations:
Pregnancy class C

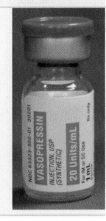

Pulseless Ventricular Tachycardia and Ventricular Fibrillation. Epinephrine and vasopressin are also indicated in pulseless VT and VF; however, electrical therapy has proven to be the most effective treatment for patients in cardiac arrest with these rhythms. If a patient in pulseless VT or VF does not respond to defibrillation, epinephrine or vasopressin should be administered as previously indicated. If the patient's rhythm does not change after two or three shocks and administration of a vasopressor, consider administration of amiodarone. If amiodarone is unavailable, lidocaine may be used as a substitute.

REVIEW QUESTIONS

1. Why is electrical therapy preferred over drug administration for the initial therapy of cardiac arrest and some arrhythmias?
2. Explain the effect of atropine on the vagus nerve in a patient with bradycardia.
3. What is the half-life of adenosine?
4. List three classes of antiarrhythmic agents.
5. To what drug class do calcium channel blockers belong, and what are their effects on the heart?
6. Explain how beta blockers decrease cardiac output.
7. What is the drug of choice for most ventricular arrhythmias?
8. What drug is indicated for the treatment of torsades de pointes?
9. What is the status of the heart's electrical and mechanical activity in pulseless electrical activity? What is the status of the heart's electrical and mechanical activity in asystole?

REFERENCES

1. Cobb LA, et al: Influence of cardiopulmonary resuscitation prior to defibrillation in patients with out-of-hospital ventricular fibrillation, *JAMA* 281:1182, 1999.
2. Katzung, BG: *Basic and clinical pharmacology,* ed 8, New York, 2000, McGraw-Hill.
3. Tamariz LJ, Bass EB: Pharmacological rate control of atrial fibrillation, *Cardiol Clin* 22(1):35-45, 2004.
4. Bunch TJ, et al: Effect of beta-blocker therapy on mortality rates and future myocardial infarction rates in patients with coronary artery disease but no history of myocardial infarction or congestive heart failure, *Am J Cardiol* 95:827, 2005.
5. Borrello F, et al: Reappraisal of beta-blocker therapy in the acute and chronic post-myocardial infarction period, *Am J Cardiol* 93: 21B, 2004.
6. American Heart Association: *Handbook of emergency cardiovascular care for healthcare providers,* Dallas, 2006, American Heart Association.
7. Deedwania PC, et al: Spontaneous conversion and maintenance of sinus rhythm by amiodarone in patients with heart failure and atrial fibrillation: observations from the Veterans Affairs Congestive Heart Failure Trial of Antiarrhythmic Therapy (CHF-STAT), *Circulation* 98:2574, 1998.

8. Atkins DL, et al: Treatment of tachyarrhythmias, *Ann Emerg Med* 37:S91-109, 2001.

9. Wayne MA, et al: Prehospital management of cardiac arrest: how useful are vasopressor and antiarrhythmic drugs? *Prehosp Emerg Care* 6:72, 2002.

10. Amiodarone Trials Meta-Analysis Investigators: Effect of prophylactic amiodarone on mortality after acute myocardial infarction and in congestive heart failure: meta-analysis of individual data from 6500 patients in randomized trials, *Lancet* 350:1417, 1997.

11. Kudenchuk PJ: Amiodarone for resuscitation after out-of-hospital cardiac arrest due to ventricular fibrillation, *N Engl J Med* 341:871, 1999.

12. Dorian P: Amiodarone versus Lidocaine in Ventricular Fibrillation Evaluation (ALIVE) trial. In *NASPE 22nd Annual Scientific Sessions* [CD-ROM], Boston, 2001, North American Society of Pacing and Electrophysiology.

13. Iseri LT: Magnesium: nature's physiologic calcium blocker, *Am Heart J* 108:188, 1984.

BIBLIOGRAPHY

Clements EA, Kuhn BR: Pharmacology of antidysrhythmic agents and vasoactive medications. In Tintinelli JE, Kelen GD, Stapczynski JS, editors: *Emergency medicine: a comprehensive study guide*, ed 6, New York, 2004, McGraw-Hill.

Elkayam U, et al: Calcium channel blockers in heart failure, *J Am Coll Cardiol* 22(4 suppl A):139A, 1993.

Iseri LT: Magnesium and cardiac arrhythmias, *Magnesium* 5:111, 1986.

Moser M, Setaro J: Continued importance of diuretics and beta-adrenergic blockers in the management of hypertension, *Med Clin North Am* 88: 157, 2004.

Congestive Heart Failure

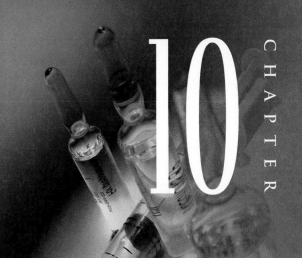

OBJECTIVES

1. Explain the concept of polypharmacy in the treatment of congestive heart failure.
2. Explain the function of a diuretic.
3. Discuss drugs used for the initial management of congestive heart failure: furosemide (Lasix), morphine sulfate, and nitroglycerin (Nitrolingual, NitroQuick, Nitro-Dur).
4. Discuss digoxin (Lanoxin) and its use in the long-term management of congestive heart failure.
5. Discuss the role of angiotensin-converting enzyme inhibitors, beta blockers, and calcium channel blockers in treating patients with congestive heart failure.

Medications that Appear in Chapter 10

Furosemide (Lasix)
Morphine sulfate
Nitroglycerin (Nitrolingual, NitroQuick, Nitro-Dur)
Digoxin (Lanoxin)
Angiotensin-Converting Enzyme (ACE) inhibitors: Captopril (Capoten), Enalapril (Vasotec), Lisinopril (Prinivil, Zestril), Ramipril (Altace)
Metoprolol (Lopressor, Toprol XL)

INTRODUCTION

Congestive heart failure (CHF) is one of the few cardiovascular disorders that continues to increase in prevalence, especially among the elderly. Currently 5 million people in the United States have heart failure, and 500,000 new cases are diagnosed each year.[1] CHF is predominantly a condition of the elderly, with 6% to 10% of all individuals older than 65 years having symptoms consistent with the disease. Paramedics are often called to assist patients with long-standing disease who are often taking multiple medications. Prehospital care providers must be familiar with the medications used for long-term therapy of CHF, as well as short-term drug therapy for exacerbations of CHF and resultant pulmonary edema.

You are dispatched to assist an elderly woman who is reporting shortness of breath. You arrive at the apartment of a 78-year-old woman who is in moderate respiratory distress. Her legs are swollen, and she reports shortness of breath that has become more severe over the past few days. She coughs when lying down and has been having difficulty sleeping for the past three nights. In fact, she tells you that her breathing has been more comfortable when she has tried to sleep in the chair in the living room. Her blood pressure is 188/92 mm Hg, heart rate is 100 beats/min, and respirations are 20 breaths/min. The patient tells you she is diabetic and hypertensive and has high cholesterol, kidney failure, and CHF. You administer high-flow oxygen with a nonrebreather ...

... face mask, establish an IV line, and administer 40 mg furosemide IV. Before leaving for the hospital, she hands you a plastic bag full of the medications she is taking. They include simvastatin (Zocor), lisinopril (Zestril), metoprolol (Lopressor, Toprol XL), furosemide (Lasix), potassium, and digoxin (Lanoxin).

OVERVIEW OF CONGESTIVE HEART FAILURE

Heart failure may be the result of ischemic heart disease, diabetes mellitus, hypertension, or disease of the heart valves. The onset of heart failure may be rather acute after a myocardial infarction or may take years to develop in conditions such as valvular heart disease, hypertension, or diabetes mellitus. Patients with heart failure may have symptoms from accumulation of excess fluid or poor peripheral perfusion and inadequate oxygen delivery to the tissues (Fig. 10-1). Signs of fluid overload include shortness of breath from pulmonary edema, as well as edema of the extremities, especially the lower legs. Poor output of the heart caused by heart failure results in an accumulation or "backing up" of fluid in the lungs, which is known as **pulmonary edema.** Other patients with heart failure may report only fatigue and weakness from poor delivery of oxygen to the tissues as a result of low cardiac output.

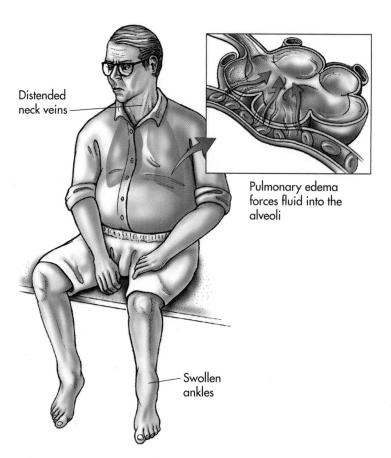

Distended neck veins

Pulmonary edema forces fluid into the alveoli

Swollen ankles

▼ Fig. 10-1   In congestive heart failure, decreased forward cardiac output by a diseased left ventricle results in the accumulation of blood in the pulmonary vasculature, leading to pulmonary edema. Pulmonary edema occurs when fluid accumulates in the alveoli. This fluid widens the gap between the alveoli and capillary membrane, which makes diffusion of oxygen and carbon dioxide less efficient.

The diagnosis of CHF is often suspected in patients with shortness of breath and peripheral edema. Shortness of breath, or dyspnea, can be caused by CHF but can also be the result of chronic obstructive pulmonary disease (COPD). CHF, as well as a variety of other conditions, can produce peripheral edema. CHF is not easily diagnosed by physical examination. Approximately 20% of patients diagnosed with CHF have no symptoms at all, and approximately 42% had only dyspnea on exertion.[2] Children with heart disease can also have heart failure and resultant pulmonary edema.

MANAGEMENT

The American Heart Association provides guidelines for the management of CHF and pulmonary edema. Long-term control of systolic and diastolic hypertension is imperative to control the symptoms seen in CHF. Patients with CHF are often taking medications for the treatment of lipid disorders. **Angiotensin-converting enzyme (ACE) inhibitors** are a class of medication recommended for patients with a history of atherosclerotic vascular disease, diabetes, and hypertension. ACE inhibitors are discussed later in this chapter. Additionally, physicians often place these patients on medications to control heart rate and treat thyroid disorders. The importance of these recommendations in prehospital management is not in the administration of these medications, but in the effects of **polypharmacy** (the administration of many drugs at the same time) on the patient with CHF who is unstable. Additionally, although these medications are often used for the treatment of CHF, drugs such as digoxin, nitrates, or ACE inhibitors may be potentially harmful in patients with CHF from valvular heart disease or with diastolic dysfunction.

The most common treatment protocols for patients with CHF in the prehospital setting include administration of oxygen, furosemide (Lasix), morphine, and nitroglycerin. The only medication that presents no harmful consequences in this setting is oxygen. Patients with symptoms consistent with CHF or pulmonary edema are treated with sublingual or mucosal nitroglycerin, IV furosemide, and IV morphine or some combination of these drugs.

DRUGS USED FOR IMMEDIATE MANAGEMENT

After the administration of oxygen, one of the principal objectives of drug therapy is reduction of pulmonary edema.

Drugs commonly used for the immediate management of CHF include furosemide, morphine sulfate, and nitroglycerin. Patients with chronic heart failure will typically be taking a diuretic such as furosemide, as well as an ACE inhibitor and a beta blocker.

Furosemide, which is a loop diuretic, is commonly used to reduce pulmonary edema. Diuretics increase urine output, and loop diuretics work by decreasing the absorption of water in the kidneys. This decrease in water absorption increases urine production and decreases intravascular volume. Loop diuretics are more effective than other diuretics in the management of acute and chronic heart failure, as well as life-threatening pulmonary edema. In the management of an adult with CHF, an initial dose of furosemide 40 mg IV push should be administered. Once administered, the diuretic effects of furosemide do not become apparent until approximately 20 minutes later. Because furosemide is not capable of providing immediate relief to the patient with CHF or dyspnea, the provider must rely on other medications for the 20 minutes of treatment.

Nitroglycerin produces vasodilation and dilates veins to a greater magnitude than it does arteries. Venodilation results in less blood returning to the heart, which produces a reduction in cardiac preload. This effect of nitroglycerin provides some early relief before the onset of the diuretic effects of furosemide. Nitroglycerin also reduces cardiac workload in patients with acute symptoms of congestive heart disease, improves blood flow to ischemic myocardium, and decreases myocardial oxygen demand.

In addition to its common uses for the treatment of pain, morphine sulfate is used in patients with CHF and pulmonary edema to relieve pulmonary congestion by venodilation. Morphine also lowers myocardial oxygen demand and reduces anxiety.

Because morphine is a respiratory depressant, paramedics need to be skilled and equipped to support the patient's airway and respirations in the event of respiratory failure.

FUROSEMIDE (LASIX)

Classification: Loop diuretic
Action: Inhibits the absorption of the sodium and chloride ions and water in the loop of Henle, as well as the convoluted tubule of the nephron. This results in decreased absorption of water and increased production of urine.
Indications: Pulmonary edema, CHF, hypertensive emergency.
Adverse Effects: Vertigo, dizziness, weakness, orthostatic hypotension, hypokalemia, thrombophlebitis. Patients with anuria, severe renal failure, untreated hepatic coma, increasing azotemia, and electrolyte depletion can develop life-threatening consequences.
Contraindications: Known sensitivity to sulfonamides or furosemide.
Dosage:
Congestive Heart Failure and Pulmonary Edema:
- **Adult:** 40 mg IV, IO administered slowly over a 1- to 2-minute period. If a satisfactory response is not achieved within 1 hour, an additional dose of 80 mg can be given. A maximum single IV dose is 160 to 200 mg.
- **Pediatric:** 1 mg/kg IV, IO or IM. If the response is not satisfactory, an additional dose of 2 mg/kg may be administered no sooner than 2 hours after the first dose.

Hypertensive Emergency:
- **Adult:** 40 to 80 mg IV, IO.
- **Pediatric:** 1 mg/kg IV or IM.

Special Considerations:
Onset of action for IV, IO administration occurs within 5 minutes and will peak within 30 minutes.
Furosemide is a diuretic, so the patient will likely have urinary urgency. Be prepared to help the patient void.
Pregnancy class C

MORPHINE SULFATE

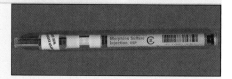

Classification: Opiate agonist, Schedule C-II
Action: Binds with opioid receptors. Morphine is capable of inducing hypotension by depression of the vasomotor centers of the brain, as well as release of the chemical histamine. In the management of angina, morphine reduces stimulation of the sympathic nervous system caused by pain and anxiety. Reduction of sympathetic stimulation reduces heart rate, cardiac work, and myocardial oxygen consumption.
Indications: Moderate to severe pain, including chest pain associated with ACS, CHF, pulmonary edema.
Adverse Effects: Respiratory depression, hypotension, nausea/vomiting, dizziness, lightheadedness, sedation, diaphoresis, euphoria, dysphoria, worsening of bradycardia and heart block in some patients with acute inferior wall MI, seizures, cardiac arrest, anaphylactoid reactions.
Contraindications: Respiratory depression, shock, known sensitivity. Use with caution in hypotension, acute bronchial asthma, respiratory insufficiency, head trauma.
Dosage:
Pain:
- **Adult:** 2.5 to 15 mg IV, IO, IM, or Sub-Q administered slowly over a period of several minutes. The dose is the same whether administered IV, IO, IM, or Sub-Q.
- **Pediatric:**
  - **6 months to 12 years:** 0.05 to 0.2 mg/kg IV, IO, IM, or Sub-Q.
  - **Younger than 6 months:** 0.03 to 0.05 mg/kg IV, IO, IM, or Sub-Q.

cont'd

MORPHINE SULFATE—CONT'D

Chest Pain Associated with Acute Coronary Syndromes, Congestive Heart Failure, and Pulmonary Edema:

Administer small doses and reevaluate the patient. Large doses may lead to respiratory depression and worsen the patient's hypoxia.

- **Adult:** 2 to 4 mg slow IV, IO over a 1- to 5-minute period with increments of 2 to 8 mg repeated every 5 to 15 minutes until patient relieved of chest pain.
- **Pediatric:** 0.1 to 0.2 mg/kg/dose IV, IO.

Special Considerations:

Monitor vital signs and pulse oximetry closely. Be prepared to support patient's airway and ventilations.

Overdose should be treated with naloxone.

Pregnancy class C

NITROGLYCERIN (NITROLINGUAL, NITROQUICK, NITRO-DUR)

Classification: Antianginal agent

Action: Relaxes vascular smooth muscle, thereby dilating peripheral arteries and veins. This causes pooling of venous blood and decreased venous return to the heart, which decreases preload. Nitroglycerin also reduces left ventricular systolic wall tension, which decreases afterload.

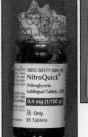
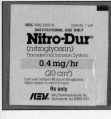
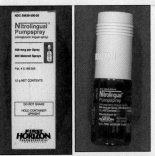

Indications: Angina, ongoing ischemic chest discomfort, hypertension, myocardial ischemia associated with cocaine intoxication.

Adverse Effects: Headache, hypotension, bradycardia, lightheadedness, flushing, cardiovascular collapse, methemoglobinemia.

Contraindications: Hypotension, severe bradycardia or tachycardia, increased ICP, intracranial bleeding, patients taking any medications for erectile dysfunction (such as sildenafil [Viagra], tadalafil [Cialis], or vardenafil [Levitra]), known sensitivity to nitrates. Use with caution in anemia, closed-angle glaucoma, hypotension, postural hypotension, uncorrected hypovolemia.

Dosage:

- **Adult:**
  - **Sublingual tablets:** 1 tablet (0.3-0.4 mg) at 5-minute intervals to a maximum of 3 doses.
  - **Translingual spray:** 1 (0.4 mg) spray at 5-minute intervals to a maximum of 3 sprays.
  - **Ointment:** 2% topical (Nitro-Bid ointment): Apply 1 to 2 inches of paste over the chest wall, cover with transparent wrap, and secure with tape.
  - **IV:**
    - **Bolus:** 12.5 to 25 mcg
    - **Infusion:** 5 mcg/min; may increase rate by 5 to 10 mcg/min every 5 to 10 minutes as needed. End points of dose titration for nitroglycerin include a drop in the blood pressure of 10%, relief of chest pain, and return of ST segment to normal on a 12-lead ECG.
  - **Pediatric IV infusion:** The initial pediatric infusion is 0.25 to 0.5 mcg/kg/min IV, IO titrated by 0.5 to 1 mcg/kg/min. Usual required dose is 1 to 3 mcg/kg/min to a maximum dose of 5 mcg/kg/min.

Special Considerations:

Administration of nitroglycerin to a patient with right ventricular MI can result in hypotension.

Pregnancy class C

DRUGS USED FOR LONG-TERM MANAGEMENT

Common medications used for the long-term management of patients with CHF include digoxin, lisinopril, and metoprolol. Although these medications are not likely to be administered by prehospital providers, many patients with heart disease take some or all of them. Paramedics must be familiar with these medications because patients can experience ill effects from them that the paramedic may need to recognize and treat.

Digoxin is used in patients with CHF to increase myocardial contractility and often to slow the heart rate. Digoxin may also be used in patients with chronic atrial fibrillation. Simply put, digoxin helps the heart beat stronger and slower. When the heart beats fast, less time is available for the ventricle to fill with blood, which means less blood can fill the ventricle; therefore cardiac output is decreased. When the heart rate is slowed, the ventricles are given more time to fill, and cardiac output is increased.

Blood delivering oxygen to the cells of the heart travels through the coronary arteries. When the heart contracts (systole), the coronary arteries are also squeezed; that action prevents oxygen-rich blood from moving forward. The only time that blood can carry oxygen to the heart is between contractions (diastole). By slowing the heart rate, cardiac consumption of oxygen is reduced, and blood flow to the heart is increased. In summary, the benefits of a drug-induced reduction of heart rate include the following:

- Decreased myocardial oxygen consumption
- Improved stroke volume, increasing cardiac output
- Prolonged diastolic coronary blood flow

A rapid heart rate (especially atrial fibrillation) reduces the filling of the heart, leading to decreased cardiac output and blood pressure.

Lisinopril is an ACE inhibitor. When angiotensin is inhibited, production of the most powerful vasoconstrictor in the body (**angiotensinogen**) halts. As a result, the patient will have a decrease in blood pressure and mild diuresis. ACE inhibitors also reduce cardiac ischemic events, mortality rate, and hospital admissions for individuals with CHF.

Metoprolol, a beta blocker, binds to beta adrenergic receptors and decreases blood pressure and heart rate, which are beneficial to the diseased heart. Metoprolol is a cardioselective beta blocker used to control hypertension and decrease cardiac workload in the patient with CHF. Adding a beta blocker to an ACE inhibitor has been shown to decrease mortality rate and hospital admissions in symptomatic patients with heart failure.[3]

DIGOXIN (LANOXIN)

Classification: Cardiac glycoside

Action: Inhibits sodium-potassium-adenosine triphosphatase membrane pump, resulting in an increase in calcium inside the heart muscle cell, which causes an increase in the force of contraction of the heart.

Indications: CHF, to control the ventricular rate in chronic AF and atrial flutter, narrow-complex PSVT.

Adverse Effects: Headache, weakness, GI disturbances, arrhythmias, nausea/vomiting, diarrhea, vision disturbances.

Contraindications: Digitalis allergy, VT and VF, heart block, sick sinus syndrome, tachycardia without heart failure, pulse lower than 50 to 60 beats/min, MI, ischemic heart disease, patients with preexcitation AF or atrial flutter (i.e., a delta wave, characteristic of Wolff-Parkinson-White syndrome, visible during normal sinus rhythm).

Dosage: Dosage is individualized.

Special Considerations:

Low levels of serum potassium can lead to digoxin toxicity and bradycardia. Conditions such as administration of steroids or diuretics or vomiting and diarrhea can produce low levels of potassium and subsequent digoxin toxicity.

Pregnancy class C

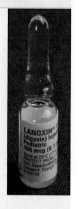

ANGIOTENSIN-CONVERTING ENZYME INHIBITORS, BETA BLOCKERS, AND CALCIUM CHANNEL BLOCKERS

Angiotensin-Converting Enzyme Inhibitors

Many patients with CHF are prescribed ACE inhibitors. This class of drugs blocks, or antagonizes, the enzyme responsible for the production of the hormone **angiotensin II.** Angiotensin II is a vasoconstrictor that is 40 times more powerful than norepinephrine. In addition to being a vasoconstrictor, angiotensin II also has positive inotropic and chronotropic properties. Therefore drugs that block the production of angiotensin II (ACE inhibitors) reduce blood pressure, decrease cardiac afterload, reduce heart rate, and reduce the force of contraction of the heart. ACE inhibitors reduce the mortality rate in patients with moderate and severe CHF.

ANGIOTENSIN-CONVERTING ENZYME (ACE) INHIBITORS: CAPTOPRIL (CAPOTEN), ENALAPRIL (VASOTEC), LISINOPRIL (PRINIVIL, ZESTRIL), RAMIPRIL (ALTACE)

Classification: ACE inhibitors
Action: Blocks the enzyme responsible for the production of angiotensin II, resulting in a decrease in blood pressure.
Indications: Congestive heart failure, hypertension, post–myocardial infarction.
Adverse Effects: Headache, dizziness, fatigue, depression, chest pain, hypotension, palpitations, cough, dyspnea, upper respiratory infection, nausea/vomiting, rash, pruritus, angioedema, renal failure.
Contraindications: Angioedema related to previous treatment with an ACE inhibitor, known sensitivity. Use with caution in aortic stenosis, bilateral renal artery stenosis, hypertrophic obstructive cardiomyopathy, pericardial tamponade, elevated serum potassium levels, acute kidney failure.
Dosage:
  · **Adult:** Medication is administered orally. Dosage is individualized.
  · **Pediatric:** Medication is administered orally. Dosage is individualized.
Special Considerations:
Pregnancy class D

Beta Blockers

Beta blockers are helpful in the long-term management of patients with CHF; however, beta blockers should be avoided in patients who are unstable or have decompensated CHF. In the management of a patient with chronic heart failure, the dose of beta blockers is slowly and progressively increased over a prolonged period.

METOPROLOL (LOPRESSOR, TOPROL XL)

Classification: Beta adrenergic antagonist, antianginal, antihypertensive, class II antiarrhythmic
Action: Inhibits the strength of the heart's contractions, as well as heart rate. This results in a decrease in cardiac oxygen consumption. Also saturates the beta receptors and inhibits dilation of bronchial smooth muscle (beta$_2$ receptor).
Indications: ACS, hypertension, SVT, atrial flutter, AF, thyrotoxicosis.
Adverse Effects: Tiredness, dizziness, diarrhea, heart block, bradycardia, bronchospasm, drop in blood pressure.
Contraindications: Cardiogenic shock, AV block, bradycardia, known sensitivity. Use with caution in hypotension, chronic lung disease (asthma and COPD).
Dosage:
Cardiac Indications:
  · **Adult:** 5 mg slow IV, IO over a 5-minute period; repeat at 5-minute intervals up to a total of three infusions totaling 15 mg IV, IO.
  · **Pediatric:** Not recommended for pediatric patients; no studies available.

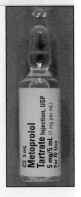

cont'd

METOPROLOL (LOPRESSOR, TOPROL XL)—CONT'D

Special Considerations:
Blood pressure, heart rate, and ECG should be monitored carefully.
Use with caution in patients with asthma.
Pregnancy class C

Calcium Channel Blockers

Certain calcium channel blockers such as verapamil, diltiazem, and nifedipine should be avoided in patients with CHF because they have been shown to increase morbidity and mortality rates in patients with left ventricular systolic dysfunction from heart failure.[4]

REVIEW QUESTIONS

1. What are some medical conditions that may predispose a patient to develop CHF?
2. What is the function of a diuretic?
3. How is morphine beneficial in the treatment of heart failure?
4. What are the benefits to the heart of preventing tachycardia when treating someone with heart disease?
5. What is the role of digoxin in the treatment of CHF?
6. Explain the effects of ACE inhibitors on the heart.
7. What precautions should be followed in administering beta blockers to a patient with CHF?

REFERENCES

1. American Heart Association: *Heart disease and stroke statistics: 2005 update,* Dallas, 2005, American Heart Association.
2. Marantz PR, et al: The relationship between left ventricular systolic function and congestive heart failure diagnosed by clinical criteria, *Circulation* 77:607, 1988.
3. The Cardiac Insufficiency Bisoprolol Study II (CIBIS-II): a randomized trial, *Lancet* 353:9, 1999.
4. O'Conner CM, et al: Effect of amlodipine on mode of death among patients with advanced heart failure in the PRAISE trial. Prospective Randomized Amlodipine Survival Evaluation, *Am J Cardiol* 82:881, 1998.

BIBLIOGRAPHY

Ahmed A: American College of Cardiology/American Heart Association: Chronic heart failure evaluation and management guidelines: relevance to the geriatric practice, *J Am Geriatr Soc* 51:123, 2003.

Cesario DA, Fonarow GC: Beta-blocker therapy for heart failure: the standard of care, *Rev Cardiovasc Med* 3:14, 2002.

Chatterjee K: Congestive heart failure: what should be the initial therapy and why? *Am J Cardiovasc Drugs* 2:1, 2002.

Cummins RO: Guidelines 2000 for cardiopulmonary resuscitation and emergency cardiovascular care, *Circulation* 102:I112, 2000.

Dominguez OJ: Breathless, *Emerg Med Serv* 31:87, 2002.

Kahn MG: *Cardiac drug therapy,* ed 5, Oxford, 1999, WB Saunders.

Lange C: Dyspnea and cough in an elderly woman with diabetes and CHF, *Clin Advisor* 8:106, 2005.

Mosesso VN, Dunford J, Blackwell T, et al: Prehospital therapy for acute congestive heart failure: state of the art, *Prehosp Emerg Care* 7:13, 2003.

Shapiro SE: Evidence review: emergency medical services treatment of patient with congestive heart failure/acute pulmonary edema: do risks outweigh benefits? *J Emerg Nurs* 31:51, 2005.

Yamaguchi S, Bocock JM: Acute dyspnea. In Hamilton GC, et al: *Emergency medicine: an approach to clinical problem-solving,* ed 2, Philadelphia, 2003, WB Saunders.

Endocrine Emergencies

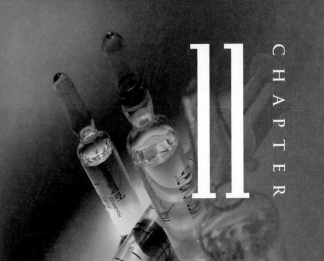

CHAPTER 11

OBJECTIVES

1. Differentiate type 1 and type 2 diabetes.
2. Explain the roles of glucagon, glycogen, and glucose in hypoglycemia.
3. Discuss the following medications for the treatment of hypoglycemia: dextrose (50% dextrose, 25% dextrose), thiamin (vitamin B_1), and glucagon.
4. Define diabetic ketoacidosis and the complications associated with this condition for diabetic patients.
5. Discuss the effect of insulin in diabetic ketoacidosis.
6. Identify the causes of acute adrenal insufficiency, and discuss how hydrocortisone (Cortef, Solu-Cortef) is used to treat this condition.
7. Discuss the medications used in the treatment of thyrotoxicosis: esmolol (Brevibloc), labetalol (Trandate, Normodyne), and metoprolol (Lopressor).

Medications that Appear in Chapter 11

Dextrose (Dextrose 50%, Dextrose 25%, Dextrose 10%)
Glucagon
Thiamine (Vitamin B_1)
Insulin, Regular (Humulin R, Novolin R)
Hydrocortisone sodium succinate (Cortef, Solu-Cortef)
Esmolol (Brevibloc)
Labetalol (Normodyne, Trandate)
Metoprolol (Lopressor, Toprol XL)

INTRODUCTION

This chapter describes pharmacologic treatment of the most common endocrine emergencies, including diabetic emergencies such as hypoglycemia, hyperglycemia, and diabetic ketoacidosis. Thyroid and adrenal emergencies, including thyrotoxicosis and adrenal insufficiency, are also addressed.

You are called to a local supermarket in response to a 63-year-old man who was found unconscious. He has a history of heart disease and type 2 diabetes. He takes a beta blocker and glyburide, an oral hypoglycemic medication. The patient's wife states that he has not eaten much today. On arrival you find him on the floor, and his mental status is depressed. His airway is patent, and he is breathing with no obstruction. His blood pressure is 120/95 mm Hg, and his heart rate is 120 beats/min. He appears pale and feels clammy to the touch. A glucometer reveals a blood sugar level of 52 mg/dL. IV access is obtained, and IV 50% dextrose is administered. He begins to awaken and a maintenance IV with D_5W is begun. Ten minutes after the bolus of dextrose, the patient's repeat blood sugar is 138 mg/dL. His heart rate is improving at 90 beats/min, and his blood pressure is stable.

OVERVIEW OF DIABETES

Diabetes is a disease manifested by a dysfunctional pancreas. Insulin is required to convert sugars into energy for use by the body. Diabetes takes two different forms, **type 1 diabetes** and **type 2 diabetes.** Patients with type 1 diabetes do not produce insulin. Without insulin, the cells of the body are not able to take sugar into the cell to be used for energy by that cell. Sugar is the main fuel of the cells, and like a car without gasoline, the cells of the body are not able to run without sugar. Patients with type 2 diabetes are capable of making insulin; however, the insulin is not used properly by the body, a condition known as *insulin resistance*. The majority of people with diabetes have type 2.

Insulin is used in patients with type 1 diabetes and some patients with type 2 diabetes. Insulin stimulates the uptake of glucose by the cells of the body and lowers the level of sugar in the blood (Fig. 11-1). Insulin allows glucose to enter cells, and potassium follows in turn. Oral hypoglycemic medications are used to manage most patients with type 2 diabetes. These agents act at a receptor on the insulin-producing cells of the pancreas. Some oral hypoglycemic agents also act by improving insulin's action on cells around the body. Oral hypoglycemic medications have a tendency to contribute to hypoglycemia, especially in certain groups of patients such as the elderly and those with liver and kidney disease.

Diabetes is a common disease, and paramedics routinely will encounter patients who take various forms of insulin. These various forms differ in their onset and duration of

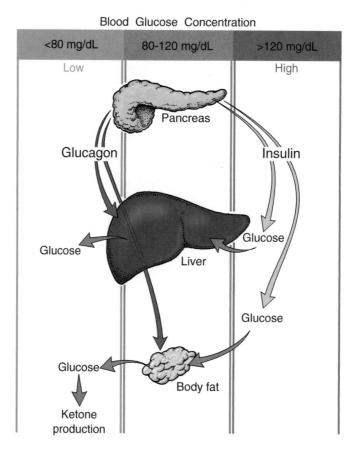

▼ **Fig. 11-1**   The interaction of the hormones insulin and glucagon in the body in relation to blood glucose levels. A rise in blood glucose levels stimulates insulin release from the pancreas. Insulin allows glucose to enter the liver and allows entry of amino acids into muscle and free fatty acids into fat tissue. A low glucose level in the blood stimulates glucagon production in the pancreas. When glucagon is present, glucose is released from its stored form in the liver to make it available for the body's cells. (From Pons P, Cason D, editors: *Paramedic field care, a complaint-based approach,* St Louis, 1997, Mosby.)

action. Although prehospital providers are exposed to several different forms of insulin, if a paramedic administers insulin to a patient, it will most likely be regular insulin. Several types of insulin are on the market. What distinguishes these different types are the time of onset and the duration of action. Some forms of insulin have a fast onset of action that may last only a few hours. In contrast, other, longer-acting insulins may have a slower onset but last as long as 24 hours. A patient's blood sugar level changes throughout the day. It may be lower between meals or overnight. After a meal or a snack, blood sugar increases (Fig. 11-2). To provide reasonable control of blood sugar, a patient may be taking several different forms of insulin.

Diabetes is an increasingly common disease process. Diabetic emergencies, in particular, are commonly encountered by paramedics. These emergencies typically represent complications of a blood sugar level that is too high (hyperglycemia, resulting in ketoacidosis) or too low (hypoglycemia, resulting in seizure or coma).

HYPOGLYCEMIA

Hypoglycemia (low blood sugar) is the most common complication experienced by patients with diabetes and is a life-threatening emergency. It is often referred to as *insulin shock*. Research has shown that diabetic patients have fewer long-term complications when they maintain tight control of their blood sugar. However, with the increased effort toward improved blood glucose control can come an increased risk of hypoglycemia. In fact, as a patient's average blood sugar approaches 120 mg/dL, the incidence of hypoglycemia increases threefold.[1]

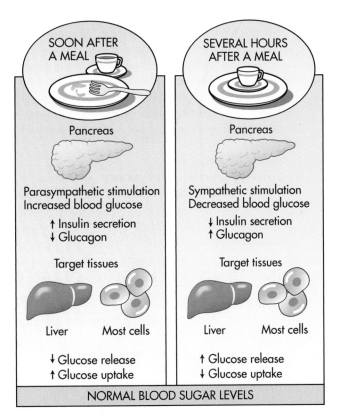

▼ Fig. 11-2 Diagram of the counterregulatory mechanisms of glucose metabolism with insulin and glucagon. Several hours after a meal, decreased blood glucose levels will inhibit insulin and stimulate glucagon, as well as the sympathetic nervous system. These changes allow glycogen to release glucose from the liver and decrease glucose uptake by the muscles, making glucose rise in the bloodstream. Immediately after a meal, blood glucose levels rise, stimulating insulin release, decreasing glucagon, and stimulating parasympathetic signals. These changes allow the formation of glycogen and storage of glucose into the liver and peripheral tissues. (From Sanders M: *Mosby's paramedic textbook,* ed 3 rev, St Louis, 2007, Mosby.)

Mild hypoglycemia commonly occurs in patients with diabetes and can simply be treated with oral glucose. However, moderate hypoglycemia can lead to serious hypoglycemia; that is, low blood sugar that requires intervention by someone other than the patient. The cause of hypoglycemia is not always recognized, and the patient can have little warning to intervene and prevent worsening of the situation. This is particularly true for patients who have had diabetes for several years because they can lose the ability to recognize symptoms of hypoglycemia, such as tachycardia, pallor, sweating, and anxiety. This is referred to as **hypoglycemic unawareness.**

Hypoglycemia is often caused by the insufficient intake of sugar from inadequacies in the diet or by excessive insulin from inaccurate dosing or excessive action of the medication. Both factors typically contribute to hypoglycemia. Increased utilization of glucose by the body, such as occurs during and after exercise or strenuous physical activity, can cause blood sugar to drop rapidly, resulting in hypoglycemia.

The patient in the previous scenario had a hypoglycemic episode, most likely from the oral hypoglycemic medication used to treat his type 2 diabetes. Remember, oral hypoglycemic medications work by increasing insulin secretion. This increased insulin release, combined with the fact that the patient had not eaten much that day, likely resulted in the patient's episode of hypoglycemia.

During hypoglycemia, the body's defenses include secretion of certain hormones and activation of the sympathetic nervous system in an attempt to increase blood sugar. **Glucagon** is secreted by the pancreas in response to low blood sugar. Glucagon mobilizes glucose stored in the liver and muscle in the form of **glycogen.** Glycogen is a molecule that acts as a storage form of glucose. When the body needs additional glucose, such as in exercise or stress, the pancreas releases glucagon. Glucagon stimulates the breakdown of glycogen, producing glucose. Epinephrine, a catecholamine from the adrenal gland, ultimately stimulates an increase in blood sugar. The release of epinephrine also produces an increase in blood pressure, tachycardia, diaphoresis, and anxiety. Recall that the patient in our scenario had all these symptoms.

In the scenario, beta blockers may have prevented a rise in heart rate and blood pressure. For diabetic patients, beta blockers can mask the symptoms of hypoglycemia, and these patients can be more prone to blunted hypoglycemic unawareness.

Management

Hypoglycemia requires prompt treatment. When possible, the treatment of choice is oral glucose. If the patient is conscious, oral glucose can result in an immediate improvement. Oral glucose is available as either a glucose gel or tablet. Glucose gel is easier to tolerate and can prevent the risk of choking in the event of an altered level of consciousness.

 ## ADMINISTRATION OF ORAL GLUCOSE

Equipment Needed:
Medicine, gloves, tongue depressor or other appropriate applicator, PPE
Procedure:
1. Observe universal precautions.
2. Verify drug order.
3. Confirm right patient, right medication, right dose, right route, and right time.
4. Confirm with the patient that he or she has no allergies to the medication, and document allergies to any other medication.
5. When possible, explain to the patient what medication you are going to administer and why.
6. Ensure the patient is responsive and able to swallow.
7. Place the glucose on a tongue depressor and administer the full tube between the patient's cheek and gum.
8. Record the time of drug administration in the patient care record.

9. Evaluate the patient for desired effects of the medication, as well as any adverse effects.

If the patient has an altered or depressed level of consciousness, as in the previous scenario, or if an adequate airway is not established, parenteral administration of glucose is more appropriate. This is achieved by using IV dextrose. Dextrose is available as 50% dextrose solution. That means that 100 mL of a solution has 50 g of dextrose. The pre-loaded syringe of 50% dextrose used in most emergency situations is a 50-mL syringe (25 g dextrose in 50 mL solution). Twenty-five percent dextrose has 25 g of dextrose in 100 mL of solution, and 10% dextrose has 10 g of dextrose in 100 mL of solution. Ten percent dextrose is prepared by diluting 50% dextrose 1:4 with IV fluid.

Dextrose solutions that are more concentrated than 5% solutions are considered hypertonic and can cause irritation and pain when injected too rapidly. To avoid this irritation to the vein, any dextrose solution more concentrated than 5% should be slowly injected into a large vein. Concentrated dextrose solutions should not be administered IM or Sub-Q.

Treatment of hypoglycemia depends on the patient's level of consciousness. If IV access were not possible in the patient in the scenario, the next step would be to administer IM glucagon. This would mobilize glycogen stores from the liver and elevate blood glucose levels rather rapidly. However, a common side effect is vomiting because glucagon delays gastric emptying. Patients who have been fasting for days may not show a pronounced effect because of low glycogen levels in the liver.

Patients with hypoglycemia require close monitoring of the airway, and blood glucose should be checked every 30 minutes. In the previous scenario, even though the first repeat blood sugar was elevated, the glucose should not be lowered too aggressively with insulin because the patient has been using an oral agent whose action can last for several hours. The patient's glucose can potentially be lowered to hypoglycemic levels. In addition, if he is not able to take an oral form of glucose, the use of IV glucose may need to be continued until he can be stabilized.

Patients with depressed mental status who are alcoholics or malnourished may have a deficiency of thiamine. If given dextrose before thiamine administration, such patients can develop a brain condition **(Wernicke-Korsakoff syndrome)** that manifests itself by amnesia, confabulation, attention deficit, disorientation, and vision impairment. To prevent Wernicke-Korsakoff syndrome, administer thiamine before dextrose in malnourished or alcoholic patients.

DEXTROSE (DEXTROSE 50%, DEXTROSE 25%, DEXTROSE 10%)

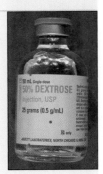

Classification: Antihypoglycemic
Action: Increases blood glucose concentrations.
Indications: Hypoglycemia
Adverse Effects: Hyperglycemia, warmth, burning from IV infusion. Concentrated solutions may cause pain and thrombosis of the peripheral veins.
Contraindications: Intracranial and intraspinal hemorrhage, delirium tremens, solution is not clear, seals are not intact.
Dosage:
Hyperkalemia:
· **Adult:** 25 g of dextrose 50% IV, IO.
· **Pediatric:** 0.5 to 1 g/kg IV, IO.
Hypoglycemia:
· **Adult:** 10 to 25 g of dextrose 50% IV (20 to 50 mL of dextrose solution).
· **Pediatric:**
  · **Older than 2 years:** 2 mL/kg of dextrose 50%.
  · **Younger than 2 years:** 2 to 4 mL/kg of dextrose 10%.
Special Considerations:
Pregnancy class C

GLUCAGON

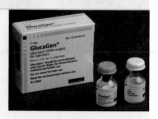

Classification: Hormone
Action: Converts glycogen to glucose.
Indications: Hypoglycemia, beta blocker overdose.
Adverse Effects: Nausea/vomiting, rebound hyperglycemia, hypotension, sinus tachycardia.
Contraindications: Pheochromocytoma, insulinoma, known sensitivity.
Dosage:
Hypoglycemia:
- **Adult:** 1 mg IM, IV, IO, or Sub-Q.
- **Pediatric (<20 kg):** 0.5 mg IM, IV, IO, or Sub-Q.
Beta blocker overdose:
- **Adult:** 2 to 5 mg IV, IO over a 1-minute period, followed by a second dose of 10 mg IV if the symptoms of bradycardia and hypotension recur. (Note that this dose is much higher than the dose required to treat hypoglycemia.)
- **Pediatric:** For patients weighing <20 kg, the dose is 0.5 mg.
Special Considerations:
Pregnancy class B

THIAMINE (VITAMIN B₁)

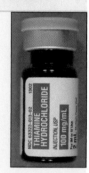

Classification: Vitamin B₁
Action: Thiamine combines with adenosine triphosphate to produce thiamine diphosphate, which acts as a coenzyme in carbohydrate metabolism.
Indications: Wernicke-Korsakoff syndrome, beriberi, nutritional supplementation.
Adverse Effects: Itching, rash, pain at injection site.
Contraindications: Known sensitivity.
Dosage:
Wernicke-Korsakoff Syndrome:
- **Adult:** 100 mg IV, IO.
- **Pediatric:** Not recommended for pediatric patients.
Special Considerations:
Pregnancy class A

DIABETIC KETOACIDOSIS

You are called to respond to a 10-year-old girl who has had vomiting and intermittent diarrhea for the past 6 days. The child's parents state that she has lost 15 pounds in 3 weeks. She is thin, with tachypnea and a fruity odor to her breath. Her heart rate is 180 beats/min, and her blood pressure is 90/60 mm Hg. Her weight is estimated at 50 pounds. IV access is obtained, and Ringer's lactate solution is begun at a maintenance rate (approximately 65 mL/hr). The glucometer reading is 560 mg/dL. Her pulse oximetry reading is 99% on room air despite rapid breathing. Her airway is patent and she is stable, although she continues to breathe rapidly. You start the patient on some oxygen by nasal cannula and place her on a cardiac monitor. ...

Diabetic ketoacidosis (DKA) occurs most commonly in patients with type 1 diabetes, although it can also occur in patients with type 2 diabetes. The key problem in DKA is lack of insulin. In diabetic patients, too little insulin prevents the cells of the body from using glucose and, consequently, blood glucose rises. The cells cannot use the glucose but still require a source of fuel. Therefore the glucose-starved cells start to break down fat, producing acid and chemicals known as **ketone bodies.**

Patients with DKA have metabolic acidosis, dehydration, and electrolyte abnormalities. The type of acidosis that these patients have is known as **ketoacidosis,** which is distinct from lactic acidosis. Ketoacidosis occurs when the body uses alternative fuel sources for energy production because of the inability to burn glucose from the lack of insulin. Conversely, **lactic acidosis** occurs in shock states when oxygen is lacking; the cellular machinery uses an inefficient energy-generating process known as *anaerobic metabolism*. The product of anaerobic metabolism is lactate; hence patients generate lactic acidosis. These two forms of acidosis are not related.

> The purpose of a car's fuel pump is to deliver fuel from the tank to the injectors of the engine. In the absence of a functional fuel pump, the car's engine can be starved of fuel despite having a tank full of gasoline. In this example, insulin is the fuel pump, and gasoline is glucose. The problem with a car's bad fuel pump is not the amount of the gasoline in the tank, but the inability to deliver that fuel to the engine. In DKA, the problem is not the elevated glucose levels but the inability to deliver that fuel (glucose) to the cellular machinery because of the lack of insulin.

High blood glucose levels often result in loss of glucose in the urine, and patients can become dehydrated. Within the kidney, glucose is filtered into the tubules that collect the urine produced. As the fluid passes through the tubules of the kidney, the glucose is reabsorbed. In cases in which the concentration of the blood glucose is elevated, the amount of glucose passed into the kidney tubules exceeds the kidney's ability to reabsorb the glucose back into the bloodstream, and glucose is spilled into the urine. The spilling of glucose into the urine typically occurs at a serum blood glucose of approximately 300 mg/dL. In Chapter 5 the concept of osmosis was discussed. The glucose molecule in the urine also decreases the reabsorption of water by the kidney and the patient rapidly becomes dehydrated. In this situation, patients have symptoms of increased thirst, increased urination, racing of the heart, and vomiting. The breath of a patient in DKA is often described as "fruity" because of the presence of the ketone bodies.

The preceding scenario illustrates a case of new-onset DKA in a pediatric patient. A similar scenario can present in a known diabetic patient who has become ill or perhaps has not received adequate insulin treatment.

Management

Treatment of DKA includes correction of dehydration and acidosis with IV fluids and insulin. *However, fluid replacement needs to be undertaken slowly.* Remember that the patient in the case lost weight and deteriorated over a 3-week period. As such, IV fluid administration should not be too rapid or aggressive unless the patient has cardiovascular instability. The patient is demonstrating tachycardia (heart rate of 180 beats/min), so an initial bolus of 10 mL/kg would be reasonable. Remember, conditions that quickly develop should be quickly corrected, and situations that slowly develop should be slowly corrected.

> ... After starting an IV line, you prepare to administer a fluid bolus. You determine that with her magnitude of hypovolemia, the patient should receive some intravascular fluid resuscitation. The patient weighs approximately 50 pounds (22 kg). You plan to administer a fluid bolus of approximately 10 mL/kg (22 kg × 10 mL/kg = 220 mL). You start a 250-mL fluid bolus of Ringer's lactate solution. Next you calculate her maintenance IV fluid rate at 62 mL/hr. After the fluid bolus, you plan to run the IV fluids at a maintenance rate of 1.5 times, or approximately 93 mL/hr (maintenance rate × 1.5 = 62 mL/hr × 1.5 = 93 mL).

Often IV fluids administered at maintenance to 1.5 times the maintenance rate are adequate for initial stabilization with the initial fluid bolus. (See Box 11-1 for pediatric maintenance rates.) The IV fluid of choice initially should not include potassium replacement

---

BOX 11-1

PEDIATRIC MAINTENANCE FLUIDS

To determine the appropriate rate of maintenance fluid, the provider must know or estimate the child's weight in kilograms. Remember that 1 kg equals approximately 2.2 pounds.

For the first 10 kg of weight, the IV fluid rate is 4 mL/hr per kilogram.

▶ A 5-kg child has an IV rate of 20 mL/hr (4 mL/hr per kilogram × 5 kg)

▶ A 10-kg child has an IV rate of 40 mL/hr (4 mL/hr per kilogram × 10 kg)

For the second 10 kg of weight (10 to 20 kg of body weight), add 2 mL/kg for each additional kilogram.

▶ For a 12-kg child, start with an IV rate of 40 mL/hr for the first 10 kg of body weight and then add 4 mL/hr for the remaining 2 kg. The IV rate then is 44 mL/hr.

· 10 kg × 4 mL/kg per hour = 40 mL/hr

· 2 kg × 2 mL/kg per hour = 4 mL/hr

· Total maintenance rate = 44 mL/hr

To calculate the IV maintenance rate for children larger than 20 kg, add an additional 1 mL/hr per kilogram.

▶ A 25-kg child will have an IV maintenance rate of:

· First 10 kg=40 mL/hr

· Second 10 kg=20 mL/hr

· Remaining 5 kg=1 mL/kg per hour × 5 kg=5 mL/hr

Therefore the total maintenance rate is 65 mL/hr.

---

because the presence of ketoacidosis suggests an elevated potassium level. (Once urine output is ensured and electrolyte status can be determined at a hospital, potassium replacement becomes increasingly important.) Treatment of DKA with insulin, as well as correction of the acidosis, moves potassium into cells and rapidly lowers blood potassium levels. Prehospital treatment should include an isotonic solution such as normal saline or Ringer's lactate. The use of bicarbonate is controversial and should be avoided except when ordered by medical direction in extreme situations.[2]

The patient's rapid breathing is the result of **ketonemia** (the presence of recognizable concentrations of ketone bodies in the plasma), acidosis, and the body's attempt to relieve itself of carbon dioxide. The fruity odor to her breath is also consistent with the presence of ketones. Her elevated heart rate is the result of a combination of responses to the body's detection of low plasma volume from dehydration, as well as the release of catecholamines such as epinephrine and norepinephrine. Patients with hyperkalemia need to be monitored for peaked T waves on the ECG. Compared with adults, children are less likely to have cardiovascular complications as potassium levels rise; however, monitoring cardiovascular status in all patients with DKA is still necessary.

Aggressive hydration, particularly with hypotonic fluids, has been shown to contribute to complications of therapy, such as cerebral edema or swelling of the brain. Conservative fluid management is therefore key!

If a patient's cardiovascular condition requires an IV fluid bolus, volume resuscitation should be conservative. In pediatric patients, boluses should be limited to 10 mL/kg at a time with fluids such as normal saline and Ringer's lactate and not repeated unless significant instability exists. Vital signs (blood pressure, heart rate, and respiratory rate) should be closely monitored, and neurologic status should be assessed. If a hypovolemic patient with DKA is resuscitated too quickly, the patient can develop cerebral edema (swelling of the brain). Therefore patients should be monitored for changes in their neurologic status.[3] A classic mistake made when caring for these patients is the addition of dextrose-containing solutions (D_5W, D_5NS, D_5 Ringer's lactate) to IV fluids. Once the patient with DKA is admitted to intensive care and the blood sugar level approaches 250 to 300 mg/dL, he or she will be switched to fluids that contain low concentrations of dextrose, such as D_5 Ringer's lactate solution. The reason to start glucose at this level of blood sugar (250 to 300 mg/dL) is to prevent the development of hypoglycemia while the blood sugar is lowered with insulin and to protect against the development of cerebral edema.

Insulin. Many EMS agencies do not carry insulin; simple IV fluid administration is often sufficient to improve hyperglycemia and help correct the metabolic acidosis until the patient can be transported and treated at a medical facility. If insulin is available and appropriate, it can be given as a bolus or drip.[4] The use of IV bolus insulin has been debated and remains a less-desirable method of treating hyperglycemia in DKA than an insulin infusion.

IV insulin has been shown to be significantly more effective than IM or Sub-Q administration, at least in the initial treatment of DKA.[4] In a patient with poor perfusion from hypovolemia or shock, subcutaneous insulin may not absorb appropriately, leading to a slow onset of action. Blood sugar should be monitored every 30 to 60 minutes while the patient is on an insulin drip or after a Sub-Q injection of insulin. The desired response should be a decrease in blood sugar by 10% per hour, or no faster than approximately 50 mg/dL per hour. Conversely, if the rate of decrease exceeds 50 mg/dL per hour, the insulin infusion may need to be decreased to prevent hypoglycemia. Acidosis often persists for several hours and can require up to 24 hours to resolve once the hyperglycemia has been corrected. Hydration and reestablishment of renal function are also critical.

INSULIN, REGULAR (HUMULIN R, NOVOLIN R)

Classification: Hormone
Action: Binds to a receptor on the membrane of cells and facilitates the transport of glucose into cells.
Indications: Hyperglycemia, insulin-dependent diabetes mellitus, hyperkalemia.
Adverse Effects: Hypoglycemia, tachycardia, palpitations, diaphoresis, anxiety, confusion, blurred vision, weakness, depression, seizures, coma, insulin shock, hypokalemia.
Contraindications: Hypoglycemia, known sensitivity.
Dosage:

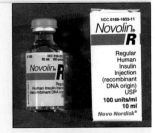

Diabetic Ketoacidosis:

- **Adult:** 0.1 U/kg IV, IO, or Sub-Q. Because of poor perfusion of the peripheral tissues, Sub-Q administration is much less effective than the IV, IO route. IV, IO insulin has a very short half-life; therefore IV, IO insulin without an infusion is not that effective. The rate for an insulin infusion is 0.05 to 0.1 U/kg/hr IV, IO. When dosing insulin, use a U-100 insulin syringe to measure and deliver the insulin. The time from administration to action, as well as the duration of action, varies greatly among different individuals, as well as at different times in the same individual.

Hyperkalemia:

- **Adult:** 10 U IV, IO of regular insulin (Insulin R), coadministered with 50 mL of $D_{50}W$ over 5 minutes.
- **Pediatric:** 0.1 U/kg Insulin R IV, IO.

Special Considerations:
Only regular insulin can be given IV, IO.
Pregnancy class B

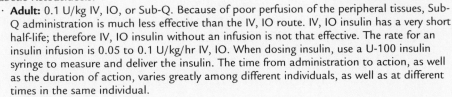

Rapid-acting insulins

Although paramedics will likely not use insulin analogs in the field, an understanding of the newer forms of rapid-acting insulins is important because many patients take these products.

Insulin lispro (Humalog), insulin aspart (NovoLog), and insulin glulisine (Apidra) are three forms of synthetic insulin whose molecular structure makes them optimal for use in the treatment of type 1 diabetes. Onset of action occurs within 10 minutes and peak action is 90 minutes, with a duration of action of 2 to 4 hours in some patients.

These insulin products do not require a 30-minute wait when administered subcutaneously before a meal. They can even be administered immediately after a meal in some patients. This is desirable in the pediatric patient in particular, whose eating habits are variable; often their insulin doses are based on their carbohydrate intake.

OVERVIEW OF ACUTE ADRENAL INSUFFICIENCY

You are called to the home of a 54-year-old man who was found unconscious on his bathroom floor. According to his wife, he had a pituitary tumor resection 6 months ago. His medications include levothyroxine (Levothroid) and hydrocortisone (Cortef). He has had the flu for the past 4 days, with a fever of 101° F, vomiting, and diarrhea. He has not eaten much in the past few days and has had no oral intake today according to his wife. Assessment reveals a weak-appearing man lying on his side. No evidence of acute trauma is visible. He is pale and his eyes appear sunken. He is breathing rapidly but without audible wheezes. His blood pressure is 100/60 mm Hg, heart rate is 140 beats/min, and respiratory rate is 30 breaths/min. He weighs approximately 70 kg, and his blood glucose is 48 mg/dL. You obtain peripheral IV access immediately and administer 50% dextrose at 2 mL/kg (approximately 140 mL in this patient). A repeat blood sugar reading after the dextrose bolus is 95 mg/dL. A bolus of normal saline is then begun at 1 L over a 1-hour period, and blood sugar is monitored every 15 to 30 minutes. The next blood sugar reading is 90 mg/dL, and the fluid is changed to D_5W. IV hydrocortisone is given at a dose of 100 mg. The patient arrives at the local emergency department approximately 55 minutes later by your ambulance. His blood pressure has increased to 110/70 mm Hg, heart rate is now 100 beats/min, and respiratory rate is 20 breaths/min. A repeat blood glucose reading is 120 mg/dL.

Acute adrenal insufficiency is a life-threatening emergency that is often underdiagnosed and undertreated. However, treatment cannot be delayed because the patient's cardiovascular and metabolic status will rapidly deteriorate. The adrenal glands are located on top of each of the kidneys and are responsible for the production and secretion of several important hormones. The **adrenal medulla** produces catecholamines such as epinephrine and norepinephrine, which help the body respond during times of stress. The adrenal cortex, or outer layer of the gland, produces **steroid hormones,** including those responsible for electrolyte stability (called **mineralocorticoids**) and antiinflammatory stress hormones (called **glucocorticoids** or **cortisol**). In addition to its antiinflammatory function, cortisol contributes to the body's stress response, particularly during times of severe illness, surgery, and trauma. Blood pressure, heart rate, and blood glucose all increase in response to cortisol action.

In some patients, adrenal insufficiency results from the lack of an enzyme, which renders them unable to produce cortisol sufficiently, such as in **congenital adrenal hyperplasia (CAH).** Adrenal insufficiency can also result from infection, injury, and an autoimmune reaction of the gland (such as the result of tuberculosis, trauma, or Addison's disease). Sometimes the adrenal glands are unable to produce adequate stress hormones because of a lack of central input from the pituitary gland. The pituitary gland secretes a hormone called **adrenocorticotropin (ACTH),** which in turn stimulates the necessary signaling at the adrenal gland and results in the production and release of cortisol and other adrenal hormones. Patients who are treated with steroids for chronic conditions (e.g., COPD, asthma, and connective tissue diseases) may develop acute adrenal insufficiency when their steroids are interrupted or during periods of illness or injury.

MANAGEMENT

Patients with adrenal insufficiency usually are treated regularly with the physiologic replacement of cortisone (Cortone). Solu-Cortef is the parenteral form of hydrocortisone, and Cortef is the enteral form. Patients are typically instructed how to increase their dosage at times of illness or surgery to achieve the normal stress levels that the body naturally would produce during these situations. Many patients have access to an "emergency kit" of IM hydrocortisone (Cortef, Solu-Cortef) to administer the necessary medication when oral tablets cannot be taken.

In the previous scenario, the patient has adrenal insufficiency. Despite having functioning adrenal glands, he does not have the correct input from the pituitary gland to stimulate adrenal production and release cortisol during stressful times, such as fever and illness. In patients without adrenal insufficiency, cortisol is secreted at three to four times the normal levels during periods of stress. This patient has a history of hydrocortisone (Cortef, Solu-Cortef) replacement, which should have been increased during illness or in conjunction with surgery to simulate the body's increased needs. The oral increase in medication is limited during periods of vomiting. In addition, intravascular volume is depleted, contributing to the patient's hypotension. If IV access cannot be obtained, IM hydrocortisone can be administered.

HYDROCORTISONE SODIUM SUCCINATE (CORTEF, SOLU-CORTEF)

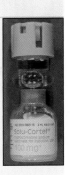

Classification: Corticosteroid
Action: Reduces inflammation by multiple mechanisms. As a steroid, it replaces the steroids that are lacking in adrenal insufficiency.
Indications: Adrenal insufficiency, allergic reactions, anaphylaxis, asthma, COPD.
Adverse Effects: Leukocytosis, hyperglycemia, increased infection, decreased wound healing, increased rate of death from sepsis.
Contraindications: Cushing's syndrome, known sensitivity to benzyl alcohol. Use with caution in diabetes, hypertension, CHF, known systemic fungal infection, renal disease, idiopathic thrombocytopenia, psychosis, seizure disorder, GI disease, glaucoma, known sensitivity.
Dosage:
Anaphylactic Shock:
· **Adult:** 100 to 500 mg IV, IO, or IM.
· **Pediatric:** 2 to 4 mg/kg/day IV, IO, or IM (max: 500 mg).
Adrenal Insufficiency:
· **Adult:** 100 to 500 mg IV, IO, or IM.
· **Pediatric:** 1 to 2 mg/kg IV, IO, or IM.
Asthma and Chronic Obstructive Pulmonary Disease:
· **Adult:** 100 to 500 mg IV, IO, IM.
· **Pediatric:** 1 mg/kg IV, IO. The dose may be reduced for infants and children, but it is governed more by the severity of the condition and response of the patient than by age or body weight. Dose should not be less than 25 mg daily.
Special Considerations:
Pregnancy class C

OVERVIEW OF THYROTOXICOSIS

You are called to the scene of a 64-year-old woman who is having a panic attack. She has a history of increased appetite, diarrhea, itching, irritability, and 10-pound weight loss over the past month. She has had insomnia for the past 2 to 3 weeks. Her husband states that she has always been healthy and is currently taking no medications. She has no history of substance abuse and no allergies. The patient appears nervous and fidgety. Her heart rate is 145 beats/min, blood pressure is 140/80 mm Hg, and respiratory rate is 30 breaths/min. Her face is reddened, and she has swelling in her neck that appears to be a goiter. Her upper eyelids are slightly swollen and retracted. She is breathing rapidly but without effort, and her lung sounds are clear. The ECG shows sinus tachycardia. IV access is obtained.

The thyroid gland is a small gland found in the neck over the voice box. The thyroid produces hormones commonly called *thyroid hormones*. Thyroid hormones are important in regulating the body's metabolic rate. When the body produces excessive amounts of thyroid hormone, the metabolic rate is increased. Elevated blood levels of thyroid hormone can result in a state known as **thyrotoxicosis.** Thyrotoxicosis is caused by autoimmune disease, infections, and cancer. Patients with thyrotoxicosis commonly experience tachycardia, tremor, diaphoresis, weight loss, and intolerance for warm rooms and environments.

MANAGEMENT

Treatment of thyrotoxicosis is aimed at protecting the various organ systems from the action of excessive thyroid hormone. Antithyroid agents are used for long-term management of thyroid disorders. These medications act within the thyroid gland to prevent production of thyroid hormone. **Thionamide agents** (propylthiouracil and methimazole) are oral antithyroid medications commonly used for the long-term management of hyperthyroidism. However, these agents inhibit the synthesis—not the release—of thyroid hormone. Therefore other medications should be used for the short-term treatment of thyrotoxicosis.

Thyroid hormone affects the cardiovascular system by sensitizing it to catecholamines, resulting in significant elevations of blood pressure and heart rate. Beta blockers can be used to treat hypertension, tachycardia, and other symptoms experienced by a patient with thyroid toxicity.[4] Beta blockers work by inhibiting the binding of catecholamines to the receptor site. Symptoms such as tremulousness, anxiety, palpitations, sweating, eyelid retraction, and tachycardia are improved with this treatment. Examples of beta blockers used to treat thyrotoxicosis include esmolol (Brevibloc), labetalol (Trandate, Normodyne), and metoprolol (Lopressor). A thorough discussion of dosing and details of beta blockers can be found in Chapter 12.

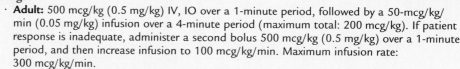

ESMOLOL (BREVIBLOC)

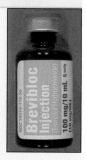

Classification: Beta adrenergic antagonist, class II antiarrhythmic
Action: Inhibits the strength of the heart's contractions, as well as heart rate, resulting in a decrease in cardiac oxygen consumption.
Indications: ACS, MI, acute hypertension, supraventricular tachyarrhythmias, thyrotoxicosis.
Adverse Effects: Hypotension, sinus bradycardia, AV block, cardiac arrest, nausea/vomiting, hypoglycemia, injection site reaction.
Contraindications: Acute bronchospasm, COPD, second- or third-degree heart block, bradycardia, cardiogenic shock, pulmonary edema, sick sinus syndrome, known sensitivity. Use with caution in patients with pheochromocytoma, Prinzmetal's angina, cerebrovascular disease, stroke, poorly controlled diabetes mellitus, hyperthyroidism, thyrotoxicosis, renal disease.
Dosage:
- **Adult:** 500 mcg/kg (0.5 mg/kg) IV, IO over a 1-minute period, followed by a 50-mcg/kg/min (0.05 mg/kg) infusion over a 4-minute period (maximum total: 200 mcg/kg). If patient response is inadequate, administer a second bolus 500 mcg/kg (0.5 mg/kg) over a 1-minute period, and then increase infusion to 100 mcg/kg/min. Maximum infusion rate: 300 mcg/kg/min.
- **Pediatric:** 500 mcg/kg (0.5 mg/kg) IV, IO over a 1-minute period, followed by an infusion at 25 to 200 mcg/kg/min.

Special Considerations:
Half-life 5 to 9 minutes
Any adverse effects caused by administration of esmolol are brief because of the drug's short half-life.
Resolution of effects usually within 10 to 20 minutes.
Pregnancy class C

LABETALOL (NORMODYNE, TRANDATE)

Classification: Beta adrenergic antagonist, antianginal, antihypertensive

Action: Binds with both the beta$_1$ and beta$_2$ receptors and alpha$_1$ receptors in vascular smooth muscle. Inhibits the strength of the heart's contractions, as well as heart rate. This results in a decrease in cardiac oxygen consumption.

Indications: ACS, SVT, severe hypertension.

Adverse Effects: Usually mild and transient; hypotensive symptoms, nausea/vomiting, bronchospasm, arrhythmia, bradycardia, AV block.

Contraindications: Hypotension, cardiogenic shock, acute pulmonary edema, heart failure, severe bradycardia, sick sinus syndrome, second- or third-degree heart block, asthma or acute bronchospasm, cocaine-induced ACS, known sensitivity. Use caution in pheochromocytoma, cerebrovascular disease or stroke, poorly controlled diabetes, with hepatic disease. Use with caution at lowest effective dose in chronic lung disease.

Dosage:

Cardiac Indications: Note: Monitor blood pressure and heart rate closely during administration.

Adult: 10 mg IV, IO over a 1- to 2-minute period. May repeat every 10 minutes to a maximum dose of 150 mg or give initial bolus and then follow with infusion at 2 to 8 mg/min.

Pediatric: 0.4 to 1 mg/kg/hr to a maximum dosage of 3 mg/kg/hr.

Severe Hypertension:

· **Adult:** Initial dose is 20 mg IV, IO slow infusion over a 2-minute period. After the initial dose, blood pressure should be checked every 5 minutes. Repeat doses can be given at 10-minute intervals. The second dose should be 40 mg IV, IO, and subsequent doses should be 80 mg IV, IO, to a maximum total dose of 300 mg. The effect on blood pressure typically will occur within 5 minutes from the time of administration. Alternatively, may be administered via IV infusion at 2 mg/min to a total maximum dose of 300 mg.

· **Pediatric:** 0.4 to 1 mg/kg/hr IV, IO infusion with a maximum dose of 3 mg/kg/hr.

Special Considerations:

Pregnancy class C

METOPROLOL (LOPRESSOR, TOPROL XL)

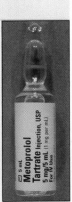

Classification: Beta adrenergic antagonist, antianginal, antihypertensive, class II antiarrhythmic

Action: Inhibits the strength of the heart's contractions, as well as heart rate. This results in a decrease in cardiac oxygen consumption. Also saturates the beta receptors and inhibits dilation of bronchial smooth muscle (beta$_2$ receptor).

Indications: ACS, hypertension, SVT, atrial flutter, AF, thyrotoxicosis.

Adverse Effects: Tiredness, dizziness, diarrhea, heart block, bradycardia, bronchospasm, drop in blood pressure.

Contraindications: Cardiogenic shock, AV block, bradycardia, known sensitivity. Use with caution in hypotension, chronic lung disease (asthma and COPD).

Dosage:

Cardiac Indications:

· **Adult:** 5 mg slow IV, IO over a 5-minute period; repeat at 5-minute intervals up to a total of three infusions totaling 15 mg IV, IO.

· **Pediatric:** Not recommended for pediatric patients; no studies available.

Special Considerations:

Blood pressure, heart rate, and ECG should be monitored carefully.

Use with caution in patients with asthma.

Pregnancy class C

REVIEW QUESTIONS

1. Explain the difference between patients with type 1 diabetes and type 2 diabetes in regard to their ability to produce insulin.
2. What is the risk of beta blockers in patients with diabetes?

3. What adverse effects is a patient likely to experience after administration of glucagon for hypoglycemia?
4. When treating a patient with DKA, what is the complication of aggressive fluid resuscitation with hypotonic fluids?
5. Can a prehospital provider treat DKA without the administration of insulin?
6. In times of stress, what are some of the actions of cortisol?
7. What are the manifestations of the increased metabolic rate during thyrotoxicosis?

REFERENCES

1. Diabetes Control and Complications Trial Research Group: Hypoglycaemia in the Diabetes Control and Complication Trial, *Diabetes* 46:271, 1997.
2. Morris L, Murphy M, Kitabchi A: Bicarbonate therapy in severe diabetic ketoacidosis, *Ann Intern Med* 105:836, 1986.
3. Harris G, et al: Minimizing the risk of brain herniation during treatment of diabetic ketoacidemia: a retrospective and prospective study, *J Pediatr* 117:22, 1990.
4. Kitabchi A, Wall B: Diabetic ketoacidosis, *Med Clin North Am* 79:9, 1995.

BIBLIOGRAPHY

Clinical practice recommendations, *Diabetes Care* 28:S1, 2005.
Rady MY, et al: Influence of individual characteristics on outcome of glycemic control in intensive care unit patients with or without diabetes mellitus, *Mayo Clin Proc* 80:1558, 2005.
Van den Berghe G, et al: Intensive insulin therapy in critically ill patients, *N Engl J Med* 345:1359, 2001.

Hypertensive Emergencies

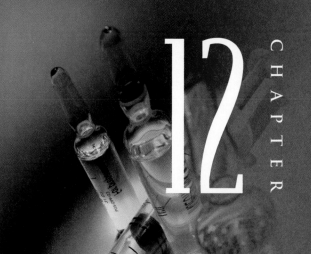

CHAPTER 12

OBJECTIVES

1. Define hypertensive urgency and hypertensive emergency.
2. Discuss the use of the following medications for the treatment of hypertensive encephalopathy, hypertensive intracranial hemorrhage, and pulmonary edema with hypertension: esmolol (Brevibloc), nicardipine (Cardene), furosemide (Lasix), sodium nitroprusside (Nipride), and labetalol (Trandate, Normodyne).
3. Discuss the use of aspirin and nitroglycerin (Nitrolingual, NitroQuick, Nitro-Dur) in the treatment of myocardial ischemia with hypertension.
4. Discuss medications used in the treatment of preeclampsia and eclampsia: magnesium sulfate and hydralazine (Apresoline).
5. Discuss medications used in the treatment of hypertension with seizure: diazepam (Valium) and phentolamine (Regitine).

Medications that Appear in Chapter 12

Esmolol (Brevibloc)
Nicardipine (Cardene)
Furosemide (Lasix)
Sodium nitroprusside (Nipride, Nitropress)
Labetalol (Normodyne, Trandate)
Aspirin, ASA
Nitroglycerin (Nitrolingual, NitroQuick, Nitro-Dur)
Magnesium sulfate
Hydralazine (Apresoline)
Diazepam (Valium)
Phentolamine (Regitine)

INTRODUCTION

More than 50 million people in the United States have hypertension. This disease is often called "the silent killer" because its victims may have no symptoms until the condition advances to the point of damaging organs and threatening the patient's life. Hypertensive emergencies require rapid identification and management by prehospital care providers. Specific emergencies often respond better to certain antihypertensive medications, which are explained in this chapter.

You are called to the home of a 52-year-old man who is unresponsive. His wife states that he has had high blood pressure for 3 years and diabetes since his 20s. He has been diagnosed with depression, for which he takes phenelzine (Nardil). He stopped taking his blood pressure medications a few months ago. She came home from shopping and found him unresponsive on the floor of their kitchen. His vital signs are blood pressure, 240/140 mm Hg; pulse, 128 beats/min; and respirations, 32 breaths/min. He is drooling. You note bilateral rales in his posterior lung fields. His right pupil is fixed and dilated. ...

In most cases, **hypertension,** or high blood pressure, has no identifiable cause, which is referred to as **essential hypertension.** Other identifiable causes of hypertension include kidney disease, arterial disease, steroids, and some endocrine tumors.

The systolic and diastolic pressures that have defined chronic hypertension have varied over the years. Historically, more emphasis was placed on systolic blood pressure, but diastolic hypertension has been determined to perhaps be more damaging in the long term. Systolic hypertension is dangerous for the elderly because it can lead to the development of strokes. For most patients with hypertension, treatment is long term and requires multiple drug therapies.

When hypertension is not diagnosed or treatment recommendations are not followed, hypertensive emergencies can arise. These can present as hypertensive urgency or hypertensive emergency. **Hypertensive urgency** is a severe elevation of the blood pressure without evidence of organ damage. **Hypertensive emergency,** also known as **malignant hypertension,** is a severe elevation in blood pressure complicated by evidence of end-organ damage. End-organ damage can occur in the kidneys (kidney failure), heart (heart failure), and brain (intracranial bleed or altered level of consciousness). Patients experiencing hypertensive emergencies can present with reports of headache, visual changes, altered level of consciousness, or heart failure. Specific hypertensive emergencies include the following:

- Hypertensive encephalopathy
- Hypertensive intracranial hemorrhage
- Pulmonary edema with hypertension
- Myocardial ischemia with hypertension
- Preeclampsia and eclampsia (hypertension with proteinuria in pregnancy)

Precipitating factors for hypertensive emergencies are listed in Box 12-1.

BOX 12-1

PRECIPITATING FACTORS FOR HYPERTENSIVE EMERGENCIES

Renal vascular hypertension
Renal disease
Connective tissue diseases (e.g., scleroderma)
Drug abuse (sympathomimetics, cocaine, PCP)
Withdrawal from antihypertensives
Tyramine ingestion while taking a monoamine oxidase inhibitor
Preeclampsia, eclampsia
Pheochromocytoma
Head injury
Tumor-secreting vasoconstricting hormones

OVERVIEW OF HYPERTENSIVE ENCEPHALOPATHY, HYPERTENSIVE INTRACRANIAL HEMORRHAGE, AND PULMONARY EDEMA WITH HYPERTENSION

The patient in the previous scenario is experiencing a hypertensive emergency, most likely hypertensive encephalopathy or possibly intracranial hemorrhage. This is an absolute emergency that, if not rapidly treated, can result in coma and death. Hypertensive encephalopathy is acute in onset and reversible. Patients often have severe headache, vomiting, and altered mental status. Intracranial bleeds are caused by a rupture of a blood vessel from elevated blood pressure. This diagnosis is confirmed by both physical examination and history. Findings include history of hypertension, abrupt cessation of antihypertensive medication, and use of a monoamine oxidase inhibitor—in the preceding scenario, phenelzine (Nardil). Physical findings include elevated blood pressure, pulmonary rales, and an altered mental status.

When determining which pharmacologic agent to use in the treatment of this emergency, the cause should be considered. This patient has risk factors for hypertensive encephalopathy and an intracranial bleed.

MANAGEMENT

Patients in a hypertensive emergency require a decrease in their blood pressure. However, do not reduce a patient's blood pressure to normal levels (e.g., 120/80 mm Hg). A too-rapid reduction of blood pressure or one at too great of a magnitude can result in ischemia of the brain or retina, leading to a stroke or blindness. The objective of the treatment of a hypertensive emergency is to reduce the diastolic blood pressure by 10% to 15% or to a diastolic pressure of 110 mm Hg. The reduction of blood pressure should be accomplished over a period of 30 to 60 minutes.

The drugs chosen to treat a particular hypertensive emergency vary by the cause of the rise of blood pressure. The patient in the previous scenario has either an intracranial hemorrhage or hypertensive encephalopathy. Many providers mistakenly think that nitroglycerin is a good drug to use in hypertensive emergencies. Nitroglycerin is a potent venodilator. Only at high doses does nitroglycerin act as an arterial dilator. Nitroglycerin decreases blood pressure by venodilation, which decreases the blood returning to the right side of the heart, which decreases the cardiac preload, which in turn decreases the patient's cardiac output. If a patient is having a hypertensive emergency resulting in decreased blood flow to the brain, a decrease in cardiac output would be undesirable. In patients having a hypertensive emergency in which the affected end organ is the brain with a possible cerebral vascular accident (stroke), the best choice of drug therapy is either a beta blocker or nicardipine (Cardene).

Esmolol (Brevibloc) is a rapid, short-acting beta$_1$ blocker. A unique property of esmolol is that it has little effect on the blood pressure of individuals who are not hypertensive. Esmolol also has a very short half-life of 9 minutes. If, after administration of esmolol, a patient's blood pressure is too low, the effect will not be prolonged. This drug is an excellent choice for the patient in the preceding scenario. Labetalol (Trandate, Normodyne) would be another potential choice of a beta blocker to use in this scenario. Labetalol has a half-life of 5 to 8 hours. Therefore, if labetalol causes an adverse effect, the duration will be much longer.

Nicardipine (Cardene) is another example of a calcium channel blocker with a number of desirable properties, including rapid onset of action, lack of toxic metabolites, and ease of titration to desired effect. Thus nicardipine effects resemble those of nitroprusside in terms of onset, duration, and offset of action. Nicardipine is a good option in the management of severe hypertension with or without target-organ damage.

Furosemide (Lasix) is a potent **diuretic.** Commonly referred to as "water pills," diuretics are medications that help reduce circulating intravascular volume by promoting an increase in urine production by the kidney. The mechanism of action of furosemide is to block salt and fluid reabsorption in the kidney, which results in a significant increase in urine output. This process is referred to as **diuresis.**

... This patient with a hypertensive emergency has two organs that are affected: the brain and lungs. Given the depressed mental status and dilated pupil, you are suspicious that he has suffered an intracranial hemorrhage. The rales or crackles in his lungs indicate that he also has some degree of pulmonary edema. The patient is protecting his airway adequately and has spontaneous respirations. You place the patient on supplemental oxygen, start an IV line, and place him on a cardiac monitor. You discuss the patient with medical direction and receive orders to administer furosemide 40 mg IV push and to give a bolus and start an infusion of esmolol.

Sodium nitroprusside (Nipride) is a common medication used for patients in a hypertensive emergency. Nipride is a potent drug, and the onset of action is within 1 minute of administration. Its action is quickly terminated when the infusion is discontinued. Nitroprusside works by dilating both the arteries and veins. The pressure receptors (**baroreceptors**) located in the walls of some blood vessels sense the drop in blood pressure and compensate for the decrease by increasing the heart rate. An increase in heart rate can be quite damaging for a patient with coronary artery disease. Remember that the patient in this scenario has a heart rate of 128 beats/min.

This drug can increase a patient's intracranial pressure (ICP). In this scenario, the patient has an altered mental status and a right pupil that is fixed and dilated. Given the history and physical findings, the patient may have had an intracranial hemorrhage. Because nitroprusside could increase the ICP and worsen the patient's brain injury, it would not be an appropriate drug choice for this patient. Additionally, assess whether the cause for the hypertension is an acute myocardial infarction (AMI); if the patient has had a myocardial infarction, nitroglycerin is the preferred drug.

> When using sodium nitroprusside, exercise great caution not to drop the blood pressure too rapidly or by too great of a magnitude.

Labetalol (Trandate, Normodyne) is a selective $alpha_1$ blocker and nonselective beta blocker. As an alpha-blocking agent, labetalol decreases blood pressure by blocking alpha-mediated contraction of vascular smooth muscle. As a drug with $beta_1$-blocking properties, it also acts on the heart to decrease heart rate, contractility, and blood pressure. Labetalol is often a first choice for treating intracranial bleeds because it does not negatively affect cerebral perfusion pressure. The use of labetalol for hypertension is perhaps more safe than nitroprusside because labetalol does not cause a rapid and uncontrolled drop in blood pressure. However, the patient in this scenario has rales that are audible in both lung fields. Labetalol should be used with caution in this patient. Hypertension and rales indicating pulmonary edema are signs of impending congestive heart failure. In that case, using furosemide (Lasix) to help control the pulmonary edema with a beta blocker would be an effective alternative. (Lasix is also discussed in Chapter 10.)

ESMOLOL (BREVIBLOC)

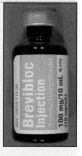

Classification: Beta adrenergic antagonist, class II antiarrhythmic
Action: Inhibits the strength of the heart's contractions, as well as heart rate, resulting in a decrease in cardiac oxygen consumption.
Indications: ACS, MI, acute hypertension, supraventricular tachyarrhythmias, thyrotoxicosis.
Adverse Effects: Hypotension, sinus bradycardia, AV block, cardiac arrest, nausea/vomiting, hypoglycemia, injection site reaction.
Contraindications: Acute bronchospasm, COPD, second- or third-degree heart block, bradycardia, cardiogenic shock, pulmonary edema, sick sinus syndrome, known sensitivity. Use with caution in patients with pheochromocytoma, Prinzmetal's angina, cerebrovascular disease, stroke, poorly controlled diabetes mellitus, hyperthyroidism, thyrotoxicosis, renal disease.
Dosage:
- **Adult:** 500 mcg/kg (0.5 mg/kg) IV, IO over a 1-minute period, followed by a 50-mcg/kg/min (0.05 mg/kg) infusion over a 4-minute period (maximum total: 200 mcg/kg). If patient response is inadequate, administer a second bolus 500 mcg/kg (0.5 mg/kg) over a 1-minute period, and then increase infusion to 100 mcg/kg/min. Maximum infusion rate: 300 mcg/kg/min.
- **Pediatric:** 500 mcg/kg (0.5 mg/kg) IV, IO over a 1-minute period, followed by an infusion at 25 to 200 mcg/kg/min.

cont'd

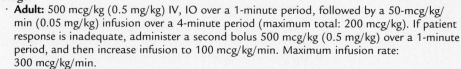

ESMOLOL (BREVIBLOC)—CONT'D

Special Considerations:
Half-life 5 to 9 minutes
Any adverse effects caused by administration of esmolol are brief because of the drug's short half-life.
Resolution of effects usually within 10 to 20 minutes.
Pregnancy class C

NICARDIPINE (CARDENE)

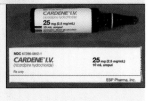

Classification: Calcium channel blocker
Action: Blocks calcium movement into the smooth muscle of the blood vessel walls, causing vasodilation.
Indications: Hypertension
Adverse Effects: Edema, headaches, flushing, sinus tachycardia, hypotension.
Contraindications: Aortic stenosis, hypotension, known sensitivity.
Use with caution in heart failure, cardiac conduction abnormalities, cerebrovascular disease, depressed AV node conduction.
Dosage:
- **Adult:** 5 mg/hr IV, IO; may increase by 2.5 mg/hr every 5 to 15 minutes (max dose: 15 mg/hr). Once the patient has achieved the desired blood pressure, decrease infusion to a maintenance dose of 3 mg/hr.
- **Pediatric:** 0.5 to 1 mcg/kg/min IV, IO infusion.

Special Considerations:
Pregnancy class C

FUROSEMIDE (LASIX)

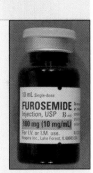

Classification: Loop diuretic
Action: Inhibits the absorption of the sodium and chloride ions and water in the loop of Henle, as well as the convoluted tubule of the nephron. This results in decreased absorption of water and increased production of urine.
Indications: Pulmonary edema, CHF, hypertensive emergency.
Adverse Effects: Vertigo, dizziness, weakness, orthostatic hypotension, hypokalemia, thrombophlebitis. Patients with anuria, severe renal failure, untreated hepatic coma, increasing azotemia, and electrolyte depletion can develop life-threatening consequences.
Contraindications: Known sensitivity to sulfonamides or furosemide.
Dosage:
Congestive Heart Failure and Pulmonary Edema:
- **Adult:** 40 mg IV, IO administered slowly over a 1- to 2-minute period. If a satisfactory response is not achieved within 1 hour, an additional dose of 80 mg can be given. A maximum single IV dose is 160 to 200 mg.
- **Pediatric:** 1 mg/kg IV, IO or IM. If the response is not satisfactory, an additional dose of 2 mg/kg may be administered no sooner than 2 hours after the first dose.
Hypertensive Emergency:
- **Adult:** 40 to 80 mg IV, IO.
- **Pediatric:** 1 mg/kg IV or IM.

Special Considerations:
Onset of action for IV, IO administration occurs within 5 minutes and will peak within 30 minutes.
Furosemide is a diuretic, so the patient will likely have urinary urgency. Be prepared to help the patient void.
Pregnancy class C

SODIUM NITROPRUSSIDE (NIPRIDE, NITROPRESS)

Classification: Antihypertensive agent
Action: Causes direct relaxation of both arteries and veins.
Indications: Hypertensive emergencies.
Adverse Effects: Cyanide or thiocyanate toxicity, nausea/vomiting, dizziness, headache, restlessness, abdominal pain, methemoglobinemia.
Contraindications: Hypotension, increased ICP, cerebrovascular disease, coronary artery disease, hepatic disease, renal disease, pulmonary disease.

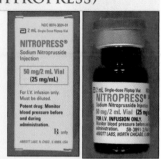

Dosage:
- **Adult:** 0.3 to 10 mcg/kg/min IV, IO. Titrate to desired blood pressure.
- **Pediatric:** Same as adult dosing.

Special Considerations:
Nitroprusside will break down when exposed to ultraviolet light. Therefore the infusion should be shielded from light by wrapping the bag with aluminum foil.
Pregnancy class C

LABETALOL (NORMODYNE, TRANDATE)

Classification: Beta adrenergic antagonist, antianginal, antihypertensive
Action: Binds with both the beta$_1$ and beta$_2$ receptors and alpha$_1$ receptors in vascular smooth muscle. Inhibits the strength of the heart's contractions, as well as heart rate. This results in a decrease in cardiac oxygen consumption.
Indications: ACS, SVT, severe hypertension.
Adverse Effects: Usually mild and transient; hypotensive symptoms, nausea/vomiting, bronchospasm, arrhythmia, bradycardia, AV block.
Contraindications: Hypotension, cardiogenic shock, acute pulmonary edema, heart failure, severe bradycardia, sick sinus syndrome, second- or third-degree heart block, asthma or acute bronchospasm, cocaine-induced ACS, known sensitivity. Use caution in pheochromocytoma, cerebrovascular disease or stroke, poorly controlled diabetes, with hepatic disease. Use with caution at lowest effective dose in chronic lung disease.
Dosage:
Cardiac Indications: Note: Monitor blood pressure and heart rate closely during administration.
- **Adult:** 10 mg IV, IO over a 1- to 2-minute period. May repeat every 10 minutes to a maximum dose of 150 mg or give initial bolus and then follow with infusion at 2 to 8 mg/min.
- **Pediatric:** 0.4 to 1 mg/kg/hr to a maximum dosage of 3 mg/kg/hr.
Severe Hypertension:
- **Adult:** Initial dose is 20 mg IV, IO slow infusion over a 2-minute period. After the initial dose, blood pressure should be checked every 5 minutes. Repeat doses can be given at 10-minute intervals. The second dose should be 40 mg IV, IO, and subsequent doses should be 80 mg IV, IO, to a maximum total dose of 300 mg. The effect on blood pressure typically will occur within 5 minutes from the time of administration. Alternatively, may be administered via IV infusion at 2 mg/min to a total maximum dose of 300 mg.
- **Pediatric:** 0.4 to 1 mg/kg/hr IV, IO infusion with a maximum dose of 3 mg/kg/hr.
Special Considerations:
Pregnancy class C

OVERVIEW OF MYOCARDIAL ISCHEMIA WITH HYPERTENSION

You are dispatched to a 63-year-old man with chest pain. The patient describes the discomfort as a pressure on the left side of his chest, with some radiation to the jaw and left arm. He also reports feeling short of breath. You observe that the patient appears to be quite anxious and is sweating profusely. The patient's daughter tells you that he had a heart attack approximately 1 month ago. When he was in the hospital, he had a cardiac catheterization, with a stent placed in one of his coronary arteries. Shortly after being discharged from the hospital, the patient lost his insurance coverage and stopped taking his "heart pills." At this point the patient protests and reports that he is still taking aspirin every day. You learn that he has a history of urinary retention, diabetes, hypertension, and hyperlipidemia, and he has smoked for more than 40 years. On physical examination, his pulse is 110 beats/min, blood pressure is 200/148 mm Hg, respirations are 24 breaths/min with bilateral rales, and his skin is moist. The pulse oximeter is reading 93%. ...

This patient's history is classic for acute myocardial ischemia and infarction (see Chapter 6). However, he has the added complication of experiencing a hypertensive emergency and thus requires immediate treatment. The patient's significant risk factors for AMI include diabetes, hypertension with abrupt cessation of medications, hyperlipidemia (high cholesterol), and a significant smoking history. He also recently had an AMI with stent placement, which is significant because coronary stents can reocclude.

MANAGEMENT

This patient needs to be treated for his AMI, but this chapter focuses on blood pressure management in the face of ischemia and infarction.

After initial management of this patient with high-flow oxygen, initiation of IV, and placement of a cardiac monitor, one 325-mg nonenteric coated aspirin should be administered, followed by nitroglycerin.

Aspirin is most commonly used to reduce pain, fever, and inflammation. Another benefit of aspirin is that it prohibits platelets from adhering to one another. Inhibiting platelet aggregation with the use of aspirin has been proven to reduce the mortality rate of patients having an AMI. In the scenario presented, aspirin will not treat the hypertension, but it will limit growth of a clot in the coronary artery stent if it is occluded and possibly preserve cardiac muscle.

Nitroglycerin is a vasodilating agent that dilates venules to a greater degree than it does arterioles. Dilation of veins reduces blood return to the heart, which decreases cardiac preload. Reduced preload reduces cardiac output, which lowers blood pressure. In addition, reducing preload decreases the actual tension of the myocardial wall. The amount of work (energy input) required by the heart muscle is also decreased; therefore the demand for oxygen is less, which helps balance oxygen supply and demand. Arterial dilation is significantly less than venous dilation. When the arterioles dilate, the coronary vessels increase in diameter; subsequently, the heart muscle receives more oxygen-enriched blood flow. These properties make nitroglycerin a desirable choice for AMI or myocardial ischemia.

After aspirin and nitroglycerin, beta blockers such as labetalol and esmolol are excellent choices. The benefits of beta blockers are that they reduce the stress to the injured heart by reducing the heart rate and force of contraction. Beta blockers improve survival in patients with myocardial ischemia. Metoprolol is a beta blocker commonly used in scenarios such as that presented previously.

ASPIRIN, ASA

Classification: Antiplatelet, nonnarcotic analgesic, antipyretic
Action: Prevents the formation of a chemical known as thromboxane A_2, which causes platelets to clump together, or aggregate, and form plugs that cause obstruction or constriction of small coronary arteries.
Indications: Fever, inflammation, angina, acute MI, and patients complaining of pain, pressure, squeezing, or crushing in the chest that may be cardiac in origin.
Adverse Effects: Anaphylaxis, angioedema, bronchospasm, bleeding, stomach irritation, nausea/vomiting.
Contraindications: GI bleeding, active ulcer disease, hemorrhagic stroke, bleeding disorders, children with chickenpox or flulike symptoms, known sensitivity.
Dosage: Note: "Baby aspirin" 81 mg, standard adult aspirin dose 325 mg.

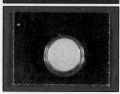

Myocardial Infarction:
- **Adult:** 160 to 325 mg PO (alternatively, four 81-mg baby aspirin are often given), 300-mg rectal suppository.
- **Pediatric:** 3 to 5 mg/kg/day to 5 to 10 mg/kg/day given as a single dose.

Pain or Fever:
- **Adult:** 325 to 650 mg PO (1 to 2 adult tablets) every 4 to 6 hours.
- **Pediatric:** 60 to 90 mg/kg/day in divided doses every 4 to 6 hours.

Special Considerations:
Pregnancy class C except the last 3 months of pregnancy, when aspirin is considered pregnancy class D.

NITROGLYCERIN (NITROLINGUAL, NITROQUICK, NITRO-DUR)

Classification: Antianginal agent
Action: Relaxes vascular smooth muscle, thereby dilating peripheral arteries and veins. This causes pooling of venous blood and decreased venous return to the heart, which decreases preload. Nitroglycerin also reduces left ventricular systolic wall tension, which decreases afterload.
Indications: Angina, ongoing ischemic chest discomfort, hypertension, myocardial ischemia associated with cocaine intoxication.
Adverse Effects: Headache, hypotension, bradycardia, lightheadedness, flushing, cardiovascular collapse, methemoglobinemia.
Contraindications: Hypotension, severe bradycardia or tachycardia, increased ICP, intracranial bleeding, patients taking any medications for erectile dysfunction (such as sildenafil [Viagra], tadalafil [Cialis], or vardenafil [Levitra]), known sensitivity to nitrates. Use with caution in anemia, closed-angle glaucoma, hypotension, postural hypotension, uncorrected hypovolemia.

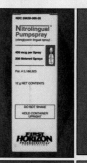
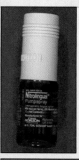
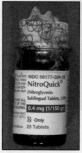
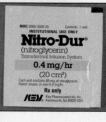

Dosage:
- **Adult:**
  - **Sublingual tablets:** 1 tablet (0.3-0.4 mg) at 5-minute intervals to a maximum of 3 doses.
  - **Translingual spray:** 1 (0.4 mg) spray at 5-minute intervals to a maximum of 3 sprays.
  - **Ointment:** 2% topical (Nitro-Bid ointment): Apply 1 to 2 inches of paste over the chest wall, cover with transparent wrap, and secure with tape.
  - **IV:**
    - **Bolus:** 12.5 to 25 mcg

cont'd

NITROGLYCERIN (NITROLINGUAL, NITROQUICK, NITRO-DUR)—CONT'D

- · **Infusion:** 5 mcg/min; may increase rate by 5 to 10 mcg/min every 5 to 10 minutes as needed. End points of dose titration for nitroglycerin include a drop in the blood pressure of 10%, relief of chest pain, and return of ST segment to normal on a 12-lead ECG.
- · **Pediatric IV infusion:** The initial pediatric infusion is 0.25 to 0.5 mcg/kg/min IV, IO titrated by 0.5 to 1 mcg/kg/min. Usual required dose is 1 to 3 mcg/kg/min to a maximum dose of 5 mcg/kg/min.

Special Considerations:
Administration of nitroglycerin to a patient with right ventricular MI can result in hypotension. Pregnancy class C

... You place the patient on oxygen, start an IV line, and place him on a cardiac monitor. Given the patient's history, you are concerned that he has myocardial ischemia with resultant hypertension. You give the patient a 325-mg nonenteric coated aspirin and tell him to bite and swallow the tablet. You then administer a 0.3-mg nitroglycerin tablet. The first nitroglycerin tablet does little to reduce his blood pressure or relieve the chest pain. Therefore 5 minutes later you administer a second 0.3-mg tablet of nitroglycerin, which improves the blood pressure.

OVERVIEW OF PREECLAMPSIA AND ECLAMPSIA

You are called to attend to a 34-year-old woman who is 36 weeks pregnant. She is actively seizing. On arrival, you see an obviously gravid female in a tonic-clonic seizure. Her husband states that she had been complaining of a headache and blurry vision. She was seizing for 5 minutes before your arrival. The patient's vital signs are blood pressure, 220/158 mm Hg; pulse, 124 beats/min; respirations, labored; and skin, warm and moist.

The patient in this scenario has an obstetric emergency known as **eclampsia.** The cause of this vasospastic form of hypertension is unique to pregnant women, and the cause is not known. Without appropriate treatment, the risk of death to the mother and fetus is significant. (Note in this scenario that the ultimate treatment is delivery of the baby.) Preeclampsia (also known as *toxemia* and *pregnancy-induced hypertension*) consists of high blood pressure, protein in the urine, and edema (swelling) of the extremities. This condition can rapidly become severe, with very high blood pressure, visual disturbances, failing kidneys, and liver damage. In rare cases, preeclampsia develops into eclampsia, in which potentially fatal convulsions occur. It also can become **HELLP syndrome,** which consists of *h*emolysis, or the breaking down of red blood cells; *el*evated liver enzymes; and *l*ow *p*latelet count. HELLP is potentially fatal to both the mother and her unborn child or children.

MANAGEMENT

Benzodiazepines typically have been used for seizure control. However, eclampsia warrants a different approach for seizure control, including administration of magnesium sulfate and hydralazine.

Magnesium sulfate acts as a membrane stabilizer and cerebral vasodilator. These effects are believed to reduce the chance of ischemia to brain tissue. With adequate dosing of magnesium, many patients with eclampsia have relief from the seizure and hypertension. Magnesium sulfate is the drug of choice for seizure control in eclampsia.

Hydralazine (Apresoline) is a vasodilating agent that selectively dilates the arteries. It can be used in the treatment of any hypertensive crisis and is often used for the treatment of preeclampsia and eclampsia. Administration of hydralazine produces a decrease in arterial pressure, so blood pressure is lowered. Additionally, a reflex tachycardia occurs once the baroreceptors sense this drop in pressure, and thus heart rate increases. Therefore this drug would not be a good choice in an individual with heart disease because of the associated increase in heart rate. Hydralazine is the drug of choice for hypertension in eclampsia if magnesium fails. Nitroprusside and labetalol have been used and determined to be safe.

Magnesium Sulfate

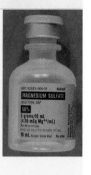

Classification: Electrolyte, tocolytic, mineral
Action: Required for normal physiologic functioning. Magnesium is a cofactor in neurochemical transmission and muscular excitability. Magnesium sulfate controls seizures by blocking peripheral neuromuscular transmission. Magnesium is also a peripheral vasodilator and an inhibitor of platelet function.
Indications: Torsades de pointes, cardiac arrhythmias associated with hypomagnesemia, eclampsia and seizure prophylaxis in preeclampsia, status asthmaticus.
Adverse Effects: Magnesium toxicity (signs include flushing, diaphoresis, hypotension, muscle paralysis, weakness, hypothermia, and cardiac, CNS, or respiratory depression).
Contraindications: AV block, GI obstruction. Use with caution in renal impairment.
Dosage:
Pulseless Ventricular Fibrillation/Ventricular Tachycardia with Torsades de Pointes or Hypomagnesemia:
- **Adult:** 1 to 2 g in 10 mL D$_5$W IV, IO administered over 5 to 10 minutes.
- **Pediatric:** 25 to 50 mg/kg IV, IO over 10 to 20 minutes; may administer faster for torsades de pointes (max single dose: 2 g).
Torsades de Pointes with a Pulse or Cardiac Arrhythmias with Hypomagnesemia:
- **Adult:** 1 to 2 g in 50 to 100 mL D$_5$W IV, IO administered over 5 to 60 minutes. Follow with 0.5 to 1 g/hr IV, IO titrated to control torsades de pointes.
- **Pediatric:** 25 to 50 mg/kg IV, IO over 10 to 20 minutes (max single dose: 2 g).
Eclampsia and Seizure Prophylaxis in Preeclampsia:
- **Adult:** 4 to 6 g IV, IO over 20 to 30 minutes, followed by an infusion of 1 to 2 g/hr.
Status Asthmaticus:
- **Adult:** 1.2 to 2 g slow IV, IO (over 20 minutes).
- **Pediatric:** 25 to 50 mg/kg (diluted in D$_5$W) slow IV, IO (over 10 to 20 minutes).
Special Considerations:
Pregnancy class A

Hydralazine (Apresoline)

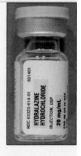

Classification: Antihypertensive agent, vasodilator
Action: Directly dilates the peripheral blood vessels.
Indications: Hypertension associated with preeclampsia and eclampsia, hypertensive crisis.
Adverse Effects: Headache, angina, flushing, palpitations, reflex tachycardia, anorexia, nausea/vomiting, diarrhea, hypotension, syncope, peripheral vasodilation, peripheral edema, fluid retention, paresthesias.
Contraindications: Patients taking diazoxide or MAOIs, coronary artery disease, stroke, angina, dissecting aortic aneurysm, mitral valve and rheumatic heart diseases.
Dosage:
Preeclampsia and Eclampsia:
- **Adult:** 5 to 10 mg IV, IO. Repeat every 20 to 30 minutes until systolic blood pressure of 90 to 105 mm Hg is attained.
Acute Hypertension Not Associated with Preeclampsia:
- **Adult:** 10 to 20 mg IV, IO, or IM.
- **Pediatric:**
  - **1 month to 12 years:** 0.1 to 0.6 mg/kg IV, IO, or IM (max: 20 mg/dose).
Special Considerations:
Pregnancy class C

OVERVIEW OF HYPERTENSION WITH SEIZURE

You are called to the scene of a 24-year-old man who is unresponsive. You arrive to find a young man who is seizing and still unresponsive. His wife indicates that he has just started regularly using cocaine. On examination, you find that the patient's blood pressure is 260/168 mm Hg; pulse is 124 beats/min; respirations are 24 breaths/min; and skin is red, hot, and moist. The patient's pupils are dilated, and he is drooling.

Cocaine is a sympathomimetic drug that stimulates the adrenergic nervous system. Persons who use cocaine can present with an overstimulation of the nervous system and potentially end-organ damage. These individuals are prone to cardiac arrhythmias, hypertensive emergencies, and chest pain. In this scenario, the patient has a significantly elevated blood pressure with seizure activity. This indicates end-organ damage and a severe hypertensive emergency.

MANAGEMENT

Hypertensive emergencies caused by a drug such as cocaine are treated differently from other hypertensive emergencies. Beta blockers are contraindicated in such scenarios because they can worsen coronary vasoconstriction. When a beta blocker is used, unopposed stimulation of the peripheral alpha receptors occurs from the catecholamine (cocaine), which can lead to an increase in blood pressure and make symptoms worse.

Diazepam (Valium) is a benzodiazepine used to help induce sleep, relieve anxiety, and relax muscle spasm. This drug is quite effective in the treatment of seizures and is indicated for use in seizures caused by cocaine.

Diazepam works in a number of ways. It promotes relaxation of muscle, actually restoring tone to the peripheral nervous system that had been inhibited by the cocaine, limiting myocardial oxygen demand, and causing peripheral vasodilation and a drop in blood pressure.

Phentolamine (Regitine) is both an $alpha_1$ and $alpha_2$ blocker. It blocks the receptors of the adrenergic sympathetic nervous system. It is most commonly used in pheochromocytoma and states of excessive catecholamines (e.g., increased levels of epinephrine and norepinephrine). It is the drug of choice for cocaine-induced hypertension.

DIAZEPAM (VALIUM)

Classification: Benzodiazepine; Schedule C-IV
Action: Binds to the benzodiazepine receptor and enhances the effects of GABA. Benzodiazepines act at the level of the limbic, thalamic, and hypothalamic regions of the CNS and can produce any level of CNS 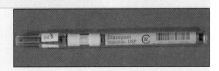 depression required (including sedation, skeletal muscle relaxation, and anticonvulsant activity).
Indications: Anxiety, skeletal muscle relaxation, alcohol withdrawal, seizures.
Adverse Effects: Respiratory depression, drowsiness, fatigue, headache, pain at the injection site, confusion, nausea, hypotension, oversedation.
Contraindications: Children younger than 6 months, acute-angle glaucoma, CNS depression, alcohol intoxication, known sensitivity.
Dosage:
Anxiety:
- **Adult:**
  - **Moderate:** 2 to 5 mg slow IV, IM.
  - **Severe:** 5 to 10 mg slow IV, IM (administer no faster than 5 mg/min).
  - **Low:** Low dosages are often required for elderly or debilitated patients.
- **Pediatric:** 0.04 to 0.3 mg/kg/dose IV, IM every 4 hours to a maximum dose of 0.6 mg/kg.

cont'd

DIAZEPAM (VALIUM)—CONT'D

Delirium Tremens from Acute Alcohol Withdrawal:
- **Adult:** 10 mg IV

Seizure:
- **Adult:** 5 to 10 mg slow IV, IO every 10 to 15 minutes; maximum total dose 30 mg.
- **Pediatric:**
  - **IV, IO:**
    - **5 years and older:** 1 mg over a 3-minute period every 2 to 5 minutes to a maximum total dose of 10 mg.
    - **Older than 30 days to younger than 5 years:** 0.2 to 0.5 mg over a 3-minute period; may repeat every 2 to 5 minutes to a maximum total dose of 5 mg.
    - **Neonate:** 0.1 to 0.3 mg/kg/dose given over a 3- to 5-minute period; may repeat every 15 to 30 minutes to a maximum total dose of 2 mg. (Not a first-line agent due to sodium benzoic acid in the injection.)
  - **Rectal administration:** If vascular access is not obtained, diazepam may be administered rectally to children.
    - **12 years and older:** 0.2 mg/kg.
    - **6 to 11 years:** 0.3 mg/kg.
    - **2 to 5 years:** 0.5 mg/kg.
    - **Younger than 2 years:** Not recommended.

Special Considerations:
Make sure that IV, IO lines are well secured. Extravasation of diazepam causes tissue necrosis. Diazepam is insoluble in water and must be dissolved in propylene glycol. This produces a viscous solution; give slowly to prevent pain on injection.
Pregnancy class D

PHENTOLAMINE (REGITINE)

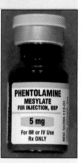

Classification: Alpha antagonist, antihypertensive
Action: Blocks alpha adrenergic receptors, causing vasodilation.
Indications: Hypertensive emergencies and hypertension caused by pheochromocytoma, cocaine-induced vasospasm of the coronary arteries.
Adverse Effects: Sinus tachycardia, angina, dizziness, orthostatic hypotension, prolonged hypotensive episodes, nausea/vomiting, diarrhea, weakness, flushing, nasal congestion.
Contraindications: Known sensitivity. Use with caution in acute MI, angina, coronary insufficiency, evidence suggestive of coronary artery disease, peptic ulcer disease.
Dosage:
Hypertensive Crisis:
- **Adult:** 5 to 15 mg IV, IO or IM.
- **Pediatric:** Not recommended for pediatric patients.

Cocaine-Induced Vasospasm:
- **Adult:** 5 mg IV, IO or IM.
- **Pediatric:** Not recommended for pediatric patients.

Special Considerations:
Pregnancy class C

REVIEW QUESTIONS

1. List five types of specific hypertensive emergencies.
2. When treating a patient with malignant hypertension, what is the maximal safe amount that a paramedic should attempt to decrease the blood pressure?
3. List contraindications for the use of nitroprusside.
4. Which antihypertensive medication needs to be protected from light? Why?
5. By what mechanism does labetalol decrease blood pressure?
6. For what drug intoxication is the use of labetalol contraindicated? Why?
7. What is the preferred drug to reduce blood pressure in a patient having an AMI?
8. What is the drug of choice when treating seizures from eclampsia?

9. How does hydralazine affect a patient's heart rate?
10. List three contraindications for the use of beta blockers.

BIBLIOGRAPHY

Chobanian AV, et al: The seventh report of the Joint National Committee on Prevention, Detection, Evaluation, and Treatment of High Blood Pressure: the JNC 7 report, *JAMA* 289:2560, 2003.

Neutel JM, et al: A comparison of intravenous nicardipine and sodium nitroprusside in the immediate treatment of severe hypertension, *Am J Hypertens* 7:623, 1994.

Schulz V: Clinical pharmacokinetics of nitroprusside, cyanide, thiosulphate and thiocyanate, *Clin Pharmacokinet* 9:239, 1984.

Vaughan CJ, Delanty N: Hypertensive emergencies, *Lancet* 356:411, 2000.

Poisonings, Overdoses, and Intoxications

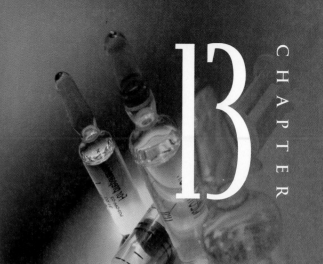

OBJECTIVES

1. Discuss the use of activated charcoal in the treatment of poisonings.
2. List treatment options for acetaminophen overdose.
3. List clinical manifestations of cyclic antidepressant overdose.
4. Discuss medications used in the treatment of cyclic antidepressant overdose: sodium bicarbonate, magnesium sulfate, phenylephrine (Neo-Synephrine), norepinephrine (Levophed), diazepam (Valium), and phenytoin (Dilantin).
5. Discuss medications used in the treatment of beta blocker overdose: atropine sulfate and glucagon.
6. Discuss the use of benzodiazepines and haloperidol (Haldol) in the treatment of amphetamine and methamphetamine intoxication.
7. Discuss medications used in the treatment of cocaine intoxication: benzodiazepines, nitroglycerin (Nitrolingual, NitroQuick, Nitro-Dur), aspirin, morphine sulfate, and phentolamine (Regitine).
8. Discuss the use of naloxone (Narcan) in the treatment of a narcotic overdose.
9. Discuss medications used in the treatment of organophosphate and nerve agent exposure: atropine sulfate and pralidoxime (2-PAM).

Medications that Appear in Chapter 13

Activated charcoal
Sodium bicarbonate
Magnesium sulfate
Phenylephrine (Neo-Synephrine)
Norepinephrine (Levophed)
Diazepam (Valium)
Phenytoin (Dilantin)
Atropine sulfate
Glucagon
Midazolam (Versed)
Lorazepam (Ativan)
Haloperidol (Haldol)
Nitroglycerin (Nitrolingual, NitroQuick, Nitro-Dur)
Aspirin, ASA
Morphine sulfate
Phentolamine (Regitine)
Thiamine (Vitamin B$_1$)
Dextrose (Dextrose 50%, Dextrose 25%, Dextrose 10%)
Naloxone (Narcan)
Pralidoxime (2-PAM, Protopam)

INTRODUCTION

Poisonings and overdoses account for a significant percentage of admissions to hospital intensive care units in the United States. Yet only a few drugs and chemicals are responsible for approximately 90% of all intoxications. In adults, poisonings are usually the result of a psychiatric disorder or recreational drug use. Children younger than 6 years are another group commonly treated for intoxications or poisonings. A third group of patients with toxin exposure are victims of biologic or chemical terrorism.

This chapter addresses the following poisonings, overdoses, and intoxications:

- Acetaminophen overdose
- Cyclic antidepressant overdose
- Beta blocker overdose
- Amphetamine and methamphetamine intoxication
- Cocaine intoxication
- Narcotic overdose
- Organophosphate and nerve agent exposure

SYRUP OF IPECAC AND ACTIVATED CHARCOAL

The objectives of any emergency provider caring for a poisoning victim are simple and straightforward. The initial priorities are the same as those in all emergencies: patency of the airway, adequate ventilation, and sufficient perfusion of blood to the critical organs. The next goal is to prevent or reduce absorption of the toxin, which can require removal of any particulate matter in the case of skin absorption, removal of the patient to a safe environment when dealing with toxic fumes, and possible administration of **activated charcoal** for ingested poisons.

For decades, administration of **syrup of ipecac** was advocated for the home and prehospital treatment of poisoning. The objective of giving ipecac is to reduce absorption of the ingested poison by inducing the patient to vomit the toxin. Ipecac induces vomiting in approximately 90% of individuals 10 to 20 minutes after administration.[1,2] After the administration of ipecac, the patient typically vomits one to eight times in the first half hour.

Although administration of ipecac was once thought to reduce the need for emergency department treatment and improve outcomes in poisonings, research has failed to demonstrate any improved benefits with ipecac administration. Ipecac is contraindicated for caustic substances because of possible damage to the esophagus when the substance is regurgitated. Recently the American Academy of Pediatrics recommended that ipecac no longer be administered.[3-5] However, because syrup of ipecac has been advocated as a home therapy for poisoning for so long, prehospital providers may encounter patients who have received ipecac before their arrival on the scene.

The first pharmacologic intervention in poisoning cases is the administration of activated charcoal. Activated charcoal reduces the absorption of the ingested poison by providing a large surface area to which the ingested poison can bind. A 1-g dose of activated charcoal provides approximately 300 to 2000 m^2 of surface area to which the toxin can adhere, limiting absorption.[6]

Activated charcoal causes patients to have nausea and vomiting. More frequent, smaller doses of activated charcoal can decrease the frequency of vomiting associated with charcoal administration. Before administration, the provider should evaluate the patient's level of consciousness and ability to cooperate with the therapy.

Despite widespread support for its use, evidence that activated charcoal reduces the rate of complications or deaths in patients who have been poisoned is lacking.[7] Activated charcoal is not recommended in all ingestions. Some ingested substances are not absorbed by activated charcoal, such as iron, lithium, alcohols, ethylene glycol, organophosphates, acids and bases, and cyanide. See Box 13-1 for a list of agents that are not well bound to activated charcoal and those drugs cleared by hemoperfusion and hemodialysis.

BOX 13-1

METHODS OF REMOVAL OF VARIOUS DRUGS

Agents Not Well Bound to Activated Charcoal

- Bromides
- Caustics
- Cyanide
- Ethylene glycol
- Iron
- Isopropyl alcohol
- Lithium
- Methanol

Agents Cleared by Hemoperfusion

- Acetaminophen
- Theophylline
- Methotrexate
- Phenylbutazone
- Procainamide
- Quinidine

Agents Cleared by Hemodialysis

- Ammonium chloride
- Amphetamine
- Atenolol
- Phenobarbital
- Procainamide
- Sotalol
- Ethanol
- Methanol
- Ethylene glycol
- Isopropanol
- Aspirin
- Lithium
- Arsenic

ACTIVATED CHARCOAL

Classification: Antidote, adsorbent
Action: When certain chemicals and toxins are in proximity to the activated charcoal, the chemical will attach to the surface of the charcoal and become trapped.
Indications: Toxic ingestion
Adverse Effects: Nausea/vomiting, constipation, or diarrhea. If aspirated into the lungs, charcoal can induce a potentially fatal form of pneumonitis.
Contraindications: Ingestion of acids, alkalis, ethanol, methanol, cyanide, ferrous sulfate or other iron salts, lithium; coma; GI obstruction.
Dosage:
- **Adult:** 50 to 100 g/dose.
- **Pediatric:** 1 to 2 g/kg.

Special Considerations:
Pregnancy class C

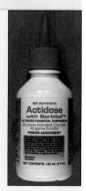

ACETAMINOPHEN OVERDOSE

You are called to provide assistance to a distraught young woman who has recently broken up with her boyfriend. When you arrive, her mother tells you that she thinks her daughter ingested approximately 40 tablets (500 mg/tablet) of acetaminophen. You find a 16-year-old girl who is crying and reporting cramping abdominal pain. Her vital signs are stable.

Acetaminophen (Tylenol) is one of the most commonly used drugs in intentional overdoses. In children the typical presentation of an acetaminophen overdose is abdominal pain, nausea, and vomiting. These symptoms are often absent in adults, even after large ingestions. In fact, the clinical symptoms of such an overdose can be absent for days before deterioration of liver function.

MANAGEMENT

Although acetaminophen overdose is a common intoxication, prehospital care is only supportive. The initial care for this patient after a poisoning or overdose is the same as for any other critically ill or injured patient. The airway may require assistance or intervention to stay open. Patients may have an altered mental status and not be able to maintain a patent airway, or the airway may be obstructed with emesis. Supplemental oxygen should be administered. An IV line should be placed, and an IV infusion should be started. Hypotension should be treated with a bolus of dextrose-free IV fluids. If the patient requires emergency administration of phenytoin, an IV line containing dextrose will result in precipitation of the phenytoin.

> When treating overdoses, avoid IV fluids such as 5% dextrose in normal saline or 5% dextrose in Ringer's lactate solution. If the patient has a seizure, the administration of phenytoin will result in precipitation of the drug.

CYCLIC ANTIDEPRESSANT OVERDOSE

> You are called to the apartment of a 25-year-old woman who was found by her roommate to have a depressed level of consciousness. The roommate is concerned that the patient overdosed on her antidepressant medication. You assess the patient and find that her heart rate is 134 beats/min. Her skin is dry, and she responds by groaning and turning away from you. You place her on oxygen and the cardiac monitor, and your partner starts an IV of normal saline. ...

Overdose from antidepressants is a common cause of overdose deaths.[8] The clinical manifestations of cyclic antidepressant overdose include the following:

- Depressed level of consciousness
- Wide-complex cardiac arrhythmias
- Hypotension
- Seizures

MANAGEMENT

After the provision of initial supportive care, the first step is administration of activated charcoal if no contraindications exist. In this scenario, the patient's decreased level of consciousness would contraindicate the administration of activated charcoal.

Cardiac arrhythmias are the most life-threatening manifestation of the symptoms of cyclic antidepressant overdose. Widening of the QRS complex to greater than 100 ms and progression to frank ventricular tachycardia are likely to occur early after ingestion. If the patient has a wide-complex QRS rhythm, treatment with sodium bicarbonate is appropriate. Some patients develop the cardiac rhythm torsades de pointes, which is treated with magnesium sulfate injection.

SODIUM BICARBONATE

Classification: Electrolyte replacement
Action: Counteracts existing acidosis.
Indications: Acidosis, drug intoxications (e.g., barbiturates, salicylates, methyl alcohol).
Adverse Effects: Metabolic alkalosis, hypernatremia, injection site reaction, sodium and fluid retention, peripheral edema.
Contraindications: Metabolic alkalosis.
Dosage:
Metabolic Acidosis during Cardiac Arrest:
  · **Adult:** 1 mEq/kg slow IV, IO; may repeat at 0.5 mEq/kg in 10 minutes.
  · **Pediatric:** Same as adult dosing.
Metabolic Acidosis Not Associated with Cardiac Arrest:
  · **Adult:** Dosage should be individualized.
  · **Pediatric:** Dosage should be individualized.

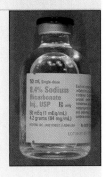

cont'd

SODIUM BICARBONATE—CONT'D

Special Considerations:
Do not administer into an IV, IO line in which another medication is being given.
Because of the high concentration of sodium within each ampule of sodium bicarbonate, use with caution in patients with CHF and renal disease.
Pregnancy class C

MAGNESIUM SULFATE

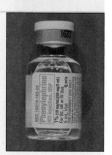

Classification: Electrolyte, tocolytic, mineral
Action: Required for normal physiologic functioning. Magnesium is a cofactor in neurochemical transmission and muscular excitability. Magnesium sulfate controls seizures by blocking peripheral neuromuscular transmission. Magnesium is also a peripheral vasodilator and an inhibitor of platelet function.
Indications: Torsades de pointes, cardiac arrhythmias associated with hypomagnesemia, eclampsia and seizure prophylaxis in preeclampsia, status asthmaticus.
Adverse Effects: Magnesium toxicity (signs include flushing, diaphoresis, hypotension, muscle paralysis, weakness, hypothermia, and cardiac, CNS, or respiratory depression).
Contraindications: AV block, GI obstruction. Use with caution in renal impairment.
Dosage:
Pulseless Ventricular Fibrillation/Ventricular Tachycardia with Torsades de Pointes or Hypomagnesemia:
- **Adult:** 1 to 2 g in 10 mL D_5W IV, IO administered over 5 to 10 minutes.
- **Pediatric:** 25 to 50 mg/kg IV, IO over 10 to 20 minutes; may administer faster for torsades de pointes (max single dose: 2 g).
Torsades de Pointes with a Pulse or Cardiac Arrhythmias with Hypomagnesemia:
- **Adult:** 1 to 2 g in 50 to 100 mL D_5W IV, IO administered over 5 to 60 minutes. Follow with 0.5 to 1 g/hr IV, IO titrated to control torsades de pointes.
- **Pediatric:** 25 to 50 mg/kg IV, IO over 10 to 20 minutes (max single dose: 2 g).
Eclampsia and Seizure Prophylaxis in Preeclampsia:
- **Adult:** 4 to 6 g IV, IO over 20 to 30 minutes, followed by an infusion of 1 to 2 g/hr.
Status Asthmaticus:
- **Adult:** 1.2 to 2 g slow IV, IO (over 20 minutes).
- **Pediatric:** 25 to 50 mg/kg (diluted in D_5W) slow IV, IO (over 10 to 20 minutes).
Special Considerations:
Pregnancy class A

Many patients who have overdosed on cyclic antidepressants have hypotension that does not respond to aggressive administration of IV fluids. This hypotension is best treated with phenylephrine or norepinephrine.

PHENYLEPHRINE (NEO-SYNEPHRINE)

Classification: Adrenergic agonist
Action: Stimulates the alpha receptors, causing vasoconstriction, which results in increased blood pressure.
Indications: Neurogenic shock, spinal shock, cases of shock in which the patient's heart rate does not need to be increased, drug-induced hypotension.
Adverse Effects: Hypertension, VT, headache, excitability, tremor, MI, exacerbation of asthma, cardiac arrhythmias, reflex bradycardia, soft tissue necrosis.
Contraindications: Acute MI, angina, cardiac arrhythmias, severe hypertension, coronary artery disease, pheochromocytoma, narrow-angle glaucoma, cardiomyopathy, MAOI therapy, known sensitivity to phenylephrine or sulfites.

cont'd

PHENYLEPHRINE (NEO-SYNEPHRINE)—CONT'D

Dosage:
- **Adult:** 100 to 180 mcg/min IV, IO. Once the blood pressure has been stabilized, the dose can be reduced to 40 to 60 mcg/min.
- **Pediatric (2 to 12 years):** 5 to 20 mcg/kg IV, IO followed by 0.1 to 0.5 mcg/kg/min IV, IO (max dose: 3 mcg/kg/min IV, IO).

Special Considerations:
Pregnancy class C

NOREPINEPHRINE (LEVOPHED)

Classification: Adrenergic agonist, inotropic, vasopressor
Action: Norepinephrine is an alpha$_1$, alpha$_2$, and beta$_1$ agonist. Alpha-mediated peripheral vasoconstriction is the predominant clinical result of administration, resulting in increasing blood pressure and coronary blood flow. Beta adrenergic action produces inotropic stimulation of the heart and dilates the coronary arteries.
Indications: Cardiogenic shock, septic shock, severe hypotension.
Adverse Effects: Dizziness, anxiety, cardiac arrhythmias, dyspnea, exacerbation of asthma.
Contraindications: Patients taking MAOIs, known sensitivity. Use with caution in hypovolemia.

Dosage:
- **Adult:** Add 4 mg to 250 mL of D$_5$W or D$_5$NS, but not normal saline alone. 0.5 to 1 mcg/min as IV, IO, titrated to maintain systolic blood pressure >80 mm Hg. Refractory shock may require doses as high as 30 mcg/min.
- **Pediatric:** 0.05 to 2 mcg/kg/min IV, IO infusion, to a maximum dose of 2 mcg/kg/min.

Special Considerations:
Do not administer in same IV line as alkaline solutions.
Half-life 1 minute
Pregnancy class C

Seizures are also a common manifestation of a cyclic antidepressant overdose. Seizure activity can run the spectrum from brief and self-limiting to intractable. In some cases seizure activity can precede ventricular tachycardia.[9] The seizures can be treated with diazepam (Valium) or another benzodiazepine. Diazepam is usually effective, and these seizures are often of short duration. Phenytoin (Dilantin) can also be used; however, data are conflicting regarding its effectiveness in the treatment of cyclic antidepressant overdoses.

... After obtaining the patient's vital signs, you attempt to gain some additional history from her. While answering the questions, she stops speaking mid-sentence, stares, and then does not respond to your questioning. She then begins to exhibit generalized tonic-clonic seizure activity. Your partner grabs the patient's head to prevent her from banging her head and harming herself. Her airway is patent, and respirations are spontaneous and nonlabored. You administer diazepam 5 mg IV. Shortly after administration the seizures stop. The patient is groggy and disoriented. While repeating your assessment and vital signs, you note that she has widening of her QRS complex. You notify medical direction about the seizure and the ECG findings. You request to administer sodium bicarbonate. You receive an order to administer 50 mEq sodium bicarbonate IV push. Through the remainder of the transport to the hospital, the patient remains somnolent but answers all your questions and follows all commands. Her vital signs are stable, and her QRS duration seems to have returned to normal.

DIAZEPAM (VALIUM)

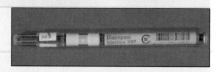

Classification: Benzodiazepine; Schedule C-IV
Action: Binds to the benzodiazepine receptor and enhances the effects of GABA. Benzodiazepines act at the level of the limbic, thalamic, and hypothalamic regions of the CNS and can produce any level of CNS depression required (including sedation, skeletal muscle relaxation, and anticonvulsant activity).
Indications: Anxiety, skeletal muscle relaxation, alcohol withdrawal, seizures.
Adverse Effects: Respiratory depression, drowsiness, fatigue, headache, pain at the injection site, confusion, nausea, hypotension, oversedation.
Contraindications: Children younger than 6 months, acute-angle glaucoma, CNS depression, alcohol intoxication, known sensitivity.
Dosage:
Anxiety:
- **Adult:**
  - **Moderate:** 2 to 5 mg slow IV, IM.
  - **Severe:** 5 to 10 mg slow IV, IM (administer no faster than 5 mg/min).
  - **Low:** Low dosages are often required for elderly or debilitated patients.
- **Pediatric:** 0.04 to 0.3 mg/kg/dose IV, IM every 4 hours to a maximum dose of 0.6 mg/kg.
Delirium Tremens from Acute Alcohol Withdrawal:
- **Adult:** 10 mg IV
Seizure:
- **Adult:** 5 to 10 mg slow IV, IO every 10 to 15 minutes; maximum total dose 30 mg.
- **Pediatric:**
  - **IV, IO:**
    - **5 years and older:** 1 mg over a 3-minute period every 2 to 5 minutes to a maximum total dose of 10 mg.
    - **Older than 30 days to younger than 5 years:** 0.2 to 0.5 mg over a 3-minute period; may repeat every 2 to 5 minutes to a maximum total dose of 5 mg.
    - **Neonate:** 0.1 to 0.3 mg/kg/dose given over a 3- to 5-minute period; may repeat every 15 to 30 minutes to a maximum total dose of 2 mg. (Not a first line agent due to sodium benzoic acid in the injection.)
  - **Rectal administration:** If vascular access is not obtained, diazepam may be administered rectally to children.
    - **12 years and older:** 0.2 mg/kg.
    - **6 to 11 years:** 0.3 mg/kg.
    - **2 to 5 years:** 0.5 mg/kg.
    - **Younger than 2 years:** Not recommended.
Special Considerations:
Make sure that IV, IO lines are well secured. Extravasation of diazepam causes tissue necrosis.
Diazepam is insoluble in water and must be dissolved in propylene glycol. This produces a viscous solution; give slowly to prevent pain on injection.
Pregnancy class D

PHENYTOIN (DILANTIN)

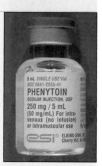

Classification: Anticonvulsant
Action: Depresses seizures by affecting the movement of sodium and calcium into neural tissue.
Indications: Generalized tonic-clonic seizures.
Adverse Effects: Nausea/vomiting, depression of cardiac conduction, sedation, nystagmus, tremors, ataxia, dysarthria, gingival hypertrophy, hirsutism, facial coarsening, hypotension.
Contraindications: Sinus bradycardia, sinoatrial block, second- and third-degree heart block, Adams-Stokes syndrome, known sensitivity to hydantoins.
Dosage:
- **Adult:** 15 to 20 mg/kg IV, IO should be administered slowly at a rate not exceeding 50 mg/min. (This requires approximately 20 minutes in a 70-kg patient.)
- **Pediatric:** 15 to 20 mg/kg IV, IO, administered at a rate of 1 to 3 mg/kg/min.
Special Considerations:
Continuously monitor the ECG and blood pressure during administration.
Pregnancy class D

BETA BLOCKER OVERDOSE

You are called to assist a 78-year-old woman who has been diagnosed with depression after the recent death of her husband of 50 years. The patient's daughter found the patient with an empty bottle of labetalol. The date on the bottle indicates that the prescription of 40 tablets was refilled only 3 days ago. Your assessment of the patient reveals an elderly woman who is minimally responsive. Her heart rate is 42 beats/min, and blood pressure is 74/44 mm Hg. Her skin is cool and dry.

As seen in this scenario, patients who have overdosed on beta blockers usually have bradycardia, heart block, and hypotension.[10,11] Some beta blockers can also cause delirium, seizures, and coma when taken in excessive doses. Patients typically will manifest these symptoms within 6 hours of ingestion.

MANAGEMENT

The initial treatment for bradycardia is administration of atropine and IV fluids. In most cases of beta blocker overdose, atropine therapy is often inadequate. Administration of atropine after the overdose of beta blockers is only symptomatic therapy. If atropine increases the heart rate, the effect of the atropine is often brief and the bradycardia will recur. The main goal of therapy is to improve the patient's perfusion. This increase in perfusion can occur even when the patient still has some degree of bradycardia.

Atropine is the initial treatment for bradycardia from beta blockers, but glucagon is considered the antidote for beta blocker overdose. However, glucagon's success is variable. In some cases it works immediately, but other patients have no response at all. Glucagon, which typically is used to treat diabetic emergencies, can increase the heart rate and blood pressure after beta blocker overdose. Glucagon works by increasing the concentration of an energy-storing chemical inside the cells known as **cyclic adenosine monophosphate (cAMP).** The increased concentration of cAMP results in the heart beating stronger (inotropy) and faster (chronotropy).[12]

If a patient reverts to a shocklike state with bradycardia despite repeated dosing of glucagon, physicians at the hospital may elect to place the patient on an infusion or drip of glucagon. Although this is not a prehospital intervention, paramedics may be exposed to this therapy when transporting patients between facilities as a member of a critical care transport or flight service team.

Drugs commonly used to treat bradycardia and hypotension, such as epinephrine, norepinephrine, and dopamine, are not successful in the treatment of beta blocker overdose.

ATROPINE SULFATE

Classification: Anticholinergic (antimuscarinic)
Action: Competes reversibly with acetylcholine at the site of the muscarinic receptor. Receptors affected, in order from the most sensitive to the least sensitive, include salivary, bronchial, sweat glands, eye, heart, and GI tract.
Indications: Symptomatic bradycardia, asystole or PEA, nerve agent exposure, organophosphate poisoning.
Adverse Effects: Decreased secretions resulting in dry mouth and hot skin temperature, intense facial flushing, blurred vision or dilation of the pupils with subsequent photophobia, tachycardia, restlessness. Atropine may cause paradoxical bradycardia if the dose administered is too low or if the drug is administered too slowly.

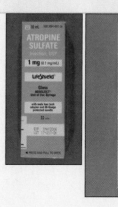

cont'd

ATROPINE SULFATE—CONT'D

Contraindications: Acute MI; myasthenia gravis; GI obstruction; closed-angle glaucoma; known sensitivity to atropine, belladonna alkaloids, or sulfites. Will not be effective for infranodal (type II) AV block and new third-degree block with wide QRS complex.

Dosage:

Symptomatic Bradycardia:
- **Adult:** 0.5 mg IV, IO every 3 to 5 minutes to a maximum dose of 3 mg.
- **Adolescent:** 0.02 mg/kg (minimum 0.1 mg/dose; maximum 1 mg/dose) IV, IO up to a total dose of 2 mg.
- **Pediatric:** 0.02 mg/kg (minimum 0.1 mg/dose; maximum 0.5 mg/dose) IV, IO, to a total dose of 1 mg.

Asystole/Pulseless Electrical Activity:
- 1 mg IV, IO every 3 to 5 minutes, to a maximum dose of 3 mg. May be administered via ET tube at 2 to 2.5 mg diluted in 5 to 10 mL of water or normal saline.

Nerve Agent or Organophosphate Poisoning:
- **Adult:** 2 to 4 mg IV, IM; repeat if needed every 20 to 30 minutes until symptoms dissipate. In severe cases, the initial dose can be as large as 2 to 6 mg administered IV. Repeat doses of 2 to 6 mg can be administered IV, IM every 5 to 60 minutes.
- **Pediatric:** 0.05 mg/kg IV, IM every 10 to 30 minutes as needed until symptoms dissipate.
- **Infants <15 lb:** 0.05 mg/kg IV, IM every 5 to 20 minutes as needed until symptoms dissipate.

Special Considerations:

Half-life 2.5 hours

Pregnancy class C; possibly unsafe in lactating mothers.

Atropine used for treatment of bradycardia has a maximum dose of 3 mg or 0.04 mg/kg. However, when treating organophosphate poisoning, atropine dosing should be repeated until secretions are dried.

GLUCAGON

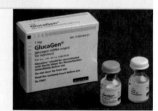

Classification: Hormone

Action: Converts glycogen to glucose.

Indications: Hypoglycemia, beta blocker overdose.

Adverse Effects: Nausea/vomiting, rebound hyperglycemia, hypotension, sinus tachycardia.

Contraindications: Pheochromocytoma, insulinoma, known sensitivity.

Dosage:

Hypoglycemia:
- **Adult:** 1 mg IM, IV, IO, or Sub-Q.
- **Pediatric (<20 kg):** 0.5 mg IM, IV, IO, or Sub-Q.

Beta blocker overdose:
- **Adult:** 2 to 5 mg IV, IO over a 1-minute period, followed by a second dose of 10 mg IV if the symptoms of bradycardia and hypotension recur. (Note that this dose is much higher than the dose required to treat hypoglycemia.)
- **Pediatric:** For patients weighing <20 kg, the dose is 0.5 mg.

Special Considerations:

Pregnancy class B

The dose of glucagon used to treat beta blocker overdose is significantly higher than the dose required to treat hypoglycemia.

Most patients will have nausea and vomiting after glucagon administration. Be prepared with a basin and suction to keep the airway patent.

AMPHETAMINE AND METHAMPHETAMINE INTOXICATION

You are dispatched to the local police department to evaluate a 24-year-old man who is currently in police custody. You arrive to find the patient in an agitated and restless state. He is extremely diaphoretic. His heart rate is 130 beats/min, and blood pressure is 182/110 mm Hg. With some effort you are able to establish an IV line and administer diazepam 5 mg IV. The patient yanks the IV out and remains agitated and threatening to everyone in the vicinity. Next you administer haloperidol 10 mg IM. After several minutes the patient begins to calm down and you are able to get him onto the ambulance stretcher without physical force or restraints.

Drugs such as amphetamines and methamphetamines increase the body's levels of circulating epinephrine and norepinephrine—the "fight-or-flight" hormones. These elevated levels of epinephrine and norepinephrine are responsible for the observed tachycardia, hypertension, hyperthermia, agitation, and mydriasis (pupil dilation). Because of supernormal levels of the catecholamines, patients with amphetamine and methamphetamine overdoses can also have myocardial ischemia, cardiac arrhythmia, seizure, stroke, intracranial hemorrhage, and death.

MANAGEMENT

Neither gastric lavage nor activated charcoal has a role in managing these intoxications, because most of the drug has been absorbed by the time the patient is seen by a prehospital provider. Benzodiazepines (diazepam, midazolam, and lorazepam) can be used to control agitation, and haloperidol can be administered to those who do not respond to benzodiazepine therapy.

Activated charcoal is not used in amphetamine overdose, because most of the drug is absorbed by the time EMS arrives at the hospital.

Benzodiazepines work by binding with a benzodiazepine receptor. Gamma-aminobutyric acid (GABA), a naturally occurring neurotransmitter in the body, binds to the same receptors. When either a benzodiazepine or GABA binds to this receptor, it allows additional chloride ions to enter the cell that bears the receptor. The net effect is that the influx of chloride causes the cell to be less excitable. Clearly this is a desirable effect when these receptors are on the cells of the brain and nervous tissue and the patient is agitated, anxious, or seizing. Haloperidol (Haldol) is a potent antipsychotic agent often used to treat agitation. This drug has a low incidence of sedation and hypotension.

MIDAZOLAM (VERSED)

Classification: Benzodiazepine, Schedule C-IV
Action: Binds to the benzodiazepine receptor and enhances the effects of the brain chemical (neurotransmitter) GABA. Benzodiazepines act at the level of the limbic, thalamic, and hypothalamic regions of the CNS to produce short-acting CNS depression (including sedation, skeletal muscle relaxation, and anticonvulsant activity).
Indications: Sedation, anxiety, skeletal muscle relaxation.
Adverse Effects: Respiratory depression, respiratory arrest, hypotension, nausea/vomiting, headache, hiccups, cardiac arrest.
Contraindications: Acute-angle glaucoma, pregnant women, known sensitivity.
Dosage:
Sedation:
Note: The dose of midazolam needs to be individualized. Every dose should be administered slowly over a period of 2 minutes. Allow 2 minutes to evaluate the clinical effect of the dose given.

cont'd

MIDAZOLAM (VERSED)—CONT'D

- **Adult:**
  - **Healthy and younger than 60 years:** *Some patients require as little as 1 mg IV, IO. No more than 2.5 mg should be given over a 2-minute interval.* If additional sedation is required, continue to administer small increments over 2-minute periods (max dose: 5 mg). If the patient also has received a narcotic, he or she will typically require 30% less midazolam than the same patient not given the narcotic.
  - **60 years and older and debilitated or chronically ill patients:** This group of patients has a higher risk of hypoventilation, airway obstruction, and apnea. The peak clinical effect can take longer in these patients; therefore dose increments should be smaller, and the rate of injection should be slower. *Some patients require a dose as small as 1 mg IV, IO, and no more than 1.5 mg should be given over a 2-minute period.* If additional sedation is required, additional midazolam should be given at a rate of no more than 1 mg over a 2-minute period (max dose: 3.5 mg). If the patient also has received a narcotic, he or she will typically require 50% less midazolam than the same patient not given the narcotic.
  - **Continuous infusion:** Continuous infusions can be required for prolonged transport of intubated, critically ill, and injured patients. After an initial bolus dose, the adult patient will require a maintenance infusion dose of 0.02 to 0.1 mg/kg/hr (1-7 mg/hr).
- **Pediatric (weight-based):** Pediatric patients typically require higher doses of midazolam than do adults on the basis of weight (in mg/kg). Younger pediatric patients (younger than 6 years) require higher doses (in mg/kg) than older pediatric patients. Midazolam takes approximately 3 minutes to reach peak effect; therefore wait at least 2 minutes to determine effectiveness of drug and need for additional dosing.
  - **12 to 16 years:** Same as adult dosing. Some patients in this age group require a higher dose than that used in adults, but rarely does a patient require more than 10 mg.
  - **6 to 12 years:** 0.025 to 0.05 mg/kg IV, IO up to a total dose of 0.4 mg/kg. Exceeding 10 mg as total dose usually is not necessary.
  - **6 months to 5 years:** 0.05 to 0.1 mg/kg IV, IO up to a total dose of 0.6 mg/kg. Exceeding 6 mg as total dose usually is not necessary.
  - **Younger than 6 months:** Dosing recommendations for this age group is unclear. Because this age group is especially vulnerable to airway obstruction and hypoventilation, use small increments with frequent clinical evaluation. Dose: 0.05 to 0.1 mg/kg IV, IO.

Special Considerations:
Patients receiving midazolam require frequent monitoring of vital signs and pulse oximetry. Be prepared to support patient's airway and ventilation.
Pregnancy class D

LORAZEPAM (ATIVAN)

Classification: Benzodiazepine; Schedule C-IV
Action: Binds to the benzodiazepine receptor and enhances the effects of the brain chemical GABA, an inhibitory transmitter, and may result in a state of sedation, hypnosis, skeletal muscle relaxation, anticonvulsant activity, coma.
Indications: Preprocedure sedation induction, anxiety, status epilepticus.
Adverse Effects: Headache, drowsiness, ataxia, dizziness, amnesia, depression, dysarthria, euphoria, syncope, fatigue, tremor, vertigo, respiratory depression, paradoxical CNS stimulation.
Contraindications: Known sensitivity to lorazepam, benzodiazepines, polyethylene glycol, propylene glycol, or benzyl alcohol; COPD; sleep apnea (except while being mechanically ventilated); shock; coma; acute closed-angle glaucoma.

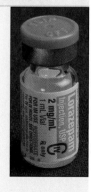

Dosage: Note: IV, IO lorazepam needs to be administered slowly.
Analgesia and Sedation:
- **Adult:** 2 mg or 0.44 mg/kg IV, IO, whichever is smaller. This dosage will provide adequate sedation in most patients and should not be exceeded in patients older than 50 years.
- **Pediatric:** 0.05 mg/kg IV, IO. Each dose should not exceed 2 mg IV, IO.

cont'd

LORAZEPAM (ATIVAN)—CONT'D

Seizures:
- **Adult:** 4 mg IV, IO given over 2 to 5 minutes; may repeat in 10 to 15 minutes (max total dose: 8 mg in a 12-hour period).
- **Pediatric:**
  - **Adolescents:** 0.07 mg/kg slow IV, IO given over 2 to 5 minutes (max single dose: 4 mg). May repeat in 10 to 15 minutes (max dose: 8 mg in a 12-hour period).
  - **Children and infants:** 0.1 mg/kg slow IV, IO given over 2 to 5 minutes (max single dose: 4 mg). May repeat at half the original dose in 10 to 15 minutes if seizure activity resumes.
  - **Neonates:** 0.05 mg/kg slow IV, IO given over 2 to 5 minutes. May repeat in 10 to 15 minutes.

Special Considerations:
Be prepared to support the patient's airway and ventilation.
Pregnancy class D

HALOPERIDOL (HALDOL)

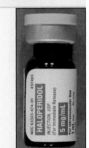

Classification: Antipsychotic agent
Action: Selectively blocks postsynaptic dopamine receptors.
Indications: Psychotic disorders, agitation.
Adverse Effects: Extrapyramidal symptoms, drowsiness, tardive dyskinesia, hypotension, hypertension, VT, sinus tachycardia, QT prolongation, torsades de pointes.
Contraindications: Depressed mental status, Parkinson's disease.
Dosage:
- **Adult:**
  - **Mild agitation:** 0.5 to 2 mg PO or IM.
  - **Moderate agitation:** 5 to 10 mg PO or IM.
  - **Severe agitation:** 10 mg PO or IM.
- **Pediatric:** Not recommended for pediatric patients.

Special Considerations:
Pregnancy class C

COCAINE INTOXICATION

You are called to an office tower to assist a 35-year-old man reporting chest pain. You enter an office suite where a party is taking place with caterers and a live band. You and your partner are quickly escorted to a large office in the rear, where you find the patient. He is sitting on the floor and appears extremely agitated. He is rocking back and forth and is covered in sweat. A co-worker of the patient tells you that he looks terrible and is reporting chest pain. Upon additional questioning by your partner, she admits that she and the patient were doing cocaine before the patient exhibited these symptoms. On your examination, the patient is warm and diaphoretic. His heart rate is 142 beats/min and blood pressure is 182/108 mm Hg. His lungs are clear. He is alert and oriented to date and place but remains agitated and aggressive. The patient has no motor or sensory deficits, but his pupils are 8 mm and reactive to light. ...

MANAGEMENT

Intoxication with cocaine results in an adrenergic response, with the resultant clinical findings of tachycardia, hypertension, dilated pupils, hyperthermia, and agitation. The initial treatment for the agitation includes the use of benzodiazepines such as diazepam (Valium), midazolam (Versed), or lorazepam (Ativan). Haloperidol (Haldol) is the second-line drug used in patients who do not respond to the benzodiazepines or who are psychotic.

Cocaine can produce serious cardiovascular complications such as tachycardia, hypertension, chest pain, and myocardial ischemia.[13] The chest pain associated with cocaine intoxication is ischemic in nature. The patient initially should be given a benzodiazepine such as diazepam. In fact, up to this point the treatment for cocaine intoxication is similar to therapy for amphetamine use.

> ... You administer 5 mg Valium to the patient, and he becomes less agitated. You place him on supplemental oxygen and provide three doses of sublingual nitroglycerin and one aspirin. Despite these drug interventions, the patient still reports chest pain that rates as a 7 on a scale of 1 to 10.

Because the chest pain seen with cocaine intoxication is often ischemic in nature, the drug therapy used in other forms of chest pain is indicated—administration of nitroglycerin.[14,15]

NITROGLYCERIN (NITROLINGUAL, NITROQUICK, NITRO-DUR)

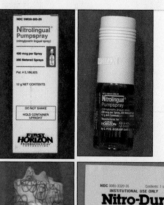

Classification: Antianginal agent

Action: Relaxes vascular smooth muscle, thereby dilating peripheral arteries and veins. This causes pooling of venous blood and decreased venous return to the heart, which decreases preload. Nitroglycerin also reduces left ventricular systolic wall tension, which decreases afterload.

Indications: Angina, ongoing ischemic chest discomfort, hypertension, myocardial ischemia associated with cocaine intoxication.

Adverse Effects: Headache, hypotension, bradycardia, lightheadedness, flushing, cardiovascular collapse, methemoglobinemia.

Contraindications: Hypotension, severe bradycardia or tachycardia, increased ICP, intracranial bleeding, patients taking any medications for erectile dysfunction (such as sildenafil [Viagra], tadalafil [Cialis], or vardenafil [Levitra]), known sensitivity to nitrates. Use with caution in anemia, closed-angle glaucoma, hypotension, postural hypotension, uncorrected hypovolemia.

Dosage:

- **Adult:**
  - **Sublingual tablets:** 1 tablet (0.3-0.4 mg) at 5-minute intervals to a maximum of 3 doses.
  - **Translingual spray:** 1 (0.4 mg) spray at 5-minute intervals to a maximum of 3 sprays.
  - **Ointment:** 2% topical (Nitro-Bid ointment): Apply 1 to 2 inches of paste over the chest wall, cover with transparent wrap, and secure with tape.
  - **IV:**
    - **Bolus:** 12.5 to 25 mcg
    - **Infusion:** 5 mcg/min; may increase rate by 5 to 10 mcg/min every 5 to 10 minutes as needed. End points of dose titration for nitroglycerin include a drop in the blood pressure of 10%, relief of chest pain, and return of ST segment to normal on a 12-lead ECG.
- **Pediatric IV infusion:** The initial pediatric infusion is 0.25 to 0.5 mcg/kg/min IV, IO titrated by 0.5 to 1 mcg/kg/min. Usual required dose is 1 to 3 mcg/kg/min to a maximum dose of 5 mcg/kg/min.

Special Considerations:
Administration of nitroglycerin to a patient with right ventricular MI can result in hypotension. Pregnancy class C

The patient in the preceding scenario has ischemic chest pain. Therefore the administration of aspirin should be considered. Aspirin reduces the effectiveness of platelets to form clots. Platelets are formed elements of the blood that, when activated, are responsible for the formation of small plugs that seal blood vessels, such as in the case of a laceration. In the case of ischemic chest pain, the activated platelets form small plugs that occlude the flow of blood vessels in the heart. The spasm of the coronary arteries and occlusion with platelet plugs result in the heart muscle not receiving the critical amount of oxygen. Administering aspirin inhibits the enzyme cyclooxygenase and impairs platelet function for the life of the platelet, which is 7 days.

If the patient's chest pain persists after treatment with benzodiazepines, nitroglycerin, and aspirin, the paramedic should consider administration of morphine. Phentolamine (Regitine) is another medication that may be used in this situation. Phentolamine is an alpha adrenergic blocker aimed at reducing systemic blood pressure and vasoconstriction of the coronary arteries.[16] Adrenergic receptors, when stimulated, produce the clinical responses of hypertension, tachycardia, dilated pupils, agitation, and hyperthermia. Alpha receptors result in vasoconstriction and hypertension. When the patient is given phentolamine, the drug binds to the alpha receptor, preventing the cocaine molecule from producing its clinical effects of vasoconstriction and hypertension. Alpha receptors do not produce an increase in heart rate (chronotropy) or forcefulness of heart contraction (inotropy). Those effects are mediated by beta receptors.

Hypertension from cocaine should not be treated with beta blockers because they can exacerbate the coronary artery vasoconstriction and result in an increased chance of death.[17]

> Treatment of cocaine-induced hypertension can constrict coronary arteries and produce cardiac complications and even death.

Some patients with cocaine intoxication have seizures. The best method of stopping these seizures is administrating a benzodiazepine, such as diazepam, followed by a loading dose of phenytoin.

ASPIRIN, ASA

Classification: Antiplatelet, nonnarcotic analgesic, antipyretic
Action: Prevents the formation of a chemical known as thromboxane A_2, which causes platelets to clump together, or aggregate, and form plugs that cause obstruction or constriction of small coronary arteries.
Indications: Fever, inflammation, angina, acute MI, and patients complaining of pain, pressure, squeezing, or crushing in the chest that may be cardiac in origin.
Adverse Effects: Anaphylaxis, angioedema, bronchospasm, bleeding, stomach irritation, nausea/vomiting.
Contraindications: GI bleeding, active ulcer disease, hemorrhagic stroke, bleeding disorders, children with chickenpox or flulike symptoms, known sensitivity.
Dosage: Note: "Baby aspirin" 81 mg, standard adult aspirin dose 325 mg.

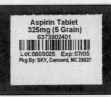

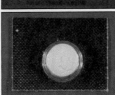

Myocardial Infarction:
- **Adult:** 160 to 325 mg PO (alternatively, four 81-mg baby aspirin are often given), 300-mg rectal suppository.
- **Pediatric:** 3 to 5 mg/kg/day to 5 to 10 mg/kg/day given as a single dose.

Pain or Fever:
- **Adult:** 325 to 650 mg PO (1 to 2 adult tablets) every 4 to 6 hours.
- **Pediatric:** 60 to 90 mg/kg/day in divided doses every 4 to 6 hours.

Special Considerations:
Pregnancy class C except the last 3 months of pregnancy, when aspirin is considered pregnancy class D.

MORPHINE SULFATE

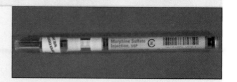

Classification: Opiate agonist, Schedule C-II

Action: Binds with opioid receptors. Morphine is capable of inducing hypotension by depression of the vasomotor centers of the brain, as well as release of the chemical histamine. In the management of angina, morphine reduces stimulation of the sympathic nervous system caused by pain and anxiety. Reduction of sympathetic stimulation reduces heart rate, cardiac work, and myocardial oxygen consumption.

Indications: Moderate to severe pain, including chest pain associated with ACS, CHF, pulmonary edema.

Adverse Effects: Respiratory depression, hypotension, nausea/vomiting, dizziness, lightheadedness, sedation, diaphoresis, euphoria, dysphoria, worsening of bradycardia and heart block in some patients with acute inferior wall MI, seizures, cardiac arrest, anaphylactoid reactions.

Contraindications: Respiratory depression, shock, known sensitivity. Use with caution in hypotension, acute bronchial asthma, respiratory insufficiency, head trauma.

Dosage:

Pain:

- **Adult:** 2.5 to 15 mg IV, IO, IM, or Sub-Q administered slowly over a period of several minutes. The dose is the same whether administered IV, IO, IM, or Sub-Q.
- **Pediatric:**
  - **6 months to 12 years:** 0.05 to 0.2 mg/kg IV, IO, IM, or Sub-Q.
  - **Younger than 6 months:** 0.03 to 0.05 mg/kg IV, IO, IM, or Sub-Q.

Chest Pain Associated with Acute Coronary Syndromes, Congestive Heart Failure, and Pulmonary Edema:

Administer small doses and reevaluate the patient. Large doses may lead to respiratory depression and worsen the patient's hypoxia.

- **Adult:** 2 to 4 mg slow IV, IO over a 1- to 5-minute period with increments of 2 to 8 mg repeated every 5 to 15 minutes until patient relieved of chest pain.
- **Pediatric:** 0.1 to 0.2 mg/kg/dose IV, IO.

Special Considerations:

Monitor vital signs and pulse oximetry closely. Be prepared to support patient's airway and ventilations.

Overdose should be treated with naloxone.

Pregnancy class C

PHENTOLAMINE (REGITINE)

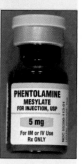

Classification: Alpha antagonist, antihypertensive

Action: Blocks alpha adrenergic receptors, causing vasodilation.

Indications: Hypertensive emergencies and hypertension caused by pheochromocytoma, cocaine-induced vasospasm of the coronary arteries.

Adverse Effects: Sinus tachycardia, angina, dizziness, orthostatic hypotension, prolonged hypotensive episodes, nausea/vomiting, diarrhea, weakness, flushing, nasal congestion.

Contraindications: Known sensitivity. Use with caution in acute MI, angina, coronary insufficiency, evidence suggestive of coronary artery disease, peptic ulcer disease.

Dosage:

Hypertensive Crisis:

- **Adult:** 5 to 15 mg IV, IO or IM.
- **Pediatric:** Not recommended for pediatric patients.

Cocaine-Induced Vasospasm:

- **Adult:** 5 mg IV, IO or IM.
- **Pediatric:** Not recommended for pediatric patients.

Special Considerations:

Pregnancy class C

OVERVIEW OF NARCOTIC OVERDOSE

Your unit is dispatched to a local rescue mission to evaluate an unconscious man who was found on the street. You arrive to find a 23-year-old man who is well known to the police as a heroin abuser. On assessment, the patient moans because of deep pain. His blood pressure is 72/52 mm Hg, heart rate is 112 beats/min, and respirations are 12 breaths/min and very shallow. On physical examination, the patient is grossly intoxicated with alcohol. His upper extremities have multiple needle tracks, as well as small, circular scars that appear to be from previous skin abscesses. As you roll the patient to inspect his back, you find a bag that contains drug paraphernalia, needles, and a substance that looks like heroin. He has no obvious external signs of traumatic injury.

Overdose can occur with any type of opiate use, in either medical or abuse settings. Opiates, or narcotics, are commonly abused medications. Heroin, a common drug of abuse and overdose, is classified as an opiate and is responsible for the majority of opiate-related overdoses.[18] Heroin is often abused by injecting the drug intervenously, known as "mainlining," although the most common method of heroin abuse is snorting the drug. In Asian countries, heroin is commonly smoked. Overdose typically occurs with heroin use because the quantity of heroin in any given sample can vary greatly. Heroin is also more soluble in fat, allowing the drug to reach higher levels in the system more rapidly than other forms of opiates.

Patients with an opiate/narcotic overdose typically have a depressed level of consciousness, hypotension, and respiratory depression. In any patient with a depressed level of consciousness, prehospital care must focus on supporting the ABCs. Even when the provider has a strong and well-founded suspicion of the cause of the patient's altered level of consciousness, as in this case, the obligation is to rule out common and easily treated metabolic conditions such as diabetic complications of hypoglycemia or diabetic ketoacidosis. In most cases, the cause of altered level of consciousness is unknown.

MANAGEMENT

On establishing an IV, the provider should immediately administer a combination of medications known as the **coma cocktail.** The coma cocktail, a mixture of thiamine, dextrose, and naloxone, can prove to be both diagnostic and therapeutic.[19] Thiamine, commonly referred to as *vitamin B₁*, is administered to prevent and possibly treat a condition known as *Wernicke-Korsakoff syndrome,* an altered mental status caused by a deficiency of the vitamin thiamine. This condition is common in chronic alcoholics.

Hypoglycemia should also be considered and, if identified, treated with dextrose. If the glucometer indicates that the patient is hypoglycemic, administer 50% dextrose. The adult patient should receive 50 g (1 ampule) of IV dextrose. Consider administration of thiamine before dextrose to avoid Wernicke-Korsakoff syndrome.[20] In the absence of hypoglycemia, do not administer dextrose.[20]

Naloxone (Narcan), a drug known as a **competitive antagonist,** binds to the opiate receptor to prevent the opiate from exerting its effects of altered mental status, hypotension, and respiratory depression.

THIAMINE (VITAMIN B₁)

Classification: Vitamin B₁
Action: Thiamine combines with adenosine triphosphate to produce thiamine diphosphate, which acts as a coenzyme in carbohydrate metabolism.
Indications: Wernicke-Korsakoff syndrome, beriberi, nutritional supplementation.
Adverse Effects: Itching, rash, pain at injection site.
Contraindications: Known sensitivity.
Dosage:
Wernicke-Korsakoff Syndrome:
· **Adult:** 100 mg IV, IO.
· **Pediatric:** Not recommended for pediatric patients.
Special Considerations:
Pregnancy class A

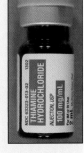

DEXTROSE (DEXTROSE 50%, DEXTROSE 25%, DEXTROSE 10%)

Classification: Antihypoglycemic
Action: Increases blood glucose concentrations.
Indications: Hypoglycemia
Adverse Effects: Hyperglycemia, warmth, burning from IV infusion. Concentrated solutions may cause pain and thrombosis of the peripheral veins.
Contraindications: Intracranial and intraspinal hemorrhage, delirium tremens, solution is not clear, seals are not intact.
Dosage:
Hyperkalemia:
  · **Adult:** 25 g of dextrose 50% IV, IO.
  · **Pediatric:** 0.5 to 1 g/kg IV, IO.
Hypoglycemia:
  · **Adult:** 10 to 25 g of dextrose 50% IV (20 to 50 mL of dextrose solution).
  · **Pediatric:**
    · **Older than 2 years:** 2 mL/kg of dextrose 50%.
    · **Younger than 2 years:** 2 to 4 mL/kg of dextrose 10%.
Special Considerations:
Pregnancy class C

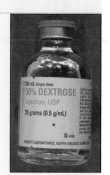

NALOXONE (NARCAN)

Classification: Opioid antagonist
Action: Binds the opioid receptor and blocks the effect of narcotics.
Indications: Narcotic overdoses, reversal of narcotics used for procedure-related anesthesia.
Adverse Effects: Nausea/vomiting, restlessness, diaphoresis, tachycardia, hypertension, tremulousness, seizures, cardiac arrest, narcotic withdrawal. Patients who have gone from a state of somnolence from a narcotic overdose to wide awake may become combative.
Contraindications: Known sensitivity to naloxone, nalmefene, or naltrexone. Use with caution in patients with supraventricular arrhythmias or other cardiac disease, head trauma, brain tumor.
Dosage:
  · **Adult:** 0.4 to 2 mg IV, IO, ET, IM, or Sub-Q. Alternatively, administer 2 mg intranasally. Higher doses (10-20 mg) may be required for overdoses of synthetic narcotics. A repeat dose of one third to two thirds the original dose is often necessary.
  · **Pediatric:**
    · **5 years or older or weight >20 kg:** 2 mg IV, IO, ET, IM, or Sub-Q.
    · **Younger than 5 years or weight <20 kg:** 0.1 mg/kg IV, IO, ET, IM, or Sub-Q; may repeat every 2 to 3 minutes.
Special Considerations:
Pregnancy class C

ORGANOPHOSPHATE AND NERVE AGENT EXPOSURE

You are dispatched to the home of a 52-year-old male farmer. The patient's wife tells you that her husband must have caught the flu because he has diarrhea and is vomiting. You assess the patient, who tells you that he was feeling great until he worked the fields that afternoon. Shortly after loading the fertilizer spreader, he began to have nausea, vomiting, and profuse sweating. You perform a physical examination. His heart rate is 144 beats/min, and he is sweating profusely. He seems to be having excessive oral secretions, and his pupils are pinpoint. On auscultation of lung sounds, he has wheezes in all lung fields. ...

Organophosphates are a class of chemicals found in insecticides and fertilizers and are common in agricultural environments. Organophosphates were originally developed in the 1930s for use as insecticides. Subsequently these chemicals were altered for use as nerve agents. The nerve gases **sarin** and **VX** are potent organophosphates. This class of chemicals can gain access to the body through inhalation, ingestion, and absorption through the skin. Sarin was released in a Tokyo subway by a terrorist group in 1995.

Organophosphates are the most commonly used insecticide in the world and are responsible for 80% of the intoxications from insecticides. Each year, more than 80,000 people are poisoned by organophosphates, and half of these victims are children. Phosphates are highly explosive and are also routinely used by the military.

Organophosphates poison the body by inhibiting the enzyme **acetylcholinesterase.** Under normal conditions, acetylcholinesterase breaks down and deactivates the neurotransmitter acetylcholine. Without acetylcholinesterase present to break it down, acetylcholine builds up and causes overstimulation of the parasympathetic nervous system. Overstimulation of the parasympathetic nervous system results in both muscarinic and nicotinic effects.

The effects of muscarinic receptor blockage can be remembered by the mnemonic **DUMBBELS.** *Muscarinic* requires *muscles*. To build muscles, one needs DUMBBELS:

*D*iarrhea
*U*rination
*M*iosis (contraction of pupils)
*B*radycardia
*B*ronchospasm and bronchorrhea
*E*mesis
*L*acrimation
*S*alivation, secretion, and sweating

The effects of nicotinic receptor blockage can be committed to memory by the mnemonic **MTWHF.** *Nicotinic* is similar to the word *nicotine*, and smokers need nicotine every day of the week (MTWHF):

*M*ydriasis (dilation of pupils)
*T*achycardia
*W*eakness
*H*ypertension and hyperglycemia
*F*asciculations (involuntary contractions, twitching)

MANAGEMENT

Symptoms of organophosphate intoxication can occur within 5 minutes of exposure. The most dangerous manifestations of organophosphate poisoning are excessive respiratory secretions (bronchorrhea), bronchospasm, and respiratory insufficiency.[21] Excessive respiratory secretions and respiratory failure make securing the airway imperative. Of critical importance is that, if intubation is performed, the rapid depolarizing agent succinylcholine (Anectine) should *not* be used because it cannot be broken down and can result in prolonged paralysis of the patient.[22] The initial drug intervention in patients intoxicated with organophosphates is the administration of atropine.

The most dangerous manifestations of organophosphate poisoning are respiratory complications.

> ... You give the patient a bolus of atropine. His wheezing stops and the secretions decrease. However, the patient remains tachycardic, with a heart rate of 140 beats/min and blood pressure of 184/105 mm Hg. He is extremely weak, as demonstrated by the inability to lift his head or arms.

As demonstrated in this case, atropine reverses the effects of the muscarinic receptors, but the nicotinic effects will persist and the patient will continue to have profound muscle weakness. To reverse the effects of organophosphates on the nicotinic receptors, the provider needs to administer pralidoxime (2-PAM).[23]

PRALIDOXIME (2-PAM, PROTOPAM)

Classification: Cholinergic agonist, antidote
Action: Reactivates cholinesterase.
Indications: Toxicity from nerve agents (organophosphates) having cholinesterase activity.
Adverse Effects: Dizziness, blurred vision, hypertension, diplopia, hyperventilation, laryngospasm, nausea/vomiting, sinus tachycardia.
Contraindications: Myasthenia gravis, renal failure, inability to control the airway.
Dosage:
· **Adult:** 1 to 2 g (dilute in 100 mL normal saline) over a 15- to 30-minute period. If this is not practical or if pulmonary edema is present, the dose should be given slowly (≥5 min) by IV as a 5% solution in water.
· **Autoinjector:** Pralidoxime is also available as an autoinjector that delivers 600 mg IM. Repeat doses can be given every 15 minutes to a total of three doses (1800 mg). Pralidoxime autoinjector is not recommended for pediatric patients.
· **Pediatric:** 20 to 50 mg/kg IV, IO over a 10-minute period.
Special Considerations:
Pregnancy class C

REVIEW QUESTIONS

1. What is the risk of vomiting and aspirating activated charcoal?
2. Activated charcoal is contraindicated in what common overdose?
3. After overdose with a cyclic antidepressant, a patient begins to show a wide-complex tachycardia. What is the initial drug of choice?
4. What is the cardiovascular effect of a too-rapid administration of phenytoin (Dilantin)?
5. What is the pharmacologic antidote for beta blocker overdose?
6. What are the effects of methamphetamine on the body?
7. Why are gastric lavage and activated charcoal not effective in treating a methamphetamine overdose?
8. What is the initial drug used for the treatment of agitation in a patient who is intoxicated with cocaine?
9. What are the medications included in the coma cocktail?
10. What are the most dangerous manifestations of organophosphate poisoning?
11. When intubating a victim of organophosphate poisoning, why should succinylcholine (Anectine) be avoided?

REFERENCES

1. Manoguerra AS, Krenzelok EP: Rapid emesis from high-dose ipecac syrup in adults and children intoxicated with antiemetics and other drugs, *Am J Hosp Pharm* 35:1360, 1978.
2. MacLean WC: A comparison of ipecac syrup and apomorphine in the immediate treatment of ingestion of poisons, *J Pediatr* 82:121, 1973.

3. Bond GR: Home syrup of ipecac use does not reduce emergency department use or improve outcome, *Pediatrics* 112:1061, 2003.
4. Shannon M: The demise of ipecac, *Pediatrics* 112:1180, 2003.
5. American Academy of Pediatrics Committee on Injury and Poison Prevention: Poison treatment in the home, *Pediatrics* 112:1182, 2003.
6. American Academy of Clinical Toxicology; European Association of Poison Centres and Clinical Toxicologists: Position statement and practice guidelines on the use of multidose activated charcoal in the treatment of acute poisoning, *J Toxicol Clin Toxicol* 37:731, 1999.
7. Menzies DG, Busuttil A, Prescott LF: Fatal pulmonary aspiration of oral activated charcoal, *Br Med J* 287:459, 1988.
8. Litovitz TL, et al: Annual report of the American Association of Poison Control Centers Toxic Exposure Surveillance System, *Am J Emerg Med* 20:391, 2001.
9. Ellison DW, Pentel PR: Clinical features and consequences of seizures due to cyclic overdose, *Am J Emerg Med* 7:5, 1989.
10. Reith DM, et al: Relative toxicity of beta blockers in overdose, *J Clin Pharmacol* 34:273, 1996.
11. Love JN, et al: Acute beta blocker overdose: factors associated with the development of cardiovascular morbidity, *J Toxicol Clin Toxicol* 38:275, 2000.
12. Taubolet P, et al: Pathophysiology and management of self-poisoning with beta-blockers, *J Toxicol Clin Toxicol* 31:531, 1993.
13. Hollander JE, Hoffman RS: Cocaine-induced myocardial infarction: an analysis and review of the literature, *J Emerg Med* 10:169, 1992.
14. Baumann BM, et al: Randomized, double-blind placebo-controlled trial of diazepam, nitroglycerin, or both for treatment of patients with potential cocaine-associated acute coronary syndromes, *Acad Emerg Med* 7:878, 2000.
15. Honderick T, et al: A prospective randomized, controlled trial of benzodiazepines and nitroglycerine or nitroglycerine alone on the treatment of cocaine-associated with acute coronary syndromes, *Am J Emerg Med* 21:31, 2003.
16. Hollander JE, Coates WA, Hoffman RS: Use of phentolamine for cocaine-induced myocardial ischemia, *N Engl J Med* 327:361, 1992.
17. Kloner RA, Hale S: Unraveling the complex effects of cocaine on the heart, *Circulation* 87:1046, 1993.
18. *Results from the 2003 National Survey on Drug Use and Health: national findings,* Washington, DC, 2004, United States Department of Health and Human Services.
19. Hoffman RS, Goldfrank LR: The poisoned patient with altered level of consciousness: controversies in the use of the "coma cocktail", *JAMA* 274:562, 1995.
20. Reuler JB, Girard DE, Cooney TG: Wernicke's encephalopathy, *N Engl J Med* 312:1035, 1985.
21. Lee P, Tai DYH: Clinical features of patients with acute organophosphate poisoning requiring intensive care, *Intens Care Med* 27:694, 2001.
22. Selden BC, Curry SC: Prolonged succinylcholine-induced paralysis in organophosphate insecticide poisoning, *Ann Emerg Med* 16:215, 1987.
23. Eddleston M, et al: Oximes in organophosphorus pesticide poisoning: a systemic review of clinical trials, *Q J Med* 95:275, 2002.

Respiratory Emergencies

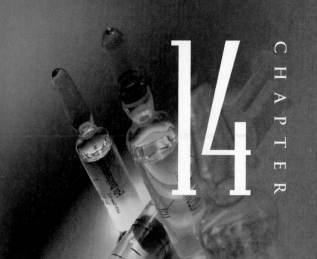

CHAPTER 14

OBJECTIVES

1. Define nasal cannula, rebreather face mask, nonrebreather face mask, and Venturi mask.
2. Discuss the use of oxygen in a respiratory emergency.
3. Describe the two types of bronchodilator agents.
4. Discuss the benefits of the metered-dose inhaler.
5. Demonstrate the proper procedure for administering medication through a metered-dose inhaler.
6. Discuss medications used in the treatment of asthma: albuterol (Proventil, Ventolin), ipratropium bromide (Atrovent), and albuterol/ipratropium (Combivent).
7. Discuss medications used as second-line therapy for acute exacerbation of asthma: methylprednisolone sodium succinate (Solu-Medrol), hydrocortisone sodium succinate (Solu-Cortef), aminophylline, magnesium sulfate, and racemic epinephrine.
8. Briefly describe the key treatment for patients with chronic obstructive pulmonary disease.

Medications that Appear in Chapter 14

Oxygen
Albuterol (Proventil, Ventolin)
Levalbuterol (Xopenex)
Ipratropium bromide (Atrovent)
Albuterol/ipratropium (Combivent)
Methylprednisolone sodium succinate (Solu-Medrol)
Hydrocortisone sodium succinate (Cortef, Solu-Cortef)
Aminophylline
Magnesium sulfate
Racemic epinephrine/racepinephrine (microNefrin, S_2)

INTRODUCTION

Respiratory distress is one of the most common patient presentations encountered by prehospital professionals. In fact, the prehospital treatment of respiratory distress has been shown to produce positive outcomes in patients—more so than in other illnesses.[1] These positive outcomes are seen in increased survival rates, shorter hospital stays, and decreased costs to the healthcare system. Acute respiratory distress affects the young and old, male and female, and individuals of all ethnicities. Although the underlying pathologic condition causing the respiratory distress may be different, with the exception of acute pulmonary edema most of the prehospital care is aimed at treatment of reversible bronchial constriction, or bronchospasm.

Y ou are dispatched to a church to assist a 72-year-old woman reporting shortness of breath. When you arrive you are escorted to a library, where you find a moderately obese woman lying on a couch. You learn that she has a medical history of diabetes, hypertension, and asthma. Her heart rate is 88 beats/min, blood pressure is 144/92 mm Hg, respiratory rate is 16 breaths/min, and oxygen saturation (SaO_2) is 87%. On physical examination the patient's breath sounds are diminished in both lungs. You place the patient on 100% oxygen with a nonrebreather mask. Shortly after placing the patient on oxygen, her SaO_2 increases to 94%.

OXYGEN

Although often overlooked as a drug, oxygen is the most commonly used medication in the prehospital setting. As with any drug, oxygen has associated risks, as well as benefits. Oxygen is used daily by basic and advanced prehospital providers, sometimes with little consideration to its pharmacologic properties.

Oxygen is a colorless and odorless gas stored in either green or aluminum cylinders at a pressure of 1800 to 2400 psi. As the oxygen passes through the attached regulator, the gas pressure is decreased to a working pressure of 60 psi. Oxygen is contained in nine different sizes of cylinders labeled alphabetically (Table 14-1). An understanding of the capacities of these cylinders is helpful to the prehospital provider in determining the duration of oxygen therapy that a given cylinder can provide (Fig. 14-1).

The quantity of oxygen delivered to a specific patient can be considered in terms of the concentration of inspired oxygen and flow. The atmosphere consists of 78% nitrogen, 21% oxygen, and a variety of other gases that compose the remaining 1%. The concentration of inspired oxygen is referred to as the **fraction of inspired oxygen (FiO_2).** Because the percentage of oxygen in the atmosphere is 21%, the FiO_2 in normal room air is 21%. When a patient has shortness of breath, chest pain, or shock, supplemental oxygen is administered to increase the concentration of oxygen breathed by the patient. Increasing the concentration of inspired oxygen increases the content of oxygen in blood and subsequently the amount of oxygen delivered to the heart and peripheral tissues.

OXYGEN DELIVERY DEVICES

Oxygen delivery devices include the **nasal cannula** and face mask. The basic principle by which these devices work is the creation of a reservoir filled with oxygen-enriched gas. When the patient inhales, he or she breathes from this oxygen-enriched reservoir. Nasal cannulas and nonrebreather face masks typically are the most commonly used noninvasive devices for delivering oxygen in the prehospital setting. However, patients involved in interfacility transfers may use additional devices, as described in this section.

TABLE 14-1

Oxygen Cylinders: Capacity and Duration of Use

Cylinder	Capacity (L)	Duration of Use at 5 L/Min	Duration of Use at 10 L/min
A	76	15 min	8 min
B	196	39 min	20 min
D	396	1.3 hr	40 min
E	659	2.1 hr	1.1 hr
F	2062	6.8 hr	3.4 hr
M	3000	10 hr	5.0 hr
G	5331	17.7 hr	8.8 hr
H	5570	18.5 hr	9.2 hr
K	7500	25 hr	12.5 hr

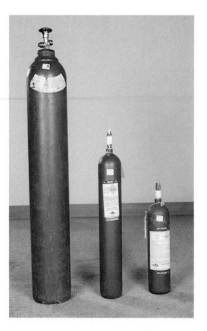

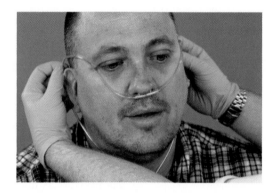

▼ **Fig. 14-1** Various sizes of oxygen cylinders: M, E, and D. (From Stoy W, Platt T, Lejeune D, and Center for Emergency Medicine: *Mosby's EMT-basic textbook revised,* ed 2, St Louis, 2007, Mosby.)

▼ **Fig. 14-2** Nasal cannula. (From Stoy W, Platt T, Lejeune D, and Center for Emergency Medicine: *Mosby's EMT-basic textbook revised,* ed 2, St Louis, 2007, Mosby.)

The nasal cannula is a noninvasive means of delivering supplemental oxygen in a low-flow and nonintrusive fashion (Fig. 14-2). Oxygen flows through two nasal prongs into the oropharynx, which acts as an oxygen reservoir, resulting in an increase in the oxygen concentration. A nasal cannula set with a flow rate of 6 L/min is capable of delivering an oxygen concentration between 35% and 45%.

Various oxygen face masks are capable of delivering an oxygen concentration based on the flow rate, reservoir of the mask, presence or absence of a reservoir bag, and side ports in the mask with directional valves. The simple oxygen face mask does not have a reservoir bag or unidirectional side ports. Room gases mix with the oxygen inside the mask. At a flow rate of 6 to 10 L/min, these masks are capable of delivering an FiO_2 between 30% and 60%.

Rebreather face masks, or **partial rebreather face masks,** have a face mask and a reservoir bag (Fig. 14-3, *A*). Oxygen accumulates in the reservoir bag. During inspiration the patient inhales oxygen in the reservoir, as well as some room air through the side ports. When the patient exhales, some of the expired breath goes back into the reservoir bag, where it is then rebreathed. Partial rebreather masks are capable of delivering 60% oxygen.

Nonrebreather face masks are similar to rebreather masks in appearance and function, with the exception of having one-way exhalation valves on the sides of the mask and on the reservoir bag (Figure 14-3, *B*). The valves on the sides of the mask prevent inhalation of room air during inspiration. The valve on the reservoir prevents any of the exhaled breath from entering the oxygen-rich reservoir. Nonrebreather face masks require a higher flow rate of 12 to 15 L/min and are capable of delivering oxygen concentrations close to 100%.

Emergency departments and hospitals often use the **Venturi mask.** Venturi masks come with a series of small plastic inserts that fit ports on the mask and regulate the concentration of oxygen that the patient can inhale (Fig. 14-4). By changing the plastic insert, the provider can, with a significant degree of precision, alter the oxygen concentration from 24% to 60%. The flow of oxygen depends on the desired FiO_2 (Table 14-2).

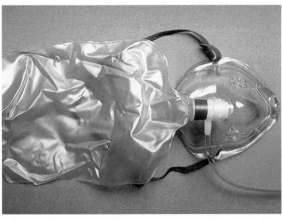 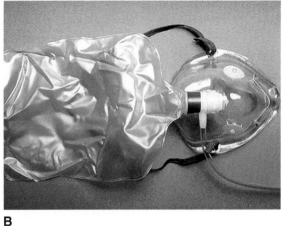

A **B**

▼ Fig. 14-3 **A,** Partial rebreather mask. This mask has an oxygen reservoir bag but no valves over the side ports. **B,** Nonrebreather mask. This mask has an oxygen reservoir bag, as well as one-way valves over the side ports. (From Aehlert B: *Mosby's comprehensive pediatric emergency care,* rev, St Louis, 2007, Mosby.)

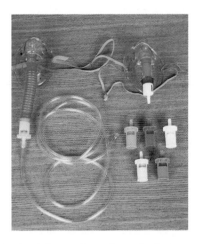

▼ Fig. 14-4 Venturi mask. On the right are the various plastic inserts that control the concentration of oxygen. (From Henry M, Stapleton E: *EMT prehospital care,* ed 3 rev, St Louis, 2007, Mosby.)

TABLE 14-2

Venturi Mask Inserts and Oxygen Flow Rates

Oxygen Delivery	Insert Color	Oxygen Flow Rate
24%	Blue	2 L/min
28%	White	4 L/min
35%	Yellow	6 L/min
40%	Red	8 L/min
60%	Green	12 L/min

 ## INITIATION OF OXYGEN THERAPY

Equipment Needed:
Oxygen source, oxygen flow meter, mask or cannula
Procedure:
1. Observe universal precautions.
2. When possible, explain to the patient what procedure you are going to perform and why.

3. Ensure the protective seal has been removed from the valve on the tank. Do not lose the washer attached to the seal, because it provides an airtight seal between the regulator and the tank. Turn the valve away from yourself or anyone else.

4. Quickly open and close the valve to blow any dirt or contaminants out of the tank opening.

5. Place the washer over the inlet port on the regulator. Line up the regulator port and pins with the tank opening and holds in the tank valve. Check the flow meter to ensure it is turned off. Tighten the screw by hand.

6. Open the tank to test for an airtight seal. If there is leakage, tighten the screw until the leak stops. Once you have made sure there are no leaks, it must be completely open or completely closed.

7. Adjust the flow meter to the desired setting.

8. When finished, turn off the flow meter and close the tank valve.

9. Open the flow meter momentarily to release the pressure from the regulator.

On occasion, prehospital providers encounter patients with **chronic obstructive pulmonary disease (COPD),** who require continuous oxygen while at home. Continuous oxygen can require a transtracheal catheter, which is inserted surgically. Transtracheal catheters, like nasal cannulas, are used for long-term oxygen therapy in patients with chronic lung disease. Some patients find that the long-term use of nasal cannulas is irritating to the nose at night; such patients may receive transtracheal catheters, which are held in place by a necklace.

OXYGEN

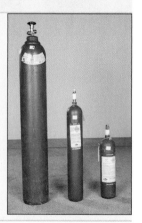

Classification: Elemental gas
Action: Facilitates cellular energy metabolism.
Indications: Hypoxia, ischemic chest pain, respiratory distress, suspected carbon monoxide poisoning, traumatic injuries, shock.
Adverse Effects: High concentrations can cause decreased level of consciousness and respiratory depression in patients with chronic carbon dioxide retention or chronic lung disease.
Contraindications: Known paraquat poisoning.
Dosage:
Low-Concentration Oxygen:
  · A dose of 1 to 4 L/min by a nasal cannula is appropriate.
High-Concentration Oxygen:
  · A dose of 10 to 15 L/min via nonrebreather mask is appropriate.
Special Considerations:
Pregnancy class A

BRONCHODILATORS

Your unit has been dispatched to a local high school for a youth having an asthma attack. The dispatcher informs you that the patient is in the gymnasium. You arrive to find a 17-year-old boy sitting in the middle of the basketball court. Several friends are standing around the patient, attempting to assist and calm him. You clear back the crowd and begin your assessment. You find an anxious young man who has rapid and somewhat labored respirations. He is moving air. The patient's respiratory rate is 32 breaths/min, heart rate is 110 beats/min, and blood pressure is 142/88 mm Hg. ...

Patients with **asthma** (an inflammatory disease of the lungs characterized by typically reversible airway obstruction) and COPD have respiratory distress from a functional narrowing of the conducting airways. As a result, these patients report that they feel as though they are breathing through a straw. Spasm of the bronchial smooth muscle, also known as **bronchospasm,** results in a decrease in the airway diameter.

Another factor that contributes to respiratory distress is edema of the mucosa that lines the respiratory tract. This inflammatory edema results in a thickening of the mucosal linings and a resultant decrease in airway diameter. Increased secretions also contribute to the distress of these patients. Any reduction of the radius of the airway, from either broncho-spasm or mucosal edema, can have a profound effect on the flow of gas.

Poiseuille's law is the law of physics that determines the resistance and flow of gas. This law states that the flow of gas through a tube is proportional to the radius of the airway to the fourth power. Therefore if the radius of an airway decreases from 4 mm to 3 mm from bronchospasm or mucosal edema, the potential flow of gas decreases by almost one third from even this small reduction in the airway.

The first thing the patient in the preceding scenario needs is supplemental oxygen. After oxygen, administration of an inhaled **bronchodilator** would be appropriate.

Bronchodilators can be divided into selective and nonselective agents. Selective agents act preferentially on the bronchial smooth muscle and improve the patient's condition while minimizing side effects. Beta$_2$ agonists are sympathomimetic medications that target the beta$_2$ receptors and cause relaxation of bronchial smooth muscle without stimulating tachycardia or hypertension. Most of these medications are selective for the beta$_2$ receptor; however, paramedics must be cautious because excessive doses can produce the undesirable effects seen with alpha and beta$_1$ stimulation (e.g., tachycardia and hypertension). Use beta$_2$ agonists with caution in patients with a history of heart disease, and always monitor the ECG during and after treatments. Examples of beta$_2$ agonists include albuterol (Proventil), terbutaline (Brethine), metaproterenol (Alupent), formoterol (Foradil), and pirbuterol (Maxair).

Nonselective agents act on alpha, beta$_1$, and beta$_2$ adrenergic receptors. Stimulation of the alpha receptors causes constriction of peripheral blood vessels and results in blood pressure elevation. Beta$_1$ receptors, which are predominantly located in cardiac tissue, increase heart rate and cardiac contractility when stimulated. Stimulation of the beta$_2$ receptors results in bronchodilation by relaxation of bronchial smooth muscle. Racemic epinephrine is an example of a nonselective bronchodilator.

INHALATION DELIVERY OF MEDICATIONS

The delivery of beta$_2$-specific medications can be accomplished by **nebulization,** parenteral administration, and oral administration. A nebulizer is an instrument that converts a liquid medication into a fine mist to be inhaled. A pneumatic nebulizer uses a gas as the driving force to make this conversion. Ultrasonic nebulizers use ultrasonic sound to convert the liquid medication to an inhalable mist. A **metered-dose inhaler (MDI)** is a pressurized medication chamber that delivers the medication by a propellant spray. By far the most common and most effective method of administration in an acute situation is nebulization. The goal of nebulization is to deliver small particles of the medication directly to the receptor sites in the lung by inhalation. To achieve this goal, many variables must be addressed. First, particle size of the nebulized medication is of critical importance. Medication particles that are too large are deposited in the oral pharynx or upper airway, and the medication never makes its way to the lung. Conversely, if the particles of medication are too small, they become suspended in the source gas, inhaled, and exhaled again—without depositing the medication at the target site.

The mechanics of delivering inhaled medications can be accomplished in two basic ways: the MDI and the pneumatically powered nebulizer.

NEBULIZATION THERAPY

Equipment Needed:
Nebulizer unit, tubing, oxygen source, medication
Procedure:
1. Observe universal precautions.
2. Verify drug order.

3. Confirm right patient, right medication, right dose, right route, and right time.
4. When possible, explain to the patient what medication you are going to administer and why.
5. Prepare all necessary equipment and the medication to be administered.
6. Expose the medication cup by unscrewing the lid. Add the medication to the cup, and reattach the lid.
7. Attach the mouthpiece and the tubing to the nebulizer.
8. Connect the oxygen-connecting hose to the appropriate connector on the nebulizer cup.
9. Attach the other end of the oxygen tubing to an oxygen source, and adjust the flow of oxygen to 6 L/min. A mist should come out of the mouthpiece.
10. Instruct the patient to hold the nebulizer mouthpiece in his or her mouth and breathe as deeply as possible. This process should be continued until the liquid has been used up.
11. Monitor the patient throughout the treatment, and reassess ventilatory adequacy and vital signs after the treatment has been completed. Compare findings with the patient's pretreatment ventilatory adequacy.
12. Repeat the treatment if needed, and provide supplemental oxygen as needed.
13. Record the time of drug administration in the patient care record.
14. Evaluate the patient for desired effects of the medication, as well as any adverse effects. Continued reevaluation should occur throughout transport.

METERED DOSE INHALER

The MDI delivers a predetermined amount of mediation in the correct particle size propelled by a small amount of gas. The MDI unit comes with two parts: the canister and mouthpiece (Fig. 14-5).

Although they may look as simple as an ordinary spray can, MDIs are more complicated. Remember, particle size is critical. If an MDI is used improperly, the medication will not reach its intended site in the lung.

Imagine driving an automobile on a curvy mountain road. Experienced drivers know that when approaching a sharp curve they need to slow down to make the curve. If they do not, the car's excessive forward speed will create a momentum that cannot be overcome; the car will hit the guardrail and slide off the road.

A similar problem can be encountered with MDIs. Often the propellant in the MDI canister jettisons the medication particles at a rapid speed. The oropharynx, like the mountain road, has several rather sharp curves. If the medication particles move too rapidly, they cannot negotiate the curves of the oropharynx and slam into the walls of the oropharynx. The result is that the medication does not reach the intended site in the lung.

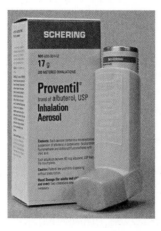

▼ **Fig. 14-5**   Metered dose inhaler. (From Stoy W, Platt T, Lejeune D, and Center for Emergency Medicine: *Mosby's EMT-basic textbook revised,* ed 2, St Louis, 2007, Mosby.)

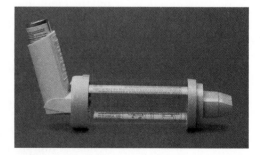

▼ **Fig. 14-6**   Metered dose inhaler with spacer. (From Henry M, Stapleton E: *EMT prehospital care,* ed 3 rev, St Louis, 2007, Mosby.)

The use of a **spacer device** can facilitate slower movement of the medication particles (Fig. 14-6). The spacer slows the forward movement of the medication particles. When a spacer device is not available, holding the MDI approximately 2 inches from the mouth also causes the particles to slow before entering the oropharynx, achieving an effect similar to that of the spacer device.

The development of MDIs has allowed patients to carry their rescue medications with them wherever they go. Many EMS systems use MDIs to care for acute bronchospasm; however, studies have shown that the particle deposition of the medications in patients with moderate to severe bronchospasm is not as effective as with use of a pneumatically powered nebulizer. This is primarily because the medication is delivered over a very short period (0.5 to 1 second), which means that higher flow rates of gas are required. Continuing with the example of driving on a mountain road, a large portion of the medication will not be able to negotiate the many sharp curves of the oropharynx. Much of the medication is deposited on the walls of the oropharynx, resulting in less medication reaching the intended target. If moderate to severe bronchospasm exists, the medication never fully reaches the target sites secondary to the bronchospasm itself. When a nebulizer is used, the flow rate of the medication is slower; therefore more of the medication is able to reach the target receptors in the lung.

METERED DOSE INHALER

Equipment Needed:
MDI with medication, PPE
Procedure:
1. Observe universal precautions.
2. Verify drug order.
3. Confirm right patient, right medication, right dose, right route, and right time.
4. Confirm with the patient that he or she has no allergies to the medication, and document allergies to any other medication.
5. When possible, explain to the patient what medication you are going to administer and why.
6. Shake the inhaler for 5 to 10 seconds.
7. Insert the outlet tube into the patient's mouth.
8. Direct the patient to squeeze the ends of the medication canister to deliver the medication.
9. Instruct the patient to inhale a slow, full, deep breath.
10. Instruct the patient to hold the breath for up to 5 seconds if possible.
11. Repeat if indicated.
12. Record the time of drug administration in the patient care record.
13. Evaluate the patient for desired effects of the medication, as well as any adverse effects. Continued reevaluation should occur throughout transport.

METERED DOSE INHALER WITH A SPACER

Equipment Needed:
MDI with medication, spacer, PPE
Procedure:
1. Observe universal precautions.
2. Verify drug order.
3. Confirm right patient, right medication, right dose, right route, and right time.
4. Confirm with the patient that he or she has no allergies to the medication, and document allergies to any other medication.
5. When possible, explain to the patient what medication you are going to administer and why.
6. Shake the inhaler for 5 to 10 seconds.
7. Insert the outlet tube into the spacer.

8. Instruct the patient to place the spacer device into his or her mouth and close the lips over it.
8. Direct the patient to squeeze the ends of the medication canister to deliver the medication.
9. Instruct the patient to inhale a slow, full, deep breath.
10. Instruct the patient to hold the breath for up to 10 seconds if possible.
11. Wait approximately 60 seconds and repeat.
12. Reassess breath sounds, vital signs, and ventilations.
12. Record the time of drug administration in the patient care record.
13. Evaluate the patient for desired effects of the medication, as well as any adverse effects. Continued reevaluation should occur throughout transport.

MDI canisters have no markings to specify the amount of medication remaining in an inhaler. The metal canister can be placed in a glass of water to help determine the amount of medication remaining. As the liquid portion of the contents (medication) is used, it is replaced by the expanding propellant gas. The more propellant gas in the inhaler, the more the inhaler will float. A full inhaler will sink to the bottom of the glass.

OVERVIEW OF ASTHMA

... You determine that the patient is having an asthma attack, likely initiated from exercise. He tells you that he has an inhaler in his gym bag, and you send the gym teacher to retrieve it. The teacher returns minutes later carrying the patient's inhaler. You inspect the label. The name on the label matches that of the patient, and the medication is albuterol. You ask the patient whether he needs your assistance to take the medication. He replies, "I think I need your help." You take the inhaler and shake it 10 times. You then tell the patient that you are going to administer the medication by MDI and instruct him to take a slow, deep breath and hold the breath for 5 seconds if he can. You administer the medication and repeat the process. The patient initially coughs after your administration of the MDI, but his respirations then begin to deepen and slow.

Although many consider asthma to be a relatively mild breathing condition that can be quickly alleviated, more than 4000 Americans die each year from asthma attacks according to the Centers for Disease Control and Prevention. Approximately 500,000 hospitalizations took place in 2002 for asthma, with 11.8 million lost work days and 14.7 million lost school days.[2]

Acute asthma attacks can affect patients of all ages. Asthma is caused by a trigger reaction. Triggers can be either **intrinsic** (within the body) or **extrinsic** (outside the body). Examples of intrinsic triggers include exertion, such as an attack triggered by exercise, and anxiety related to stress. Examples of external triggers are reactions to animal dander, dust, insect droppings, pollen, and cleaning chemicals.

MANAGEMENT

A main focus in management of asthma is for the patient to avoid the triggers that initiate attacks whenever possible and mitigate the effects of these triggers. When EMS is called, these goals have not been achieved and patient management is aimed at the reversal of acute bronchospasm. Although parenteral medications can be used to treat patients with asthma, the first line of medications is inhaled beta$_2$-specific drugs. If inhaled bronchodilators fail, IV medications are then administered to reduce bronchospasm and inflammation.

Albuterol (Proventil, Ventolin) is by far the most common inhaled drug used to treat reversible bronchospasm. Albuterol is one of several inhaled bronchodilators that have been developed to target only the beta$_2$ receptor. Prior beta$_2$ agonists had varying degrees of effect on alpha and beta$_1$ receptors, and stimulation of these sites may cause unwanted reactions in already compromised patients (Table 14-3). For example, stimulation of alpha receptors could cause unwanted vasoconstriction, and stimulation of beta₁ receptors could cause increased heart rate. As such, more time between treatments was required to compensate for the unwanted, predominantly beta₁, adverse effects.

The first-generation drugs had significant beta₁ effects along with beta₂ effects. Second-generation drugs were more beta₂ specific but would still increase heart rate and could not be given close together. Finally, third-generation medications predominantly targeted the beta₂ receptors. When given by inhalation and specifically targeting the smooth muscle in the airways, they had little or no systemic effect. Without these systemic effects, multiple and continuous treatments could be given for moderate to severe exacerbations.

Clinical trials have demonstrated that albuterol can be safely and effectively delivered by providers at the basic level.[2] Subsequent to these investigations, many states have adopted the practice of allowing basic-level providers to administer albuterol to symptomatic patients with chronic asthma.

Levalbuterol (Xopenex) is a purified form of albuterol. The early experience with this new form of albuterol is that it is as effective as albuterol in relief of symptoms and results in fewer undesirable side effects, such as tachycardia and tremors.

Ipratropium bromide (Atrovent) is used in more severe exacerbations of asthma or in cases in which the patient has a limited response to treatment with albuterol. Ipratropium bromide is not an adrenergic agent but is considered an anticholinergic. In more severe cases of bronchospasm, additional treatment with ipratropium bromide has provided greater symptomatic relief than albuterol used as a single agent. Adrenergic agents such as albuterol act more centrally in the bronchial tree, whereas cholinergic agents such as ipratropium are more effective in the peripheral airways. Adrenergic agents are more effective in asthma, whereas the peripheral action of ipratropium provides greater benefits in patients with COPD.

Albuterol/ipratropium (Combivent) is a combination product that takes advantage of the different mechanisms of action and anatomic sites of action of albuterol and ipratropium bromide to deliver both medications in a single preparation.

TABLE 14-3

Sympathomimetic Properties of Various Generations of Bronchodilators

	Alpha	Beta₁	Beta₂
Generation 1 (Isuprel)	+	+++++	+++++
Generation 2 (Bronkosol)	0	+++	++++
Generation 3 (Albuterol)	0	+	+++++
Epinephrine	++++	++++++	+++++

ALBUTEROL (PROVENTIL, VENTOLIN)

Classification: Bronchodilator, beta agonist
Action: Binds and stimulates beta₂ receptors, resulting in relaxation of bronchial smooth muscle.
Indications: Asthma, bronchitis with bronchospasm, and COPD.
Adverse Effects: Hyperglycemia, hypokalemia, palpitations, sinus tachycardia, anxiety, tremor, nausea/vomiting, throat irritation, dry mouth, hypertension, dyspepsia, insomnia, headache, epistaxis, paradoxical bronchospasm.
Contraindications: Angioedema, sensitivity to albuterol or levalbuterol. Use with caution in lactating patients, cardiovascular disorders, cardiac arrhythmias.

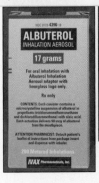
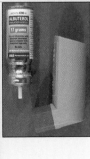

cont'd

ALBUTEROL (PROVENTIL, VENTOLIN)—CONT'D

Dosage:
Acute Bronchospasm:
- **Adult:**
  - **MDI:** 4 to 8 puffs every 1 to 4 hours may be required.
  - **Nebulizer:** 2.5 to 5 mg every 20 minutes for a maximum of three doses. After the initial three doses, escalate the dose or start a continuous nebulization at 10 to 15 mg/hr.
- **Pediatric:**
  - **MDI:**
    - **4 years and older:** 2 inhalations every 4 to 6 hours; however, in some patients, 1 inhalation every 4 hours is sufficient. More frequent administration or more inhalations are not recommended.
    - **Younger than 4 years:** Administer by nebulization.
  - **Nebulizer:**
    - **Older than 12 years:** The dose for a continuous nebulization is 0.5 mg/kg/hr.
    - **Younger than 12 years:** 0.15 mg/kg every 20 minutes for a maximum of three doses. Alternatively, continuous nebulization at 0.5 mg/kg/hr can be delivered to children younger than 12 years.

Asthma in Pregnancy:
- **MDI:** Two inhalations every 4 hours. In acute exacerbation, start with 2 to 4 puffs every 20 minutes.
- **Nebulizer:** 2.5 mg (0.5 mL) by 0.5% nebulization solution. Place 0.5 mL of the albuterol solution in 2.5 mL of sterile normal saline. Flow is regulated to deliver the therapy over a 5- to 20-minute period. In refractory cases, some physicians order 10 mg nebulized over a 60-minute period.

Special Considerations:
Pregnancy class C

LEVALBUTEROL (XOPENEX)

Classification: Beta agonist
Action: Stimulates beta$_2$ receptors, resulting in relaxation of the smooth muscle in the lungs, uterus, and vasculature that supply skeletal muscle.
Indications: Acute bronchospasm or bronchospasm prophylaxis in patient with asthma.
Adverse Effects: Hyperglycemia, hypokalemia, palpitations, sinus tachycardia, anxiety, tremor, nausea/vomiting, throat irritation, hypertension, dyspepsia, insomnia, headache.
Contraindications: Angioedema, sensitivity to albuterol or levalbuterol. Use with caution in lactating patients, cardiovascular disorders, cardiac arrhythmias. Do not use in patients taking phenothiazines because this may cause prolonged QT interval and cardiac arrhythmias. Also avoid use in patients getting sotalol

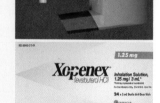

because they may decrease bronchodilating effects and cause bronchospasm, prolonged QT interval, and cardiac arrhythmias.
Dosage:
MDI:
- **Adult:** 2 inhalations every 4 to 6 hours. In some patients, 1 inhalation may be sufficient. For acute exacerbations, 4 to 8 inhalations every 20 minutes up to 4 hours, then every 1 to 4 hours as needed.
- **Pediatric:**
  - **4 to 12 years:** 2 inhalations every 4 to 6 hours. In some patients, 1 inhalation may be sufficient. For acute exacerbations, 2 to 4 inhalations every 20 minutes for 3 doses, then 2 to 4 inhalations every 1 to 4 hours as needed.
  - **Younger than 4 years:** Safe and effective use has not been established. For acute exacerbations, 2 to 4 inhalations holding a valved holding chamber and face mask every 20 minutes for 3 doses, then 2 to 4 inhalations every 1 to 4 hours as needed.
Nebulizer:
- **Adult:** Usually, 0.63 mg 3 times/day. For acute exacerbations, 1.25 to 2.5 mg every 20 minutes for 3 doses, then 1.25 to 5 mg every 1 to 4 hours as needed.

cont'd

LEVALBUTEROL (XOPENEX)—CONT'D

- **Pediatric:**
  - **6 to 11 years:** Usually, 0.31 mg 3 times/day. For acute exacerbations, 0.075 mg/kg (1.25 mg minimum) every 20 minutes for 3 doses, then 0.075 to 0.15 mg/kg (5 mg maximum) every 1 to 4 hours as needed.
  - **Younger than 6 years:** Safe and effective use has not been established. For acute exacerbations, 1.25 to 2.5 mg every 20 minutes for 3 doses, then 1.25 to 5 mg every 1 to 4 hours as needed.

Special Considerations:
Pregnancy class C

IPRATROPIUM BROMIDE (ATROVENT)

Classification: Bronchodilator, anticholinergic
Action: Antagonizes the acetylcholine receptor on bronchial smooth muscle, producing bronchodilation.
Indications: Asthma, bronchospasm associated with COPD.
Adverse Effects: Paradoxical acute bronchospasm, cough, throat irritation, headache, dizziness, dry mouth, palpitations.
Contraindications: Closed-angle glaucoma, bladder neck obstruction, prostatic hypertrophy, known sensitivity including peanuts or soybeans and atropine or atropine derivatives.

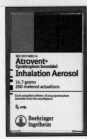 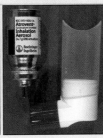

Dosage:
MDI:

- **Adult:** 4 inhalations every 10 minutes, with no more than 24 inhalations per day or closer than 4 hours apart.
- **Pediatric:**
  - **Older than 12 years:** 2 to 3 puffs inhaled every 6 to 8 hours. Maximum of 12 puffs/day.
  - **5 to 12 years:** 1 to 2 puffs inhaled every 6 to 8 hours. Maximum of 8 puffs/day.

Nebulization:

- **Adult:** 0.5 mg every 6 to 8 hours.
- **Pediatric: 5 to 14 years:** 0.25 to 0.5 mg every 20 minutes for 3 doses as needed.

Special Considerations:
Ipratropium bromide is not typically used as a sole medication in the treatment of acute exacerbation of asthma. Ipratropium bromide is commonly administered after a beta agonist.
Care should be taken to not allow the aerosol spray (especially in the MDI) to come into contact with the eyes. This can cause temporary blurring of vision that resolves without intervention within 4 hours.
Pregnancy class B

ALBUTEROL/IPRATROPIUM (COMBIVENT)

Classification: Combination bronchodilator
Action: Binds and stimulates beta$_2$ receptors, resulting in relaxation of bronchial smooth muscle, and antagonizes the acetylcholine receptor, producing bronchodilation.
Indications: Second-line treatment (if bronchodilator is ineffective) in COPD or severe acute asthma exacerbations during medical transport.
Adverse Effects: Headache, cough, nausea, arrhythmias, paradoxical acute bronchospasm.
Contraindications: Allergy to soybeans or peanuts; known sensitivity to atropine, albuterol, or their respective derivatives. Used with caution in patients with asthma, hypertension, angina, cardiac arrhythmias, tachycardia, cardiovascular disease, congenital long QT syndrome, closed-angle glaucoma.

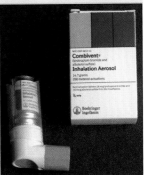

cont'd

ALBUTEROL/IPRATROPIUM (COMBIVENT)—CONT'D

Dosage:
- **Adult:** 2 puffs inhaled every 6 hours by MDI, with a maximum daily dose of 12 puffs/day.
- **Pediatric:** Not recommended for pediatric patients.

Special Considerations:
Pregnancy class C

Second-Line Therapy for Acute Exacerbation of Asthma

The clinical picture of a patient having an asthma attack or exacerbation of COPD is that of a patient gasping for breath, using accessory muscles of respiration, and wheezing. In asthma and COPD, bronchodilators provide symptomatic therapy but do not directly treat the underlying and initiating lung condition. In cases in which a prolonged transport time is likely, consider corticosteroids to treat the inflammatory processes involved in both asthma and COPD. The most commonly used corticosteroids are methylprednisolone and hydrocortisone.

Peak expiratory flow rate (PEFR) is an objective assessment that can guide a provider's determination of the severity of an exacerbation; the patient's response to therapy; and the indication for therapy, such as the start of steroids. When the initial PEFR is less than 50% of predicted, corticosteroids should be administered after ipratropium bromide administration. Corticosteroids should also be considered when the PEFR does not improve by at least 10% after bronchodilator therapy or when the PEFR is less than 70% after 1 hour of therapy.

Aminophylline and its derivatives work to reduce the smooth muscle bronchospasm associated with acute respiratory distress. Aminophylline is an effective drug that can reach therapeutic levels very quickly; however, if that therapeutic level is exceeded, even by a modest amount, unwanted side effects can develop. When a fine margin exists between effectiveness and toxicity, a drug is known to have a narrow **therapeutic index.** Aminophylline's narrow therapeutic index is one reason why this drug is used with less frequency than in years past.

Aminophylline is begun by administering a loading dose to place serum levels in the therapeutic range. Because this drug is rapidly metabolized, a maintenance infusion is required to keep it at a therapeutic level. Care must be taken in patients with renal or hepatic dysfunction because their excretion can be impaired, thus causing excessively dangerous levels to develop. Smoking or chewing tobacco increases the rate of removal of aminophylline from the body, so a higher dose is required. For these reasons, aminophylline is not commonly used in the prehospital field.

Magnesium sulfate has been demonstrated to decrease bronchospasm in a subset of asthmatic patients. Patients who do not show an adequate response to beta$_2$ agonist medications can have a favorable response to magnesium sulfate. Magnesium sulfate should not be used in all patients having an asthmatic attack; however, consider using magnesium in patients who do not improve after beta agonist therapy.

For years, epinephrine administered subcutaneously was the treatment of choice for young patients with asthma. Epinephrine does have strong and desirable beta$_2$ effects; however, it also has strong and undesirable alpha and beta$_1$ effects. Rebound bronchospasm can be a secondary problem with the administration of epinephrine in the management of an asthma attack. Although epinephrine is effective when initially administered, its effects are short lived. If considering epinephrine for use in adults with asthma, do not underestimate beta$_1$-mediated cardiac complications such as tachycardia and hypertension. For these reasons, epinephrine should be used with caution, if at all, in the treatment of the patient with asthma.

METHYLPREDNISOLONE SODIUM SUCCINATE (SOLU-MEDROL)

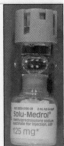

Classification: Corticosteroid
Action: Reduces inflammation by multiple mechanisms.
Indications: Anaphylaxis, asthma, COPD.
Adverse Effects: Depression, euphoria, headache, restlessness, hypertension, bradycardia, nausea/vomiting, swelling, diarrhea, weakness, fluid retention, paresthesias.
Contraindications: Cushing's syndrome, fungal infection, measles, varicella, known sensitivity (including sulfites). Use with caution in active infections, renal disease, penetrating spinal cord injury, hypertension, seizures, CHF.
Dosage:
Asthma and Chronic Obstructive Pulmonary Disease:
- **Adult:** 40 to 80 mg IV.
- **Pediatric:** 1 mg/kg (up to 60 mg) IV, IO per day in two divided doses.

Anaphylactic Shock:
- **Adult:** 1 to 2 mg/kg/dose, then 0.5 to 1 mg/kg every 6 hours.
- **Pediatric:** Same as adult dosing.

Blunt Spinal Cord Injury:
- **Adult:** 30 mg/kg IV, IO over a period of 1 hour, then as an infusion to run for the remaining 23 hours at a dose of 5.4 mg/kg/hr.
- **Pediatric:** Same as adult dosing.

Special Considerations:
May mask signs and symptoms of infection.
Pregnancy class C

HYDROCORTISONE SODIUM SUCCINATE (CORTEF, SOLU-CORTEF)

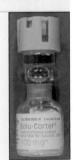

Classification: Corticosteroid
Action: Reduces inflammation by multiple mechanisms. As a steroid, it replaces the steroids that are lacking in adrenal insufficiency.
Indications: Adrenal insufficiency, allergic reactions, anaphylaxis, asthma, COPD.
Adverse Effects: Leukocytosis, hyperglycemia, increased infection, decreased wound healing, increased rate of death from sepsis.
Contraindications: Cushing's syndrome, known sensitivity to benzyl alcohol. Use with caution in diabetes, hypertension, CHF, known systemic fungal infection, renal disease, idiopathic thrombocytopenia, psychosis, seizure disorder, GI disease, glaucoma, known sensitivity.
Dosage:
Anaphylactic Shock:
- **Adult:** 100 to 500 mg IV, IO, or IM.
- **Pediatric:** 2 to 4 mg/kg/day IV, IO, or IM (max: 500 mg).

Adrenal Insufficiency:
- **Adult:** 100 to 500 mg IV, IO, or IM.
- **Pediatric:** 1 to 2 mg/kg IV, IO, or IM.

Asthma and Chronic Obstructive Pulmonary Disease:
- **Adult:** 100 to 500 mg IV, IO, IM.
- **Pediatric:** 1 mg/kg IV, IO. The dose may be reduced for infants and children, but it is governed more by the severity of the condition and response of the patient than by age or body weight. Dose should not be less than 25 mg daily.

Special Considerations:
Pregnancy class C

AMINOPHYLLINE

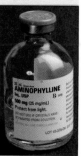

Classification: Bronchodilator
Action: Relaxes the smooth muscle of the bronchial airways and pulmonary blood vessels. May also have antiinflammatory properties.
Indications: Bronchospasm
Adverse Effects: Seizures, cardiac arrest, arrhythmias, nausea/vomiting, abdominal pain or cramping, headache, tachycardia, palpitations, anxiety, ventricular arrhythmias.
Contraindications: Known sensitivity. Use with caution in liver disease, kidney disease, seizures, cardiac arrhythmias.
Dosage: A loading dose is first administered, followed by an infusion.
· **Adult:** Load with 5 mg/kg IV, IO slowly over a 20- to 30-minute period, followed by an infusion. An infusion rate of 0.4 mg/kg/hr is effective for a nonsmoker, but a patient who smokes can require a high infusion rate at 0.8 mg/kg/hr IV, IO. When treating patients with CHF, reduce the dose to 0.2 mg/kg/hr.
· **Pediatric:** Load with 5 mg/kg slow IV, IO over a 20-minute period.
  · **Older than 12 years:** 0.4 mg/kg/hr IV, IO.
  · **10 to 12 years:** 0.7 mg/kg/hr IV, IO.
  · **1 to 9 years:** 0.8 to 1 mg/kg/hr IV, IO.
  · **6 months to 1 year:** 0.6 to 0.7 mg/kg/hr IV, IO.
  · **6 to 24 weeks:** 0.5 mg/kg/hr IV, IO.
Special Considerations:
Pregnancy class C

MAGNESIUM SULFATE

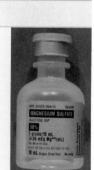

Classification: Electrolyte, tocolytic, mineral
Action: Required for normal physiologic functioning. Magnesium is a cofactor in neurochemical transmission and muscular excitability. Magnesium sulfate controls seizures by blocking peripheral neuromuscular transmission. Magnesium is also a peripheral vasodilator and an inhibitor of platelet function.
Indications: Torsades de pointes, cardiac arrhythmias associated with hypomagnesemia, eclampsia and seizure prophylaxis in preeclampsia, status asthmaticus.
Adverse Effects: Magnesium toxicity (signs include flushing, diaphoresis, hypotension, muscle paralysis, weakness, hypothermia, and cardiac, CNS, or respiratory depression).
Contraindications: AV block, GI obstruction. Use with caution in renal impairment.
Dosage:
Pulseless Ventricular Fibrillation/Ventricular Tachycardia with Torsades de Pointes or Hypomagnesemia:
· **Adult:** 1 to 2 g in 10 mL D_5W IV, IO administered over 5 to 10 minutes.
· **Pediatric:** 25 to 50 mg/kg IV, IO over 10 to 20 minutes; may administer faster for torsades de pointes (max single dose: 2 g).
Torsades de Pointes with a Pulse or Cardiac Arrhythmias with Hypomagnesemia:
· **Adult:** 1 to 2 g in 50 to 100 mL D_5W IV, IO administered over 5 to 60 minutes. Follow with 0.5 to 1 g/hr IV, IO titrated to control torsades de pointes.
· **Pediatric:** 25 to 50 mg/kg IV, IO over 10 to 20 minutes (max single dose: 2 g).
Eclampsia and Seizure Prophylaxis in Preeclampsia:
· **Adult:** 4 to 6 g IV, IO over 20 to 30 minutes, followed by an infusion of 1 to 2 g/hr.
Status Asthmaticus:
· **Adult:** 1.2 to 2 g slow IV, IO (over 20 minutes).
· **Pediatric:** 25 to 50 mg/kg (diluted in D_5W) slow IV, IO (over 10 to 20 minutes).
Special Considerations:
Pregnancy class A

RACEMIC EPINEPHRINE/RACEPINEPHRINE (MICRONEFRIN, S₂)

Classification: Bronchodilator, adrenergic agent
Action: Stimulates both alpha and beta receptors, causing vasoconstriction, reduced mucosal edema, and bronchodilation.
Indications: Bronchial asthma, croup.
Adverse Effects: Anxiety, dizziness, headache, tremor, palpitations, tachycardia, cardiac arrhythmias, hypertension, nausea/vomiting.
Contraindications: Glaucoma, elderly, cardiac disease, hypertension, thyroid disease, diabetes, known sensitivity to sulfites.
Dosage:
· **Adult:** Add 0.5 mL to nebulizer; for hand-bulb nebulizer, administer 1 to 3 inhalations; for jet nebulizer, add 3 mL of diluent, swirl the nebulizer and administer for 15 minutes.
· **Pediatric:**
  · **Older than 4 years:** Same as adult dosing.
  · **Younger than 4 years:** Safe and effective use has not been demonstrated.
Special Considerations:
Monitor blood pressure, heart rate, and cardiac rhythm for changes.
Onset of action is 1 to 5 minutes.
Pregnancy class C

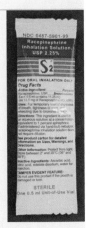

CHRONIC OBSTRUCTIVE PULMONARY DISEASE

COPD is the classification for diseases that cause obstruction in the pulmonary tree. The two most common diseases are emphysema and chronic bronchitis. Both pathologic conditions cause an increase in sputum production and resultant bronchospasm. As the increase in sputum worsens, so can the irritation and the bronchospasm. Initial treatment of mild to moderate COPD exacerbation is aimed at reducing bronchospasm and mobilizing and clearing the sputum from the airways.

MANAGEMENT

In severe exacerbations, treatment is first aimed at oxygenation and ventilation of the patient. Oxygenation needs to be provided with care. Patients with a long-standing history of COPD breathe on what is known as a **hypoxic respiratory drive.** This means that the patient requires a mild degree of hypoxia to continue breathing. If the patient is given too much oxygen, the hypoxic respiratory drive is removed, as well as the patient's stimulus for spontaneous respirations. Therefore, when monitoring these patients, an SaO_2 in the low 90s as measured by pulse oximetry is considered adequate.

Bronchodilators and steroids are used to manage COPD in a similar fashion as for the treatment of asthma. A detailed discussion of the treatment of pulmonary edema is found in Chapter 10.

REVIEW QUESTIONS

1. Explain how FiO_2 is related to the amount of oxygen delivered to the heart and tissues.
2. Explain the difference between a rebreather face mask and a nonrebreather face mask.
3. What class of drugs typically is used in the treatment of bronchospasm, and on what receptors do these drugs act?
4. What are two methods of delivering medications directly to the respiratory bronchioles?
5. What occurs when the particle size of a nebulized medication is too small or too large?
6. What is the purpose of using a spacer device with an MDI?
7. What is the main goal in the management of a patient with asthma?

8. What does it mean when a drug has a narrow therapeutic index?
9. Explain the concept of hypoxic respiratory drive in patients with COPD.

REFERENCES

1. National Center for Health Care Statistics: Asthma prevalence, health care use and mortality, 2002. In *Morbidity and mortality: 2004 chart book on cardiovascular, lung, and blood diseases,* Bethesda, Md, 2004, National Institutes of Health.
2. Centers for Disease Control and Prevention: *National Asthma Survey 2003,* Hyattsville, Md, 2003, US Department of Health and Human Services.

BIBLIOGRAPHY

Greenstone I, et al: Combination of inhaled long-acting beta$_2$-agonists and inhaled steroids versus higher dose of inhaled steroids in children and adults with persistent asthma, *Cochrane Database Syst Rev* 2005.

Murphy S, Sheffer AL, Pauwels RA: *National Asthma Education and Prevention Program: highlights of the expert panel report II: guidelines for the diagnosis and management of asthma,* Bethesda, Md, 1997, National Heart, Lung, and Blood Institute.

Nelson HS: Adrenergic bronchodilators, *N Engl J Med* 333:499, 1995.

Plotnick LH, Ducharme FM: Combined inhaled anticholinergic agents and beta-2-agonists for initial treatment of acute asthma in children, *Cochrane Database Syst Rev* CD000060, 2000.

Rodrigo GJ, Rodrigo C: The role of anticholinergics in acute asthma treatment: an evidence-based evaluation, *Chest* 121:1977, 2002.

Senthilselvan A, et al: Regular use of corticosteroids and low use of short-acting beta$_2$-agonists can reduce asthma hospitalization, *Chest* 127:1242, 2005.

Stoodley RG, Aaron SD, Dales RE: The role of ipratropium bromide in the emergency management of acute asthma exacerbation: a metaanalysis of randomized clinical trials, *Ann Emerg Med* 34:8, 1999.

Seizures

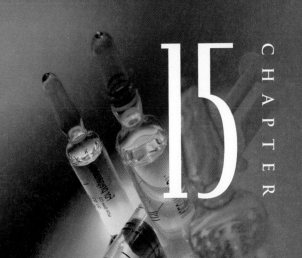

OBJECTIVES

1. Demonstrate the proper procedure for rectal administration of diazepam, and discuss why rectal administration is sometimes necessary for a patient having a seizure.
2. Discuss benzodiazepines used in the treatment of seizures: diazepam (Valium) and lorazepam (Ativan).
3. Discuss other anticonvulsants (nonbenzodiazepines) used in the treatment of seizures: phenytoin (Dilantin), carbamazepine (Tegretol), phenobarbital (Luminal), valproic acid (Depakote), gabapentin (Neurontin), and lamotrigine (Lamictal).

Medications that Appear in Chapter 15

Diazepam (Valium)
Lorazepam (Ativan)
Felbamate (Felbatol)
Phenytoin (Dilantin)
Fosphenytoin (Cerebyx)
Carbamazepine (Tegretol)
Phenobarbital (Luminal)
Valproic acid (Depakote)
Gabapentin (Neurontin)
Lamotrigine (Lamictal)

INTRODUCTION

Seizure activity is a common emergency that requires prompt management by prehospital professionals. Although most seizures stop without treatment, if a paramedic arrives on the scene of a patient in active seizure, the patient is likely to be in **status epilepticus.**[1] Status epilepticus is defined as continuous seizure activity for longer than 30 minutes or a series of seizures without full recovery of consciousness between seizures. Status epilepticus affects approximately 60,000 people in the United States each year, with the majority being children.[2] An estimated 10% of EMS calls involving children are for seizures.[3] Because prolonged seizure activity can lead to brain damage and poor functional status, one of the most important determinants of outcome is duration of seizure activity. Paramedics must know how to manage seizures.[4,5] Seizure activity is the result of chaotic, abnormal, high-

You receive a call that a 13-year-old boy was found to be unresponsive by his mother at home. According to the mother, the child has had seizures in the past but they have been controlled for the last 12 years with medication. On arrival, the boy is lying supine on the floor and making tonic-clonic, jerking movements. His eyes are rolled back in his head, and he does not respond to stimulation. His pants are wet and you smell urine. ...

frequency firing of neurons, which can cause an alteration in level of consciousness. On examination, patients having a seizure can display jerking movements referred to as **tonic-clonic seizures.** These patients often have an altered mental status, abnormal eye movement, and incontinence of bowel or bladder.

MANAGEMENT

The initial management of seizure activity in both children and adults hinges on maintaining an adequate airway and providing supplemental oxygen, as well as continually assessing that the patient is breathing adequately. Additionally, paramedics should take action to protect the patient from injury by removing the patient from an environment in which he or she is at risk for injury during convulsions. Once a patent airway has been established and adequate oxygenation and ventilation are ensured, the paramedic should attempt to secure venous access for the administration of medication to stop seizure activity.[6]

In this scenario, the initial management of this patient in the midst of active seizure activity includes turning the patient on his side to clear the airway. The next steps would be to quickly ensure that the patient is breathing adequately, administer supplemental oxygen, and obtain an initial set of vital signs. Finally, while attempting to secure vascular access to treat the seizure with IV diazepam (Valium), the provider should take a brief history from the mother to identify any significant medical history, such as diabetes with hypoglycemia; previous seizure history; known medications, including **anticonvulsants;** possible intoxicants; and recreational drugs. The management of hypoglycemia, which is a common cause of seizures, is addressed in Chapter 11.

BENZODIAZEPINES

The mainstay of management for seizure activity and status epilepticus is the administration of anticonvulsant agents. The most common class of agents used in the initial management of seizure activity, particularly in the prehospital setting, are the benzodiazepines.[7] Benzodiazepines are used as the initial class of drugs to stop seizure activity because their principal pharmacologic effects are mitigated through **gamma-aminobutyric acid (GABA),** an inhibitory neurotransmitter in the central nervous system.[8] The concept of a receptor was introduced in Chapter 1. GABA is a type of receptor in the central nervous system. When a drug such as a benzodiazepine binds with the GABA receptor, the result is inhibition or a decrease in the activity of the central nervous system. The inhibition of the nervous system is manifested as sedation or the cessation of seizures.

Two benzodiazepines commonly used to treat seizure activity are diazepam and lorazepam (Ativan). Although diazepam is considered first-line treatment, lorazepam has also been demonstrated to be safe and possibly more effective in the termination of status epilepticus when administered by appropriately trained prehospital professionals.[7]

Midazolam (Versed) can also be used to stop an active seizure, but its usefulness is limited by its short half-life. Patients can have subsequent seizures shortly after the initial dosing of midazolam, which makes this drug a poor choice when treating seizures.

The short half-life of midazolam makes this drug a poor choice when treating seizures.

Starting an IV in a patient who is actively seizing is a difficult task. Administration of diazepam rectally allows easy access to obtain a rapid blood level of this medication.

RECTAL ADMINISTRATION OF DIAZEPAM

Equipment Needed:
Two 3-mL syringes, 5F feeding tube, saline flush, water-soluble lubricant
Procedure:

1. Observe universal precautions.
2. Verify drug order.
3. Confirm right patient, right medication, right dose, right route, and right time.
4. Confirm with the patient that he or she has no allergies to the medication, and document allergies to any other medication.
5. When possible, explain to the patient what medication you are going to administer and why.
6. Draw the desired dose of the medication into a 3-mL syringe.
7. Attach a 5F feeding tube to the 3-mL syringe.
8. Into a second 3-mL syringe, draw 1 mL of normal saline to be used as a flush.
9. Ensure that the airway is controlled and patent.
10. Place the patient on his or her side with knees bent toward the chest. Alternatively, with the patient in the supine position, have someone help spread the patient's legs.
11. Apply a water-soluble lubricant (e.g., K-Y Jelly, Johnson & Johnson, New Brunswick, NJ) to the tip of the catheter.
12. Introduce the lubricated catheter into the rectum and advance approximately 1 inch.
13. Inject the diazepam through the catheter, and then flush the feeding catheter with the saline flush.
14. Withdraw the catheter and dispose of it properly.
15. Record the time of drug administration in the patient care record.
16. Evaluate the patient for desired effects of the medication, as well as any adverse effects. Continued reevaluation should occur throughout transport.

DIAZEPAM (VALIUM)

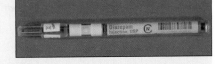

Classification: Benzodiazepine; Schedule C-IV
Action: Binds to the benzodiazepine receptor and enhances the effects of GABA. Benzodiazepines act at the level of the limbic, thalamic, and hypothalamic regions of the CNS and can produce any level of CNS depression required (including sedation, skeletal muscle relaxation, and anticonvulsant activity).
Indications: Anxiety, skeletal muscle relaxation, alcohol withdrawal, seizures.
Adverse Effects: Respiratory depression, drowsiness, fatigue, headache, pain at the injection site, confusion, nausea, hypotension, oversedation.
Contraindications: Children younger than 6 months, acute-angle glaucoma, CNS depression, alcohol intoxication, known sensitivity.
Dosage:
Anxiety:
  · **Adult:**
    · **Moderate:** 2 to 5 mg slow IV, IM.
    · **Severe:** 5 to 10 mg slow IV, IM (administer no faster than 5 mg/min).
    · **Low:** Low dosages are often required for elderly or debilitated patients.
  · **Pediatric:** 0.04 to 0.3 mg/kg/dose IV, IM every 4 hours to a maximum dose of 0.6 mg/kg.
Delirium Tremens from Acute Alcohol Withdrawal:
  · **Adult:** 10 mg IV
Seizure:
  · **Adult:** 5 to 10 mg slow IV, IO every 10 to 15 minutes; maximum total dose 30 mg.
  · **Pediatric:**
    · **IV, IO:**
      · **5 years and older:** 1 mg over a 3-minute period every 2 to 5 minutes to a maximum total dose of 10 mg.

cont'd

DIAZEPAM (VALIUM)—CONT'D

- **Older than 30 days to younger than 5 years:** 0.2 to 0.5 mg over a 3-minute period; may repeat every 2 to 5 minutes to a maximum total dose of 5 mg.
- **Neonate:** 0.1 to 0.3 mg/kg/dose given over a 3- to 5-minute period; may repeat every 15 to 30 minutes to a maximum total dose of 2 mg. (Not a first-line agent due to sodium benzoic acid in the injection.)
- **Rectal administration:** If vascular access is not obtained, diazepam may be administered rectally to children.
  - **12 years and older:** 0.2 mg/kg.
  - **6 to 11 years:** 0.3 mg/kg.
  - **2 to 5 years:** 0.5 mg/kg.
  - **Younger than 2 years:** Not recommended.

Special Considerations:
Make sure that IV, IO lines are well secured. Extravasation of diazepam causes tissue necrosis. Diazepam is insoluble in water and must be dissolved in propylene glycol. This produces a viscous solution; give slowly to prevent pain on injection.
Pregnancy class D

LORAZEPAM (ATIVAN)

Classification: Benzodiazepine; Schedule C-IV
Action: Binds to the benzodiazepine receptor and enhances the effects of the brain chemical GABA, an inhibitory transmitter, and may result in a state of sedation, hypnosis, skeletal muscle relaxation, anticonvulsant activity, coma.
Indications: Preprocedure sedation induction, anxiety, status epilepticus.
Adverse Effects: Headache, drowsiness, ataxia, dizziness, amnesia, depression, dysarthria, euphoria, syncope, fatigue, tremor, vertigo, respiratory depression, paradoxical CNS stimulation.
Contraindications: Known sensitivity to lorazepam, benzodiazepines, polyethylene glycol, propylene glycol, or benzyl alcohol; COPD; sleep apnea (except while being mechanically ventilated); shock; coma; acute closed-angle glaucoma.
Dosage: Note: IV, IO lorazepam needs to be administered slowly.
Analgesia and Sedation:
- **Adult:** 2 mg or 0.44 mg/kg IV, IO, whichever is smaller. This dosage will provide adequate sedation in most patients and should not be exceeded in patients older than 50 years.
- **Pediatric:** 0.05 mg/kg IV, IO. Each dose should not exceed 2 mg IV, IO.
Seizures:
- **Adult:** 4 mg IV, IO given over 2 to 5 minutes; may repeat in 10 to 15 minutes (max total dose: 8 mg in a 12-hour period).
- **Pediatric:**
  - **Adolescents:** 0.07 mg/kg slow IV, IO given over 2 to 5 minutes (max single dose: 4 mg). May repeat in 10 to 15 minutes (max dose: 8 mg in a 12-hour period).
  - **Children and infants:** 0.1 mg/kg slow IV, IO given over 2 to 5 minutes (max single dose: 4 mg). May repeat at half the original dose in 10 to 15 minutes if seizure activity resumes.
  - **Neonates:** 0.05 mg/kg slow IV, IO given over 2 to 5 minutes. May repeat in 10 to 15 minutes.

Special Considerations:
Be prepared to support the patient's airway and ventilation.
Pregnancy class D

... The patient's mother states that he has had seizures since he was quite young and they have been difficult to control. He has been on several medications since his seizures began. Two weeks ago, his neurologist started him on felbamate and valproic acid. The patient slowly begins to awaken and seems confused. You are able to get a set of baseline vitals and start a peripheral IV line. As you get the patient moved to the cot, he begins to have another seizure. Your partner protects the boy's head and airway while you administer diazepam 5 mg IV. The patient's seizures stop. You speak with medical direction about the boy's medical history and medications. They recommend transporting without loading with phenytoin because he is already taking felbamate and valproic acid. The remainder of the transport is without any additional events.

OTHER ANTICONVULSANTS

One major reason patients develop recurrent seizures is failure to achieve an appropriate blood plasma concentration with their prescribed medication(s). Often this is attributable to noncompliance on the part of patients in adhering to their medical regimen. For this reason, paramedics must acquire a medication history and be familiar with common anticonvulsant medications, including common adverse reactions, even though they may not administer them.

> A common cause of seizures is a patient's noncompliance with his or her prescribed medications.

Phenytoin (Dilantin) is an anticonvulsant used to control partial and generalized seizures. As with many anticonvulsant medications, drug levels are monitored to ensure that patients remain within a therapeutic range to control seizures while minimizing side effects. Because phenytoin produces some adverse effects when administered to patients, **prodrug** preparations of phenytoin can be administered. A prodrug is an inactive or less-active form of a drug that, once administered, is converted to the body in the active form of a drug. Prodrugs often have fewer adverse effects than the drug to which they are eventually converted. For example, a prodrug preparation of phenytoin is fosphenytoin (Cerebyx), which is converted to phenytoin after administration. The advantage of fosphenytoin in emergency situations is that the drug can be administered at a more rapid rate than phenytoin. Fosphenytoin can be given either IV or IM.[9,10]

Carbamazepine (Tegretol) is used to treat partial and generalized tonic-clonic seizures. Its action on the brain is similar to that of many of the other anticonvulsants in that it stabilizes the nerve membranes to decrease abnormal nerve cell firing.[11]

Phenobarbital (Luminal) belongs to the class of anticonvulsants referred to as *barbiturates*. Phenobarbital is considered a second-line therapy because of the troublesome side effects it causes, such as sedation, depression, and agitation. As with phenytoin, the liver metabolizes phenobarbital, where it induces some of the hepatic enzymes that can cause accelerated metabolism of several other medications.[12,13]

Valproic acid (Depakote) is another drug commonly used to treat seizures, as well as mood disorders. Although generally well tolerated, valproic acid does require regular monitoring of blood levels to ensure maintenance of therapeutic levels and minimize adverse drug reactions.

FELBAMATE (FELBATOL)

Classification: Anticonvulsant
Action: Although the mechanism of action is not known, it is believed that felbamate antagonizes the effects of glycine, increases the seizure threshold in absence seizures, and prevents the spread of generalized tonic-clonic and partial seizures.

Indications: Partial seizures with and without generalization in epileptic adults; partial and generalized seizures associated with Lennox-Gastaut syndrome in children.
Adverse Effects: Nausea/vomiting, suicidal ideation and behavior, depression, insomnia, dyspepsia, upper respiratory tract infection, fatigue, headache, constipation, diarrhea, rhinitis, anxiety, aplastic anemia, photosensitivity.
Contraindications: Blood dyscrasias, hepatic disease, known sensitivity to carbomates.
Dosage: Should be individualized based on condition.
Special Considerations:
Pregnancy class C

PHENYTOIN (DILANTIN)

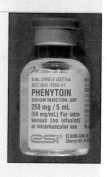

Classification: Anticonvulsant

Action: Depresses seizures by affecting the movement of sodium and calcium into neural tissue.

Indications: Generalized tonic-clonic seizures.

Adverse Effects: Nausea/vomiting, depression of cardiac conduction, sedation, nystagmus, tremors, ataxia, dysarthria, gingival hypertrophy, hirsutism, facial coarsening, hypotension.

Contraindications: Sinus bradycardia, sinoatrial block, second- and third-degree heart block, Adams-Stokes syndrome, known sensitivity to hydantoins.

Dosage:
- **Adult:** 15 to 20 mg/kg IV, IO should be administered slowly at a rate not exceeding 50 mg/min. (This requires approximately 20 minutes in a 70-kg patient.)
- **Pediatric:** 15 to 20 mg/kg IV, IO, administered at a rate of 1 to 3 mg/kg/min.

Special Considerations:
Continuously monitor the ECG and blood pressure during administration.
Pregnancy class D

FOSPHENYTOIN (CEREBYX)

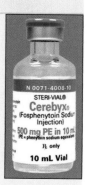

Classification: Anticonvulsant

Action: Alters the movement of sodium and calcium into nervous tissue and prevents the spread of seizure activity.

Indications: Partial and generalized seizures, status epilepticus, seizure prophylaxis.

Adverse Effects: Phenytoin can cause several adverse effects often related to drug dose, including sedation, nystagmus, tremors, ataxia, dysarthria, gingival hypertrophy, hirsutism, and facial coarsening. Too-rapid administration can cause hypotension.

Contraindications:

Bradycardia, bundle branch blocks, agranulocytosis, Adams-Stokes syndrome, hydantoin hypersensitivity.

Dosage: The dose and concentration of fosphenytoin is expressed in PE to simplify the conversion between phenytoin and fosphenytoin.
- **Adult:** The usual loading dose of fosphenytoin is 15 to 20 mg PE/kg IV, not to exceed 150 mg PE/min IV rate.
- **Pediatric:** The usual loading dose of fosphenytoin is 15 to 20 mg PE/kg IV, not to exceed 3 mg PE/kg/min (max dose: 150 mg PE/min) IV rate.

Special Considerations:
Pregnancy class D
Compatible with breast-feeding

CARBAMAZEPINE (TEGRETOL)

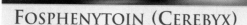

Classification: Anticonvulsant

Action: Decreases the spread of the seizure.

Indications: Partial and generalized tonic-clonic seizures.

Adverse Effects: Dizziness, drowsiness, ataxia, nausea/vomiting, blurred vision, confusion, headache, transient diplopia, visual hallucinations, life-threatening rashes.

Contraindications: AV block, bundle branch block, agranulocytosis, bone marrow suppression, MAOI therapy, hypersensitivity to carbamazepine or tricyclic antidepressants. Use with caution in petit mal, atonic, or myoclonic seizures; liver disease; patients with blood dyscrasia caused by drug therapies or blood disorders; patients with a history of cardiac disease; or patients with a history of alcoholism.

Dosage:
- **Adult:** 200 mg PO every 12 hours.
- **Pediatric:**
  - **6 to 11 years:** 100 mg PO twice daily.
  - **Younger than 6 years:** 10 to 20 mg/kg/day PO 2 or 3 times per day.

Special Considerations:
Pregnancy class D

PHENOBARBITAL (LUMINAL)

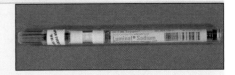

Classification: Anticonvulsant, barbiturate, Schedule C-IV

Action: Depresses seizure activity in the cortex, thalamus, and limbic system; increases threshold for electrical stimulation of motor cortex; produces state of sedation.

Indications: Seizures

Adverse Effects: Depression, agitation, respiratory depression, accelerated metabolism of several other medications.

Contraindications: Liver dysfunction, porphyria, agranulocytosis, known sensitivity to barbiturates. Use with caution with respiratory dysfunction.

Dosage:
· **Adult:** 15 to 18 mg/kg IV, IO; infuse at a rate not faster than 60 mg/min.
· **Pediatric:** 15 to 20 mg/kg IV, IO; infuse at a rate not faster than 2 mg/kg/min.

Special Considerations:
Be prepared to manage the patient's airway.
Pregnancy class D

VALPROIC ACID (DEPAKOTE)

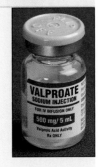

Classification: Anticonvulsant, antimanic

Action: Although the exact mechanism of action is unknown, it is suggested that valproic acid increases brain concentrations of GABA.

Indications: Seizures, mood disorders.

Adverse Effects: Tremor, transient hair loss, weight gain, weight loss.

Contraindications: Liver disease.

Dosage: Dosing is individualized.

Special Considerations:
Although generally well tolerated, valproic acid does require regular monitoring of blood levels to ensure maintenance of therapeutic levels while minimizing adverse drug reactions.
Pregnancy class D

In the past few years, several new anticonvulsants have been designed to manage seizures. Interestingly, these are the first new drugs approved since 1978, when valproic acid was approved for use.[14] As these drugs become more commonly used in patients with seizures that are difficult to control, paramedics will see them more frequently and therefore should have a general understanding of their potential side effects and toxicities. Two of these newer anticonvulsant agents are gabapentin (Neurontin) and lamotrigine (Lamictal).

Since gabapentin (Neurontin) was approved as an adjunctive medication for seizure disorders, it has become widely used for many other indications, as well. Unlike many of the other anticonvulsants, gabapentin is well absorbed orally. Gabapentin also has recently been approved for the treatment of many different neuropathic pain syndromes.[15] Gabapentin is useful for the treatment of pain because it acts on nerve cells to stabilize the cell membrane.

Lamotrigine (Lamictal) is another of the newer anticonvulsants recently approved for therapy for partial and generalized seizures.

GABAPENTIN (NEURONTIN)

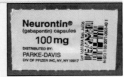

Classification: Anticonvulsant

Action: The exact mechanism of action has not been determined.

Indications: Seizures, neuropathic pain syndromes.

Adverse Effects: Dizziness, ataxia, sleepiness, gait disturbances, upset stomach.

Contraindications: Known sensitivity. Use with caution in elderly patients, renal impairment.

cont'd

GABAPENTIN (NEURONTIN)—CONT'D

Dosage:
- **Adult:** 300 to 1800 mg PO daily.
- **Pediatric:**
  - **5 to 12 years:** 25 to 35 mg/kg/day PO divided in three divided doses daily.
  - **3 to 4 years:** 40 mg/kg/day PO divided in three divided doses daily.

Special Considerations:
Pregnancy class C

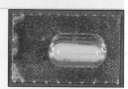

LAMOTRIGINE (LAMICTAL)

Classification: Anticonvulsant, antimanic agent
Action: The exact mechanism of action has not been determined. Studies suggest lamotrigine stabilizes neuronal membranes by acting at voltage-sensitive sodium channels, thereby decreasing presynaptic release of glutamate and aspartate, resulting in decreased seizure activity.
Indications: Seizures, bipolar disorders.
Adverse Effects: Headache, dizziness, nausea/vomiting, ataxia, diplopia.
Contraindications: Known sensitivity.
Dosage:
- **Adult:** Medication is administered orally. Dosage is individualized.
- **Pediatric:** Medication is administered orally. Dosage is individualized.

Special Considerations:
Pregnancy class C

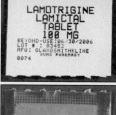
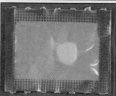

REVIEW QUESTIONS

1. Define status epilepticus.
2. Why would rectal administration of a medication be necessary in a patient having a seizure?
3. What class of drugs is used in the initial management of seizures?
4. What eye condition is a contraindication for administration of benzodiazepines?
5. Explain a prodrug and give an example.

REFERENCES

1. Rainbow J, Browne GJ, Lam LT: Controlling seizures in the prehospital setting: diazepam or midazolam? *J Paediatr Child Health* 38:582, 2002.
2. Alldredge BK, Wall DB: Effect of prehospital treatment on the outcome of status epilepticus in children, *Pediatr Neurol* 13:213, 1995.
3. Galustyan SG, et al: The short-term outcome of seizure management by prehospital personnel: a comparison of two protocols, *Pediatr Emerg Care* 19:221, 2003.
4. Karasalihoglu S, et al: Risk factors of status epilepticus in children, *Pediatr Int* 45:429, 2003.
5. Alldredge BK, Wall DB, Ferriero DM: Effect of prehospital treatment on the outcome of status epilepticus in children, *Pediatr Neurol* 12:213, 1995.
6. Alldredge BK, et al: A comparison of lorazepam, diazepam, and placebo for the treatment of out-of-hospital status epilepticus, *N Engl J Med* 345:631, 2001.
7. Goodchild CS: GABA receptors and benzodiazepines, *Br J Anaesth* 71:127, 1993.
8. Barsan WG, Ward JT, Otten EJ: Blood levels of diazepam after endotracheal administration in dogs, *Ann Emerg Med* 11:242, 1982.
9. Boucher BA, et al: The safety, tolerability, and pharmacokinetics of fosphenytoin after intramuscular and intravenous administration in neurosurgery patients, *Pharmacotherapy* 16:638, 1996.
10. Boucher BA: Fosphenytoin: a novel phenytoin prodrug, *Pharmacotherapy* 16:777, 1996.

11. Sobotka JL, Alexander B, Cook BL: A review of carbamazepine's hematologic reactions and monitoring recommendations, *DICP* 24:1214, 1990.
12. Appleton R, Martland T, Phillips B: Drug management for acute tonic-clonic convulsions including convulsive status epilepticus in children, *Cochrane Database Syst Rev* 4:CD001905, 2002.
13. Stoelting RK: Antiepileptic drugs. In Stoelting RK, editor: *Pharmacology & physiology in anesthetic practice,* Philadelphia, 1999, Lippincott-Raven, p 510.
14. Dichter MA, Brodie MJ: New antiepileptic drugs, *N Engl J Med* 334:1583, 1996.
15. Spina E, Perugi G: Antiepileptic drugs: indications other than epilepsy, *Epileptic Disord* 6:57, 2004.

BIBLIOGRAPHY

Feliciani C, et al: Skin reactions due to anti-epileptic drugs: several case-reports with long-term follow-up, *Int J Immunopathol Pharmacol* 16:89, 2003.

Schaub N, Bircher AJ: Severe hypersensitivity syndrome to lamotrigine confirmed by lymphocyte stimulation in vitro, *Allergy* 55:191, 2000.

Schlienger RG, Knowles SR, Shear NH: Lamotrigine-associated anticonvulsant hypersensitivity syndrome, *Neurology* 51:1172, 1998.

Sladden M, Mortimer N, Chave T: Toxic epidermal caused by lamotrigine, *Aust Fam Physician* 33:829, 2004.

Shock

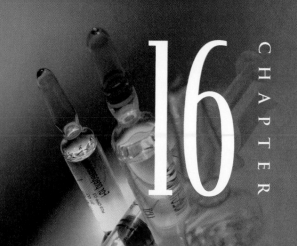

CHAPTER 16

OBJECTIVES

1. Explain the difference between compensated and uncompensated shock.
2. Differentiate among the five causes and types of shock: hypovolemic, cardiogenic, neurogenic, septic, and anaphylactic.
3. Define rapid responders, transient responders, and nonresponders.
4. List the benefits of packed red blood cell transfusion.
5. Differentiate among the four blood types: O, A, B, and AB.
6. Demonstrate the proper procedure for packed red blood cell administration for hypovolemic shock.
7. Discuss medications used in the treatment of cardiogenic shock: dobutamine (Dobutrex), dopamine (Intropin), norepinephrine (Levophed), and milrinone (Primacor).
8. Discuss the use of phenylephrine (Neo-Synephrine) in the treatment of neurogenic shock.
9. Explain why, in septic shock, the exaggerated response, not the infection, creates the shock state.

Medications that Appear in Chapter 16

Dobutamine (Dobutrex)
Dopamine (Intropin)
Norepinephrine (Levophed)
Milrinone (Primacor)
Phenylephrine (Neo-Synephrine)

INTRODUCTION

To treat shock appropriately, the prehospital professional must understand what shock is, its various causes, and the treatments for each particular type. The treatment for one type of shock may be a vasopressor, but treatment of a second type of shock may be fluid resuscitation. Failure to identify the various types of shock and match the appropriate treatment with the type of shock can cause the patient significant peril. In regard to therapy of other conditions, the provider must recognize a condition (e.g., ventricular tachycardia) and know the appropriate drug intervention (e.g., amiodarone) for that condition. When treating shock, the provider must recognize the presence of the condition and determine its cause (e.g., hypovolemia) to select the most appropriate intervention. This chapter describes the five causes of shock and their appropriate pharmacologic management.

Your unit is called to the scene of a multiple motor vehicle crash. The patient you are directed to care for is a 19-year-old man who is the driver of a car that has run off the road and come to rest in a ravine. The patient is trapped in the car by his legs. The vehicle has been stabilized from shifting, and no fuel or electrical hazards are present. The patient is awake and answering questions. His airway is patent. Respirations are rapid and shallow. His heart rate is 132 beats/min, and blood pressure is 100/84 mm Hg. He is alert and oriented. The patient has a large laceration to the forehead, and bleeding is controlled with some direct pressure. The lungs are clear, but the patient is very tender when you palpate the ribs on the left. The abdomen is tender. The patient has an obvious open left femur fracture.

OVERVIEW OF SHOCK

Shock is an abnormality of the circulatory system that results in inadequate tissue perfusion and oxygen delivery.[1] Impaired oxygen delivery can occur in the presence of low, normal, and even elevated blood pressure. Therefore a provider should not assume that only hypotensive patients can be in shock. The classic presentation of the hypotensive, tachycardic patient in shock actually occurs late in the course of shock, after a patient has lost his or her ability to compensate. Hence the hypotensive, tachycardic patient in shock is said to be in **decompensated shock.**

> Shock can occur in the presence of low, normal, and even elevated blood pressure.

Regardless of the cause of shock, before becoming unstable a patient's physiologic functioning alters to compensate. Such compensations can involve the shunting of blood from less-critical to more-critical areas, elevation of cardiac output, an increase in heart rate, and vasoconstriction. During such periods of compensation, the patient can exhibit normal mentation and only slight alterations in vital signs. As such, these patients can appear stable. However, in reality, these patients are in compensated shock.

The term "stable" is often used to describe patients with normal blood pressure. In fact, shock-related alterations in blood pressure are typically late findings in the patient in shock. The early clinical findings of shock include skin perfusion, respiratory rate, and altered mental status. Patients can have delayed capillary refill, and their skin is often cold and clammy.

> Hypotension is a late finding of shock.

In shock, a patient's respiratory rate can increase to improve minute ventilation to compensate for metabolic acidosis. Additionally, increased respiratory rate improves blood return to the heart because the respiratory apparatus serves as a bellows. Improved cardiac return results in improved cardiac output. Because the early signs of uncompensated shock can be subtle and even misleading, prehospital providers need to maintain a high index of suspicion for shock. Terms such as "stable" and "unstable" can be incorrectly interpreted as "not sick" or "sick." Therefore patients in shock should more accurately be considered as being either compensated or uncompensated.

Paramedics can rapidly determine whether a patient is in uncompensated shock without any special equipment. A widely accepted indicator of perfusion is blood pressure. Without a blood pressure cuff, a general estimation of blood pressure can be obtained by palpation of peripheral pulses. A bounding radial pulse readily indicates that the patient has an adequate blood pressure of at least 90 mm Hg. Cerebral perfusion can be rapidly determined by evaluating the patient's mental status. A patient who is thinking clearly is perfusing the brain satisfactorily; however, with marginal perfusion, clarity of thought is lost.

CAUSES OF SHOCK

Shock is not a disease process; rather, it is the *symptom* of an underlying disease process. Treatment of hypotension is relatively simple, and blood pressure can return to normal after the administration of fluids and a vasopressor. However, if the cause of hypotension is blood loss from a gastrointestinal bleed or myocardial infarction, the blood flow to vital organs actually decreases (i.e., worsening of the shock) despite a normal blood pressure. If the patient is in septic shock from a perforated colon, IV fluids and vasopressors do nothing to control the fecal contamination of the abdominal cavity. A patient with a tension pneumothorax requires only rapid decompression of the chest; fluids and drugs are not required and, in fact, can delay definitive therapy.

These examples illustrate the importance of understanding the causes of the various forms of shock to provide effective treatment. The five types of shock are hypovolemic, cardiogenic, neurogenic, septic, and anaphylactic.

When encountering a patient with hypoperfusion, determine which one of the five causes is the mostly likely source of the patient's hypoperfusion. In some cases the cause is obvious. For example, the patient with a gunshot wound to the abdomen with no radial pulse and a weak, rapid carotid pulse is in **hypovolemic shock.** A 65-year-old man with a blood pressure of 84/58 mm Hg who described chest pain before becoming disoriented is likely in cardiogenic shock.

In other cases the source of the hypotension requires critical thought. Such clinical dilemmas most commonly occur in hypotension after blunt trauma. For example, did hypoperfusion from a cardiac event cause an altered sensorium, which then resulted in a motor vehicle accident or fall?

Box 16-1 summarizes the treatment for each type of shock. Fortunately, one component of therapy is the same for all five causes of shock: IV resuscitation. Significant debate exists regarding the need for and magnitude of IV fluid resuscitation in shock, especially hypovolemic shock from penetrating trauma, which is discussed in greater detail later in the chapter.

The patient in the previous scenario is likely in hypovolemic shock. He has several possible sources of blood loss, including the scalp laceration and the open femur fracture. Other less-obvious sources of blood loss could be from rib fractures or an abdominal injury. The patient has a rapid heart rate, rapid respiration rate, and slight depression of blood pressure.

BOX 16-1

TREATMENT FOR THE FIVE CAUSES OF SHOCK

Hypovolemic: Control of hemorrhage, fluid, blood products, and perhaps surgery to definitively control any ongoing bleeding
Cardiogenic: Fluid, chronotropic drugs, inotropic drugs, vasoconstrictors, and in some cases vasodilators
Neurogenic: Fluid and vasoconstrictors
Septic: Fluid, vasoconstrictors, inotropic drugs, and eventually control of the infectious source with antibiotics and perhaps surgery
Anaphylactic: Fluids, epinephrine, antihistamines, and steroids

The appropriate therapy for this patient is administration of IV fluids with an isotonic crystalloid solution such as normal saline or Ringer's lactate solution. Controlling ongoing blood loss and administration of fluids will likely improve the vital signs and the delivery of oxygen to peripheral tissues and reverse the shock process. Administration of a vasopressor would also increase his blood pressure.

MANAGEMENT

> You respond to a 1:15 AM call to a bar known to attract a rowdy clientele. Shots have been fired, and initial reports indicate multiple casualties. A crowd has gathered outside the bar. The interior has been vacated except for the owner and staff. Two injuries are present—both patients are male and approximately 25 years old. One of the patients is sitting on the floor near the back of the bar. He is obviously intoxicated but is looking around the well-lit bar. His right thigh has a pressure dressing fashioned from towels. The dressing is almost entirely saturated with blood. He is asking about his friend, who is lying on the floor.
>
> The second patient has a dressing applied to the left lower quadrant of the abdomen that shows only a few spots of blood. He moves all four extremities as he attempts to sit upright, although he lacks the strength to sit up. As the bar staff speaks to him, he looks at them but does not seem to understand. Your partner reports a systolic blood pressure of 82 mm Hg and a heart rate of 136 beats/min.
>
> Within moments of surveying the scene, it is apparent which patient most urgently requires your attention. A closer examination of the second patient indicates that he has a rapid, weak radial pulse. His fingers are cool, and capillary refill is 4 seconds. He responds only to questions posed in a loud, commanding voice. The patient can identify himself but does not accurately describe his location. ...

HYPOVOLEMIC SHOCK

Even without a blood pressure cuff, you know the second patient in the above scenario is in shock. First, he is tachycardic. Prolonged capillary refill and cool extremities indicate peripheral vasoconstriction. His mental status may be clouded by alcohol or drugs, but his altered sensorium is likely affected by marginal cerebral perfusion. The patient's systolic blood pressure of 82 mm Hg and heart rate of 136 beats/min further confirm that he is in shock.

In this case, the circumstances of a gunshot wound to the abdomen clearly led to shock caused by hypovolemia. Cardiogenic shock can be excluded by the events preceding the shock state. Neurogenic and septic shock can be excluded by the evidence of peripheral vasoconstriction. Neurogenic shock can be considered only with interrupted spinal cord function, which limits peripheral sympathetic tone. Hypovolemic shock is typically associated with a heart rate slower than expected for the degree of hypotension. Penetrating abdominal injuries can lead to sepsis. However, sepsis from intraabdominal infection caused by a gunshot wound would require several days to develop.

A drop in blood pressure from acute hemorrhage requires a loss of approximately 30% of the circulating blood volume.[1] As a general guideline, circulating blood volume is 7% of the ideal body weight. For a patient with an ideal body weight of 80 kg, the circulating blood volume is 5600 mL ($80 \times 0.07 = 5.6$ L or 5600 mL). The circulating volume lost to cause a drop in blood pressure is 1680 mL ($5600 \times 0.30 = 1680$ mL). In other words, more than 4 U of blood (1 U of blood contains 350 mL) must be lost from the circulation before the blood pressure drops.

> A drop in blood pressure caused by acute hemorrhage requires a loss of approximately 30% of the circulating blood volume.

The initial therapy for hypovolemic shock is control of the source of hemorrhage, if possible. As control of hemorrhage is obtained, fluid resuscitation is performed. The fluid infused at initial resuscitation should be a **crystalloid,** preferably normal saline. Normal saline is nearly isotonic and is compatible with blood. Ringer's lactate solution is another crystalloid that is commonly used; however, it is not compatible with the infusion of blood. IV lines used for blood administration must be flushed with normal saline before the administration of blood.

> Normal saline is compatible to be given with infused blood; Ringer's lactate is not.

The route of fluid administration in the prehospital setting is optimally two large-bore peripheral IV sites. In cases in which peripheral veins are not accessible, IO routes should be considered (see Chapter 5). According to the principles of both Advanced Trauma Life Support (ATLS) and Prehospital Trauma Life Support (PHTLS), adults in hypovolemic shock should receive a rapid fluid bolus of 1 to 2 L of crystalloid. Pediatric patients should receive 20 mL/kg of crystalloid.

Patients who demonstrate improved perfusion, heart rate, or blood pressure with crystalloid infusion can be categorized as rapid responders, transient responders, or nonresponders. Rapid responders do not need further aggressive resuscitation. They have no ongoing hemorrhage; the source of bleeding has been controlled with pressure or the patient's normal hemostatic mechanisms. Transient responders improve as their intravascular volume is replenished. However, with ongoing manifestations of poor perfusion return, transient responders require blood transfusion and control of hemorrhage. Nonresponders have uncontrolled hemorrhage and require blood transfusion and control of bleeding.

> ... The patient lying on the floor is given normal saline. (For the sake of discussion, transport is delayed in this scenario, but this patient does require rapid transport to a trauma center.) After 15 minutes of on-scene time, the patient has received 2 L of normal saline, and he appropriately responds to your requests to remain quiet. Blood pressure is 98/60 mm Hg, and heart rate is 100 beats/min. This patient is a responder to fluid administration. Ten minutes later, with an additional 250 mL of normal saline on board, the patient is less lucid, he is more tachycardic, and his radial pulse is weaker. He has become a transient responder. ...

In this case, the paramedic does not yet have control of the source of bleeding. Should the patient's heart rate and blood pressure be returned to normal? The answer is "no." This patient would benefit from the use of **hypotensive resuscitation.** That is, the goal is not to return his vital signs to normal, but to maintain physiologic functioning until the source of hemorrhage can be controlled. Some may ask, "What can be wrong with normal vital signs? Why not infuse more normal saline, because he responded initially?" These are logical questions, and their answer lies in a more detailed examination of the nature of traumatic hypovolemic shock.

Part of the study of pharmacology is appropriate dosing. What is the appropriate dose or volume of IV fluids? Administration of IV fluids in excessive amounts or at too-rapid of a rate can cause patients to bleed more rapidly. Controversy exists in the medical literature regarding appropriate IV fluid administration in patients with penetrating torso trauma.[2] Control of hemorrhage for torso trauma requires rapid access to a trauma surgeon. In the operating room, and especially in the field, the best chance for hemostasis is the victim's clotting mechanism—in addition to direct pressure or an extremity tourniquet. Administration of IV fluids does nothing to stop the bleeding.

Although obvious, the emphasis that bleeding patients are losing blood, not saline, is still important. Saline lacks the ability to carry oxygen and the factors capable of producing clots. In fact, aggressive fluid resuscitation to restore normal blood pressure can dislodge the fragile clot and cause bleeding to resume. The platelets and coagulation proteins consumed in clot formation would then be lost, and the ability of the body to affect hemostasis would be limited as platelets and coagulation proteins become diluted with aggressive fluid resuscitation. In addition, large volumes of unwarmed fluids can predispose a patient to hypothermia. Because blood coagulation factors function within a narrow temperature range, the onset of hypothermia can render the blood coagulation system less functional and result in ongoing hemorrhage.

Hypotensive resuscitation and *limited resuscitation* are terms used to describe fluid algorithms followed to restore systolic blood pressure to subnormal levels, not normal levels. After control of hemorrhage, standard end points of resuscitation are sought.

One protocol for hypotensive resuscitation guides fluid administration to achieve and maintain adequate perfusion, as assessed by four criteria.[3] Fluid is to be administered in volumes to achieve one of the following results:

1. Consciousness, as demonstrated by ability to follow commands
2. Palpable radial pulse
3. Systolic blood pressure of 90 mm Hg
4. Mean arterial pressure of 60 mm Hg

Patients in hypovolemic shock may require transfusion of blood. Because of acute blood loss, the hypotensive patient in the scenario has a deficit of 30% of blood volume. Transient responders probably need blood, and nonresponders certainly require blood transfusion. Because most prehospital care providers do not have the availability to transfuse blood, potential delays incurred by establishing IV lines and administering fluids may benefit the patient little or not at all.

Although most ground-based prehospital providers will not find themselves in circumstances that require them to administer blood, transfusion of blood is a skill often required of air medical providers, those involved in interhospital transport, and military providers.

Even though patients hemorrhage whole blood, transfusion of whole blood is a relatively rare occurrence, even in the hospital setting. The blood product most often transfused is **packed red blood cells (pRBCs).** Standard blood banking practices involve separating donated whole blood into components. Red blood cells (RBCs), platelets, and plasma are all separated. In this manner, a single unit of blood can provide therapy for many patients.

Blood component therapy is administered to patients with specific needs. The overwhelming majority of blood donations are provided to patients who do not need the transfusion of whole blood. Blood component therapy also has a practical component. Platelets require storage at a warmer temperature than RBCs. If platelets were stored with RBCs at $4°C$, the platelets would clump with the RBCs and plasma proteins. Coagulation factors in plasma are also labile at $4°C$. Therefore storage of whole blood at the temperature required for RBCs causes significant problems.

pRBC transfusion offers two benefits: oxygen-carrying capability and volume. The most significant benefit is oxygen-carrying capacity. The oxygen dissolved in plasma is insignificant compared with the oxygen carried by hemoglobin in pRBCs. The volume of 1 U of pRBCs is approximately 350 mL.

As with any therapy, the risks and benefits must be weighed. One risk of transfusion therapy is disease transmission. Even though aggressive testing of donors is performed to minimize the risk of disease transmission, the risk of HIV and hepatitis C transmission is approximately one case per 1 million U transfused. The risk of hepatitis B transmission is approximately four cases per 1 million U transfused.[4]

In standard transfusion therapy, the greatest risk is ABO-incompatible blood transfusions. For the prehospital provider, ABO incompatibility is not a concern because only type O blood is available. Information on a patient's blood type and the testing to confirm the blood type in the field is not practical. For these reasons, only universal donor blood, type O, is available.

To review, the four blood types are O, A, B, and AB. Type A has A antigen on the RBC surface, type B has B antigen on the RBC surface, and type AB has A and B antigens on the RBC surface. Natural antibodies occur against the cell surface antigen that is not present on the RBC surface. That is, an individual with type A blood has naturally occurring antibodies against B antigen. Type B patients have antibodies against A antigen, and type AB patients have no antibodies against A or B antigen. Type O patients have antibodies against both A and B antigens. Type O individuals are universal donors because their RBC surfaces do not contain A or B antigen.

The optimal unit of pRBCs for field administration is type O Rh⁻. The Rh status of pRBCs infused is of minimal consequence to male patients or female patients without the possibility of future pregnancy. However, in women with the possibility of future pregnancy, Rh⁺ blood should be avoided. Rh⁻ patients who receive Rh⁺ blood develop antibodies against the Rh factor in approximately 80% of cases. The seroconversion that occurs can pose a risk in a subsequent pregnancy if the Rh⁻ mother becomes pregnant with an Rh⁺ fetus. The fetus can develop chronic hemolytic disease of the newborn.[3]

> ...You are a flight medic on an air ambulance who has been called to transport a gunshot victim (the second patient described in the previous scenario). After you receive the report, you decide that the patient could benefit from transfusion of pRBCs while being transported to the regional trauma center.

ADMINISTERING A BLOOD TRANSFUSION

Equipment Needed:
1 U pRBCs, blood tubing, normal saline, PPE
Procedure:
1. Observe universal precautions.
2. Confirm right patient.
3. When possible, explain to the patient what procedure you are going to perform and why.
4. Examine the refrigeration record to ensure the proper pRBC temperature has been maintained.
5. Examine the expiration date on the units. Check the pack number on the transfusion record and compare it with the pack number on the label on the blood product.
6. Confirm the blood is type O.
7. Examine the blood for evidence of leakage, clumps, or abnormal color.
8. Confirm the blood is Rh⁻ if the patient is a woman younger than 50 years. In life-threatening situations, this may be disregarded.
9. Record vital signs of the patient before transfusion and at least every 15 minutes during the transfusion.
10. Ensure all tags and labels remain attached to the unit of blood.
11. Ensure the tubing to the unit of blood is filtered.
12. Confirm the pRBCs will be infused through a line flushed with normal saline.
13. Attach the unit of pRBCs to the tubing and the open valve to begin the transfusion.
14. Closely observe the transfusion during the first 15 mL of transfusion. An acute hemolytic reaction can occur with infusion of even a small volume. If any sign of a transfusion reaction occurs, stop the transfusion immediately. Do not discard the unit; save it for further analysis on arrival to definitive care.
15. Document identifying numbers of the unit infused, infusion times, and vital signs.

CARDIOGENIC SHOCK

You are dispatched at 5:30 AM to a residence in response to a 65-year-old man with chest pain. You are met at the door by the patient's wife, who reports that her husband has a history of angina beginning 5 years ago. At that time he underwent cardiac catheterization and was found to have a critical narrowing of one of his coronary arteries. He was managed with stent placement and has been free of symptoms since that time. His wife reports that he had been feeling well until this morning. He has been faithful in taking atorvastatin (Lipitor) 20 mg orally every day for hyperlipidemia.

Your patient is found lying on the couch with his right arm hanging limply off the side. He has two pillows under his head and neck. He rouses when addressed. He tells you he has chest pressure like he has never previously had. He also reports feeling short of breath. The discomfort and sense of uneasiness woke him approximately 90 minutes ago, when he left his bedroom for the living room. His extremities are cool. His radial pulse is present. You notice prominent external jugular veins. His heart rate is 104 beats/min, blood pressure is 86/58 mm Hg, and respiratory rate is 22 breaths/min. Rales are present in the lung bases bilaterally.

It is evident that the patient in this scenario is in shock, and the task of the prehospital professional is to determine rapidly the type of shock before beginning therapy. With no suggestion of trauma or gastrointestinal blood loss, a hypovolemic source of shock can most likely be excluded. One possible source of hypovolemia would be a leaking aneurysm, but with no abdominal or back pain, blood loss from an abdominal aortic aneurysm is unlikely. The chest pain could be a manifestation of a leaking thoracic aortic aneurysm; however, hypovolemia is effectively excluded by the presence of the full neck veins. A neurogenic source can be excluded by the patient's ability to maintain lower extremity function, as confirmed by his movement to the couch from the bedroom after the onset of the chest discomfort. Sepsis as a cause of his hypotension is also unlikely. The distended neck veins and cool extremities suggest peripheral vasoconstriction and ineffectiveness of the cardiac cycle (signs seen only late in septic shock). The patient is experiencing cardiogenic shock on the basis of myocardial ischemia.

Cardiogenic shock is inadequate tissue perfusion caused by pump failure, most commonly from acute myocardial infarction.[5] In such cases the myocardium loses its ability to contract effectively. Factors other than pump failure can result in cardiogenic shock. For example, mechanical factors that result in inadequate filling of the right or left atrium can prevent effective cardiac function. **Pericardial tamponade** is an example of a mechanical source of cardiogenic shock. Other mechanical factors, such as severe cardiac valve dysfunction, can cause cardiogenic shock. In these circumstances, blood does not maintain an effective, unidirectional flow through the heart. Rather, the blood "sloshes" back and forth during the cardiac cycle across the dysfunctional valve. Tissue perfusion is negatively affected by such inefficient flow.

The major clinical feature of cardiogenic shock is evidence of inadequate tissue perfusion manifested by peripheral vasoconstriction, delayed capillary refill, and decreased mental capacity. An additional feature is pulmonary congestion or pulmonary edema. In cases of acute left ventricular dysfunction, the heart is unable to propel blood to the systemic peripheral circulation. The lower pressure right ventricle and pulmonary circulation typically are less affected by pump failure, and blood flow through the right side of the heart to the lungs continues. In the left side of the heart, cardiac emptying to the peripheral circulation is compromised. Left atrial filling pressures increase, resulting in congestion of the pulmonary vascular bed. As a consequence, oxygenation can be impaired. Tachypnea, shortness of breath, and rales are observed. In cases of acute valvular dysfunction cardiac murmurs can be heard.

The mortality rate for cardiogenic shock is between 50% and 80%.[5] Risk factors for death from cardiogenic shock complicating myocardial infarction include age, previous myocardial infarction, cold and clammy skin, and oliguria (scanty urine production).[6] The best outcomes are achieved in patients in whom the cause of the cardiac dysfunction can be quickly reversed. For patients with acute myocardial infarction, reversal is achieved by myocardial revascularization.[5]

For patients with cardiogenic shock caused by cardiac ischemia, nitroglycerin is not indicated because hypotension can be exacerbated by its vasodilatory effects. The use of beta adrenergic blockers should also be limited. These products should be initiated only after resolution of the state of hypoperfusion.[5]

Heart rate **(chronotropism),** force of cardiac contraction **(inotropism),** and systemic vascular resistance can all be manipulated by adrenergic agonists. The manipulation of these receptors by drugs that bind to them allows the provider to alter cardiac performance. As stated in Chapter 1, adrenergic receptors are categorized into four major groups: $alpha_1$, $alpha_2$, $beta_1$, and $beta_2$. Stimulation of each type of adrenergic receptor results in predominant effects.[7] A patient whose heart would benefit from positive inotropic and chronotropic effects would be well served by a medication that stimulates the $beta_1$ adrenergic receptors.

Two adrenergic agonists are most commonly used in cardiogenic shock: dobutamine and dopamine. Dobutamine is the agent of choice to improve cardiac output in cardiogenic shock for patients with systolic blood pressure greater than 80 mm Hg.[5] Dobutamine's major effect is to increase cardiac contractility and cardiac output. Although it has some $beta_1$ stimulatory effects, dobutamine does not significantly increase heart rate. Tachycardia should be avoided in cardiogenic shock to minimize the heart's oxygen demand. Dobutamine also does not raise systemic vascular resistance. Patients receiving this medication should be closely observed for tachycardia and hypotension. Specifically, dobutamine should be used with caution in atrial fibrillation.

Dopamine is another effective medication for patients in cardiogenic shock.[5] A $beta_1$-mediated increase in contractility and heart rate can improve cardiac output, but the downside of this effect is an increase in myocardial oxygen consumption. Because dopamine causes some alpha-mediated vasoconstriction, it is a good choice for the treatment of cardiogenic shock associated with hypotension (systolic blood pressure less than 80 mm Hg). As the dose of dopamine is increased, a predominantly alpha-mediated vasoconstriction occurs.

Dopamine has $beta_1$ effects, as well as $alpha_1$ effects. The $alpha_1$ stimulation produces vasoconstriction, which increases blood pressure. Dopamine can exacerbate myocardial ischemia from tachycardia and increased systemic vascular resistance.

In patients with cardiogenic shock refractory to dopamine, norepinephrine (Levophed) should be administered.[5] Norepinephrine is an $alpha_1$, $alpha_2$, and $beta_1$ agonist. Alpha-mediated peripheral vasoconstriction is the predominant clinical result of administration.

Milrinone (Primacor) is another drug used to treat cardiogenic shock by stimulating the heart to increase cardiac output. The drugs previously discussed in this chapter are medications that treat cardiogenic shock by binding various adrenergic receptors. Milrinone, however, is a member of the class of drugs known as **phosphodiesterase inhibitors,** which ultimately increase the concentration of calcium inside the cardiac cell. As such, milrinone is able to improve cardiac output independently of adrenergic receptors. Because milrinone works by a different mechanism, it can be effective in patients who do not respond to therapy with the adrenergic stimulating agents (dopamine, dobutamine, and norepinephrine).

Milrinone has a positive inotropic effect and peripheral vasodilatory action, but it has no significant chronotropic or arrhythmogenic action. Because of the vasodilatory effect, patients should be closely observed for hypotension.[5]

Special caution is required when infusing vasoactive medications, and monitoring is absolutely critical. Hypoperfusion, cardiac arrhythmias, and exacerbation of myocardial ischemia are real possibilities. Reliable venous access must be maintained. When administering vasoactive drugs, be sure that venous access is reliably secured. If an IV line becomes dislodged and the vasoactive drug infiltrates into the soft tissue, the patient may incur extensive soft tissue necrosis at the site of the drug infiltration. The risk of soft tissue damage with Sub-Q infusion of adrenergic agonists from an infiltrated IV site is great. If Sub-Q infiltration does occur, infiltration of 10 mg phentolamine mixed in 5 to 10 mL of normal saline can prevent tissue loss.[8]

DOBUTAMINE (DOBUTREX)

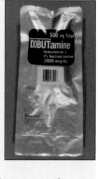

Classification: Adrenergic agent
Action: Acts primarily as an agonist at beta$_1$ adrenergic receptors with minor beta$_2$ and alpha$_1$ effects. Consequently, dobutamine increases myocardial contractility and stroke volume with minor chronotropic effects, resulting in increased cardiac output.
Indications: CHF, cardiogenic shock.
Adverse Effects: Tachycardia, PVCs, hypertension, hypotension, palpitations, arrhythmias.
Contraindications: Suspected or known poisoning/drug-induced shock, systolic blood pressure <100 mm Hg with signs of shock, idiopathic hypertrophic subaortic stenosis, known sensitivity (including sulfites). Use with caution in hypertension, recent MI, arrhythmias, hypovolemia.
Dosage:
· **Adult:** 2 to 20 mcg/kg/min IV, IO. At doses >20 mcg/kg/min, increases of heart rate of >10% may induce or exacerbate myocardial ischemia.
· **Pediatric:** Same as adult dosing.
Special Considerations:
Half-life 2 minutes
Pregnancy class C

DOPAMINE (INTROPIN)

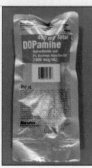

Classification: Adrenergic agonist, inotropic, vasopressor
Action: Stimulates alpha and beta adrenergic receptors. At moderate doses (2-10 mcg/kg/min), dopamine stimulates beta$_1$ receptors, resulting in inotropy and increased cardiac output while maintaining dopaminergic-induced vasodilatory effects. At high doses (>10 mcg/kg/min), alpha adrenergic agonism predominates, and increased peripheral vascular resistance and vasoconstriction result.
Indications: Hypotension and decreased cardiac output associated with cardiogenic shock and septic shock, hypotension after return of spontaneous circulation following cardiac arrest, symptomatic bradycardia unresponsive to atropine.
Adverse Effects: Tachycardia, arrhythmias, skin and soft tissue necrosis, severe hypertension from excessive vasoconstriction, angina, dyspnea, headache, nausea/vomiting.
Contraindications: Pheochromocytoma, VF, VT, or other ventricular arrhythmias, known sensitivity (including sulfites). Correct any hypovolemia with volume fluid replacement before administering dopamine.
Dosage:
· **Adult:** 2 to 20 mcg/kg/min IV, IO infusion. Starting dose 5 mcg/kg/min; may gradually increase the infusion by 5 to 10 mcg/kg/min to desired effect. Cardiac dose is usually 5 to 10 mcg/kg/min; vasopressor dose is usually 10 to 20 mcg/kg/min. Little benefit is gained beyond 20 mcg/kg/min.
· **Pediatric:** Same as adult dosing.
Special Considerations:
Half-life 2 minutes
Pregnancy class C

NOREPINEPHRINE (LEVOPHED)

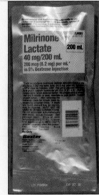

Classification: Adrenergic agonist, inotropic, vasopressor
Action: Norepinephrine is an $alpha_1$, $alpha_2$, and $beta_1$ agonist. Alpha-mediated peripheral vasoconstriction is the predominant clinical result of administration, resulting in increasing blood pressure and coronary blood flow. Beta adrenergic action produces inotropic stimulation of the heart and dilates the coronary arteries.
Indications: Cardiogenic shock, septic shock, severe hypotension.
Adverse Effects: Dizziness, anxiety, cardiac arrhythmias, dyspnea, exacerbation of asthma.
Contraindications: Patients taking MAOIs, known sensitivity. Use with caution in hypovolemia.
Dosage:
- **Adult:** Add 4 mg to 250 mL of D_5W or D_5NS, but not normal saline alone. 0.5 to 1 mcg/min as IV, IO, titrated to maintain systolic blood pressure >80 mm Hg. Refractory shock may require doses as high as 30 mcg/min.
- **Pediatric:** 0.05 to 2 mcg/kg/min IV, IO infusion, to a maximum dose of 2 mcg/kg/min.

Special Considerations:
Do not administer in same IV line as alkaline solutions.
Half-life 1 minute
Pregnancy class C

MILRINONE (PRIMACOR)

Classification: Inotropic
Action: Milrinone is a positive inotropic drug and vasodilator with minimal chronotropic effect. Milrinone inhibits an enzyme, cAMP phosphodiesterase, which results in an increase in the concentration of calcium inside the cardiac cell. The result is improvement in diastolic function and myocardial contractility.
Indications: Cardiogenic shock, CHF.
Adverse Effects: Cardiac arrhythmias, nausea/vomiting, hypotension.
Contraindications: Valvular heart disease, known sensitivity.
Dosage:
- **Adult:** 50 mcg/kg IV, IO over a period of 10 minutes, followed by an infusion of 0.375 to 0.5 mcg/kg/min (max dose: 0.75 mcg/kg/min).
- **Pediatric:** Same as adult dosing.

Special Considerations:
Pregnancy class C

NEUROGENIC SHOCK

You are a flight medic and your aircraft is dispatched to a motor vehicle crash in which one person is reported to be entrapped. You arrive to find the patient, a 17-year-old girl, trapped by her legs in the driver's seat. First responders have placed her in a cervical collar and started oxygen. The patient is talking but appears to be somewhat lethargic. Your assessment shows that her airway is clearly patent. Your partner reports a pulse oximeter reading of 93%. Her breath sounds are clear bilaterally, and she appears to be moving her chest wall equally. You note that her respirations appear to be somewhat rapid and shallow and estimate that her respiratory rate is approximately 32 breaths/min. You reach over to take her pulse and note that it is palpable but weak. Her heart rate is only 52 beats/min, and her blood pressure is 90/56 mm Hg. She tells you that she cannot move her legs and that she cannot feel anything below her nipple line.

Once her legs have been freed, you place the patient in full spinal immobilization and extricate her from the vehicle. ...

Prehospital professionals encounter **neurogenic shock** in patients who have had a spinal cord injury. When the sympathetic pathways from the spinal cord are interrupted by an injury, blood vessels dilate. When all the blood vessels of the affected area dilate, the volume of the vascular tree has enlarged but the amount of the blood filling the vasculature has remained the same, which results in relative hypovolemia. These patients may appear similar to those with hypovolemic shock, even when they have not lost blood. Complicating matters, if the lesion to the spinal cord involves the sympathetic innervation of the heart, the patient may also have bradycardia, meaning the heart will slow and aggravate the hypotension.

> Patients with neurogenic shock may also have bradycardia in addition to hypotension.

Patients with neurogenic shock lose input to the blood vessels from the nervous system. Without this input, the blood vessels dilate. Without losing a single drop of blood, the patient is initially hypovolemic.

> Imagine having a car with a 10-gallon tank. In that tank are 10 gallons of gasoline. If for some unexplained reason the tank expands to a 20-gallon capacity with the same 10 gallons of gasoline, the tank is suddenly half full. To maintain the tank's full status, the action would be twofold: try to fill the now-larger tank, and try to reduce the size of the tank.

Fluid infusion to improve preload is the initial therapy for neurogenic shock. Neurogenic shock mainly involves managing a bigger vascular container, and fluid administration simply refills that vascular container. Of note, fluids, not vasopressors, are the initial treatment for neurogenic shock. Prehospital providers encounter multiple-trauma patients who are hypotensive, with the origin being hemorrhage, spinal cord injury, or perhaps both. Do not assume that hypotension is from spinal shock and then rush to use a vasopressor. As previously mentioned, vasopressors used in hemorrhagic shock improve blood pressure but decrease tissue perfusion and oxygen delivery. The net effect is that the shock is worse.

> IV fluids, not vasopressors, are the initial treatment for neurogenic shock.

The treatment for the patient with hypotensive trauma is the same whether the cause is hemorrhage or spinal shock: IV fluid therapy. Remember, exercise moderation when providing IV fluids to a hypotensive patient with trauma. Patients with hypotension from spinal shock may not exhibit the expected tachycardia and may even have bradycardia because of a loss of cardiac sympathetic tone.

Once the volume status of the patient is adequate, consideration should be given to the use of vasopressor agents. If the patient has a low heart rate, dopamine would be the recommended vasopressor. Dopamine possesses alpha effects, which stimulate the adrenergic receptors on the blood vessels and reestablish the vascular tone lost from the interruption of sympathetic innervation. Dopamine also has beta$_1$ properties that increase the heart rate. Many patients have an adequate heart rate and require only the benefit of an agent capable of providing alpha stimulation. Phenylephrine (Neo-Synephrine) stimulates only the alpha receptor and is the most common choice for patients in neurogenic shock.

PHENYLEPHRINE (NEO-SYNEPHRINE)

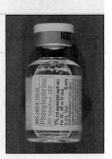

Classification: Adrenergic agonist

Action: Stimulates the alpha receptors, causing vasoconstriction, which results in increased blood pressure.

Indications: Neurogenic shock, spinal shock, cases of shock in which the patient's heart rate does not need to be increased, drug-induced hypotension.

Adverse Effects: Hypertension, VT, headache, excitability, tremor, MI, exacerbation of asthma, cardiac arrhythmias, reflex bradycardia, soft tissue necrosis.

Contraindications: Acute MI, angina, cardiac arrhythmias, severe hypertension, coronary artery disease, pheochromocytoma, narrow-angle glaucoma, cardiomyopathy, MAOI therapy, known sensitivity to phenylephrine or sulfites.

Dosage:

- **Adult:** 100 to 180 mcg/min IV, IO. Once the blood pressure has been stabilized, the dose can be reduced to 40 to 60 mcg/min.
- **Pediatric (2 to 12 years):** 5 to 20 mcg/kg IV, IO followed by 0.1 to 0.5 mcg/kg/min IV, IO (max dose: 3 mcg/kg/min IV, IO).

Special Considerations:

Pregnancy class C

... Once the patient is safely on a cot, immobilized, and placed in the helicopter, you repeat an assessment. Her airway is patent; respirations are shallow and rapid at 28 breaths/min. Heart rate is slow at 54 beats/min, and when you palpate her pulse you note that her skin is warm. Blood pressure is 88/60 mm Hg. Her neurologic status is unchanged, with no motor or sensory function below the nipple line. Your assessment is that the patient has a spinal cord injury and is in spinal shock. Because she is a multiple-trauma victim from a motor vehicle crash, you are also worried that the patient could have blood loss from injuries to internal organs such as the liver and spleen. Therefore the patient could also have an element of hypovolemic shock. You know that the initial treatment for neurogenic shock is the same as for hypovolemic shock: intravascular volume expansion. You administer a bolus of 1 L Ringer's lactate solution, and the vital signs are essentially unchanged. You administer a second liter of Ringer's lactate. She still has some bradycardia (heart rate 60 beats/min), and her blood pressure after the second liter of fluid is 92/58 mm Hg. Her skin is still warm. You consult medical direction and report your neurologic examination of no motor or sensory function below the nipple line, low blood pressure, slow heart rate, and warm skin. She has only minimal response after 2 L of fluid boluses and no obvious signs of external or internal blood loss. Your estimated time to landing at the trauma center is approximately 25 minutes. Because the patient already has bradycardia, you request to start dopamine to avoid increasing the bradycardia as a complication from the phenylephrine. You start the dopamine at 5 mcg/kg per minute. Within approximately 5 minutes the blood pressure increases to 100/64 mm Hg and the heart rate increases to 66 beats/min.

SEPTIC SHOCK

Septic shock is a state of shock or poor blood perfusion from the systemic effects of an infection. The infection can be localized to the blood, the lungs, urine, or an abscess. The body responds to the infection by a defensive inflammatory response that is exaggerated. The exaggerated response, not the infection, creates the shock state, but the infection initiates the exaggerated response. A common expression states that when falling off a cliff, it's not the fall that kills you, but the sudden stop. This is illustrative of septic shock. In most cases of septic shock, the infection is not what kills the patient; the body's response to the infection does. This simple concept is not understood by many clinicians who encounter septic shock.

In septic shock, the patient has a source of infection that initiates the complex sequence of events in the body known as a *systemic inflammatory response*. This is a massive inflammatory reaction that produces chaos in several of the body's vital organ systems. The inflammatory reaction produces toxins within the body that result in dilation of the blood vessels. Another effect of the produced toxins is that the blood vessels become "leaky," and the patient can become hypovolemic as he or she loses intravascular fluid to the extravascular space. Therefore these patients have vasodilation, such as that seen in neurogenic shock, and decreased intravascular volume, such as that seen in hypovolemic shock. As in neurogenic shock, supportive drug therapy includes intravascular volume expansion with IV fluids and the use of vasopressors after appropriate fluid resuscitation. Vasopressors such as norepinephrine can be used to provide vasopressor support while the underlying source of infection is treated.

A prehospital provider has a limited ability to have a significant effect on the actual infection. The use of IV fluids and vasopressors is supportive care until the source of the infection can eventually be identified and treated. The commonly used vasopressors (norepinephrine and dopamine) have already been discussed.

> Remember the concept introduced at the beginning of the chapter: shock is a symptom, not a disease, and the ultimate treatment of septic shock is rapid control of the infection. This can entail antibiotics or even surgery.

ANAPHYLACTIC SHOCK

The prehospital management of anaphylaxis and anaphylactic shock is described in Chapter 8.

The opinions expressed herein are the personal views of the author and should not be construed as official or reflecting the views of the U.S. Department of Defense. This is a U.S. government work and is not copyrighted.

REVIEW QUESTIONS

1. List the early signs of shock.
2. What are the five types of shock?
3. What is a common treatment for all types of shock?
4. What is the initial therapy for hypovolemic shock?
5. What type of IV fluid used in the treatment of hypovolemic shock is compatible with the infusion of blood?
6. Differentiate rapid responders from transient responders and nonresponders.
7. List the benefits of pRBC transfusions as opposed to whole blood.
8. Why should Rh$^+$ blood transfusions be avoided in female patients who may become pregnant?
9. What drug might be a good choice for the treatment of cardiogenic shock in a patient who is not responding to adrenergic agents?
10. Explain why IV fluids, not vasopressors, are the initial therapy for neurogenic shock.
11. For a patient in septic shock, explain why the exaggerated response, not the infection, creates the shock state.

REFERENCES

1. American College of Surgeons: *Advanced trauma life support for doctors, student course manual*, ed 7, Chicago, 2004, American College of Surgeons.
2. Tischerman SA, et al: Clinical practice guidelines: endpoints of resuscitation, *J Trauma* 57(4):898-912, 2004.

3. *Emergency war surgery,* ed 3, Washington, DC, 2004, United States Department of Defense.
4. Goodnaugh LT, et al: Transfusion medicine—blood transfusion, *N Engl J Med* 340:438, 1999.
5. Hollenberg S, Kavinsky C, Parrillo J: Cardiogenic shock, *Ann Intern Med* 131:47, 1999.
6. Hasdal D, et al: Cardiac shock complicating acute myocardial infarction: predictors of death, *Am Heart J* 138(1 pt 10):21, 1999.
7. Mycek MJ, et al: *Lippincott's illustrated reviews: pharmacology,* ed 2, Boston, 2000, Lippincott Williams & Wilkins.
8. Peters JI, Utset OM: Vasopressors in shock management: choosing and using wisely, *J Crit Illness* 4:62, 1989.

BIBLIOGRAPHY

Antmann EM, et al: ACC/AHA guidelines for the management of patients with ST-elevation myocardial infarction—executive summary, *J Am Coll Cardiol* 44:671, 2004.
Bickell WH, et al: Immediate versus delayed fluid resuscitation for patients with penetrating torso injuries, *N Engl J Med* 331:1105, 1994.
Braunwald E, Ross J Jr, Sonnenblick EH: *Mechanisms of contraction of the normal and failing heart,* ed 2, Boston, 1976, Little, Brown, p 77.
Capone AC, et al: Improved outcome with fluid restriction in treatment of uncontrolled hemorrhagic shock, *J Am Coll Surg* 180:49, 1995.
De Backer D, et al: Effects of dopamine, norepinephrine, and epinephrine on the splanchnic circulation in septic shock: which is best? *Crit Care Med* 31:1659, 2003.
Dutton RP, Mackenzie CF, Scalea TM: Hypotensive resuscitation during active hemorrhage: impact on in-hospital mortality, *J Trauma* 52:1141, 2002.
Hardy JF, De Moerloose P, Samama M: Massive transfusion and coagulopathy: pathophysiology and implications for clinical management, *Can J Anaesth* 51:293, 2004.
Hochman JS, et al: One-year survival following early revascularization for cardiogenic shock, *JAMA* 285:190, 2001.
Kwan I, Bunn F, Roberts I: Timing and volume of fluid administration for patients with bleeding, *Cochrane Database Syst Rev* CD002245, 2003.
McKinley BA, Valdivia A, Moore FA: Goal-oriented shock resuscitation for major torso trauma: what are we learning? *Curr Opin Crit Care* 9:292, 2003.
Michard F, Teboul JL: Predicting fluid responsiveness in ICU patients: a critical analysis of the evidence, *Chest* 121:2000, 2002.
Mueller HS, et al: ACC expert consensus document. Present use of bedside right heart catheterization in patients with cardiac disease, *J Am Coll Cardiol* 32:840, 1998.
Mullner M, et al: Vasopressors for shock, *Cochrane Database Syst Rev* CD003709, 2004.
Stainsby D, et al: Guidelines on the management of massive blood loss, *Br J Haematol* 135:634, 2006.
Steel A, Bihari D: Choice of catecholamine: does it matter? *Curr Opin Crit Care* 6:347, 2000.

Traumatic Brain Injury and Spinal Cord Injury

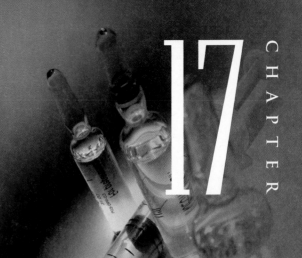

OBJECTIVES

1. Define the two types of trauma to the brain: primary brain injury and secondary brain injury.
2. List two goals of the treatment of severe traumatic brain injury.
3. Discuss medications used in the treatment of traumatic brain injury: mannitol (Osmitrol) and hypertonic saline (3% saline).
4. Discuss the use of methylprednisolone sodium succinate (Solu-Medrol) in the treatment of blunt spinal cord injury.

Medications that Appear in Chapter 17

Mannitol (Osmitrol)
Hypertonic saline (3% saline)
Methylprednisolone sodium succinate (Solu-Medrol)

INTRODUCTION

Head injury, also known as **traumatic brain injury,** is one of the leading causes of death and disability after trauma. Every year in the United States, approximately 1.6 million persons incur a traumatic brain injury. Of that number, 80,000 have some permanent neurologic impairment and 52,000 die.[1] The role of the prehospital professional in improving outcomes in this group of patients is monumental. Simple interventions initiated in the field have profound effects on the patient in the hours and weeks to follow.

Your unit is dispatched to the scene of a gunshot wound. Police have already arrived and secured the scene. On your arrival, law enforcement reports that the victim appears to have been cleaning his handgun when the weapon discharged, shooting the man in the head. You find a 58-year-old man lying supine on the floor, holding a bath towel over the bleeding wound on his forehead. You immediately evaluate his ABCs. His airway is patent, he is breathing spontaneously, and he is perfusing well. He is conscious, answers questions, and moves all four extremities on command. You do not identify any motor or sensory deficits. His heart rate is 88 beats/min, blood pressure is 148/92 mm Hg, respiratory rate is 16 breaths/min, and pulse oximeter reading is 94%. You place the patient on oxygen by a nonrebreather face mask, apply a sterile dressing to the wound, and ask your partner to hold pressure on the wound while you start an IV line.

TRAUMATIC BRAIN INJURY

Any type of head injury involves one of two types of trauma to the brain. **Primary brain injury** occurs directly to the brain from mechanical forces at the time of the initial insult. **Secondary brain injury** occurs hours after the time of the injury. In a significant number of head-injured patients, secondary brain injury leads to delayed death and disability.

The brain is contained in a bony, boxlike structure—the skull. With secondary brain injury the brain swells, resulting in a decrease in blood flow to the injured brain (Fig. 17-1, *A*). Therefore the brain experiences additional swelling, resulting in even less blood flow. And so continues the cycle of increased swelling, reduced blood flow, and increased secondary brain injury. As the brain swells, the pressure inside the skull increases; this is known as intracerebral hypertension or **intracranial pressure (ICP)** (Fig. 17-1, *B*). **Hypotension** and **hypoxia** have been noted to double the death rate after head trauma from secondary brain injury.[2]

No specific interventions can prevent primary brain injury, but secondary brain injury is preventable and somewhat treatable. The two most important interventions to avoid secondary brain injury are to prevent hypoxia and hypotension. *Hypotension,* defined as a blood pressure less than 90 mm Hg, is seen in approximately 35% of patients with severe head trauma; hypotension increases the mortality rate in these patients from 27% to 50%.[2] Therefore the prehospital provider's priorities for patient treatment in a scenario such as the previous one are to ensure patency of the airway, deliver high-flow oxygen, monitor oxygen saturation, apply pressure to the wound to preserve blood volume, and maintain adequate blood pressure with IV fluids.

> Two conditions should be avoided in the head-injured patient: hypoxia and hypotension.

> You and your partner are dispatched to a motor vehicle crash in which the driver is reported to be entrapped. You arrive to find a 19-year-old woman trapped in the driver's seat. She appears to be unconscious and has sonorous respirations. A first responder has gained access to the rear seat of the vehicle and has immobilized the patient's cervical spine. The extrication crew informs you that they should have the patient out of the vehicle in a few minutes. You evaluate the patient and find that she does have spontaneous respirations, but they appear to be somewhat labored. Her chest rise and breath sounds are equal. She has a weak radial pulse of approximately 120 beats/min by palpation. On your secondary examination, you discover that the patient has a significant number of facial fractures, a large laceration on her posterior scalp, and unequal pupils. You determine that her other injuries include a right femur fracture. ...

MANAGEMENT

The treatment of severe traumatic brain injury has two goals. The first is to identify as quickly as possible an intracranial injury that may require surgery. Such injuries include **epidural, subdural,** and **intraparenchymal hematomas.** These brain injuries can be referred to as the primary brain injury. The second goal is to prevent those conditions that result in secondary brain injury: hypoxia and hypotension.[3] Secondary brain injury results in swelling of the brain, which increases the ICP, which reduces blood flow to the brain and oxygen delivery to the brain tissue. Often the swelling of the brain (secondary brain injury) is more lethal than the primary brain injury.

> Good prehospital care may reduce the mortality rate and improve outcome in head-injured patients in the days to weeks after the injury.

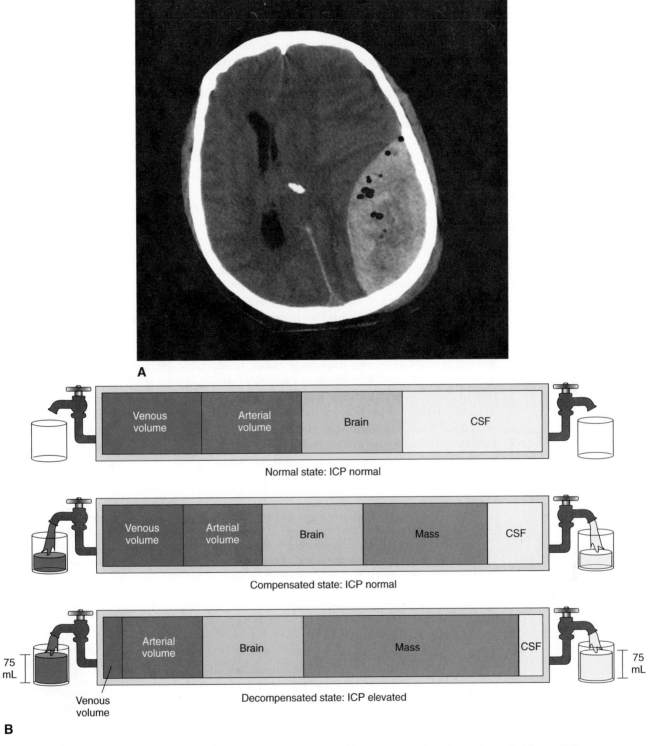

▼ **Fig. 17-1   A,** Severe traumatic brain injury with epidural hematoma and cerebral edema. **B,** Monro-Kellie doctrine. *Normal conditions:* The skull contains the brain, arterial blood, venous blood, and cerebrospinal fluid (CSF). *Compensated state, ICP normal:* With an intracranial mass from an intracranial hematoma, the body compensates by decreasing the volume of CSF. *Decompensated state, ICP elevated:* With ongoing expansion of the mass or swelling of the brain, the volumes of venous or arterial blood decrease. The result is an elevation of ICP. (From Prehospital Trauma Life Support Committee of the National Association of Emergency Medical Technicians in Cooperation with the Committee on Trauma of The American College of Surgeons: *Prehospital trauma life support,* ed 6, St Louis, 2007, Mosby.)

The primary brain injury occurs before any EMS responder arrives on the scene of an emergency. The early care that the head-injured patient receives before arrival at a trauma center or evaluation by a neurosurgeon often determines whether a patient survives and the magnitude of impairment.

The pharmacologic management of traumatic brain injuries is focused on reducing the magnitude of the secondary brain swelling, decreasing the ICP, and improving the blood flow to the brain.

Mannitol (Osmitrol) is an **osmotic diuretic** that principally works in the injured brain by dehydrating the brain and thereby decreasing swelling. Osmotic diuretics pull fluid out of tissues and cells and move it into the vascular space, where excessive fluids can be filtered out in urine. Mannitol expands the intravascular volume and reduces the viscosity of blood, improving blood flow in the injured brain.[4] Research has shown that prehospital mannitol administration does not result in a drop in the systolic blood pressure.[5]

Hypertonic saline works in a similar fashion as mannitol to decrease brain swelling and ICP by dehydrating the brain. Hypertonic saline has a significantly greater concentration of sodium than normal or physiologic saline (0.9%). (The concentration of hypertonic saline can vary in different regions.) The effect of increased sodium concentration is that water is pulled from brain tissue toward the elevated sodium concentration in the vascular space. This movement of water toward a high sodium concentration is an example of osmosis. The result is dehydration of the brain and a reduction of ICP.

Animal studies have shown that hypertonic saline is as effective in reducing increased ICP as is mannitol.[6] It has been shown to decrease brain swelling in patients with traumatic brain injury who demonstrate secondary brain injury.[7] When studied in a prehospital setting, resuscitation with hypertonic saline produced a greater systolic blood pressure than traditional crystalloid resuscitative fluids.[8] Additional research specifically looking at patients with traumatic brain injury concluded that patients who received hypertonic saline were twice as likely to survive as patients who had received traditional therapy with crystalloid fluids.[9] In addition to the reduction of brain edema, hypertonic saline benefits the injured brain by improving blood flow and reducing blood vessel spasm.

> ... The patient is extricated, her spine is immobilized, and she is intubated. You are en route to the hospital. The patient's left pupil is enlarged and nonreactive to light, and she exhibits flexion posturing. You are concerned that the patient has elevated ICP. Your transport time is 35 minutes to the local trauma center, and the weather does not permit helicopter transport. You communicate your concerns to medical direction and obtain permission to administer mannitol.

MANNITOL (OSMITROL)

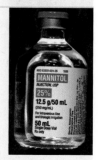

Classification: Osmotic diuretic
Action: Facilitates the flow of fluid out of tissues (including the brain) and into interstitial fluid and blood, thereby dehydrating the brain and reducing swelling. Reabsorption by the kidney is minimal, consequently increasing urine output.
Indications: Increased ICP.
Adverse Effects: Pulmonary edema, headache, blurred vision, dizziness, seizures, hypovolemia, nausea/vomiting, diarrhea, electrolyte imbalances, hypotension, hypertension, sinus tachycardia, PVCs, angina, phlebitis.
Contraindications: Active intracranial bleeding, CHF, pulmonary edema, severe dehydration. Use with caution in hypovolemia, renal failure.
Dosage:
- **Adult:** 0.5 to 2 g/kg IV, IO followed by 0.25 to 1 g/kg administered every 4 hours.
- **Pediatric:** 0.25 to 1 g/kg IV, IO followed by 0.25 to 0.5 g/kg every 4 hours.
Special Considerations:
Mannitol should not be given in the same IV, IO line as blood.
Pregnancy class C

HYPERTONIC SALINE (3% SALINE)

Classification: Volume expander, electrolyte solution
Action: The hypertonic nature of this fluid pulls extravascular fluid into the vascular space. Hypertonic saline may therefore be used as a volume expander in cases of hypovolemia or to reduce the edema of the swollen brain. Three percent saline has an electrolyte concentration of 514 mEq/L sodium.
Indications: Reduction of increased intracranial pressure resulting from traumatic brain injury, hypovolemic shock.
Adverse Effects: Increased rate of bleeding, alteration of blood clotting ability, osmotic demyelination syndrome.
Contraindications: Pulmonary congestion, pulmonary edema, known sensitivity. Hypertonic saline should not be administered by the IO route.
Dosage: Note: Hypertonic saline is available in several concentrations from 3% to 5%.
  · **Adult:** 250-mL bag of hypertonic saline infused IV slowly over a 1-hour period.
  · **Pediatric:** 6.5 to 10 mL/kg infused slowly IV over a 2-hour period.
Special Considerations:
Hypertonic saline can cause damage to the vein in which it is administered.
Pregnancy class C

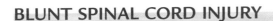

BLUNT SPINAL CORD INJURY

Your unit has been assigned to stand by at a local Fourth of July fireworks display. Shortly after the fireworks begin, you are called to assist a 28-year-old man who fell from a tree. When you arrive, you learn that the patient was climbing a tree to get a better view of the fireworks. A tree branch broke and the patient fell, striking several large tree branches on his way to the ground. You find the patient lying supine under a tree. He appears grossly intoxicated and reports severe pain in the center of his back. The patient is controlling his airway, and his respirations are not labored. His blood pressure is 92/66 mm Hg, heart rate is 74 beats/min, respirations are 16 breaths/min, and arterial oxygen saturation is 95%. Your physical examination is remarkable in that the patient cannot feel or move his lower extremities and has no sensation below the level of his umbilicus. His skin is warm, with a brisk capillary refill.

MANAGEMENT

The presentation of the patient in the above scenario is highly suspicious for a spine fracture with spinal cord injury. Since the early 1990s, the use of high-dose IV methylprednisolone (Solu-Medrol) has been the standard of care for the treatment of blunt spinal cord injury.[10,11] The mechanism of action by which steroids assist in blunt spinal cord injury remains unknown. Steroids may decrease the production of damaging oxygen-free radicals, improve blood flow, and limit swelling of the spinal cord.[12-14] Methylprednisolone should not be used in cases in which the spinal cord is injured from penetrating trauma because administration provides no benefit. The administration of steroids at high doses is controversial and associated with a high risk for infection. Refer to local protocols and local medical direction for guidance.

METHYLPREDNISOLONE SODIUM SUCCINATE (SOLU-MEDROL)

Classification: Corticosteroid
Action: Reduces inflammation by multiple mechanisms.
Indications: Anaphylaxis, asthma, COPD.
Adverse Effects: Depression, euphoria, headache, restlessness, hypertension, bradycardia, nausea/vomiting, swelling, diarrhea, weakness, fluid retention, paresthesias.
Contraindications: Cushing's syndrome, fungal infection, measles, varicella, known sensitivity (including sulfites). Use with caution in active infections, renal disease, penetrating spinal cord injury, hypertension, seizures, CHF.

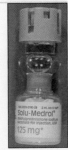

cont'd

METHYLPREDNISOLONE SODIUM SUCCINATE (SOLU-MEDROL)—CONT'D

Dosage:
Asthma and Chronic Obstructive Pulmonary Disease:
- **Adult:** 40 to 80 mg IV.
- **Pediatric:** 1 mg/kg (up to 60 mg) IV, IO per day in two divided doses.

Anaphylactic Shock:
- **Adult:** 1 to 2 mg/kg/dose, then 0.5 to 1 mg/kg every 6 hours.
- **Pediatric:** Same as adult dosing.

Blunt Spinal Cord Injury:
- **Adult:** 30 mg/kg IV, IO over a period of 1 hour, then as an infusion to run for the remaining 23 hours at a dose of 5.4 mg/kg/hr.
- **Pediatric:** Same as adult dosing.

Special Considerations:
May mask signs and symptoms of infection.
Pregnancy class C

REVIEW QUESTIONS

1. Differentiate primary brain injury and secondary brain injury.
2. What are the effects of hypotension and hypoxia on survival from brain injury?
3. List two goals of the treatment of severe traumatic brain injury.
4. How does mannitol decrease brain swelling?
5. When administrating hypertonic saline, should the infusion be administered rapidly or slowly, and why?
6. What is the primary medication used in the treatment of blunt spinal cord injury?

REFERENCES

1. Gabriel EJ, et al: *Guidelines for the prehospital management of traumatic brain injury,* New York, 2000, Brain Trauma Foundation.
2. Miller JD, Becker DB: Secondary insults to the injured brain, *J Royal Coll Surg* 27:292, 1982.
3. Chesnut RM: Avoidance of hypotension: conditio sine qua non of successful severe head-injury management, *J Trauma* 42:S4, 1997.
4. Barry K, Berman A: Mannitol infusion. Part III. The acute effect of the intravenous infusion of mannitol on blood and plasma volume, *N Engl J Med* 264:1085, 1961.
5. Sayre M, et al: Out-of-hospital administration of mannitol to head-injured patients does not change systolic blood pressure, *Acad Emerg Med* 3:840, 1996.
6. Freshman SH, et al: Hypertonic saline versus mannitol: a comparison for treatment of acute head injuries, *J Trauma* 35:344, 1993.
7. Hartl R, et al: Hypertonic/hyperoncotic saline reliably reduces ICP in severely head-injured patients with intracranial hypertension, *Acta Neurochirugia* 70:126, 1997.
8. Mattox KL, et al: Prehospital hypertonic saline/dextran infusion for post-traumatic hypotension, *Ann Surg* 213:482, 1991.
9. Wade CE, et al: Individual patient cohort analysis of the efficacy of hypertonic saline/dextran in patients with traumatic brain injury and hypotension, *J Trauma* 42:561, 1997.
10. Bracken MB, Shepard MJ, Collins WF: A randomized, controlled trial methylprednisolone or naloxone in the treatment of acute spinal-cord injury, *N Engl J Med* 322:1405, 1990.
11. Bracken MB, et al: Methylprednisolone or naloxone treatment after acute spinal cord injury: 1 year follow-up data, *J Neurosurg* 76:23, 1992.
12. Amar PA, Levy ML: Pathogenesis and pharmacological strategies for mitigating secondary damage in acute spinal cord injury, *Neurosurgery* 44(5):1027-1039, 1999.
13. Tator CH: Experimental and clinical studies of the pathophysiology and management of acute spinal cord injury, *J Spinal Cord Med* 19:206, 1996.
14. Zeidman SM, et al: Clinical applications of pharmacologic therapies for spinal cord injury, *J Spinal Disord* 9:367, 1996.

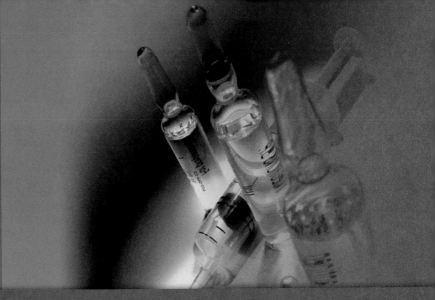

PART

III

Special Considerations and Procedures

Critical Care Transport

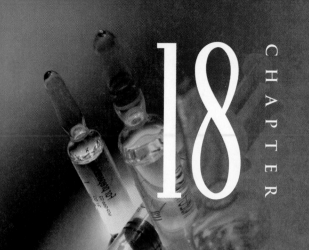

OBJECTIVES

1. Define the following transport equipment: intravenous lines, flow controllers, pressure bags, infusion sets, intravenous pumps, drug calculators, and fluid warmers.
2. Discuss medications used in transport for the treatment of HELLP syndrome: dexamethasone (Decadron), magnesium sulfate, phenytoin (Dilantin), hydralazine (Apresoline), and labetalol (Trandate, Normodyne).
3. Discuss medications used in transport for treatment after cardiac arrest or myocardial infarction: vecuronium (Norcuron), amiodarone (Cordarone), midazolam (Versed), and eptifibatide (Integrilin).
4. Discuss medications used in transport for the treatment of closed-head injury: propofol (Diprivan), fentanyl citrate (Sublimaze), and mannitol (Osmitrol).
5. Describe the Parkland formula, the Wallace rule of nines, and the rule of palms in treating patients with burn injury.
6. List signs and symptoms of a blood transfusion reaction.

Medications that Appear in Chapter 18

Dexamethasone (Decadron)
Magnesium sulfate
Phenytoin (Dilantin)
Hydralazine (Apresoline)
Labetalol (Normodyne, Trandate)
Midazolam (Versed)
Amiodarone (Cordarone)
Eptifibatide (Integrilin)
Vecuronium (Norcuron)
Insulin, Regular (Humulin R, Novolin R)
Propofol (Diprivan)
Fentanyl citrate (Sublimaze)
Mannitol (Osmitrol)

INTRODUCTION

Critical care transport can include air medical transport from the scene, as well as ground and air transport from one facility to another. Paramedics typically are quite familiar with the transport of patients from the scene to the hospital. However, interfacility transport involves different patient management strategies, multiple medications, and advanced procedures. Although paramedics are not expected to know every drug used in the medical field, familiarity with commonly used critical care drugs encountered during transport is beneficial. This chapter pulls together the challenges of prolonged transport of critically ill patients and incorporates concepts of drug therapy, safety of administration, medication math, and medication administration equipment.

TRANSPORT EQUIPMENT

Familiarity with equipment is an important aspect of critical care transport. This includes IV lines, flow controllers, pressure bags, infusions sets, and IV pumps. (Although some of this equipment may also be presented elsewhere in this text, its inclusion here is specific to the discussion of critical care transport.)

INTRAVENOUS LINES

IV lines are available in several forms. A **peripheral line** is a 14- to 24-gauge catheter inserted into a peripheral vein. A **central venous catheter** (also known as a *central line*) is a special IV catheter inserted into a central vein to allow the quick administration of medications and large volumes of fluid.

The most common central line is a **triple-lumen catheter (TLC)** (Fig. 18-1). It has three ports that are typically color coded: distal, medial, and proximal. Because these catheters are made by several manufacturers, the ends of the catheters must be read to determine their placement. The distal port is the end of the catheter. This port can be used for central venous pressure monitoring, as well. The medial port is between the distal and proximal ports. The proximal port is at the end of the catheter closest to the exit from the patient.

Peripherally inserted central catheters (PICC lines) are also common (Fig. 18-2). This catheter's entry point usually is an upper extremity, with the end of the catheter in a central vein. PICC lines must be regularly flushed to prevent clotting. Some patients have implantable devices, such as MediPorts (Bard Access Systems, Salt Lake City, Utah) or Portacaths (Smiths Medical, Colonial Way, Watford [UK]). These types of catheters typically are inserted in patients with a chronic medical condition that requires frequent administration of IV medications. A common indication would be a patient with a malignancy needing chemotherapy. A **Huber needle** is a special needle that must be used to access these ports (Fig. 18-3).

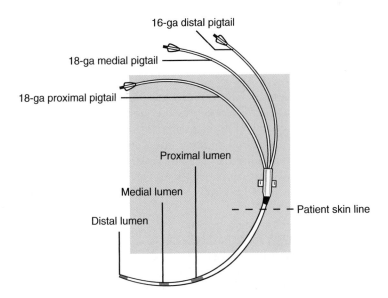

▼ **Fig. 18-1** Triple-lumen catheter (TLC). (From Macklin D, Chernecky C: *Real world nursing survival guide: IV therapy,* St Louis, 2004, Saunders.)

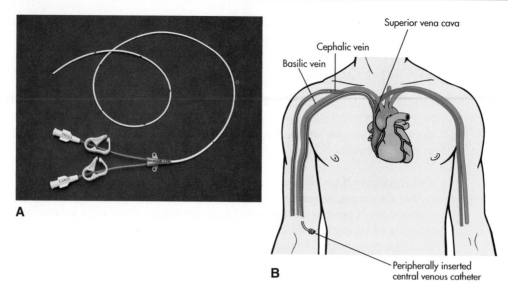

▼ **Fig. 18-2** **A,** PICC line. **B,** Placement of PICC line. (**A** from Aehlert B: *Mosby's comprehensive pediatric emergency care,* rev, St Louis, 2007, Mosby. **B** from Perry AG, Potter PA: *Clinical nursing skills and techniques,* ed 6, St Louis, 2006, Mosby.)

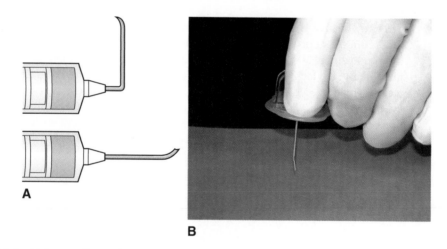

▼ **Fig. 18-3** Huber needle used to access implantable devices such as MediPorts and Portacaths. **A,** Two Huber needles used to enter implanted part. **B,** Insertion of Huber needle. (From Perry AG, Potter PA: *Clinical nursing skills and techniques,* ed 6, St Louis, 2006, Mosby.)

Patients occasionally have an **arterial line** in place, which is an invasive line used for continuous blood pressure monitoring. The set includes pressurized tubing, a transducer, and a bag of normal saline inside a **pressure bag.** The pressure bag is required to prevent the backflow of blood into the tubing from the arterial system. If you transport a patient with an arterial line but your monitor does not have the capability to monitor invasive blood pressure, simply prepare the patient with the attached pressure bag. Arterial lines are used only for monitoring. Do not administer any medications or fluids into these lines.

FLOW CONTROLLERS

Flow controllers that are not part of a traditional infusion pump are sometimes used during critical care transport. The most commonly used flow controller is the Dial-A-Flo (Cardinal Health, Inc., San Diego, Calif.) (Fig. 18-4), which can be connected to the IV tubing as an extension set, allowing the paramedic to adjust a dial and ultimately deliver a set volume of fluid.

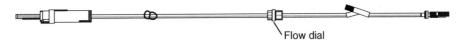

▼ **Fig. 18-4** Dial-A-Flo flow controller. (Flow regulator set distributed by Cardinal Health, Inc., San Diego, Calif.)

PRESSURE BAGS

A pressure bag can be used in several different ways. By inflating a pressure bag over IV fluids, the paramedic can increase the amount of volume delivered to the patient at any given time. For example, when transporting a burn victim who needs increased fluids to maintain a normotensive blood pressure, the fluids can be placed in a pressure bag. Pressure bags are used to increase the rate of IV administration beyond what is possible with simply placing the IV bag to wide-open flow with only gravity. When high IV flow rates are required, a pressure bag is often necessary. A patient need not be hypotensive to require a pressure bag.

Two types of pressure bags allow the paramedic to accommodate either 500-mL or 1000-mL bags of fluid. The setup of both bags is the same: a slot for placement of the IV fluid, a connector from the bag to a balloon pump, a valve regulator, and an attached stopcock (Fig. 18-5). The stopcock must be in the lateral (perpendicular to the tubing) position to inflate the bag. Once the bag is inflated to the desired pressure of 300 mm Hg, a green regulator valve appears. If the bag is overinflated, a red regulator valve appears, prompting a decrease in pressure. The stopcock must be turned upward to maintain the pressure in the bag. When the bag is ready to be deflated, simply turn it downward.

> When administering IV fluids with a pressure bag, aspirate any air from the IV fluid bag to avoid an air embolism.

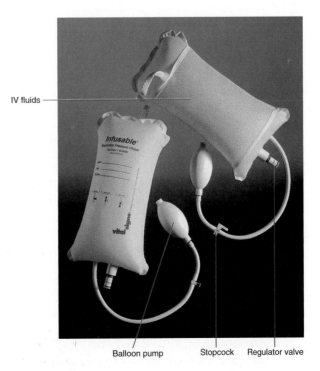

▼ **Fig. 18-5** A 1000-mL pressure bag. (Courtesy Vital Signs, Inc., Totowa, NJ.)

INFUSION SETS

Paramedics must be familiar with the different types of **infusion sets** that may be used in an interfacility transport. Infusion sets are used in the administration of IV fluids through peripheral or central venous catheters. The four main types of infusion sets are **macrodrip, microdrip, blood tubing sets,** and **volume-control chamber** sets. Each of these infusion sets can also be packaged for use as an infusion pump. In addition, infusion sets can be vented or nonvented. **Multidrip infusion sets** are widely used.

Macrodrip Infusion Sets

Macrodrip infusion sets allow the administration of 1 mL of fluid in 10 to 15 drops, depending on the set (Fig. 18-6, *A*). They are used to administer rapid infusions and basic maintenance fluids such as normal saline and Ringer's lactate solution.

Microdrip Infusion Sets

Microdrip infusion sets can administer 1 mL of fluid in 60 drops, which makes drug calculations easier for administration without the use of a pump (Fig. 18-6, *B*). For example, 1 mL/min equals 60 drops in 1 minute (or 1 drop every second). For use in practice, determine the number of milliliters needed per minute to determine drip rate.

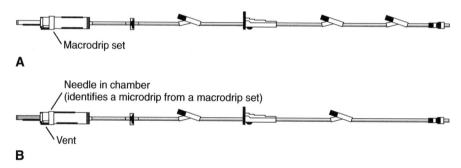

A, Macrodrip set

Needle in chamber
(identifies a microdrip from a macrodrip set)

B, Vent

▼ Fig. 18-6   **A,** Macrodrip infusion set. **B,** Microdrip infusion set. (Courtesy Cardinal Health, Inc., San Diego, Calif.)

> When you grab an infusion set during an emergency, remember this: a needle in the middle of the drip chamber means it is a *micro* set (which makes calculations easier). No needle means it is a *macro* set.

Blood Tubing Sets

Blood tubing sets are usually found as Y-type blood sets. They deliver approximately 10 drops/mL with an integrated blood filter. The Y-type set allows the administration of an infusion of both normal saline and blood at the same time.

> Normal saline is the only IV fluid compatible with the administration of blood.

Volume-Control Chamber Sets

Volume-control chamber sets are used to prevent fluid overloading in patients (Fig. 18-7). For example, a volume-control chamber set can be used when transporting a pediatric patient to prevent the administration of excessive amounts of fluids. To use a volume-control chamber set properly, first fill it with the desired amount of fluid. Then set the clamp between the IV fluid and the volume-control chamber for the remainder of the administration. The clamp between the volume-control chamber and the patient can now be opened for safe administration of fluids or medications. IV infusions can be injected in the volume-control chamber and diluted with the IV fluids to be administered over a specific period.

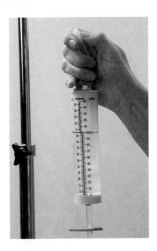

▼ **Fig. 18-7**   The volume-control chamber provides an additional level of safety to avoid inadvertent infusion of fluids to a pediatric patient or other volume-sensitive patient. (From Potter PA, Perry AG: *Fundamentals of nursing*, ed 7, St Louis, 2009, Mosby.)

Vented and Nonvented Infusion Sets

Vented infusion sets are necessary for the administration of fluids packaged in glass containers, such as nitroglycerin, eptifibatide (Integrilin), propofol (Diprivan), and albumin. To distinguish vented and nonvented sets, look at the tubing itself. Vented sets have a side port at the drip chamber that can be opened to allow air to flow into the closed fluid container. **Nonvented infusion sets** do not have a port for air to flow into the closed fluid container. Nonvented sets are used for fluids not packaged in glass containers, such as crystalloid solutions. Medications packaged in glass containers must be administered with a vented set so that the tubing line can be primed with the medication because of the vacuum created from the fluid.

You just grabbed a nonvented set and are hanging mannitol. What should you do? Insert an 18- to 20-gauge needle into the spike insertion port on the glass bottle, allowing air into the bottle so that the fluid can flow with gravity.

Multidrip Infusion Sets

A new infusion set being widely used is the multidrip infusion set (Fig. 18-8). The most widely used set is the SELEC-3 system (Biomedix Inc., St. Paul, Minn.). This system allows the paramedic to alternate among a 10-, 15-, and 60-drop set on one system. It is a quick, easy, and cost-effective way to make changes to the infusion rate without changing drip sets. The drop number can be changed by twisting the drip chamber to the desired drip set.

INTRAVENOUS PUMPS

The most commonly used **IV pump** for critical care transport is a three-channel pump, which allows the administration of three separate drugs. Multichannel pumps are lightweight devices that are easier to transport (Fig. 18-9). They are equipped with technology that integrates a drug calculator into the system. The Minimed system (Baxter, Deerfield, Ill.), which typically is used with a three-channel pump, can be used with two types of infusion sets. The first is a traditional spike set with a pump chamber, known as a *whole set*. The second set has a pump chamber without a spike set, known as a *half set*. Half sets can be used with a 60-mL syringe and attached to the carrying case for the infusion pump.

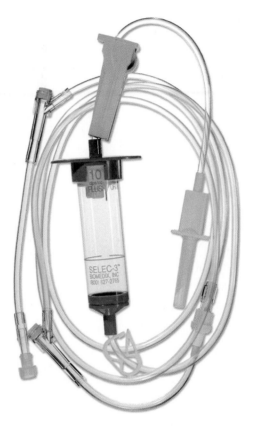

▼ **Fig. 18-8**   Biomedix SELEC-3 IV system multidrip infusion set. (Courtesy Biomedix, Inc., St. Paul, Minn.)

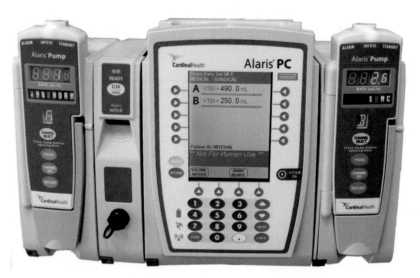

▼ **Fig. 18-9**   Multichannel infusion system. (Courtesy Cardinal Health, Inc., Dublin, Ohio.)

Of note, when using a syringe for the administration of medications, an alarm may sound. The pump will ask for confirmation that the pulling pressures are appropriate. Once the pulling pressures are adequate, a checkmark appears on the display screen for the malfunctioned channel.

A syringe system is helpful to decrease bulk when transporting a patient. A syringe system uses a large syringe containing the medication. The entire syringe is placed in a pump calibrated to compress the plunger of the syringe slowly and deliver the medication at the desired infusion rate. The syringe decreases the risk involved with transporting a patient on multiple drips supplied in glass bottles. However, when using the syringe with the half set, note the time of transport. If necessary, draw up an additional syringe while at the transferring facility to ensure enough of the desired medication is available during transport—or revert to the spike set. The half set with syringe helps decrease the number of air bubbles in the tubing by gently pushing the fluid through the system.

If problems arise while using any pump system, most systems provide on-screen, step-by-step instructions to resolve the problem. Infusion pumps are quite sensitive to air, so all air must be removed from the IV tubing before inserting the pump chamber on the tubing in the system. This is most commonly avoided with syringes so that the fluid is pushed through the tubing to clear the line. Because each infusion pump is different, knowledge of the infusion sets, setup procedures, and maintenance of your particular system is vital.

A wide variety of pumps and infusion sets used in the hospital setting are not frequently seen in EMS. EMS systems and other healthcare agencies use both non-needle and needle administration infusion sets. Paramedics in critical care transport must be prepared for both types of injection ports. As detailed in this chapter, filter needles are necessary for the safe administration of certain medications. A filter needle looks like a conventional needle but has the added ability to filter out solid material that may be floating in the fluids. Filter needles can be used when inline IV tubing filters are not available. They are also used to draw medications from glass ampules.

USE OF A VOLUMETRIC SYRINGE

Equipment needed:
Volumetric pump, syringe, IV tubing, sharps, PPE, medication, gloves
Procedure:
1. Observe universal precautions.
2. Verify drug order.
3. Confirm right patient, right medication, right dose, right route, and right time.
4. Confirm with the patient that he or she has no allergies to the medication, and document allergies to any other medication.
5. When possible, explain to the patient what medication you are going to administer and why.
6. Turn the pump on, and calculate the required amount of fluid to be infused during transport. For a portable unit, turn on the pump and check its battery life before beginning medication administration. If the battery is low, plug in the pump.
7. Draw the medication into the syringe, expelling all of the air.
8. Attach the syringe to a port on the tubing that does not have a drip set.
9. Place the syringe into the pump you are using, and administer the medication.
10. Record the time of drug administration in the patient care record.
11. Evaluate the patient for desired effects of the medication, as well as any adverse effects. Continued reevaluation should occur throughout transport.

USE OF A VOLUMETRIC PUMP

Equipment needed:
Volumetric pump, medication, gloves, IV tubing
Procedure:
1. Observe universal precautions.
2. Verify drug order.
3. Confirm right patient, right medication, right dose, right route, and right time.
4. Confirm with the patient that he or she has no allergies to the medication, and document allergies to any other medication.

5. When possible, explain to the patient what medication you are going to administer and why.
6. Turn the pump on, and prime the medication tubing to ensure all air is out of the system so that no alarms sound. For a portable unit, turn on the pump and check its battery life before beginning medication administration. If the battery is low, plug in the pump.
7. Select the channel to administer the medication. Then insert the cassette into the channel on the pump.
8. Close the channel door, and then select the channel from the main menu.
9. Choose the infusion type, either drug calculator or rate, and volume to be infused.
10. Select the rate, and program that number into the pump. Select the volume to be infused, and program that number into the pump.
11. Attach the tubing to the patient, and begin infusion.
12. Record the time of drug administration in the patient care record.
13. Evaluate the patient for desired effects of the medication, as well as any adverse effects. Continued reevaluation should occur throughout transport.

DRUG CALCULATORS

Because most infusion systems integrate drug calculators, knowledge of how to access the calculators and configure the pump for transport is important. Although the drug calculator includes information on only a limited number of medications, it can be quite advantageous. The drug calculator can make titration of critical medication quicker and easier, which also helps prevent medication administration errors.

FLUID WARMERS

Patients who require rapid fluid resuscitation or large amounts of transfused blood are at risk for developing hypothermia.[1] A **fluid warmer** can help prevent hypothermia in such situations (Figure 18-10). If your unit does not carry a fluid warmer, request that your service obtain a soft-sided cooler and heating pad.

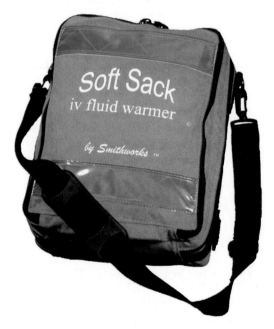

▼ **Fig. 18-10**   Fluid warmer. (Courtesy Smithworks, Clarkston, Wash.)

COMMON CRITICAL CARE TRANSPORT SCENARIOS

Several common scenarios exist in which a paramedic can be called to assist in the care of critical patients during transport between hospitals. These scenarios include **HELLP**

syndrome, status following cardiac arrest or myocardial infarction, diabetic ketoacidosis, closed-head injury, burn injury, and blood administration.

HELLP SYNDROME

HELLP syndrome is an acronym for a condition characterized by *h*emolysis, *e*levated *l*iver enzymes, and *l*ow *p*latelets. The syndrome, which is believed to be a variant of pre-eclampsia, occurs during the second half of pregnancy. The cause of HELLP syndrome is not well understood, but the result is deposition of fibrin in the lumen of blood vessels and the production of several endogenous factors that can result in multiorgan dysfunction.[2,3]

Management

Treatment considerations are primarily geared toward correcting the low platelet count and hypertension and preventing seizures.[4] The treatment that the paramedic provides during transport likely is based on laboratory findings identified at the referring hospital. Drugs often used in this treatment include dexamethasone, magnesium sulfate, phenytoin, hydralazine, and labetalol.

Dexamethasone (Decadron) is central in the treatment of HELLP syndrome. The appropriate dosage of steroids is a controversial subject in the reviewed literature. Historically, dexamethasone at a dosage of 10 mg IV every 12 hours has been shown to improve blood pressure, urine output, platelet count, and liver function. On the other hand, studies have suggested that high-dose steroids decrease the acuity of the syndrome and concurrently reduce the need for additional treatments. Further research is needed to investigate the efficiency of low-dose versus high-dose steroid therapy.[2] Some research suggests that corticosteroids have no effect on the outcome of the mother but may help accelerate lung development in the fetus. Prehospital professionals may encounter the administration of both high-dose and low-dose therapy and must be familiar with both indications. Ultimately, the administration of steroids helps prolong the time to delivery of the baby, which allows the transfer of the patient to a tertiary care center. In addition, maturation of the fetal lungs has been shown to improve with the administration of steroids.

DEXAMETHASONE (DECADRON)

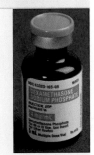

Classification: Corticosteroid
Action: Reduces inflammation and immune responses.
Indications: Various inflammatory conditions, adrenal insufficiency, nonresponsive forms of shock.
Adverse Effects: Nausea/vomiting, edema, hypertension, hyperglycemia, immunosuppression.
Contraindications: Fungal infections, known sensitivity.
Dosage:
  · **Adult:** 1 to 6 mg/kg IV to a maximum dose of 40 mg.
  · **Pediatric:** 0.03 to 0.3 mg/kg IV, IO divided into doses every 6 hours.
Special Considerations:
Pregnancy class C

Seizures are commonly associated with the development of HELLP syndrome, and the treatment of choice for seizures from eclampsia is magnesium sulfate. Therefore magnesium sulfate is administered for the prophylactic treatment of seizures in these patients. Magnesium can cause toxicity in patients, and certain aspects must be monitored during transport, such as urine output, deep tendon reflexes, and respiratory depression. Magnesium is superior to phenytoin for the prevention and treatment of eclampsia and associated seizures. However, if magnesium sulfate is contraindicated in the patient, phenytoin (Dilantin) is the alternative drug of choice. The patient's blood pressure and heart rate must be monitored at least every 5 minutes for associated side effects of phenytoin. The therapeutic range is narrow for this drug, and adverse effects can develop.

MAGNESIUM SULFATE

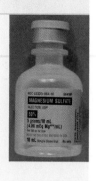

Classification: Electrolyte, tocolytic, mineral

Action: Required for normal physiologic functioning. Magnesium is a cofactor in neurochemical transmission and muscular excitability. Magnesium sulfate controls seizures by blocking peripheral neuromuscular transmission. Magnesium is also a peripheral vasodilator and an inhibitor of platelet function.

Indications: Torsades de pointes, cardiac arrhythmias associated with hypomagnesemia, eclampsia and seizure prophylaxis in preeclampsia, status asthmaticus.

Adverse Effects: Magnesium toxicity (signs include flushing, diaphoresis, hypotension, muscle paralysis, weakness, hypothermia, and cardiac, CNS, or respiratory depression).

Contraindications: AV block, GI obstruction. Use with caution in renal impairment.

Dosage:

Pulseless Ventricular Fibrillation/Ventricular Tachycardia with Torsades de Pointes or Hypomagnesemia:

- **Adult:** 1 to 2 g in 10 mL D_5W IV, IO administered over 5 to 10 minutes.
- **Pediatric:** 25 to 50 mg/kg IV, IO over 10 to 20 minutes; may administer faster for torsades de pointes (max single dose: 2 g).

Torsades de Pointes with a Pulse or Cardiac Arrhythmias with Hypomagnesemia:

- **Adult:** 1 to 2 g in 50 to 100 mL D_5W IV, IO administered over 5 to 60 minutes. Follow with 0.5 to 1 g/hr IV, IO titrated to control torsades de pointes.
- **Pediatric:** 25 to 50 mg/kg IV, IO over 10 to 20 minutes (max single dose: 2 g).

Eclampsia and Seizure Prophylaxis in Preeclampsia:

- **Adult:** 4 to 6 g IV, IO over 20 to 30 minutes, followed by an infusion of 1 to 2 g/hr.

Status Asthmaticus:

- **Adult:** 1.2 to 2 g slow IV, IO (over 20 minutes).
- **Pediatric:** 25 to 50 mg/kg (diluted in D_5W) slow IV, IO (over 10 to 20 minutes).

Special Considerations:

Pregnancy class A

PHENYTOIN (DILANTIN)

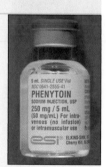

Classification: Anticonvulsant

Action: Depresses seizures by affecting the movement of sodium and calcium into neural tissue.

Indications: Generalized tonic-clonic seizures.

Adverse Effects: Nausea/vomiting, depression of cardiac conduction, sedation, nystagmus, tremors, ataxia, dysarthria, gingival hypertrophy, hirsutism, facial coarsening, hypotension.

Contraindications: Sinus bradycardia, sinoatrial block, second- and third-degree heart block, Adams-Stokes syndrome, known sensitivity to hydantoins.

Dosage:

- **Adult:** 15 to 20 mg/kg IV, IO should be administered slowly at a rate not exceeding 50 mg/min (this requires approximately 20 minutes in a 70-kg patient).
- **Pediatric:** 15 to 20 mg/kg IV, IO, administered at a rate of 1 to 3 mg/kg/min.

Special Considerations:

Continuously monitor the ECG and blood pressure during administration. Pregnancy class D

The hypertension associated with HELLP syndrome must be treated to improve the prognosis of both mother and baby. A decrease in blood pressure reduces the risk of placental abruption, seizure activity, and maternal cerebral hemorrhage. Hydralazine (Apresoline) is a commonly used medication for the treatment of maternal hypertension. It should be initiated with a systolic blood pressure greater than 160 mm Hg or a diastolic pressure greater than 105 mm Hg.[4] Labetalol is an alternative medication that can cause less maternal hypotension than hydralazine. A detailed discussion of hydralazine and other medications used in pregnancy-related hypertension is found in Chapter 19.

HYDRALAZINE (APRESOLINE)

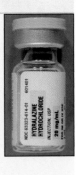

Classification: Antihypertensive agent, vasodilator
Action: Directly dilates the peripheral blood vessels.
Indications: Hypertension associated with preeclampsia and eclampsia, hypertensive crisis.
Adverse Effects: Headache, angina, flushing, palpitations, reflex tachycardia, anorexia, nausea/vomiting, diarrhea, hypotension, syncope, peripheral vasodilation, peripheral edema, fluid retention, paresthesias.
Contraindications: Patients taking diazoxide or MAOIs, coronary artery disease, stroke, angina, dissecting aortic aneurysm, mitral valve and rheumatic heart diseases.
Dosage:
Preeclampsia and Eclampsia:
· **Adult:** 5 to 10 mg IV, IO. Repeat every 20 to 30 minutes until systolic blood pressure of 90 to 105 mm Hg is attained.
Acute Hypertension Not Associated with Preeclampsia:
· **Adult:** 10 to 20 mg IV, IO, or IM.
· **Pediatric:**
  · **1 month to 12 years:** 0.1 to 0.6 mg/kg IV, IO, or IM (max: 20 mg/dose).
Special Considerations:
Pregnancy class C

LABETALOL (NORMODYNE, TRANDATE)

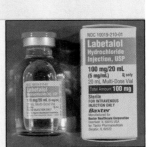

Classification: Beta adrenergic antagonist, antianginal, antihypertensive
Action: Binds with both the beta$_1$ and beta$_2$ receptors and alpha$_1$ receptors in vascular smooth muscle. Inhibits the strength of the heart's contractions, as well as heart rate. This results in a decrease in cardiac oxygen consumption.
Indications: ACS, SVT, severe hypertension.
Adverse Effects: Usually mild and transient; hypotensive symptoms, nausea/vomiting, bronchospasm, arrhythmia, bradycardia, AV block.
Contraindications: Hypotension, cardiogenic shock, acute pulmonary edema, heart failure, severe bradycardia, sick sinus syndrome, second- or third-degree heart block, asthma or acute bronchospasm, cocaine-induced ACS, known sensitivity. Use caution in pheochromocytoma, cerebrovascular disease or stroke, poorly controlled diabetes, with hepatic disease. Use with caution at lowest effective dose in chronic lung disease.
Dosage:
Cardiac Indications: Note: Monitor blood pressure and heart rate closely during administration.
  Adult: 10 mg IV, IO over a 1- to 2-minute period. May repeat every 10 minutes to a maximum dose of 150 mg or give initial bolus and then follow with infusion at 2 to 8 mg/min.
  Pediatric: 0.4 to 1 mg/kg/hr to a maximum dosage of 3 mg/kg/hr.
Severe Hypertension:
· **Adult:** Initial dose is 20 mg IV, IO slow infusion over a 2-minute period. After the initial dose, blood pressure should be checked every 5 minutes. Repeat doses can be given at 10-minute intervals. The second dose should be 40 mg IV, IO, and subsequent doses should be 80 mg IV, IO, to a maximum total dose of 300 mg. The effect on blood pressure typically will occur within 5 minutes from the time of administration. Alternatively, may be administered via IV infusion at 2 mg/min to a total maximum dose of 300 mg.
· **Pediatric:** 0.4 to 1 mg/kg/hr IV, IO infusion with a maximum dose of 3 mg/kg/hr.
Special Considerations:
Pregnancy class C

Y ou arrive at a small community hospital to transport a 22-year-old woman who is 8 months pregnant and has been diagnosed with HELLP syndrome. The patient is receiving an infusion of dexamethasone, magnesium sulfate, and hydralazine. You have a multichannel infusion pump. The patient has a 20-gauge IV in her right hand, and all three medications are infusing through this site. ...

Two questions arise from the previous scenario: Are the three medications compatible? Does the paramedic need additional access?

Magnesium sulfate is not compatible with either of the other medications. When administering multiple medications, paramedics should consult a drug compatibility reference. Additional access is needed. After the initiation of an 18-gauge IV in the left antecubital fossa, the paramedic would be ready to transfer the medications to the infusion pump. A syringe and half set could be used. The paramedic would label the syringe with the medication and concentration to calculate a drip rate in the event of a pump failure.

> ... During transport, the patient has decreased level of consciousness with decreased respiratory rate, decreased urine output by Foley catheter, and absent deep tendon reflexes.

Magnesium sulfate toxicity is the likely culprit in the previous scenario. The treatment for magnesium toxicity includes the administration of 10 to 20 mL of 10% calcium gluconate IV push. Calcium gluconate should be on board when an interfacility patient being infused with magnesium is transported. When transporting a patient receiving a specific medication, be familiar with the adverse effects and how to reverse them.[4]

TREATMENT AFTER CARDIAC ARREST OR INFERIOR MYOCARDIAL INFARCTION

> Your helicopter has been dispatched for the interfacility transport of a 55-year-old man who sustained an inferior myocardial infarction with a ventricular fibrillation arrest approximately 1 hour ago. The patient has been resuscitated. You arrive to find the patient intubated, chemically sedated, and paralyzed. The following infusions are running: vecuronium (Norcuron), midazolam (Versed), amiodarone (Cordarone), and eptifibatide (Integrilin). You are transporting the patient to a tertiary care center 30 minutes away by air for an immediate cardiac catheterization. The patient weighs 220 lb. ...

Management

Because this patient has myocardial ischemia and a dangerous cardiac arrhythmia, the goals of the paramedic during transport are to prevent additional cardiac ischemia with eptifibatide (Integrilin), prevent additional cardiac arrhythmias with amiodarone (Cordarone), and continue appropriate sedation with a midazolam (Versed) infusion and neuromuscular paralysis with vecuronium (Norcuron).

The patient is currently receiving four drug infusions; when multichannel pumps are used, only three medications can be connected to the electronic pump. Therefore in the above scenario, one of the medications should be put on a Dial-A-Flo or converted to an IV bolus. During air transport, a Dial-A-Flo works only with the addition of pressure to the system because of the decrease in atmospheric pressure and the close proximity of the bag to the patient.

An aircraft has no room for IV poles; both rotor and fixed-wing aircraft have profound space limitations. Therefore the IV bag may rest directly on the patient or be elevated only inches above the patient. However, when in an ambulance, hang the IV bag several feet above the patient.

> Next time you start an IV on a patient, watch how the drip rate increases when you elevate the bag and how it decreases when you lower the IV bag. This concept is the same one that led cities to build water towers on hills.

In the previous case study, the paramedic could use a pressure bag. Continuing the scenario, you administer midazolam (Versed), amiodarone (Cordarone), and eptifibatide (Integrilin) by electronic pump. The vecuronium (Norcuron) infusion will run without a pump. To maintain the vecuronium infusion, you place the medication bag into a pressure bag and add a Dial-A-Flo. A vecuronium infusion traditionally is mixed in a 100-mL bag of fluid, which would make the use of a pressure bag quite difficult. One dose of vecuronium as a bolus is easier to administer than the use of additional equipment. Vecuronium has a duration of action of approximately 25 to 40 minutes. Because this will last the duration of the flight, giving the paralytic medication as a bolus rather than an infusion would be more beneficial.

Other transport considerations include the use of half versus full administration sets. Because eptifibatide (Integrilin) is packaged in a glass container, syringes would be beneficial.

MIDAZOLAM (VERSED)

Classification: Benzodiazepine, Schedule C-IV
Action: Binds to the benzodiazepine receptor and enhances the effects of the brain chemical (neurotransmitter) GABA. Benzodiazepines act at the level of the limbic, thalamic, and hypothalamic regions of the CNS to produce short-acting CNS depression (including sedation, skeletal muscle relaxation, and anticonvulsant activity).
Indications: Sedation, anxiety, skeletal muscle relaxation.
Adverse Effects: Respiratory depression, respiratory arrest, hypotension, nausea/vomiting, headache, hiccups, cardiac arrest.
Contraindications: Acute-angle glaucoma, pregnant women, known sensitivity.
Dosage:
Sedation:
Note: The dose of midazolam needs to be individualized. Every dose should be administered slowly over a period of 2 minutes. Allow 2 minutes to evaluate the clinical effect of the dose given.

- **Adult:**
  - **Healthy and younger than 60 years:** *Some patients require as little as 1 mg IV, IO. No more than 2.5 mg should be given over a 2-minute interval.* If additional sedation is required, continue to administer small increments over 2-minute periods (max dose: 5 mg). If the patient also has received a narcotic, he or she will typically require 30% less midazolam than the same patient not given the narcotic.
  - **60 years and older and debilitated or chronically ill patients:** This group of patients has a higher risk of hypoventilation, airway obstruction, and apnea. The peak clinical effect can take longer in these patients; therefore dose increments should be smaller, and the rate of injection should be slower. *Some patients require a dose as small as 1 mg IV, IO, and no more than 1.5 mg should be given over a 2-minute period.* If additional sedation is required, additional midazolam should be given at a rate of no more than 1 mg over a 2-minute period (max dose: 3.5 mg). If the patient also has received a narcotic, he or she will typically require 50% less midazolam than the same patient not given the narcotic.
  - **Continuous infusion:** Continuous infusions can be required for prolonged transport of intubated, critically ill, and injured patients. After an initial bolus dose, the adult patient will require a maintenance infusion dose of 0.02 to 0.1 mg/kg/hr (1-7 mg/hr).
- **Pediatric (weight-based):** Pediatric patients typically require higher doses of midazolam than do adults on the basis of weight (in mg/kg). Younger pediatric patients (younger than 6 years) require higher doses (in mg/kg) than older pediatric patients. Midazolam takes approximately 3 minutes to reach peak effect; therefore wait at least 2 minutes to determine effectiveness of drug and need for additional dosing.
  - **12 to 16 years:** Same as adult dosing. Some patients in this age group require a higher dose than that used in adults, but rarely does a patient require more than 10 mg.
  - **6 to 12 years:** 0.025 to 0.05 mg/kg IV, IO up to a total dose of 0.4 mg/kg. Exceeding 10 mg as total dose usually is not necessary.
  - **6 months to 5 years:** 0.05 to 0.1 mg/kg IV, IO up to a total dose of 0.6 mg/kg. Exceeding 6 mg as total dose usually is not necessary.
  - **Younger than 6 months:** Dosing recommendations for this age group is unclear. Because this age group is especially vulnerable to airway obstruction and hypoventilation, use small increments with frequent clinical evaluation. Dose: 0.05 to 0.1 mg/kg IV, IO.

Special Considerations:
Patients receiving midazolam require frequent monitoring of vital signs and pulse oximetry. Be prepared to support patient's airway and ventilation.
Pregnancy class D

AMIODARONE (CORDARONE)

Classification: Antiarrhythmic, class III
Action: Acts directly on the myocardium to delay repolarization and increase the duration of the action potential.
Indications: Ventricular arrhythmias; second-line agent for atrial arrhythmias.
Adverse Effects: Burning at the IV site, hypotension, bradycardia.
Contraindications: Sick sinus syndrome, second- and third-degree heart block, cardiogenic shock, when episodes of bradycardia have caused syncope, sensitivity to benzyl alcohol and iodine.
Dosage:
Ventricular Fibrillation and Pulseless Ventricular Tachycardia:
- **Adult:** 300 mg IV, IO. May be followed by one dose of 150 mg in 3 to 5 minutes.
- **Pediatric:** 5 mg/kg (max dose: 300 mg); may repeat 5 mg/kg IV, IO up to 15 mg/kg.

Relatively Stable Patients with Arrhythmias such as Premature Ventricular Contractions or Wide-Complex Tachycardias with a Strong Pulse:
- **Adult:** 150 mg in 100 mL D$_5$W IV, IO over a 10-minute period; may repeat in 10 minutes up to a maximum dose of 2.2 g over 24 hours.
- **Pediatric:** 5 mg/kg very slow IV, IO (over 20 to 60 minutes); may repeat in 5-mg/kg doses up to 15 mg/kg (max dose: 300 mg).

Special Considerations:
Pregnancy class D

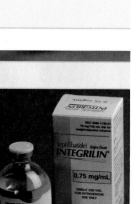

EPTIFIBATIDE (INTEGRILIN)

Classification: GP IIb/IIIa inhibitor
Action: Prevents the aggregation of platelets by binding to the GP IIb/IIIa receptor.
Indications: UA/NSTEMI—to manage medically and for those undergoing percutaneous coronary intervention.
Adverse Effects: Bleeding from the GI tract, internal bleeding, intracranial hemorrhage, hypotension, stroke, anaphylactic shock.
Contraindications: Bleeding from any source, severe uncontrolled hypertension, surgery or trauma within the previous 6 weeks, stroke within the previous 30 days, renal failure, thrombocytopenia.
Dosage:
- **Adult:** Loading dose: 180 mcg/kg IV, IO (max dose: 22.6 mg) over 1 to 2 minutes, then 2 mcg/kg/min IV, IO infusion (max dose: 15 mg/hr).
- **Pediatric:** No current dosing recommendations exist for pediatric patients.

Special Considerations:
Half-life approximately 90 to 120 minutes
Pregnancy class B

VECURONIUM (NORCURON)

Classification: Neuromuscular blocker, nondepolarizing
Action: Antagonizes acetylcholine at the motor end plate, producing skeletal muscle paralysis.
Indications: To induce neuromuscular blockade for the facilitation of ET intubation.
Adverse Effects: Muscle paralysis, apnea, dyspnea, respiratory depression, sinus tachycardia, urticaria.
Contraindications: Known sensitivity to bromides. Use with caution in heart disease, liver disease.
Dosage:
- **Adult:** 0.08 to 0.1 mg/kg IV, IO.
- **Pediatric:** Dosage is individualized.

Special Considerations:
Pregnancy class C

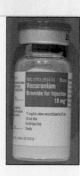

... You are in the middle of transport when a pump channel failure occurs. You are administering midazolam (Versed), amiodarone (Cordarone), and eptifibatide (Integrilin).

In this situation, the best solution would be to convert the midazolam infusion to intermittent boluses. This would continue accurate dosing of the antiarrhythmic and antiplatelet medications for the duration of the flight. If additional pump failures occur, the appropriate dosage should be calculated with a microdrip set.

Eptifibatide (Integrilin) is packaged as 0.75 mg/mL and 2 mg/mL. For the following example, the 0.75 mg/mL preparation is used. The dose is typically 2 mcg/kg per minute before a coronary catheterization. The infusion pump is running at 16 mL/hr.

Calculate the drip rate. This patient should receive 200 mcg/min, or 12,000 mcg/hr or 12 mg/hr.

$$2 \text{ mcg/kg/min} \times 100 \text{ kg} = 200 \text{ mcg/min}$$

$$200 \text{ mcg/min} \times 60 \text{ min/hr} = 12,000 \text{ mcg/hr}$$

$$\text{Convert units: } 12,000 \text{ mcg} \times 1 \text{ mg/1000 mcg} = 12 \text{ mg}$$

Infusion rate:

$$12 \text{ mg/hr} \times 1 \text{ mL/0.75 mg} = 16 \text{ mL/hr}$$

Drip rate:

$$200 \text{ mcg/min} \times 60 \text{ gtt/1 mL} \times 1 \text{ mL/750 mcg} =$$
$$(200 \times 60)/750 = 16 \text{ gtt/min (canceling units: gtt/min; remember, } 0.75 \text{ mg/mL} = 750 \text{ mcg/mL)}$$

With a microdrip set, you would administer 16 gtt/min.

DIABETIC KETOACIDOSIS

You work on a fixed-wing aircraft (airplane) and are called to a small rural hospital in Florida to transfer a 5-year-old girl to Tennessee. The child was on vacation with her parents when she became sick. The only history you have on the patient is that she was diagnosed with type 1 diabetes 6 months ago. Her blood glucose level is currently 450 mg/dL. Her parents have requested that she be transferred to her pediatric endocrinologist in Tennessee. When you arrive at the emergency department (ED), the nurse practitioner notifies you that the patient has been diagnosed with diabetic ketoacidosis (DKA). Her potassium level is 5.0, and pH is 7.28. She is currently on oxygen at 4 L/min by nasal cannula. A left subclavian TLC was placed before your arrival. ...

In the following section, some of the logistical problems of caring for a child in DKA for several hours are identified and explained. A more detailed discussion of DKA and its pharmacologic treatment is found in Chapter 11.

... The patient weighs 25 kg. The nurse practitioner has given her a 250-mL bolus of normal saline for initial hypotension, started insulin at 5.0 U/hr, and initiated normal saline with 20 mEq potassium chloride (KCl). You realize that you need to administer KCl 40 mEq/L of fluid, but the hospital stocks only normal saline with 20 mEq KCl. ...

Management

You need to make some decisions on how to manage the fluids during transport. Next you must decide how to transport the fluids. You typically would use a volume-control chamber, also known as a *buretrol* or *volutrol set* (Baxter, Deerfield, Ill.), to administer fluids to a pediatric patient. Therefore you can use a volume-control chamber set manufactured to fit into an infusion pump or a volume-control chamber that flows strictly to gravity.

Volume-control chamber sets are manufactured in such a way as to provide additional protection against the accidental administration of excessive fluid. In pediatric patients the amount of fluid being administered must be closely monitored to prevent complications of fluid overload. If a volume-control chamber is filled with the desired amount of fluid and clamped off to the bag of fluid, accidental administration of excessive fluid as a result of pump malfunctions is virtually impossible. This type of simple safety device commonly is used to prevent the complication of inadvertent volume overload or drug overdose in children's hospitals and pediatric intensive care units.

Insulin can be drawn into a syringe and infused with a half set through the infusion pump. Insulin is usually mixed at a 1:1 concentration of medication and fluid (e.g., a 100-mL bag of fluids would have 100 U = 1 U/mL). Therefore consider how long the patient will be traveling so that enough medication is on hand. In the previous scenario, the air and travel time to and from the airport is approximately 4.5 hours. Therefore, if insulin is run at 5 U/hr, at least 23 mL are needed for transport (5 U/hr × 4.5 hours = 22.5 U). Filling the syringe to 50 mL to prevent running out of insulin would be wise.

> ... You have safely arrived at the aircraft, and the patient is loaded. Forty-five minutes have passed getting from the hospital to the airport, and you have not checked the patient's blood glucose level. A fingerstick test reveals a glucose level of 380 mg/dL. You have exceeded the 10% per hour of reduction in blood glucose that is safe for the patient (450 × 0.10 = 45, and 450 − 45 = 405). You realize that the hospital did not correctly calculate the insulin infusion and set the pump at a higher dose than 0.1 U/kg per hour. ...

In this situation, the drip must be gradually titrated to reduce the patient's blood glucose level. Based on the patient's weight, the infusion should be delivered at 2.5 U/hr. Suppose you started the pump as a basic infusion, and now you cannot get the pump to use decimals. If the pump has an integrated drug calculator, you should be able to enter the drug calculator, input the appropriate information, and titrate the drip accordingly. If insulin is not integrated into the pump, you can use the dosage calculator. Input your concentration of the drug, weight, and desired dose.

> ... The remainder of the transport goes smoothly until you check the patient's glucose level and realize that it has dropped below 250 mg/dL.

In this situation, you must add dextrose to the IV fluids. However, if you do not have dextrose on board, you can make D_5NS. D_5 is 5 g dextrose per 100 mL fluid. Therefore inject a syringe of D_{50} into a 1-L bag of saline and infuse at the maintenance rate.

In this scenario the paramedic should notify the receiving medical team that the transfer took 4.5 hours and that the potassium level before transfer was 5.0 mg/dL. The receiving team will quickly draw a basic metabolic panel and an arterial blood gas reading to determine whether the patient's hyperkalemia and acidosis are resolving.

INSULIN, REGULAR (HUMULIN R, NOVOLIN R)

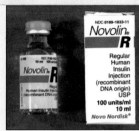

Classification: Hormone
Action: Binds to a receptor on the membrane of cells and facilitates the transport of glucose into cells.
Indications: Hyperglycemia, insulin-dependent diabetes mellitus, hyperkalemia.
Adverse Effects: Hypoglycemia, tachycardia, palpitations, diaphoresis, anxiety, confusion, blurred vision, weakness, depression, seizures, coma, insulin shock, hypokalemia.
Contraindications: Hypoglycemia, known sensitivity.
Dosage:
Diabetic Ketoacidosis:
  · **Adult:** 0.1 U/kg IV, IO, or Sub-Q. Because of poor perfusion of the peripheral tissues, Sub-Q administration is much less effective than the IV, IO route. IV, IO insulin has a very short half-life; therefore IV, IO insulin without an infusion is not that effective. The rate for an insulin infusion is 0.05 to 0.1 U/kg/hr IV, IO. When dosing insulin, use a U-100 insulin syringe to measure and deliver the insulin. The time from administration to action, as well as the duration of action, varies greatly among different individuals, as well as at different times in the same individual.
Hyperkalemia:
  · **Adult:** 10 U IV, IO of regular insulin (Insulin R), coadministered with 50 mL of $D_{50}W$ over 5 minutes.
  · **Pediatric:** 0.1 U/kg Insulin R IV, IO.
Special Considerations:
Only regular insulin can be given IV, IO.
Pregnancy class B

CLOSED-HEAD INJURY

> You are dispatched to transport a 25-year-old man who was involved in an all-terrain vehicle accident. He was not wearing a helmet. He has a closed-head injury with cerebral edema and a left femur fracture immobilized in a traction splint. The patient must be taken by ground because of icy conditions that prevent air transport. You arrive at the hospital to find the patient intubated and sedated with propofol. Mannitol, fentanyl, and a 1-L bolus of Ringer's lactate are infusing, as well. The patient weighs 220 lb. ...

Management

Transporting a patient with a traumatic brain injury (TBI) can be complex. The most concerning TBI is the closed-head injury with increased intracranial pressure (ICP). In these patients the goal of treatment is to help decrease swelling while supporting the patient's physiologic status. Increased cerebral edema can result in herniation, but it can also cause a decrease in the amount of perfusion to the brain.

Monitoring blood pressure is essential in the transport of a patient with a closed-head injury. Cerebral blood flow is calculated by the difference between the mean arterial pressure (MAP) and the ICP divided by the cerebral vascular resistance. Cerebral perfusion averages 50 mL of blood per 100 g of brain tissue per minute. Because of the difficulty in calculating the cerebral blood flow clinically, the cerebral perfusion pressure (CPP) is used. CPP is calculated from the MAP and ICP. A goal of 70 for the CPP is needed to ensure adequate cerebral perfusion. Therefore increases in ICP and decreases in MAP can result in insufficient blood flow to the brain.[5] A systolic blood pressure of at least 110 mm Hg is needed to ensure minimal blood flow to the brain. In cases in which high ICP is suspected, systolic blood pressure must be higher.

MAP is determined by the following formula:

$$(1/3\ SBP - DBP) + DBP = MAP$$

where SBP is systolic blood pressure and DBP is diastolic blood pressure. Cerebral perfusion pressure is determined by the following formula:

$$MAP - ICP = CPP$$

MAP can be calculated from the blood pressure or given as a digital readout from an automatic blood pressure machine. ICP is typically measured with an external ventricular drain. Because measuring ICP is impractical during transport, rough estimates can be determined by observing patients for signs and symptoms. Altered mental status, nausea, projectile vomiting, and unequal pupils can be signs of increasing ICP.

The Brain Trauma Foundation has issued recommendations for the prehospital transport of patients with TBI. A MAP of greater than 90 mm Hg with an ICP of 20 mm Hg results in a CPP of at least 70 mm Hg. If a patient has a systolic blood pressure less than 110 mm Hg, fluid resuscitation is necessary. Sedation and neuromuscular blocking agents may be needed to help control oxygenation and ventilation to ensure an appropriate carbon dioxide level. Continuous oxygen saturation monitoring is recommended, with a desired level of greater than 90%. In an unresponsive patient with extensor posturing and flaccidity, the recommended ventilation rates are 20 breaths/min for adults, 30 breaths/min for children, and 35 to 40 breaths/min for infants. According to the Brain Trauma Foundation, this is considered hyperventilation. In the absence of signs of herniation, avoid hyperventilation. In patients without posturing or flaccidity, a carbon dioxide level of 35 to 40 mm Hg is desired. Use end-tidal carbon dioxide monitoring to calculate the patient's carbon dioxide level. However, keep in mind that expired carbon dioxide is 3 to 5 mm Hg lower than arterial carbon dioxide.[6]

... The patient's blood pressure is 90/40 mm Hg. This translates into an MAP of 57 mm Hg and a possible CPP of 37 mm Hg. Therefore the patient is receiving a fluid bolus to improve the blood pressure. ...

Propofol (Diprivan) is the hypnotic medication of choice for patients with closed-head injuries because it decreases cerebral metabolism, thus decreasing oxygen consumption. It is also easily titrated and has a short half-life, allowing an accurate neurologic examination at the hospital. Propofol is a phenol derivative classified as an anesthetic. It is used for induction and maintenance of anesthesia, as well as sedation in intubated patients in intensive care. The mechanism of action is dose dependent and causes central nervous system depression resembling that caused by benzodiazepines and barbiturates, with rapid hypnosis and minimal excitation. Onset of action is approximately 10 to 40 seconds, and duration is 3 to 10 minutes. Propofol is a medication with limited application in prehospital care.

PROPOFOL (DIPRIVAN)

Classification: Anesthetic

Action: Produces rapid and brief state of general anesthesia.

Indications: Anesthesia induction.

Adverse Effects: Apnea, cardiac arrhythmias, asystole, hypotension, hypertension, pain at injection site.

Contraindications: Hypovolemia, known sensitivity (including soybean oil, eggs).

Dosage: A general induction dose used to produce a state of unconsciousness rapidly is 1.5 to 3 mg/kg IV, IO.

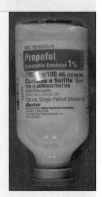

cont'd

PROPOFOL (DIPRIVAN)—CONT'D

Patient Group	Dosage	Rate of Administration (10 mg/mL)
Healthy adults younger than 55 years	2 to 2.5 mg/kg IV, IO	40 mg every 10 seconds
Elderly or debilitated patients	1 to 1.5 mg/kg IV, IO	20 mg every 10 seconds
Cardiac patients	0.5 to 1.5 mg/kg IV, IO	20 mg every 10 seconds
Patients with head injuries	1 to 2 mg/kg IV, IO	20 mg every 10 seconds
Pediatric (3 to 16 years)	2.5 to 3.5 mg/kg IV, IO	20 mg every 10 seconds

After the induction bolus, the patient must be given intermittent boluses or a maintenance infusion. For an average adult, an intermittent dose is 20 to 50 mg as needed. Alternatively, a propofol infusion may be ordered. Maintenance of anesthesia with a propofol infusion can be achieved by following the following protocols:
- **Adult patients:** 25 to 75 mcg/kg/min IV, IO.
- **Elderly, debilitated, or head-injured patients:** Use approximately 80% of the normal adult dose.
- **Pediatric:** 125 to 300 mcg/kg/min IV, IO.

Special Considerations:

Propofol should be administered only by personnel trained and equipped to manage the patient's airway and provide mechanical ventilation. In elderly and debilitated patients, avoid rapid administration to prevent hypotension, apnea, airway obstruction, and/or oxygen desaturation. Continue to monitor the patient's oxygenation and vital signs and try to limit use of propofol to patients who are intubated. Propofol should not be administered through the same IV catheter as blood or plasma. Pain can occur at the site of injection, which can be minimized by use of larger veins, slower rates of administration, and administration of 1 mL 1% lidocaine before propofol administration.

Propofol is listed as a pregnancy class B; however, propofol should be avoided in pregnant women because it crosses the placenta and can cause neonatal depression.

Because patients with closed-head injuries have undergone a traumatic experience, pain is a serious issue. The use of fentanyl citrate (Sublimaze) can potentiate propofol, with minimal hemodynamic effects. Mannitol (Osmitrol), an osmotic diuretic, is specifically used for cerebral edema. It expands the intravascular volume while decreasing the viscosity of blood. Both mechanisms can help improve cerebral blood flow. Mannitol can crystallize in cold temperatures, which requires special considerations in the field.

FENTANYL CITRATE (SUBLIMAZE)

Classification: Narcotic analgesic; Schedule C-II
Action: Binds to opiate receptors, producing analgesia and euphoria.
Indications: Pain
Adverse Effects: Respiratory depression, apnea, hypotension, nausea/vomiting, dizziness, sedation, euphoria, sinus bradycardia, sinus tachycardia, palpitations, hypertension, diaphoresis, syncope, pain at injection site.
Contraindications: Known sensitivity. Use with caution in traumatic brain injury, respiratory depression.
Dosage: Note: Dosage should be individualized.
- **Adult:** 50 to 100 mcg/dose (0.05 to 0.1 mg) IM or slow IV, IO (administered over 1 to 2 minutes).
- **Pediatric:** 1 to 2 mcg/kg IM or slow IV, IO (administered over 1 to 2 minutes).

Special Considerations:
Pregnancy class B

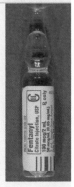

MANNITOL (OSMITROL)

Classification: Osmotic diuretic
Action: Facilitates the flow of fluid out of tissues (including the brain) and into interstitial fluid and blood, thereby dehydrating the brain and reducing swelling. Reabsorption by the kidney is minimal, consequently increasing urine output.
Indications: Increased ICP.
Adverse Effects: Pulmonary edema, headache, blurred vision, dizziness, seizures, hypovolemia, nausea/vomiting, diarrhea, electrolyte imbalances, hypotension, hypertension, sinus tachycardia, PVCs, angina, phlebitis.
Contraindications: Active intracranial bleeding, CHF, pulmonary edema, severe dehydration. Use with caution in hypovolemia, renal failure.
Dosage:
· **Adult:** 0.5 to 2 g/kg IV, IO followed by 0.25 to 1 g/kg administered every 4 hours.
· **Pediatric:** 0.25 to 1 g/kg IV, IO followed by 0.25 to 0.5 g/kg every 4 hours.
Special Considerations:
Mannitol should not be given in the same IV, IO line as blood.
Pregnancy class C

You use a multichannel pump to administer Ringer's lactate, fentanyl, propofol, and mannitol. The Ringer's lactate solution can hang by gravity. Should half or whole sets be used? The first bottle of mannitol is currently hanging, and each bottle will run over a 15-minute period. Based on the patient's weight, he will need four bottles (100 kg × 0.5 g = 50 g). The propofol is infusing at 1.8 mL/hr. The concentration is 100 mg/mL. The nurse tells you that the patient is receiving 30 mcg/kg per minute (30 mcg/100 kg per minute = 3000 mcg/min, or 180 mg/hour; 180 mg/100 mg per milliliter = 1.8 mL/hr). Both propofol and mannitol are packaged in glass bottles, so you administer them with a half set and syringe. With a ground transport time of 1 hour, the amount of fluids and syringe should be sufficient. The fentanyl infusion is running at 100 mcg/hr. Fentanyl is mixed as 50 mcg/mL, resulting in an infusion of 2 mL/hr. ...

When administering medication, be sure to label the syringes with the medication and concentration of the drug. This is especially important in the event of pump failure. The pump should have a drug calculator for the propofol so that the drug can be titrated as necessary during transport. In addition, a filter for the administration of mannitol is important. In cold temperatures, crystals in the patient can be avoided by inserting a filter needle where the mannitol enters the IV tubing. Although mannitol is infused by a pump, the medication can still crystallize between the IV pump and the patient.

... During transport, you are withdrawing mannitol for administration when you see crystals in the bottle.

With cold ambient temperatures, mannitol crystallization is not uncommon. According to the manufacturer's instructions, mannitol should be warmed to revert the medication to its previous fluid state without precipitation. If a fluid warmer is available, store the mannitol with the fluids until time for administration. If not, activate a disposable heat pack and wrap it around the mannitol. After the fluid is warmed, shake it vigorously to clear the crystals.

BURN INJURY

You are working as a flight paramedic and have been called to transfer a patient from a rural hospital to a regional burn center. You arrive and learn you are transporting a 47-year-old man who sustained full-thickness burns in a house fire. The ED has placed a 7.5 endotracheal tube, Foley catheter, and left femoral TLC. The patient arrived at the ED approximately 1 hour ago by EMS immediately from the scene. A dose of 500 mL Ringer's lactate has been infused. The patient weighs 175 lb. ...

Management

Fluid replacement is essential in preventing hypovolemia in critically ill burn patients. Major fluid shifts and losses occur during the first 24 hours of a burn injury. Fluid resuscitation is crucial during this period. Large amounts of crystalloid must be administered to replace the intravascular fluid loss that results from shifts to the interstitial spaces.

Parkland Formula of Burn Resuscitation. The Parkland formula is the most commonly used resuscitative formula. It is a pure crystalloid formula that helps replace fluids within the first 24 hours of a burn. According to the American Burn Association, the following formula can be used to calculate fluid needs in a major burn patient:

$$2 \text{ to } 4 \text{ mL} \times \text{Weight in kilograms} \times \text{Total body surface area burned}$$

Half the total fluid is administered in the first 8 hours, and the remaining half is administered over the following 16 hours. Therefore paramedics must know how to calculate the total body surface area (TBSA) burned to provide adequate fluid resuscitation to the patient. Additionally, a maintenance fluid of D_5 Ringer's lactate (D_5LR) is administered to children because of their decreased glycogen stores and needed replacement of glucose.[7]

For example, an 8-year-old child who weighs 42 kg has a TBSA burn of 25%. Time since injury is 1 hour, and the patient has received 500 mL Ringer's lactate. Maintenance fluids of D_5LR and resuscitation fluids of Ringer's lactate for this patient are shown in Tables 18-1 and 18-2.

The total amount of resuscitative fluids administered in the first 24 hours is 3150 mL. Half this volume (1575 mL) must be administered in the first 8 hours *from the time of injury.* The second half of the fluid must be given in the remaining 16 hours.

$$\text{Total volume of resuscitation fluids} = 3150 \text{ mL}$$

$$\text{First 8 hours: } 3150 \text{ mL}/2 = 1575 \text{ mL}$$

Because the patient has already received 500 mL, subtract 500 from 1575 mL:

$$1575 \text{ mL} - 500 \text{ mL} = 1075 \text{ mL}$$

This amount must be administered in the first 8 hours from the time of injury, not the first 8 hours of your care. One hour has already passed since the time of injury. Divide the amount of fluids by 7.

$$1075 \text{ mL}/7 \text{ hours} = 154 \text{ mL/hr for the next 7 hours}$$

To calculate the rate of resuscitation fluids for the remaining 16 hours, take the total 24-hour resuscitative fluid requirements (3150 mL), divide that number by 2, then divide that number by 16.

TABLE 18-1

Maintenance Fluids of D_5LR

Weight (kg)	mL/kg	Calculation	Total
First 10 kg	100 mL	10 × 100	1000 mL
Second 10 kg	50 mL	10 × 50	500 mL
Each kilogram >20 kg	20 mL	22 × 20	440 mL
			1940 mL as D_5LR

Hourly infusion of 81 mL/hr of D_5LR for the first 24 hours.

TABLE 18-2

Resuscitation Fluids of Ringer's Lactate

3-4 mL × Weight (kg)	TBSA	Fluid Resuscitation
3 × 42 = 126	126 × 25	3150 mL

Total 24-hour resuscitative fluid requirements = 3150 mL

Amount of fluids to be given from hours 9 to 24: 3150 mL/2 = 1575 mL

Hourly rate for fluids for hours 9 to 24 = 1575 mL/16 hr = 98 mL/hr

Therefore total fluids are D_5LR at 81 mL for 24 hours and Ringer's lactate at 154 mL/hr for 7 hours followed by Ringer's lactate at 98 mL/hr for the next 16 hours. Administration with a volume-control chamber set would be appropriate.

Urine output is closely monitored in burn patients to help determine whether patients are receiving an adequate amount of resuscitative fluid. The urine output in adult patients should total 0.5 mL/kg per hour, and the urine output for pediatric patients should be 1 mL/kg per hour if they weigh less than 30 kg. Therefore the insertion of a Foley catheter and/or strict intake and output recording is recommended if the patient has sustained a burn large enough to require fluid resuscitation.

Wallace Rule of Nines and Rule of Palms. The Wallace rule of nines is the most commonly used method of estimating the TBSA of large burn injuries. The rule of nines divides the patient's body surface area into units divisible by nine. This calculation is accurate for adult patients but not for children because of the disproportion of their body surface area. A modification to the rule of nines has been developed for children. The Wallace rule of nines for adults is shown in Table 18-3 and Figure 18-11.

TABLE 18-3

The Wallace Rule of Nines

Body Part	Adult
Head and neck (front and back)	9%
Each arm (front and back)	9%
Each leg (front and back)	18%
Anterior trunk (chest and abdomen)	18%
Posterior trunk (including the buttocks)	18%
Perineum	1%

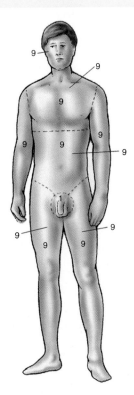

▼ **Fig. 18-11**   The Wallace rule of nines. (From Aehlert B: *Mosby's comprehensive pediatric emergency care,* rev, St Louis, 2007, Mosby.)

The rule of palms is an accurate method of estimating burns that are either scattered or comprise less than 10% TBSA. This estimation is based on the patient's palm as representative of 1% of TBSA. The palm does not include the fingers.

The Lund-Browder chart (Figure 18-12) is the more accurate calculator of TBSA, but it is not commonly used in the field because the rule of nines and rule of palms are faster and simpler. When using these methods of estimating TBSA, calculate only the areas of partial and full-thickness burns for TBSA. Do not use superficial areas for estimation.

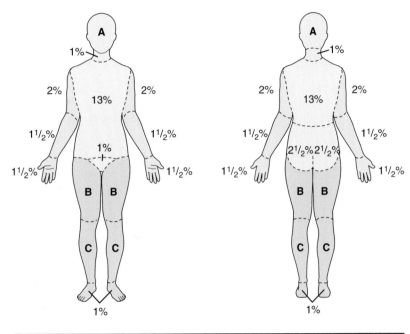

Area	Age 0	1	5	10	15	Adult
A - $1/2$ of head	$9^1/_2$%	$8^1/_2$%	$6^1/_2$%	$5^1/_2$%	$4^1/_2$%	$3^1/_2$%
B - $1/2$ of one thigh	$2^3/_4$%	$3^1/_4$%	4%	$4^1/_4$%	$4^1/_2$%	$4^1/_4$%
C - $1/2$ of one leg	$2^1/_2$%	$2^1/_2$%	$2^3/_4$%	3%	$3^1/_4$%	$3^1/_2$%

▼ **Fig. 18-12** Lund-Browder chart. (From Prehospital Trauma Life Support Committee of the National Association of Emergency Medical Technicians in Cooperation with the Committee on Trauma of the American College of Surgeons: *Prehospital trauma life support,* ed 6, St Louis, 2007, Mosby.)

A new method of determining burn size, as well as fluid resuscitation, has been developed that is easily applied in the prehospital setting. Alternative to the rule of nines, this method uses what the author refers to as the "rule of ones" and the "burn size score."

Using the old traditional methods, the burn size is estimated using the rule of nines, followed by mathematical calculation of a fluid resuscitation rate. Completion of this calculation requires two multiplication and two division operations. In an often chaotic environment while caring for a critically injured patient, this is a low priority.

By comparison, the rule of ones uses a resuscitation index with reference to a table to complete determination of fluid needs in a more simplified operation.[8] Fluid resuscitation needs are determined quickly by adding a few numbers (Figure 18-13) and referring to a simple table (Table 18-4).

The first step is using the burn size score (BSS). Using the same anatomic regions as the rule of nines, assign a score of one if more than 50% of that region is burned, and use a score of one half if a region is burned less than 50%. Add all the points to obtain the BSS, and round up the total. Cross-reference the patient's weight and BSS to determine the fluid rate.

Consider the following example:

A 70-kg victim with burns to both legs, anterior chest, and the abdomen and half the left arm. First, calculate the BSS:

▶ Right leg, 2
▶ Left leg, 2
▶ Anterior abdomen, 1
▶ Anterior chest, 1
▶ Half the left arm, 0.5

BSS = 2 + 2 + 1 + 1 + 0.5 = 6.5 (Round up to BSS of 7.)

Look at the 70-kg row on Table 18-4, and then the BSS column of 7. From the chart, you determine the fluid rate of 1103 mL/hr. A similar chart is available for pediatric patients.

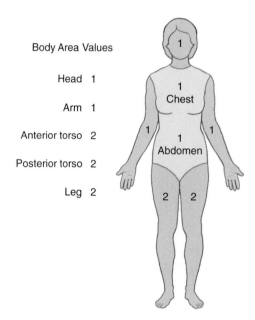

Body Area Values

Head 1

Arm 1

Anterior torso 2

Posterior torso 2

Leg 2

▼ **Fig. 18-13** Body diagram used for the determination of burn index. (From Prehospital Trauma Life Support Committee of the National Association of Emergency Medical Technicians in Cooperation with the Committee on Trauma of the American College of Surgeons: *Prehospital trauma life support,* ed 6, St Louis, 2007, Mosby.)

TABLE 18-4

Resuscitation Table Used for Determination of Fluid Resuscitation Using the Burn Resuscitation Index.

Initial IV Resuscitation Rate (Ringer's Lactate)

Patient Weight		Burn Size Score (BSS)									
lb	kg	1	2	3	4	5	6	7	8	9	10	11
88	40	90	180	270	360	450	540	630	720	810	900	990
110	50	113	225	338	450	563	675	788	900	1013	1125	1238
132	60	135	270	405	540	675	810	945	1080	1215	1350	1485
154	70	158	315	473	630	788	945	1103	1260	1418	1575	1733
176	80	180	360	540	720	900	1080	1260	1440	1620	1800	1980
198	90	203	405	608	810	1013	1215	1418	1620	1823	2025	2228
220	100	225	450	675	900	1125	1350	1575	1800	2025	2250	2475
242	110	248	495	743	990	1238	1485	1733	1980	2228	2475	2723
264	120	270	540	810	1080	1350	1620	1890	2160	2430	2700	2970
286	130	293	585	878	1170	1463	1755	2048	2340	2633	2925	3218
308	140	315	630	945	1260	1575	1890	2205	2520	2835	3150	3465
330	150	338	675	1013	1350	1688	2025	2363	2700	3038	3375	3713

> ... You assess the patient and find full-thickness burns to his entire head, anterior trunk, posterior trunk, and bilateral upper extremities circumferentially. You must determine the TBSA of this patient, as well as how much Ringer's lactate is required in the first 8 hours of resuscitation. ...

The TBSA of this patient is 63% according to the Wallace rule of nines. The patient requires 5040 mL in the first 8 hours of resuscitation when multiplying by two. Calculate TBSA as follows:

- Entire head = 9%
- Anterior trunk = 18%
- Posterior trunk = 18%
- Bilateral upper extremities circumferentially = 9% × 2 = 18%
- TBSA = 63%

According to the Parkland formula, the amount of fluid resuscitation needed is as follows:

- Amount of fluid needed in 24 hours = 2 to 4 mL × weight in kilograms × TBSA of burn injury
- Amount of fluid needed in 24 hours = 2 mL × 80 kg (convert pounds to kilograms) × 63
- Amount of fluid needed in 24 hours = 10,080 mL

Half the fluid needed in 24 hours is given in the first 8 hours. Therefore the patient requires 5040 mL in the first 8 hours. The patient has already received 500 mL before arriving at the hospital. Now the fluid to be administered is 4540 mL, and it has been 1 hour since the injury. How much fluid is initially needed must be assessed to help guide the amount needed during transport.

$$4540/7 = 649 \text{ mL/hr for the next 7 hours}$$

Changes to the formula can be made if urine output decreases or the patient becomes hypovolemic. Simply recalculate the Parkland formula but multiply by three.

> ... You are ready to transfer the patient to the burn center. You wrap the wounds in sterile sheets or bandages. You do not place sterile water or normal saline on the bandages for transport because the cool solution could cause the patient to become hypothermic. Also, this patient has circumferential burns to his bilateral upper extremities, so you frequently check his peripheral pulses to assess for compartment syndrome and the need for escharotomies.

BLOOD ADMINISTRATION

> You are called to transport a victim of multiple trauma from a local hospital to a level 1 trauma center. You arrive on the scene to find a 35-year-old man who was involved in a two-vehicle, head-on collision with ejection and rollover. He has a ruptured spleen, grade III liver laceration, and fractured pelvis. His blood pressure is 84/45 mm Hg, heart rate is 132 beats/min, and respiratory rate is 24 breaths/min. The hospital has initiated two 14-gauge IVs in the bilateral antecubitals. Blood tubing is prepared with normal saline. The hospital has requested 2 U of O⁻ blood. You are expected to prepare the patient and begin administering the blood en route to the trauma center.

The administration of blood and blood products is an important aspect of critical care transport. Because paramedics are introduced to blood administration only during critical care transports, this procedure is not typically emphasized during EMS education. For this reason, blood administration may seem intimidating. However, blood is no different from other medications administered. Blood also has adverse effects and signs and symptoms to observe. The following section provides an overview of information needed for safe blood administration.

The following factors must be considered when administering blood products: compatible fluids, filtration, time, and transfusion reactions.

The only IV fluid compatible with blood is normal saline. Ringer's lactate, although a more efficient volume expander, cannot be administered with blood because the calcium causes clotting. Any solutions that include dextrose also must not be used with blood because of the risk of hemolysis. In fact, no additional medications should be administered into a line with blood because of the risks of hemolysis.

Blood tubing incorporates a filter to allow easy administration of blood products. The filter prevents the administration of cells that have clotted in the tubing. The Y portion of the blood tubing allows a bag of normal saline to be infused after the blood administration to prevent wasting blood in the tubing. When administering blood through smaller-bore IV catheters, such as a 20-gauge catheter, saline may be needed to help dilute the blood and prevent complications in the catheter tip.[9]

In addition to the fluids, degradation of blood components must be prevented. Blood must be administered within 30 minutes of removal from the refrigerator. If a unit of blood reaches 10° C (50° F), the red blood cells degrade and the blood must be discarded. Pooled platelets also require the blood to be discarded.[9]

Monitoring for Transfusion Reactions

Transfusion reactions are the most dangerous aspect of blood administration. Table 18-5 summarizes the types, causes, and signs and symptoms of transfusion reactions. Monitoring vital signs (including temperature), patient symptoms, and respiratory status are vital in patients who receive blood products. If a transfusion reaction is suspected, stop the transfusion and flush the line with saline.

Blood Products

With the increasing risk of blood transfusions and lack of donor blood supply, the need for an additional blood product has risen. This topic is particularly important in the prehospital setting, as well as in rural areas without immediate access to blood banks. Blood substitutes, or oxygen carriers, are currently in phase II and phase III clinical trials. Two classes of these products are currently being developed: hemoglobin-based oxygen carriers and perfluorocarbon-based products. Research with the perfluorocarbon-based oxygen carriers is limited. However, hemoglobin-based products look promising for the future. The most well known of these products are PolyHeme and Hemospan. These products provide the following specific advantages:

TABLE 18-5

Identifying a Transfusion Reaction

Type	Cause	Signs and Symptoms
Acute hemolytic	ABO incompatibility	Fever, chills, low back pain, flushing, tachycardia, hypotension, cardiac arrest
Acute nonhemolytic	Reaction to donor white blood cells, platelets, plasma proteins	Headache, muscle aches, respiratory distress, cardiac arrhythmias, fever, chills
Anaphylactic	Anti–immunoglobulin A reaction to donor	Hives, urticaria, fever, flushing, itching
Circulatory overload	Rapid blood transfusion	Pulmonary congestion, restlessness, cough, shortness of breath, hypertension, distended neck veins
Bacteremia	Contaminated blood	Chills, fever, hypotension, vomiting, diarrhea, septic shock

From Meyers E: *Nurse's clinical pocket guide,* Philadelphia, 2005, FA Davis Company.

 ▶ Eliminate the risk of bloodborne pathogens
 ▶ Eliminate the need to cross-match patients
 ▶ Have a long shelf life that does not require special handing or storage
 ▶ Pharmacologically alter oxygen transport
 ▶ Improve microcirculation by reducing the risks of small clots
 ▶ Prevent the adverse effects of blood that has begun to degrade from an increased shelf life

The increased presence of these substances is expected in the future and may have a profound effect on the prehospital care of patients.[10]

REVIEW QUESTIONS

1. Name four types of infusion sets.
2. You are transporting a patient with the infusion pump set at 30 mL/hr. A pump failure occurs. What is the drip rate on a microdrip (60 gtt) set?
3. Why are steroids such as dexamethasone helpful during the transport of a patient with HELLP syndrome?
4. When transporting a patient on a magnesium drip, what should be available on board? Why?
5. What is the role of amiodarone in transporting a patient with myocardial ischemia?
6. Explain how fast you should decrease the blood glucose level in a patient with DKA and when you should initiate dextrose in the fluids.
7. In a patient with a closed-head injury, how is the CPP calculated?
8. Why is immediate fluid replacement critical in treating patients with burn injuries?
9. Explain the Wallace rule of nines.
10. What should you do if you suspect a patient is having a reaction to a blood transfusion?

REFERENCES

1. Kelley D: Hypovolemic shock: an overview, *Crit Care Nurs Q* 28:2, 2005.
2. Baxter JK, Weinstein L: HELLP syndrome: the state of the art, *Obstet Gynecol Surv* 59:838, 2004.
3. Everett M, Martin J: Twelve steps to optimal management of HELLP syndrome, *Clin Obstet Gynecol* 42:532, 1999.
4. Padden MO: HELLP syndrome: recognition and perinatal management, *Am Fam Physician* 60:829, 1999.
5. Marik PE, Varon J, Trask T: Management of head trauma, *Chest* 122:699, 2002.
6. Gabriel EJ, Ghajar J, Jagoda A: *Guidelines for prehospital management of traumatic brain injury,* Washington, DC, 2005, Brain Trauma Foundation, United States Department of Transportation.
7. *Advanced burn life support course provider manual,* Chicago, 2005, American Burn Association.
8. Lentz CW, Younan DS, Reid DJ: Burn resuscitation index: a tool for initiating fluid resuscitation, *J Burn Care Rehabil* 25:S49, 2004.
9. Meyers E: *Nurse's clinical pocket guide,* Philadelphia, 2005, FA Davis Company.
10. Habib FA, Cohn SM: Blood substitutes, *Curr Opin Anaesthesiol* 17:139, 2004.

BIBLIOGRAPHY

Schreiber D: *Spinal cord injuries,* www.emedicine.com/emerg/topic553.htm. Accessed June 23, 2005.

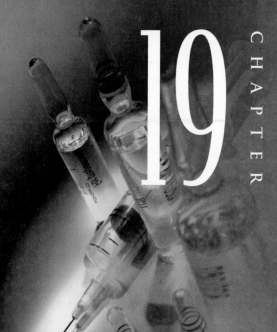

Special Considerations: Pregnancy, Pediatrics, Geriatrics, and Renal Failure

OBJECTIVES

1. Explain how physiologic changes in pregnancy can alter the pharmacologic mechanisms of a drug.
2. Differentiate the five categories in the Pregnancy Safety Category system: A, B, C, D, and X.
3. Discuss medications used for the treatment of asthma during pregnancy: albuterol (Proventil, Ventolin), terbutaline (Brethine), ipratropium bromide (Atrovent), prednisone, methylprednisolone sodium succinate (Solu-Medrol), and hydrocortisone sodium succinate (Solu-Cortef).
4. Explain the difference between chronic hypertension and gestational hypertension.
5. Discuss medications used in the treatment of hypertensive conditions during pregnancy: labetalol (Normodyne, Trandate), hydralazine (Apresoline), and magnesium sulfate.
6. Explain the impact of diabetic ketoacidosis in the pregnant patient.
7. Explain why blood pressure is not a good early indicator of perfusion in pediatric patients in shock.
8. Discuss why intraosseous lines are a beneficial alternative to IV lines in gaining vascular access in pediatric patients.
9. Explain why pediatric drug dosages are often determined by weight.
10. Discuss medications used in the treatment of pediatric bradycardia: epinephrine and atropine sulfate.
11. Discuss medications used in the treatment of pediatric tachycardia: adenosine (Adenocard) and amiodarone (Cordarone).
12. Define polypharmacy and its impact on the treatment of elderly patients.
13. Explain hemodialysis and peritoneal dialysis in the treatment of patients in end-stage renal disease.

Medications that Appear in Chapter 19

Diphenhydramine hydrochloride (Benadryl)
Albuterol (Proventil, Ventolin)
Terbutaline (Brethine)
Ipratropium bromide (Atrovent)
Prednisone
Methylprednisolone sodium succinate (Solu-Medrol)
Hydrocortisone sodium succinate (Cortef, Solu-Cortef)
Labetalol (Normodyne, Trandate)
Hydralazine (Apresoline)
Magnesium sulfate
Insulin, Regular (Humulin R, Novolin R)
Epinephrine
Atropine sulfate
Adenosine (Adenocard)
Amiodarone (Cordarone)
Procainamide (Pronestyl)
Lidocaine (Xylocaine)

INTRODUCTION

Drug therapy in certain groups of patients requires special considerations regarding route of administration, dosage, adverse effects, and drug metabolism and elimination. When caring for a pregnant woman, the prehospital provider must be mindful that he or she is caring for two patients, the mother and the fetus. Medication administered to the mother is also administered to the fetus. Therefore medications administered to pregnant women should be known to not adversely affect the physiology or development of the unborn child. IV access is more difficult to achieve in pediatric patients, who may require different routes of drug administration. In addition, given their smaller body mass, pediatric patients require dose adjustment based on their body weight. The elderly may have a gradual to profound deterioration in function of the heart, lungs, kidneys, and liver. An additional factor in the care of the elderly patient is the number of medications that these patients take on a long-term basis. The daily use of several medications (polypharmacy) can produce several potentially severe drug interactions that may cause or contribute to the initial call to EMS or result from a medication administered by a prehospital provider. Patients with renal failure are unable to excrete drugs that require excretion by the kidneys. Therefore the patients typically require smaller doses and must be monitored more closely for the development of toxicity from active drug metabolites that cannot be adequately removed by the kidneys.

SPECIAL CONSIDERATIONS IN PREGNANCY

Caring for an ill or injured pregnant patient can evoke a great deal of anxiety and apprehension in a prehospital provider. With pregnant patients, care is being provided to both the mother and her unborn child. An additional pressure is the vulnerability of the fetus to any medication administered to the mother; the administration of an inappropriate medication could lead to harm to or malformation of the fetus.

PHYSIOLOGIC CHANGES

To properly care for pregnant patients, prehospital providers must understand the normal physiologic changes that occur during pregnancy (Box 19-1). Many of these changes are capable of altering the absorption, distribution, breakdown, and elimination of medications.

Nausea and vomiting, commonly referred to as *morning sickness*, is caused by a hormone-induced delay in gastric emptying. Although pregnancy does not alter the absorption of a given drug, the delay in gastric emptying results in a delay from the time a patient takes an oral medication to the time the drug is delivered to the intestine, where it is absorbed.

BOX 19-1

NORMAL PHYSIOLOGIC ADAPTATIONS TO PREGNANCY

Cardiovascular

↑ Blood volume; plasma volume expansion increases to greater degree than red cell mass expansion, leading to a physiologic anemia of pregnancy

↓ Total peripheral resistance; decreases in blood pressure readings occur

↑ CO; results from increased blood volume; slight increase in heart rate to compensate for peripheral relaxation

↑ Oxygen consumption

Physiologic edema related to decreased COP and increased venous capillary hydrostatic pressure

Hematologic

↑ Clotting factors; predisposes to DIC and clotting

↓ Serum albumin results in decreases in COP; predisposes to pulmonary edema

Renal

↑ Renal plasma flow and glomerular filtration rate

Endocrine

↑ Estrogen produced results in increased renin-angiotension II-aldostrone secretion

↑ Progesterone production blocks aldosterone effect (slight decrease in sodium)

↑ Vasodilator prostaglandins result in resistance to angiotensin II (slight decrease in blood pressure)

CO, Cardiac output; *COP,* colloid osmotic pressure; *DIC,* disseminated intravascular coagulation.
Reprinted from Wong D, Perry S, Hockenberry-Eaton M: Maternal child nursing care, *ed 3, St Louis, 2006, Mosby.*

Respiratory drugs are rapidly effective in pregnant women because of increased minute ventilation.

Pregnant women have higher minute ventilation than nonpregnant women, so inhaled medications result in systemic effects more rapidly than in nonpregnant women. For pregnant women, drugs delivered by inhalation are absorbed at a much more rapid rate than are oral medications.

The weight gain of pregnancy alters an individual's body composition. Pregnancy increases the percentage of body fat, which creates a larger volume of distribution for fat-soluble drugs. The increase in the proportion of body fat also decreases the concentration of albumin in the blood. Serum Albumin is a major protein in blood plasma and is important in maintaining colloid osmotic pressure of the blood. A reduction in serum albumin affects drug distribution and plasma levels.

Pregnancy also induces a decrease in liver function and an increase in renal function. As a result, the breakdown of a drug by the liver can be slowed, but the excretion of that drug's by-products can be increased by an improvement in kidney function.

MEDICATION RISKS

The **placenta** is the lifeline between the mother and fetus. Oxygen, nutrients, and medications cross from the mother to the fetus via the placenta. An administered medication that has no effect on the mother can have a profound toxic effect on the fetus. The mother's circulatory system delivers medication to the fetus, but the fetus must break down and excrete the drug unassisted by the mother. Because the fetal liver and kidneys are immature, a dose of a given medication can have potentially toxic effects on the fetus.

In general, emergency medical care is complicated by the lack of reliable historical information from patients when they are confused, when they experience altered mental status, or even when they are unconscious. For this reason, providers should assume that all women of reproductive age are potentially pregnant. In addition, some women are not yet aware that they are pregnant. Therefore medication should be given only to a patient who is obviously pregnant or potentially pregnant when the benefit of that medication outweighs the potential risks.

Teratogenic drugs are medications that can result in a characteristic set of malformations in the fetus. The greatest period of vulnerability for the development of malformations is between the fourth and twelfth weeks after the last menstrual period. Teratogenic drugs typically affect the development of an organ system at a particular period of vulnerability.

The U.S. Food and Drug Administration (FDA) classifies drugs into several categories based on their risk to the fetus (Table 19-1). Drugs are categorized as A, B, C, D, or X. A is the safest, with B, C, and D noting progressively more dangerous drugs. Category X drugs are the most dangerous to use in pregnancy and should be avoided. The Pregnancy Safety Category system is limited in its usefulness because the majority of research studies conducted to determine a drug's safety have used animals. Furthermore, a large number of medications have not yet been rated. The assignment of a category to a medication is made by the manufacturer and not the government or other regulatory or safety agency. In addition, assignments to the FDA safety categories are made when a drug is new and little is known about its safety.

For a drug to affect a fetus, it must cross the placenta and enter the fetal circulation. Generally, the greater the effect of a medication on the mother, the greater the probability that it will cross the placenta and act on the fetus. Drugs that have large molecular weights are less likely to cross the placenta than are drugs with smaller molecular weights. Two common medications with large molecular weights are heparin and **insulin.** Neither of these medications can be given in an oral form because their large molecular size prevents absorption from the gastrointestinal tract, and neither of these medications can cross the placenta. However, most medications have a low molecular weight and can readily cross the placenta.

Lipophilic drugs are soluble in fat. Because the placenta is largely composed of fatty tissue, lipophilic medications are more likely to cross the placenta. In contrast, **lipophobic** medications, those that are not fat soluble, have a more difficult time crossing the placenta. For example, diphenhydramine (Benadryl) and loratadine (Claritin) are antihistamine drugs that can be used to treat allergic symptoms in nonpregnant adults. Diphenhydramine is a lipophilic drug that can rapidly cross the placenta. Loratadine is not fat soluble and has difficulty crossing the placenta; it is therefore safer for use during pregnancy.

Drugs with short half-lives are also safer for pregnant patients than are those with long half-lives. A drug with a long half life results in higher maternal serum levels for a longer period. The longer the drug remains in the mother's bloodstream, the greater the opportunity that it will cross the placenta into the fetal bloodstream.

TABLE 19-1

FDA Pregnancy Safety Categories

Category	Description
A	Controlled studies show no risk to the fetus.
B	Animal findings show risk to the fetus, although human studies do not; *or,* if no human studies are available, animal studies show no risk.
C	No human studies are available, and animal studies either show fetal risk or are not available.
D	Some investigational evidence shows risk of harm to the fetus, but potential benefits may outweigh the risks.
X	Animal or human studies or postmarketing investigations show fetal risk that outweighs possible benefits.

DIPHENHYDRAMINE HYDROCHLORIDE (BENADRYL)

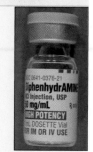

Classification: Antihistamine
Action: Binds and blocks H_1 histamine receptors.
Indications: Anaphylactic reactions
Adverse Effects: Drowsiness, dizziness, headache, excitable state (children), wheezing, thickening of bronchial secretions, chest tightness, palpitations, hypotension, blurred vision, dry mouth, nausea/vomiting, diarrhea.
Contraindications: Acute asthma, which thickens secretions; patients with cardiac histories; known sensitivity.
Dosage:
  · **Adult:** 25 to 50 mg IV, IO, IM.
  · **Pediatric: 2 to 12 years:** 1 to 1.25 mg/kg IV, IO, IM.
Special Considerations:
Pregnancy class B

ASTHMA

Your unit is dispatched to the home of a 28-year-old woman reporting shortness of breath. While en route, the dispatcher informs you that the patient is 32 weeks pregnant and is having an asthma attack. You arrive on the scene, and the husband leads you and your partner into the family room. He tells you that the patient has a history of asthma. She tested herself with a peak flowmeter and found that her peak expiratory flow rate (PEFR) was 45% of her baseline. When you reach the patient, you find an obviously pregnant woman sitting in a chair and appearing to be in respiratory distress. Your partner places the patient on oxygen and a pulse oximeter as you begin the assessment. The patient's respirations are labored with a rate of 32 breaths/min, heart rate of 88 beats/min, blood pressure of 102/76 mm Hg, and pulse oximeter reading of 94%. She is using the accessory muscles of her neck to breathe. On examination, she appears to have rhonchi and wheezes in all lung fields, heart sounds are normal, and her abdomen is remarkable for a gravid uterus. Neurologically she is following all commands and has no detectable motor or sensory deficits. Her skin is warm and moist. You determine that the patient would benefit from pharmacologic intervention for the treatment of her asthma. ...

Asthma is a reasonably common condition during pregnancy. Women with a long-standing history of asthma may note that the condition is exacerbated by pregnancy, whereas other women have their first occurrence of asthma during pregnancy. As in all conditions encountered during pregnancy, the fetus benefits by the mother's receipt of excellent care. If left untreated, asthma can have significantly negative results for both mother and fetus. It is safer for a pregnant woman to take medications than to have exacerbations of asthma.

Management
The initial therapy for a pregnant woman having an asthma attack includes oxygen and a bronchodilator. Beta$_2$ agonists commonly used for the treatment of asthma are listed as Category C medications. Research using a large number of pregnant women has demonstrated that the medications typically used for the treatment of asthma can be used without noted perinatal complications.[1]

Asthma is a common condition of pregnancy, and treatment medications can be used without perinatal complications.

The beta agonist albuterol (Proventil, Ventolin) is the first-line therapy for treatment of asthma in pregnant women. In fact, pregnant patients who have asthma should be instructed to carry albuterol with them at all times. Albuterol is most commonly administered by a metered-dose inhaler (MDI) with a spacer or as a nebulization therapy. Nebulization is a common method of albuterol administration used by many prehospital providers. Some providers argue that nebulization is inefficient because of the large size of the particles and the loss of medication from the expiratory port of the nebulization system. MDIs with spacers can obtain similar clinical improvement in the asthma with smaller doses of medication.[2,3] Four to six MDI inhalations with a spacer are roughly equivalent to one nebulization therapy.

An alternative medication to treat asthma in pregnant patients is Sub-Q terbutaline (Brethine). A third treatment option is Sub-Q epinephrine.

ALBUTEROL (PROVENTIL, VENTOLIN)

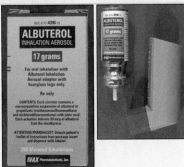

Classification: Bronchodilator, beta agonist
Action: Binds and stimulates beta$_2$ receptors, resulting in relaxation of bronchial smooth muscle.
Indications: Asthma, bronchitis with bronchospasm, and COPD.
Adverse Effects: Hyperglycemia, hypokalemia, palpitations, sinus tachycardia, anxiety, tremor, nausea/vomiting, throat irritation, dry mouth, hypertension, dyspepsia, insomnia, headache, epistaxis, paradoxical bronchospasm.
Contraindications: Angioedema, sensitivity to albuterol or levalbuterol. Use with caution in lactating patients, cardiovascular disorders, cardiac arrhythmias.
Dosage:
Acute Bronchospasm:
- **Adult:**
  - **MDI:** 4 to 8 puffs every 1 to 4 hours may be required.
  - **Nebulizer:** 2.5 to 5 mg every 20 minutes for a maximum of three doses. After the initial three doses, escalate the dose or start a continuous nebulization at 10 to 15 mg/hr.
- **Pediatric:**
  - **MDI:**
    - **4 years and older:** 2 inhalations every 4 to 6 hours; however, in some patients, 1 inhalation every 4 hours is sufficient. More frequent administration or more inhalations are not recommended.
    - **Younger than 4 years:** Administer by nebulization.
  - **Nebulizer:**
    - **Older than 12 years:** The dose for a continuous nebulization is 0.5 mg/kg/hr.
    - **Younger than 12 years:** 0.15 mg/kg every 20 minutes for a maximum of three doses. Alternatively, continuous nebulization at 0.5 mg/kg/hr can be delivered to children younger than 12 years.
Asthma in Pregnancy:
- **MDI:** Two inhalations every 4 hours. In acute exacerbation, start with 2 to 4 puffs every 20 minutes.
- **Nebulizer:** 2.5 mg (0.5 mL) by 0.5% nebulization solution. Place 0.5 mL of the albuterol solution in 2.5 mL of sterile normal saline. Flow is regulated to deliver the therapy over a 5- to 20-minute period. In refractory cases, some physicians order 10 mg nebulized over a 60-minute period.
Special Considerations:
Pregnancy class C

TERBUTALINE (BRETHINE)

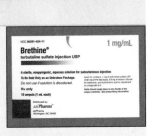

Classification: Adrenergic agonist
Action: Stimulates the beta$_2$ receptor, producing relaxation of bronchial smooth muscle and bronchodilation.
Indications: Prevention and reversal of bronchospasm.
Adverse Effects: Cardiac arrhythmias, arrhythmia exacerbation, angina, anxiety, headache, tremor, palpitations, dizziness.
Contraindications: Known sensitivity to sympathomimetics. Use with caution in hypertension, cardiac disease, cardiac arrhythmias, diabetes, elderly, MAOI therapy, pheochromocytoma, thyrotoxicosis, seizure disorder.
Dosage:
- **Adult:** 0.25 mg Sub-Q every 20 minutes for 3 doses. The usual site for the Sub-Q injection is the lateral deltoid.
- **Pediatric:** 0.01 mg/kg Sub-Q every 20 minutes for 3 doses.
Special Considerations:
Pregnancy class B

> ... You administer an albuterol nebulization therapy over a 20-minute period, with a plan to repeat the therapy every 20 minutes if the patient does not demonstrate satisfactory improvement. With an initial PEFR of less than 50%, you determine that the patient is having a severe exacerbation of her asthma and warrants additional drug therapy. ...

The next drug used to treat a pregnant patient having a severe exacerbation of asthma with a PEFR of less than 50% would be ipratropium bromide (Atrovent). Ipratropium bromide is used in severe exacerbations of asthma and in cases in which the patient has an unsatisfactory response to treatment with albuterol. In more severe cases of asthma, additional treatment with ipratropium bromide has provided greater symptomatic relief than albuterol used as a single agent.

IPRATROPIUM BROMIDE (ATROVENT)

Classification: Bronchodilator, anticholinergic
Action: Antagonizes the acetylcholine receptor on bronchial smooth muscle, producing bronchodilation.
Indications: Asthma, bronchospasm associated with COPD.
Adverse Effects: Paradoxical acute bronchospasm, cough, throat irritation, headache, dizziness, dry mouth, palpitations.
Contraindications: Closed-angle glaucoma, bladder neck obstruction, prostatic hypertrophy, known sensitivity including peanuts or soybeans and atropine or atropine derivatives.

Dosage:
MDI:
- **Adult:** 4 inhalations every 10 minutes, with no more than 24 inhalations per day or closer than 4 hours apart.
- **Pediatric:**
  - **Older than 12 years:** 2 to 3 puffs inhaled every 6 to 8 hours. Maximum of 12 puffs/day.
  - **5 to 12 years:** 1 to 2 puffs inhaled every 6 to 8 hours. Maximum of 8 puffs/day.
Nebulization:
- **Adult:** 0.5 mg every 6 to 8 hours.
- **Pediatric: 5 to 14 years:** 0.25 to 0.5 mg every 20 minutes for 3 doses as needed.

Special Considerations:
Ipratropium bromide is not typically used as a sole medication in the treatment of acute exacerbation of asthma. Ipratropium bromide is commonly administered after a beta agonist.
Care should be taken to not allow the aerosol spray (especially in the MDI) to come into contact with the eyes. This can cause temporary blurring of vision that resolves without intervention within 4 hours.
Pregnancy class B

> ... After administration of ipratropium bromide, the patient shows some improvement in her dyspnea, but she is still wheezing. Given the magnitude of the PEFR reduction and the persistent symptoms, you determine she could potentially benefit from corticosteroid therapy.

Asthma is a condition characterized by bronchospasm and inflammation of the airway. Corticosteroids should be administered in cases of severe exacerbations and certainly for impending respiratory failure. Prednisone, methylprednisolone (Solu-Medrol), and hydrocortisone (Solu-Cortef) are the steroids most commonly used in the treatment of asthma. The decision to administer corticosteroids can be made by monitoring the PEFR. When the initial PEFR is less than 50% of predicted, corticosteroids should be administered after ipratropium bromide (Box 19-2). Corticosteroids should also be considered when the PEFR does not improve by at least 10% after bronchodilator therapy or if the PEFR is lower than 70% after 1 hour of therapy.[4]

BOX 19-2

INDICATIONS FOR THE USE OF STEROIDS IN ASTHMA

PEFR <50% of predicted after ipratropium bromide (Atrovent) administration
PEFR does not improve by >10% after bronchodilator administration
PEFR <70% predicted after 1 hour of therapy

The beneficial effects of corticosteroids may not become apparent for several hours after administration. An IV preparation of a steroid may be used in an emergency when oral dosing is not practical. Orally administered steroids are rapidly absorbed, with nearly complete bioavailability. More is not necessarily better in the case of systemic corticosteroids, and large doses of corticosteroids have not been demonstrated to be any more beneficial than smaller doses. A review of several published investigations has shown that higher doses of steroids do not provide a benefit in either lung function or preventing respiratory failure.[5] The uses of inhaled steroids have been debated regarding their effectiveness in acute asthma exacerbations; some investigations have shown equivalent benefit with oral prednisone, whereas other inquiries have reached the opposite conclusion.[6,7]

PREDNISONE

Classification: Corticosteroid
Action: Reduces inflammation
Indications: Inflammatory conditions, such as asthma with bronchospasm.
Adverse Effects: Many adverse effects of steroid use are not related to short-term use but typically are seen with long-term use and during withdrawal.
Contraindications: Cushing's syndrome, fungal infections, measles, varicella, known sensitivity.
Dosage:
  · **Adult:** Dosage must be individualized.
  · **Pediatric:** Dosage must be individualized.
Special Considerations:
Pregnancy class C

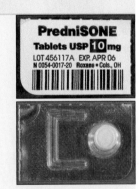

METHYLPREDNISOLONE SODIUM SUCCINATE (SOLU-MEDROL)

Classification: Corticosteroid
Action: Reduces inflammation by multiple mechanisms.
Indications: Anaphylaxis, asthma, COPD.
Adverse Effects: Depression, euphoria, headache, restlessness, hypertension, bradycardia, nausea/vomiting, swelling, diarrhea, weakness, fluid retention, paresthesias.
Contraindications: Cushing's syndrome, fungal infection, measles, varicella, known sensitivity (including sulfites). Use with caution in active infections, renal disease, penetrating spinal cord injury, hypertension, seizures, CHF.
Dosage:
Asthma and Chronic Obstructive Pulmonary Disease:
  · **Adult:** 40 to 80 mg IV.
  · **Pediatric:** 1 mg/kg (up to 60 mg) IV, IO per day in two divided doses.
Anaphylactic Shock:
  · **Adult:** 1 to 2 mg/kg/dose, then 0.5 to 1 mg/kg every 6 hours.
  · **Pediatric:** Same as adult dosing.

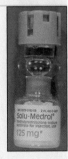

cont'd

METHYLPREDNISOLONE SODIUM SUCCINATE (SOLU-MEDROL)—CONT'D

Blunt Spinal Cord Injury:
- **Adult:** 30 mg/kg IV, IO over a period of 1 hour, then as an infusion to run for the remaining 23 hours at a dose of 5.4 mg/kg/hr.
- **Pediatric:** Same as adult dosing.

Special Considerations:
May mask signs and symptoms of infection.
Pregnancy class C

HYDROCORTISONE SODIUM SUCCINATE (CORTEF, SOLU-CORTEF)

Classification: Corticosteroid
Action: Reduces inflammation by multiple mechanisms. As a steroid, it replaces the steroids that are lacking in adrenal insufficiency.
Indications: Adrenal insufficiency, allergic reactions, anaphylaxis, asthma, COPD.
Adverse Effects: Leukocytosis, hyperglycemia, increased infection, decreased wound healing, increased rate of death from sepsis.
Contraindications: Cushing's syndrome, known sensitivity to benzyl alcohol. Use with caution in diabetes, hypertension, CHF, known systemic fungal infection, renal disease, idiopathic thrombocytopenia, psychosis, seizure disorder, GI disease, glaucoma, known sensitivity.

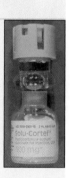

Dosage:
Anaphylactic Shock:
- **Adult:** 100 to 500 mg IV, IO, or IM.
- **Pediatric:** 2 to 4 mg/kg/day IV, IO, or IM (max: 500 mg).

Adrenal Insufficiency:
- **Adult:** 100 to 500 mg IV, IO, or IM.
- **Pediatric:** 1 to 2 mg/kg IV, IO, or IM.

Asthma and Chronic Obstructive Pulmonary Disease:
- **Adult:** 100 to 500 mg IV, IO, IM.
- **Pediatric:** 1 mg/kg IV, IO. The dose may be reduced for infants and children, but it is governed more by the severity of the condition and response of the patient than by age or body weight. Dose should not be less than 25 mg daily.

Special Considerations:
Pregnancy class C

HYPERTENSIVE CRISIS

You work for an EMS agency in a rural area. The closest hospital is a 25-bed facility with a two-bed emergency department (ED). Because of severe storms in the region, you and your partner have had a slow afternoon. You are dispatched to the local hospital to transfer a pregnant woman to a regional university hospital 120 miles away. You arrive at the ED and obtain a report from the emergency physician. She walks you over to the bed, where you meet a 26-year-old woman who is 35 weeks pregnant. The patient arrived at the ED slightly more than 1 hour before your arrival. She reported a headache that lasted all day, and her husband states that she seemed to become more somnolent as the day progressed. When they first admitted the patient to the ED, her blood pressure was 180/110 mm Hg. One week ago the patient was seen by her family physician, who determined her blood pressure was normal at that time. Today, with the report of headache and a significantly elevated blood pressure, the emergency physician obtained blood and urine tests in an attempt to confirm the diagnosis of preeclampsia. The high-risk obstetrician at the university hospital has accepted the patient, but because of inclement weather she will need to be transported by ground. You and your partner will care for this patient over the next several hours during transport. ...

Hypertension is a relatively common condition during pregnancy, with an incidence of 10% to 15%.[8] Hypertension in pregnancy is such a serious problem that it accounts for 15% of all pregnancy-related deaths.[9] Several types of hypertension can occur during pregnancy, ranging from benign to life-threatening in their course.

Chronic hypertension occurs when the patient has a history of hypertension that precedes the pregnancy. Preeclampsia and eclampsia are hypertensive conditions that can occur as a result of pregnancy. Preeclampsia is a life-threatening condition characterized by hypertension, protein in the urine, edema, and other diagnostic criteria not apparent to prehospital providers. Eclampsia occurs when a woman experiencing preeclampsia has seizures. **Gestational hypertension** is elevated blood pressure that first occurs during pregnancy but does not meet the diagnostic criteria of eclampsia.

Management

In the case of severe hypertension, the mother should be treated with antihypertensive agents in an effort to reduce maternal complications. However, the blood pressure threshold at which a pregnant woman should be treated remains controversial. One suggested threshold for treatment is a diastolic blood pressure greater than 105 mm Hg or a systolic blood pressure greater than 160 mm Hg. Clearly the young woman in the scenario exceeds both thresholds.[10]

... You perform an initial evaluation. The patient currently is resting comfortably, and her blood pressure is 140/94 mm Hg. She reports some improvement in her headache but tells you she prefers the lights off to avoid aggravating her headache. You load her into the ambulance and begin the several-hour trip down the highway. Approximately 20 minutes into the trip, the patient states that her head is starting to bother her again. You retake her blood pressure, which is 176/112 mm Hg. You are worried about the severity of her hypertension and the return of her symptoms. You believe her blood pressure should be treated. ...

Patients should be considered candidates for pharmacologic therapy for hypertension when their systolic blood pressure exceeds 160 mm Hg or diastolic pressure exceeds 105 mm Hg. If the patient's blood pressure exceeds these measurements, the prehospital provider should consult with medical direction or follow standing local protocols. The two drugs often used to treat hypertensive conditions during pregnancy are labetalol (Normodyne, Trandate) and hydralazine (Apresoline).

An excellent medication used for the treatment of hypertensive crisis in pregnancy is the beta blocker labetalol. Hydralazine is another common antihypertensive medication used during pregnancy. Evaluation of research trials that used hydralazine determined that hydralazine can result in a greater likelihood of inducing maternal hypotension, and the drug should not be used as a first-line agent for the acute treatment of hypertension.[11,12] Nitroglycerin is another effective antihypertensive drug. One advantage of nitroglycerin (as previously discussed in Chapter 12) is its short half-life of only 1 to 3 minutes.

The danger in using any antihypertensive agent is dropping the blood pressure to the point at which placental blood flow decreases. With labetalol, another concern is fetal bradycardia.

LABETALOL (NORMODYNE, TRANDATE)

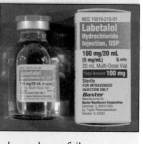

Classification: Beta adrenergic antagonist, antianginal, antihypertensive

Action: Binds with both the beta$_1$ and beta$_2$ receptors and alpha$_1$ receptors in vascular smooth muscle. Inhibits the strength of the heart's contractions, as well as heart rate. This results in a decrease in cardiac oxygen consumption.

Indications: ACS, SVT, severe hypertension.

Adverse Effects: Usually mild and transient; hypotensive symptoms, nausea/vomiting, bronchospasm, arrhythmia, bradycardia, AV block.

Contraindications: Hypotension, cardiogenic shock, acute pulmonary edema, heart failure, severe bradycardia, sick sinus syndrome, second- or third-degree heart block, asthma or acute bronchospasm, cocaine-induced ACS, known sensitivity. Use caution in pheochromocytoma, cerebrovascular disease or stroke, poorly controlled diabetes, with hepatic disease. Use with caution at lowest effective dose in chronic lung disease.

Dosage:

Cardiac Indications: Note: Monitor blood pressure and heart rate closely during administration.

    Adult: 10 mg IV, IO over a 1- to 2-minute period. May repeat every 10 minutes to a maximum dose of 150 mg or give initial bolus and then follow with infusion at 2 to 8 mg/min.

    Pediatric: 0.4 to 1 mg/kg/hr to a maximum dosage of 3 mg/kg/hr.

Severe Hypertension:

- **Adult:** Initial dose is 20 mg IV, IO slow infusion over a 2-minute period. After the initial dose, blood pressure should be checked every 5 minutes. Repeat doses can be given at 10-minute intervals. The second dose should be 40 mg IV, IO, and subsequent doses should be 80 mg IV, IO, to a maximum total dose of 300 mg. The effect on blood pressure typically will occur within 5 minutes from the time of administration. Alternatively, may be administered via IV infusion at 2 mg/min to a total maximum dose of 300 mg.
- **Pediatric:** 0.4 to 1 mg/kg/hr IV, IO infusion with a maximum dose of 3 mg/kg/hr.

Special Considerations:

Pregnancy class C

HYDRALAZINE (APRESOLINE)

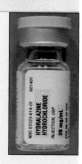

Classification: Antihypertensive agent, vasodilator

Action: Directly dilates the peripheral blood vessels.

Indications: Hypertension associated with preeclampsia and eclampsia, hypertensive crisis.

Adverse Effects: Headache, angina, flushing, palpitations, reflex tachycardia, anorexia, nausea/vomiting, diarrhea, hypotension, syncope, peripheral vasodilation, peripheral edema, fluid retention, paresthesias.

Contraindications: Patients taking diazoxide or MAOIs, coronary artery disease, stroke, angina, dissecting aortic aneurysm, mitral valve and rheumatic heart diseases.

Dosage:

Preeclampsia and Eclampsia:

- **Adult:** 5 to 10 mg IV, IO. Repeat every 20 to 30 minutes until systolic blood pressure of 90 to 105 mm Hg is attained.

Acute Hypertension Not Associated with Preeclampsia:

- **Adult:** 10 to 20 mg IV, IO, or IM.
- **Pediatric:**
  - **1 month to 12 years:** 0.1 to 0.6 mg/kg IV, IO, or IM (max: 20 mg/dose).

Special Considerations:

Pregnancy class C

> ... You repeat the blood pressure measurement to ensure no error occurred. The second blood pressure reading is 180/108 mm Hg. The patient tells you that her headache is 8 on a pain scale of 1 to 10. She asks you to turn off the lights in the compartment because they are aggravating her headache. After consultation with medical direction, you administer labetalol 20 mg IV. After a few minutes, you measure her blood pressure again. No improvement has occurred with the labetalol. After 20 minutes, still no improvement in the patient's blood pressure or symptoms has occurred. You administer labetalol 40 mg IV, wait several minutes, and then retake the blood pressure. The blood pressure has decreased to 146/94, and the patient seems to have some relief from her headache.

The definitive treatment for eclampsia is delivery of the fetus, which is generally avoided in the prehospital setting. Prehospital providers often are required to participate in the interhospital transfer to a specialty facility of a woman with eclampsia or preeclampsia. One of the goals of therapy is to prevent or treat the seizures. The agent of choice for prevention and treatment of eclamptic seizures is magnesium sulfate. Magnesium is indicated when the diastolic blood pressure is greater than 100 mm Hg and signs of an impending seizure are present.

MAGNESIUM SULFATE

Classification: Electrolyte, tocolytic, mineral
Action: Required for normal physiologic functioning. Magnesium is a cofactor in neurochemical transmission and muscular excitability. Magnesium sulfate controls seizures by blocking peripheral neuromuscular transmission. Magnesium is also a peripheral vasodilator and an inhibitor of platelet function.
Indications: Torsades de pointes, cardiac arrhythmias associated with hypomagnesemia, eclampsia and seizure prophylaxis in preeclampsia, status asthmaticus.
Adverse Effects: Magnesium toxicity (signs include flushing, diaphoresis, hypotension, muscle paralysis, weakness, hypothermia, and cardiac, CNS, or respiratory depression).
Contraindications: AV block, GI obstruction. Use with caution in renal impairment.
Dosage:
Pulseless Ventricular Fibrillation/Ventricular Tachycardia with Torsades de Pointes or Hypomagnesemia:
  · **Adult:** 1 to 2 g in 10 mL D_5W IV, IO administered over 5 to 10 minutes.
  · **Pediatric:** 25 to 50 mg/kg IV, IO over 10 to 20 minutes; may administer faster for torsades de pointes (max single dose: 2 g).
Torsades de Pointes with a Pulse or Cardiac Arrhythmias with Hypomagnesemia:
  · **Adult:** 1 to 2 g in 50 to 100 mL D_5W IV, IO administered over 5 to 60 minutes. Follow with 0.5 to 1 g/hr IV, IO titrated to control torsades de pointes.
  · **Pediatric:** 25 to 50 mg/kg IV, IO over 10 to 20 minutes (max single dose: 2 g).
Eclampsia and Seizure Prophylaxis in Preeclampsia:
  · **Adult:** 4 to 6 g IV, IO over 20 to 30 minutes, followed by an infusion of 1 to 2 g/hr.
Status Asthmaticus:
  · **Adult:** 1.2 to 2 g slow IV, IO (over 20 minutes).
  · **Pediatric:** 25 to 50 mg/kg (diluted in D_5W) slow IV, IO (over 10 to 20 minutes).
Special Considerations:
Pregnancy class A

DIABETIC KETOACIDOSIS

Despite intensive control of diabetes during pregnancy, approximately 5% of pregnant women with diabetes develop diabetic ketoacidosis (DKA).[13] DKA is a state of insulin deficiency that produces a condition of hyperglycemia, dehydration, and metabolic acidosis. A detailed discussion is found in Chapter 11. DKA in pregnancy can be fatal for the fetus, with fetal mortality rates approaching 50%. Elevated maternal blood glucose levels result in osmotic diuresis and electrolyte shifts. The loss of circulatory blood volume and electrolyte shifts in the mother result in a drop in placental blood flow and oxygen content.

Management

In addition to the initial treatment priorities of maintaining the airway, breathing, and circulatory status, the paramedic should administer 1 L of an isotonic fluid (0.9% saline or Ringer's lactate) over a 1-hour period. After this initial fluid bolus, the IV infusion should continue at a rate of 250 to 500 mL/hr. This strategy of fluid resuscitation with isotonic fluids should continue until the patient's blood glucose level is approximately 250 mg/dL. Once the blood sugar level is less than 250 mg/dL, the fluid should be changed to an IV fluid that contains 5% dextrose. This addition of 5% dextrose prevents a too-rapid and perhaps dangerous decline in the serum glucose concentration.

Many EMS agencies do not carry insulin because of its need for refrigeration; however, paramedics may see insulin-dependent patients during interhospital transfers. If ordered, an initial insulin bolus of 0.1 U/kg IV should be given. This typically is followed by an insulin infusion running at a dose of 0.05 to 0.1 U/kg per hour. During an insulin infusion, blood glucose measurements are taken hourly or every other hour. If the blood glucose level does not decrease by 25% after 2 hours, the paramedic should double the initial insulin infusion dose. Once the blood glucose level reaches 250 mg/dL, the IV fluid should be changed to one containing 5% dextrose and the insulin infusion rate should be decreased by one half. Once the blood glucose level has reached 150 mg/dL, the insulin infusion rate should be decreased to 1 to 2 U/hr.

INSULIN, REGULAR (HUMULIN R, NOVOLIN R)

Classification: Hormone
Action: Binds to a receptor on the membrane of cells and facilitates the transport of glucose into cells.
Indications: Hyperglycemia, insulin-dependent diabetes mellitus, hyperkalemia.
Adverse Effects: Hypoglycemia, tachycardia, palpitations, diaphoresis, anxiety, confusion, blurred vision, weakness, depression, seizures, coma, insulin shock, hypokalemia.
Contraindications: Hypoglycemia, known sensitivity.
Dosage:
Diabetic Ketoacidosis:
- **Adult:** 0.1 U/kg IV, IO, or Sub-Q. Because of poor perfusion of the peripheral tissues, Sub-Q administration is much less effective than the IV, IO route. IV, IO insulin has a very short half-life; therefore IV, IO insulin without an infusion is not that effective. The rate for an insulin infusion is 0.05 to 0.1 U/kg/hr IV, IO. When dosing insulin, use a U-100 insulin syringe to measure and deliver the insulin. The time from administration to action, as well as the duration of action, varies greatly among different individuals, as well as at different times in the same individual.

Hyperkalemia:
- **Adult:** 10 U IV, IO of regular insulin (Insulin R), coadministered with 50 mL of $D_{50}W$ over 5 minutes.
- **Pediatric:** 0.1 U/kg Insulin R IV, IO.

Special Considerations:
Only regular insulin can be given IV, IO.
Pregnancy class B

SPECIAL CONSIDERATIONS FOR PEDIATRIC PATIENTS

The following section discusses the pediatric population and special issues that must be considered in their treatment. It is often said that children are not little adults, and in many ways this is true. Regarding IV access; fluid management; and the treatment of shock, pain, and cardiac and neurologic emergencies, several key differences between pediatric and adult patients are critical to keep in mind when delivering care to children.

DRUG DOSING

In addition to being smaller than adults, the body composition of infants and children is dramatically different from that of adults. The various body compartments, as described in Chapter 5, have different relative sizes than those of the adult. In adults, 60% of the body, based on total body mass, is water. The percentage of total body water of an infant is approximately 80%, a proportion that decreases to approximately 60% by adulthood. In the first year of life, the percentage of fat nearly doubles in infants. Infants have a much smaller percentage of muscle mass than adults, but they have much larger brains and livers in relation to their total body weight. Infants and children also have large volumes of distribution and rapid metabolic rates. Because of differences in a child's metabolism during the various stages of development, a simple linear reduction of an adult drug dose is not appropriate.

Information on pediatric drug dosing is usually given on the basis of age, weight, or body surface area of the child. In most cases, drugs for pediatric use usually recommend a particular dose in milligrams per kilogram or pound. For many drugs, the recommended weight-based dose (or weight-normalized dose) is presented for children of different ages or weight groups. For many drugs, the weight-normalized dose increases as the weight of the child decreases. A dose appropriate for an 8-year-old may be too small for a 2-year-old.

> The provider must be mindful that the calculated pediatric dose should not exceed the recommended adult dose.

You are called to the home of an 18-month-old boy who has had vomiting and diarrhea for 4 days. He has not had urine output since the night before, and the parents state that he has been sleepy and poorly responsive to normal stimuli. When you arrive, you find a pale boy sleeping in his mother's arms. His heart rate is 120 beats/min, and his blood pressure is 90/70 mm Hg. The mother tells you that the child normally weighs approximately 24 pounds; she believes he has lost 4 pounds since he became ill. His breathing is shallow, and his eyes appear sunken. You are in a rural area, and the transport time to the nearest hospital is approximately 40 minutes. You examine the patient's extremities and find that his pulses are weak. Few veins are visible, and IV access is critical at this point. You decide that intraosseous access is necessary. Once secured, you administer a bolus of 0.9% normal saline (10 mL/kg, or approximately 100 mL). You reassess vital signs, and his heart rate is now 110 beats/min. Blood pressure remains unchanged. You maintain IV infusion at 60 mL/hr and transport the patient on a monitor.

HYPOVOLEMIC SHOCK

When assessing a child in shock, a critical point to realize is that blood pressure is not the primary vital sign that indicates the patient's status. In most pediatric patients a drop in blood pressure is the last sign of deterioration; therefore blood pressure is not a good indicator of the child's perfusion. When assessing a child for shock, palpate peripheral pulses and evaluate temperature and capillary refill of the distal extremities.

> In hypovolemic pediatric patients, blood pressure is a late sign of deterioration.

Cardiac output (CO) is determined by the stroke volume (SV) of the heart multiplied by the heart rate (HR):

$$CO = HR \times SV$$

Stroke volume is the amount of blood ejected by the heart with each heartbeat. An adult has some variability in stroke volume; however, stroke volume in a child is relatively stable.

Therefore the only mechanism that a child has to improve cardiac output in shock is an increased heart rate.

Vascular Access and Management

Vascular access is a challenge in pediatric patients because of the small size of their blood vessels, greater amount of subcutaneous fat, and unwillingness to cooperate with the provider. Vascular access is particularly difficult and time-consuming with children in shock. Each emergency response team should establish a plan for how much time should be spent attempting to obtain access to each IV site and should identify the most appropriately trained personnel to attempt access. If one or two lines are not obtained within 2 to 5 minutes, medications should be given by an alternate method so that resuscitation is not delayed.

The preferred peripheral site for IV placement in a child is the antecubital fossa. In an infant, a scalp vein or a superficial vein of an extremity can be used if larger veins are not accessible (Fig. 19-1). Additional useful equipment includes a tourniquet and 18- to 24-gauge angiocatheters. Disadvantages to a peripheral IV line include risk of the line becoming dislodged, occlusion of the line, and possible tissue injury with extravasation of irritants.

IO lines are an alternative to venous access in children when vascular access is critical but peripheral access is not achievable. A 15- to 18-gauge bone marrow needle with stylet is placed in the marrow cavity of the child's tibia (Fig. 19-2). Placement is directed perpendicular to the flat part of the proximal tibia, and the needle is inserted through the skin 1 to 3 cm (approximately one finger's width) just medial to the tibial

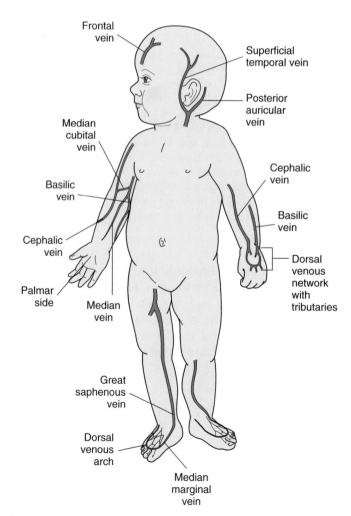

▼ **Fig. 19-1**   Various sites for placement of IV catheters in infants. (From Aehlert B: *Mosby's comprehensive pediatric emergency care*, rev, St Louis, 2007, Mosby.)

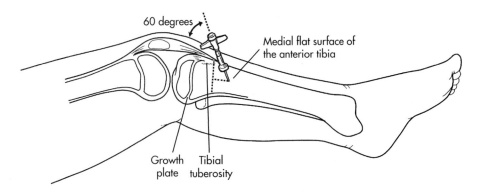

▼ **Fig. 19-2**   Anterior tibial placement of an intraosseous infusion. (From Aehlert B: *Mosby's comprehensive pediatric emergency care,* rev, St Louis, 2007, Mosby.)

tuberosity. The catheter is advanced through the bone into the marrow space, at which point a "pop" is usually felt. Successful placement is confirmed by aspiration of marrow content and easy infusion of fluid.

Alternate sites for IO catheter placement include the distal tibia and distal femur. Most fluids that can be infused through a peripheral IV can also be infused intraosseously, and absorption is rapid from the tibia bone marrow cavity. Once an IO catheter is established and fluid boluses have been administered, a peripheral IV line may be more accessible with improved hydration of the child.

Rare but significant complications of IO access include osteomyelitis, cellulitis, infiltration of fluid, anterior compartment syndrome, tibial fracture, and fat embolus. IO lines are not suitable for long-term use, and an increased incidence of leaking at the site of insertion exists. To minimize complications, IO needles should not be placed in fractured bones or at a site that was previously used. They should also not be used for prolonged periods. Additionally, an IO needle should not be placed in patients with a history of osteogenesis imperfecta, a bone condition that makes the bones brittle and susceptible to fracture.

Never place an intraosseous line in a fractured bone.

Once IV access has been obtained, fluid management and treatment of shock can begin. Remember, shock is the collapse of the body's cardiovascular system, which prevents it from providing oxygen and nutrients for the body's vital metabolic needs. Once an airway and adequate oxygenation have been secured and a functioning infusion line has been obtained, fluid resuscitation can begin. Improving the blood volume is best achieved with IV fluids, and if appropriate, blood products may be administered (such as in air medicine or a military setting). If packed red blood cells are required, the provider should transfuse 10 mL/kg of blood.

Volume expansion in children is based on weight rather than the use of a standard bolus, such as in adults. A safe rule of thumb is to give a bolus of no more than 10 to 20 mL/kg at a time, with close reassessment of vital signs between boluses. The bolus is given rapidly over minutes. Appropriate fluids for fluid resuscitation include crystalloids such as 0.9% sodium chloride or Ringer's lactate solution. After each intervention—whether fluid bolus, airway intervention, or cardiac compressions—a full reassessment of the patient's status is critical. Be sure to proceed in the appropriate ABC order so that treatment of shock is most effective. As is true for the care of any injured or ill patient, remember to check and recheck.

The volume of a fluid bolus for a pediatric patient is 10 to 20 mL/kg.

ARRHYTHMIAS

Pediatric cardiac arrhythmias are often referred to in the simple terms of "abnormal heart rate" and rhythms that are either "too fast" or "too slow." Unlike the complex rhythms more commonly found in adults, children tend to have less history of cardiac disease and symptoms more likely to represent an acute, reversible process. The more commonly presenting abnormal rhythms in pediatric patients can be grouped by age and are shown in Table 19-2. See Chapter 9 for an in-depth discussion of these arrhythmias.

The treatment of pediatric arrhythmias can also be simplified. Treatment may consist of only establishing an airway and improving circulation with IV hydration, never underemphasizing the importance of the ABCs in resuscitation.

However, when initial resuscitative measures are not adequate in stabilizing the patient, a sound knowledge of medications for the treatment of arrhythmias in pediatric patients is important.

TABLE 19-2

Common Pediatric Arrhythmias Grouped by Age

<1 year	Bradycardia, atrial fibrillation, ventricular fibrillation
1-5 years	Supraventricular tachycardia, bradycardia, atrial flutter
6-12 years	Nonspecific arrhythmia, supraventricular tachycardia, atrial flutter
13-18 years	Nonspecific arrhythmia, atrial fibrillation

From Barkin RM, Rosen P: Emergency pediatrics: a guide to ambulatory care, *ed 6, St Louis, 2003, Mosby.*

When approaching the pediatric patient with an arrhythmia, a thorough evaluation should include a history and physical assessment. Children who are at risk for arrhythmias include those with congenital heart disease or other diseases that can lead to heart failure. These patients have symptoms of cardiogenic shock with poor perfusion. They are often pale and short of breath, with irritability and changes in mental status. Remember that blood pressure is a poor indicator of shock in a child. Feel the child. Are his or her feet warm? If not, how far up the arm or leg can you detect the warmness that indicates adequate perfusion? Evaluate capillary refill in the nail beds or over the patella. In the infant or young child who is unable to communicate, the parent or guardian can relay a history of poor feeding or increased somnolence.

Too Slow

Management. The treatment of bradycardia is determined by the stability of the patient. As with all patients, evaluate and establish the airway if required. Evaluate the breathing and determine the adequacy of circulation. If the patient is stable and not hypotensive, oxygen and IV fluids are often adequate treatments until the patient can be transported to a facility for further evaluation. Hypoxia is the most common cause of bradycardia in pediatric patients. Repeated evaluation of the patient's vital signs and ABCs is vital. If the child is in cardiorespiratory distress, he or she may require mechanical compressions and drug therapy. Epinephrine is the first drug used in the treatment of pediatric bradycardia. If the patient remains bradycardic after the epinephrine, move to atropine sulfate.

EPINEPHRINE

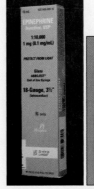
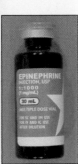

Classification: Adrenergic agent, inotropic
Action: Binds strongly with both alpha and beta receptors, producing increased blood pressure, increased heart rate, bronchodilation.
Indications: Bronchospasm, allergic and anaphylactic reactions, restoration of cardiac activity in cardiac arrest.
Adverse Effects: Anxiety, headache, cardiac arrhythmias, hypertension, nervousness, tremors, chest pain, nausea/vomiting.
Contraindications: Arrhythmias other than VF, asystole, PEA; cardiovascular disease; hypertension; cerebrovascular disease; shock secondary to causes other than anaphylactic shock; closed-angle glaucoma; diabetes; pregnant women in active labor; known sensitivity to epinephrine or sulfites.
Dosage:
Cardiac Arrest:
  · **Adult:** 1 mg (1:10,000 solution) IV, IO; may repeat every 3 to 5 minutes.
  · **Pediatric:** 0.01 mg/kg (1:10,000 solution) IV, IO; repeat every 3 to 5 minutes as needed (max dose: 1 mg).
Symptomatic Bradycardia:
  · **Adult:** 1 mcg/min (1:10,000 solution) as a continuous IV infusion; usual dosage range: 2 to 10 mcg/min IV; titrate to effect.
  · **Pediatric:** 0.01 mg/kg (1:10,000 solution) IV, IO; may repeat every 3 to 5 minutes (max dose: 1 mg). If giving epinephrine by ET tube, administer 0.1 mg/kg.
Asthma Attacks and Certain Allergic Reactions:
  · **Adult:** 0.3 to 0.5 mg (1:1000 solution) IM or Sub-Q; may repeat every 10 to 15 minutes (max dose: 1 mg).
  · **Pediatric:** 0.01 mg/kg (1:1000 solution) IM or Sub-Q (max dose: 0.5 mg).
Anaphylactic Shock:
  · **Adult:** 0.1 mg (1:10,000 solution) IV slowly over 5 minutes, or IV infusion of 1 to 4 mcg/min, titrated to effect.
  · **Pediatric:** Continuous IV infusion rate of 0.1 to 1 mcg/kg/min (1:10,000 solution); titrate to response.
Special Considerations:
Half-life 1 minute
Pregnancy class C

ATROPINE SULFATE

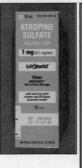
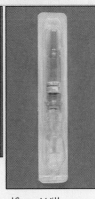

Classification: Anticholinergic (antimuscarinic)
Action: Competes reversibly with acetylcholine at the site of the muscarinic receptor. Receptors affected, in order from the most sensitive to the least sensitive, include salivary, bronchial, sweat glands, eye, heart, and GI tract.
Indications: Symptomatic bradycardia, asystole or PEA, nerve agent exposure, organophosphate poisoning.
Adverse Effects: Decreased secretions resulting in dry mouth and hot skin temperature, intense facial flushing, blurred vision or dilation of the pupils with subsequent photophobia, tachycardia, restlessness. Atropine may cause paradoxical bradycardia if the dose administered is too low or if the drug is administered too slowly.
Contraindications: Acute MI; myasthenia gravis; GI obstruction; closed-angle glaucoma; known sensitivity to atropine, belladonna alkaloids, or sulfites. Will not be effective for infranodal (type II) AV block and new third-degree block with wide QRS complex.

cont'd

ATROPINE SULFATE—CONT'D

Dosage:
Symptomatic Bradycardia:
- **Adult:** 0.5 mg IV, IO every 3 to 5 minutes to a maximum dose of 3 mg.
- **Adolescent:** 0.02 mg/kg (minimum 0.1 mg/dose; maximum 1 mg/dose) IV, IO up to a total dose of 2 mg.
- **Pediatric:** 0.02 mg/kg (minimum 0.1 mg/dose; maximum 0.5 mg/dose) IV, IO, to a total dose of 1 mg.

Asystole/Pulseless Electrical Activity:
- 1 mg IV, IO every 3 to 5 minutes, to a maximum dose of 3 mg. May be administered via ET tube at 2 to 2.5 mg diluted in 5 to 10 mL of water or normal saline.

Nerve Agent or Organophosphate Poisoning:
- **Adult:** 2 to 4 mg IV, IM; repeat if needed every 20 to 30 minutes until symptoms dissipate. In severe cases, the initial dose can be as large as 2 to 6 mg administered IV. Repeat doses of 2 to 6 mg can be administered IV, IM every 5 to 60 minutes.
- **Pediatric:** 0.05 mg/kg IV, IM every 10 to 30 minutes as needed until symptoms dissipate.
- **Infants <15 lb:** 0.05 mg/kg IV, IM every 5 to 20 minutes as needed until symptoms dissipate.

Special Considerations:
Half-life 2.5 hours
Pregnancy class C; possibly unsafe in lactating mothers.

Too Fast

Management. A heart rhythm that is too fast is also addressed beginning with the sequence of ABCs. Airway is critical because the increased heart rate can indicate respiratory compromise and its associated panic or the body's early response to poor oxygenation. Once the airway is established and oxygenation has been provided, focus attention on evaluation of the circulation. Once IVs have been established, evaluate for dehydration and other disorders that can contribute to the increased heart rate. Fever itself can cause tachycardia; however, fluids help in this situation, as well. Therefore consider the need for an IV fluid bolus with either 0.9% normal saline or Ringer's lactate at 10 to 20 mL/kg, with rapid and close reassessment of vital signs after each bolus and caution regarding the overzealous administration of fluids, such as in the case of DKA.

Evaluation of the rate, as well as the width of the QRS complex, often helps determine whether the arrhythmia is supraventricular tachycardia or ventricular tachycardia. In both cases, if the patient is unstable, cardioversion at a dose of 0.5 to 1.0 J/kg is warranted. If the patient is stable but the tachyarrhythmia is presumed to be supraventricular tachycardia and is unresponsive to the usual resuscitative measures, consider adenosine (Adenocard) administration.

Adenosine is a drug that slows the heart rate by acting at the atrioventricular node to alter the conduction of the electrical stimulation to the pacer. It has an immediate onset, and its half-life is equally as fast, taking effect in 10 seconds or less. An important but concerning fact about the use of adenosine is its ability to cause transient atrioventricular block, which can appear to be asystole for the 10-second period. In a child, this is alarming. However, the paramedic must expect and understand this possibility as the rhythm is monitored with administration of adenosine.

In cases of stable ventricular tachycardia, amiodarone (Cordarone), procainamide, or lidocaine may be appropriate treatment, followed by cardioversion. However, when a patient has unstable ventricular tachycardia, cardioversion should be used appropriately.

ADENOSINE (ADENOCARD)

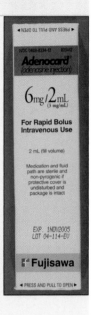

Classification: Antiarrhythmic
Action: Slows the conduction of electrical impulses at the AV node.
Indications: Stable reentry SVT. Does not convert AF, atrial flutter, or VT.
Adverse Effects: Common adverse reactions are generally mild and short-lived: sense of impending doom, complaints of flushing, chest pressure, throat tightness, numbness. Patients will have a brief episode of asystole after administration.
Contraindications: Sick sinus syndrome, second- or third-degree heart block, poison-/drug-induced tachycardia.
Dosage: Note: Adenosine should be delivered only by rapid IV bolus with a peripheral IV or directly into a vein, in a location as close to the heart as possible, preferably in the antecubital fossa. Administration of adenosine must be immediately followed by a saline flush, and then the extremity should be elevated.
  · **Adult:** Initial dose 6 mg rapid IV, IO (over a 1- to 3-second period) immediately followed by a 20-mL rapid saline flush. If the first dose does not eliminate the rhythm in 1 to 2 minutes, 12 mg rapid IV, IO, repeat a second time if required.
  · **Pediatric:**
    · **Children >50 kg:** Same as adult dosing.
    · **Children <50 kg:** Initial dose 0.1 mg/kg IV, IO (max dose: 6 mg) immediately followed by a ≥5-mL rapid saline flush; may repeat at 0.2 mg/kg (max dose: 12 mg).
Special Considerations:
Use with caution in patients with preexisting bronchospasm and those with a history of AF.
Elderly patients with no history of PSVT should be carefully evaluated for dehydration and rapid sinus tachycardia requiring volume fluid replacement rather than simply treated with adenosine.
Pregnancy class C

AMIODARONE (CORDARONE)

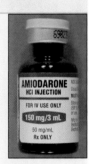

Classification: Antiarrhythmic, class III
Action: Acts directly on the myocardium to delay repolarization and increase the duration of the action potential.
Indications: Ventricular arrhythmias; second-line agent for atrial arrhythmias.
Adverse Effects: Burning at the IV site, hypotension, bradycardia.
Contraindications: Sick sinus syndrome, second- and third-degree heart block, cardiogenic shock, when episodes of bradycardia have caused syncope, sensitivity to benzyl alcohol and iodine.
Dosage:
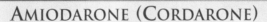
Ventricular Fibrillation and Pulseless Ventricular Tachycardia:
  · **Adult:** 300 mg IV, IO. May be followed by one dose of 150 mg in 3 to 5 minutes.
  · **Pediatric:** 5 mg/kg (max dose: 300 mg); may repeat 5 mg/kg IV, IO up to 15 mg/kg.
Relatively Stable Patients with Arrhythmias such as Premature Ventricular Contractions or Wide-Complex Tachycardias with a Strong Pulse:
  · **Adult:** 150 mg in 100 mL D₅W IV, IO over a 10-minute period; may repeat in 10 minutes up to a maximum dose of 2.2 g over 24 hours.
  · **Pediatric:** 5 mg/kg very slow IV, IO (over 20 to 60 minutes); may repeat in 5-mg/kg doses up to 15 mg/kg (max dose: 300 mg).
Special Considerations:
Pregnancy class D

PROCAINAMIDE (PRONESTYL)

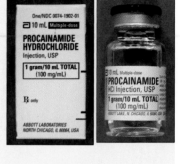

Classification: Antiarrhythmic, class IA
Action: Blocks influx of sodium through membrane pores, consequently suppresses atrial and ventricular arrhythmias by slowing conduction in myocardial tissue.
Indications: Alternative to amiodarone for stable monomorphic VT with normal QT interval and preserved ventricular function, reentry SVT if uncontrolled by adenosine and vagal maneuvers if blood pressure stable, AF with rapid rate in Wolff-Parkinson-White syndrome.
Adverse Effects: Asystole, VF, flushing, hypotension, PR prolongation, QRS widening, QT prolongation.
Contraindications: AV block, QT prolongation, torsades de pointes. Use with caution in hypotension, heart failure.
Dosage:
  · **Adult:** 20 mg/min slow IV, IO (max total dose: 17 mg/kg until one of the following occurs: arrhythmia resolves, hypotension, QRS widens by >50% of original width).
  · **Maintenance:** Infusion (after resuscitation from cardiac arrest): mix 1 g in 250 mL solution (4 mg/mL), infuse at 1 to 4 mg/min.
  · **Pediatric:** 15 mg/kg slow IV, IO over 30 to 60 minutes.
Special Considerations:
Pregnancy class C

LIDOCAINE (XYLOCAINE)

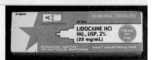

Classification: Antiarrhythmic, class IB
Action: Blocks sodium channels, increasing the recovery period after repolarization; suppresses automaticity in the His-Purkinje system and depolarization in the ventricles.
Indications: Ventricular arrhythmias, when amiodarone is not available: cardiac arrest from VF/VT, stable monomorphic VT with preserved ventricular function, stable polymorphic VT with normal baseline QT interval and preserved left ventricular function (when ischemia and electrolyte imbalance are treated), stable polymorphic VT with baseline QT prolongation suggestive of torsades de pointes.
Adverse Effects: Toxicity (signs may include anxiety, apprehension, euphoria, nervousness, disorientation, dizziness, blurred vision, facial paresthesias, tremors, hearing disturbances, slurred speech, seizures, sinus bradycardia), seizures without warning, cardiac arrhythmias, hypotension, cardiac arrest, pain at injection site.
Contraindications: AV block; bleeding; thrombocytopenia; known sensitivity to lidocaine, sulfite, or paraben. Use with caution in bradycardia, hypovolemia, cardiogenic shock, Adams-Stokes syndrome, Wolff-Parkinson-White syndrome.
Dosage:
Pulseless Ventricular Tachycardia and Ventricular Fibrillation:
  · **Adult IV, IO:** 1 to 1.5 mg/kg IV, IO; may repeat at half the original dose (0.5-0.75 mg/kg) every 5 to 10 minutes to a maximum dose of 3 mg/kg. If a maintenance infusion is warranted, the rate is 1 to 4 mg/min.
  · **Adult ET tube:** 2 to 10 mg/kg ET tube, diluted in 10 mL normal saline or sterile distilled water.
  · **Pediatric IV, IO:** 1 mg/kg IV, IO (maximum: 100 mg). If a maintenance infusion is warranted, the rate is 20 to 50 mcg/kg/min.
  · **Pediatric ET tube:** 2 to 3 mg/kg ET tube, followed by a 5-mL flush of normal saline.
Perfusing Ventricular Rhythms:
  · **Adult:** 0.5 to 0.75 mg/kg IV, IO (up to 1-1.5 mg/kg may be used). Repeat 0.5 to 0.75 mg/kg every 5 to 10 minutes to a maximum total dose of 3 mg/kg. A maintenance infusion of 1 to 4 mg/min (30-50 mcg/kg/min) is acceptable.
  · **Pediatric:** 1 mg/kg IV, IO. May repeat every 5 to 10 minutes to a maximum dose of 3 mg/kg. Maintenance infusion rate is 20 to 50 mcg/kg/min.
Special Considerations:
Half-life approximately 90 minutes
Pregnancy class B

MANAGEMENT OF DIABETIC KETOACIDOSIS

Diabetes is a common disease in children. Prehospital providers encounter children with complications of diabetes, which is discussed in Chapter 11. However, a key difference in the treatment of pediatric DKA warrants mention. The child with DKA should not receive a bolus of insulin. However, when possible, the child with DKA should receive an insulin drip in the same fashion as an adult. When treating DKA in adults, physicians and providers are often taught that the first three items are fluids, fluids, and fluids. Do not apply this philosophy to children because aggressive fluid administration in a child with DKA can result in cerebral edema. Cerebral edema has been reported in children receiving fluids in excess of 2.5 times the maintenance rate.

SPECIAL CONSIDERATIONS FOR ELDERLY PATIENTS

People continue to live longer with a higher quality of life, largely because of break-throughs in drug therapy. As a result, an increasing number of older adults take several medications concurrently. These patients are likely to be taking numerous drugs pre-scribed by several different physicians in addition to over-the-counter medications that are self-prescribed. Sometimes patients are placed on medications without sufficient regard for drug interactions or adverse effects.

Polypharmacy occurs when a patient is taking multiple medications for the treatment of several medical disorders. The danger of polypharmacy is the increased likelihood of an adverse effect or serious drug interaction. Drug interactions are a preventable cause of hospitalization and death among the elderly.[14] In fact, 70% to 80% of elderly patients have adverse drug effects at a frequency several times greater than that in younger adults.[15] Adverse drug effects and interactions are responsible for approximately 17% of hospital admissions in the elderly.[16] Ray et al. reported that 32,000 elderly patients fall and sustain hip fractures each year as a result of the adverse effects of medications.[17]

As the body ages, its ability to respond to various insults decreases. An understanding of age-related changes in anatomy and physiology is necessary to reduce drug-related complications. Older patients often lose muscle mass and total body weight. Therefore a drug dose acceptable for an adult often should be reduced in an elderly patient. Certain medications may require weight-based dosing similar to pediatric drug dosing. Despite weighing the same or even less than a large child, many older patients are prescribed standard adult dosages, and the result is drug toxicity.

Age-related physiologic changes in medication response in the elderly are attributable to changes in medication absorption, distribution, breakdown, and excretion. Absorption can be reduced by decreased motility of the stomach and reduced production of stomach acid. Breakdown or metabolism of medications from their active to nonactive forms by the liver is less effective with increasing age. Excretion is also affected. With age, the blood flow to the kidneys is often reduced, as is the ability of the kidneys to filtrate and concen-trate the urine. After the age of 30 years, adults lose approximately 6% to 10% of kidney function per decade. Therefore, by the age of 70 years, a healthy individual will have lost approximately 50% of his or her renal function compared with a younger adult.

The result of these age-related decreases in kidney function is accumulation of drugs or drug by-products. Medications that have the potential of becoming toxic in renal disease include digoxin, antibiotics, antihypertensives, and antiarrhythmics.

Altered drug effects in the elderly are also explained by alterations in the way drugs interact with their various receptors. In addition to loss of weight, the body's composition changes with age. A proportional increase in body fat and a decrease in total body water occur. With an increase in body fat, fat-soluble drugs will collect in the fat stores. A decrease in muscle mass leads to a decrease in the volume of distribution of many drugs, which can cause toxic drug levels of water-soluble drugs such as digoxin and theophylline.

In addition, poor nutrition can decrease the body's production of albumin. **Albumin,** a protein produced by the liver, is found in the blood and interstitial space. Many drugs bind to and are transported by albumin. When drugs bind to albumin, a percentage of the drug does not bind to the albumin. The portion of the drug that does not bind to the albumin is the portion that is active. With a decrease in albumin, the total amount of unbound or active drug increases. Therefore, for a given dose, the effectiveness of a drug is increased and potentially toxic.

When caring for elderly patients, prehospital providers must remember that this group of patients is often taking multiple medications and clearly at risk for polypharmacy and drug interactions. Any medication that must be administered in an emergency setting can result in an unanticipated interaction and adverse drug effect. Elderly patients may be at risk for decreased compliance with prescription medications because of problems such as depression, poor memory, dementia, and financial restrictions.

SPECIAL CONSIDERATIONS FOR PATIENTS WITH RENAL FAILURE

Renal failure is a progressive, rapidly developing, chronic disease that, in its most extreme form, results in permanent loss of kidney function. Patients with renal failure require careful management of their diet, fluid intake, and drug therapy. Acute renal failure is a rapidly developing condition that can occur in up to 10% of patients admitted to an intensive care unit. More than 260,000 people in the United States have chronic kidney disease, 48,000 await kidney transplants, and each year more than 50,000 people die from complications of renal failure. The common causes of chronic renal failure include hypertension and diabetes mellitus. Causes of renal failure include trauma, pregnancy, hemorrhage, and complications of drug therapy.

Acute renal failure is a disease that typically occurs in hospitalized patients, but prehospital providers are called to assist or transport patients with chronic renal failure. Many patients with chronic renal failure have a decline in their kidney function managed by medications, vitamins, and special diets.

The most extreme form of chronic renal failure is known as **end-stage renal disease (ESRD).** Patients with ESRD cannot make urine and require some form of renal replacement therapy or dialysis to stay alive. **Hemodialysis** is the removal of toxic substances from the bloodstream by filtering the patient's blood through a machine and then passing the blood back to the patient. Hemodialysis is an efficient means of cleansing the blood. The principal risks of hemodialysis are hypotension and arrhythmias.

Peritoneal dialysis is the process by which a special solution is delivered to the patient's abdomen through a catheter. The special solution dwells in the abdomen for a period, absorbing many of the toxic substances in the blood. After several hours, the solution is drained and the poisons are removed from the body. Although substantially less efficient than hemodialysis, peritoneal dialysis does not result in hypotension or require anticoagulation. The disadvantage of peritoneal dialysis is the length of time required for dialysis therapy and the risk of infection to the abdominal cavity.

The role of the kidney is largely to remove waste products from the blood and control the internal environment of the body. Therefore, as the kidneys fail, the internal milieu changes the effectiveness of various drugs. One of the normal functions of the kidneys is to produce natural buffers; however, as kidney function declines to less than 20% of normal, patients can develop metabolic acidosis.

The kidney's most obvious function is the creation of urine. With decreasing renal function, the kidneys lose their ability to concentrate urine. Patients usually are able to manage their own fluid balance as long as they control sodium intake. However, patients with renal failure may not be able to tolerate large volumes of IV fluids.

Maintaining potassium balance is another critical function of the kidneys. When kidney function is less than 10% of normal, the potassium balance is impaired and can accumulate to dangerous and critical levels.

In addition to removing toxic waste products, the kidneys have a role in the formation of red blood cells. The kidneys manufacture a protein known as **erythropoietin,** which stimulates the bone marrow to produce red blood cells. Patients with renal failure are not able to make erythropoietin, resulting in a decrease in the number of red blood cells in the bloodstream, or **anemia.** Patients with chronic renal failure often take epoetin alfa

(Epogen), a synthetic form of erythropoietin, to increase their blood count and treat the anemia.

When caring for a patient with renal insufficiency or renal failure, prehospital providers should question the need, dosage, and possible interaction of every medication administered. Many drugs are metabolized or excreted by the kidneys, and the dosage of these drugs needs to be reduced in renal failure. Drug dosages often need to be reduced in proportion to the degree of renal impairment.

REVIEW QUESTIONS

1. In what ways do the physiologic changes in pregnancy alter the pharmacologic mechanisms of a drug?
2. What is a teratogenic drug?
3. Name the categories of the Pregnancy Safety Category system.
4. An allergy to what food is a contraindication for use of ipratropium bromide (Atrovent)?
5. When should you consider the use of corticosteroids for the treatment of asthma?
6. How does gestational hypertension differ from chronic hypertension?
7. At what systolic and diastolic blood pressures should drug therapy be considered for the treatment of hypertension in a pregnant woman?
8. What is DKA, and what is its significance to the fetus?
9. Is blood pressure a reliable sign of pending shock in a pediatric patient?
10. What is stroke volume?
11. List the complications associated with intraosseous infusions.
12. Why are pediatric drug dosages given by weight?
13. What is the most common cause of bradycardia in children?
14. When administering adenosine in the pediatric patient, why should the prehospital care provider monitor for asystole in the first 10 seconds?
15. What is the risk of too-aggressive fluid administration in a child with DKA?
16. Define polypharmacy, and describe its danger to elderly patients.
17. In a 70-year-old patient, what percentage of kidney function is considered normal?
18. What are the causes of renal failure?
19. What are the causes of chronic renal failure?
20. What classes of drugs can become toxic in patients with kidney disease?
21. Define hemodialysis.

REFERENCES

1. Schatz M, et al: The safety of asthma and allergy medications during pregnancy, *J Allergy Clin Immunol* 100:301, 1997.
2. Turner JR, et al: Equivalence of continuous flow nebulizer and metered-dose inhaler with reservoir bag for treatment of acute airflow obstruction, *Chest* 93:476, 1988.
3. Salzman GA, et al: Aerosolized metaproterenol in the treatment of asthmatics with severe airflow obstruction. Comparison of two delivery methods, *Chest* 95:1017, 1989.
4. Murphy S, Sheffer AL, Pauwels RA: *National Asthma Education and Prevention Program: highlights of the expert panel report II: guidelines for the diagnosis and management of asthma,* Bethesda, Md, 1997, National Heart, Lung, and Blood Institute.
5. Manser R, Reid D, Abramson M: Corticosteroids for acute severe asthma in hospitalised patients, *Cochrane Database Syst Rev* (1):CD001740, 2001.
6. Edmonds ML, et al: Replacement of oral corticosteroids with inhaled corticosteroids in the treatment of acute asthma following emergency department discharge: a meta-analysis, *Chest* 121:1798, 2002.
7. Schuh S, et al: A comparison of inhaled fluticasone and oral prednisone for children with severe acute asthma, *N Engl J Med* 343:689, 2000.
8. Sherri A, et al: Preeclampsia and eclampsia revisited, *South Med J* 96:891, 2003.
9. Report of the National High Blood Pressure Education Program Working Group on High Blood Pressure in Pregnancy, *Am J Obstet Gynecol* 183:S1, 2000.
10. Lenfant C, National Education Program Working Group on High Blood Pressure in Pregnancy: Working group on high blood pressure in pregnancy, *J Clin Hypertens* 3(2):75-88, 2001.

11. Magee LA, Ornstein MP, von Dadelszen P: Fortnightly review: management of hypotension in pregnancy, *Br Med J* 318:1332, 1999.
12. Magee LA, Cham C, Waterman EJ: Hydralazine for treatment of severe hypertension in pregnancy: meta-analysis, *Br Med J* 327(7421):955-960, 2003.
13. Rodgers BD, Rodgers DE: Clinical variables associated with diabetic ketoacidosis during pregnancy, *J Reprod Med* 36:797, 1991.
14. Juurlink DN, et al: Drug-drug interactions among elderly patients hospitalized for drug toxicity, *JAMA* 289:1652, 2003.
15. Katzung BG: *Basic and clinical pharmacology,* ed 6, Norwalk, Conn, 1995, Appleton & Lange.
16. Nananda JF, Kronholm P: The role of medication noncompliance and adverse drug reactions in hospitalizations of the elderly, *Arch Intern Med* 50:841, 1990.
17. Ray WA, Griffin MR, Schaffner W: Psychotropic drug use and the risk of hip fracture, *N Engl J Med* 316:363, 1987.

Pharmacology-Assisted Intubation

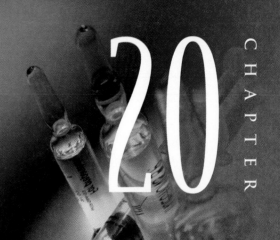

CHAPTER 20

OBJECTIVES

1. Differentiate the goals of rapid sequence induction from rapid sequence intubation.
2. List six questions to ask when preparing for rapid sequence intubation.
3. List three goals of rapid sequence intubation.
4. Discuss depolarizing paralytics used in rapid sequence intubation: succinylcholine (Anectine) and atropine sulfate.
5. Discuss nondepolarizing paralytics used in rapid sequence intubation: vecuronium (Norcuron), rocuronium (Zemuron), atracurium (Tracrium), and pancuronium (Pavulon).
6. Discuss deep sedation medications used in rapid sequence intubation: midazolam (Versed), etomidate (Amidate), ketamine (Ketalar), and flumazenil (Romazicon).
7. List the seven P's of rapid sequence intubation technique.

Medications that Appear in Chapter 20

Succinylcholine (Anectine)
Atropine sulfate
Rocuronium (Zemuron)
Vecuronium (Norcuron)
Atracurium (Tracrium)
Pancuronium (Pavulon)
Midazolam (Versed)
Flumazenil (Romazicon)
Etomidate (Amidate)
Ketamine (Ketalar)

INTRODUCTION

Although endotracheal intubation was documented as long as 1000 years ago, it has been in only the past 60 years that this procedure has been recognized as a valuable resuscitative tool for emergency medicine.[1,2] Endotracheal intubation as an advanced prehospital procedure developed over the past 25 years, paralleling the advancement and refinement of prehospital care in general.

In 1970, Stept and Safar[3] first described a 15-step technique of rapid sequence induction in which patients who had full stomachs could undergo general anesthesia with a lower risk of aspiration. Key components of this technique were the use of short-acting IV barbiturates (the induction) and muscular paralytic drugs (neuromuscular blockade).

Your unit is called to a local junior high school gymnasium for a woman who is having a seizure. When you arrive you find the woman lying supine on the floor with several bystanders. You note that there is some vomit on the floor by her head and she is not responding. On examination, you note that she has some vomit around her mouth. You attempt to suction her airway but cannot because her teeth are clenched. You administer oxygen by face mask and place a pulse oximeter. Her oxygen saturation is 82%. You once again try to clear her airway but are not successful. You perform a modified jaw thrust, but this does not improve her oxygen saturation, so you place a nasopharyngeal airway. This maneuver increases her oxygen saturation only slightly to 85%. Her mental status has not improved, but she has not had any additional motor seizure activity. The treatment priority of any emergency is protection or establishment of a patent airway. You cannot be assured that this patient's airway is not obstructed by her tongue or vomit. Jaw thrust maneuvers and nasopharyngeal airways have not rescued the patient from her hypoxia. She will require establishment of an airway with pharmacologic assistance.

Most patients encountered by paramedics present with full stomachs (as well as other obstacles to intubation, such as clenched teeth). The technique of **rapid sequence induction** was adapted for emergency use as **rapid sequence intubation.** Both techniques are known as *RSI,* but the *I* refers to induction or intubation to reflect different goals. For RS induction, the ultimate goal is a patient who is safely anesthetized; for RS intubation, the goal is a patient who is safely endotracheally intubated. RS intubation as performed by emergency physicians first emerged in the early 1980s and became well established as a standard emergency department (ED) technique by the early 1990s.[4] In this chapter, *RSI* refers only to RS intubation.

Because RSI has been shown to improve success rates for endotracheal intubation in the ED, it makes sense that RSI can also be successfully used in the prehospital environment.[4-7] In fact, Wayne and Friedland has demonstrated a 96% intubation success rate (fewer than three attempts) with the prehospital use of succinylcholine in approximately 3000 patients intubated over a 20-year period in the Bellingham, Wash., EMS system.[8,9] Other studies have also demonstrated improved intubation success rates with paramedic-administered RSI.[10]

However, some studies have demonstrated a poorer outcome for patients who underwent paramedic-administered RSI, primarily those with severe head trauma, despite the increased intubation success rate.[11,12] This poor outcome may be a result of excessive hyperventilation, which can severely lower arterial carbon dioxide (CO_2) pressures, leading to excessive constriction of the brain blood vessels and impaired delivery of oxygen, and from prolonged hypoxia during the intubation attempts.[13] Both effects were demonstrated during paramedic-performed intubations in a study conducted in the San Diego EMS system.[11] These negative effects possibly could be minimized by limiting the duration of intubation attempts, carefully monitoring pulse oximetry during and after intubation, and using end-tidal CO_2 monitoring to guide ventilation rate and volume.[14]

RAPID SEQUENCE INTUBATION GOALS

This chapter describes medications that paramedics can use to facilitate airway management, primarily those that can make endotracheal intubation easier or safer. A major portion of this chapter is dedicated to discussion of the medications needed to perform RSI. When RSI is performed correctly, the patient is chemically paralyzed, deeply sedated or anesthetized, and endotracheally intubated (Fig. 20-1).

The powerful medications discussed in this chapter allow the paramedic to assume control of the airway and breathing of a critically ill or injured patient. As such, the paramedic must ask himself or herself several questions in preparation for assuming this control, including the following:

 ▶ If I administer these drugs, will I be able to intubate the patient if he or she stops breathing?

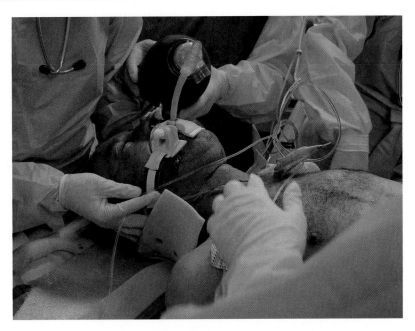

▼ **Fig. 20-1**   A endotracheally intubated patient.

▶ If I am unable to intubate the patient, will I be able to ventilate him or her?

▶ If I am unable to intubate or ventilate this patient, do I have other options?

▶ Do I have the right equipment on hand? Is the equipment assembled?

▶ Does the patient have any medical problems or conditions for which these drugs and techniques are contraindicated?

▶ If I do not act, will this patient die or have permanent brain damage?

RSI has the following three goals:

1. To overcome barriers to intubation (e.g., clenched teeth and combativeness) by establishing a condition of deep sedation and skeletal muscle relaxation while protecting against aspiration of stomach contents into the lungs

2. To provide protection against the body's normal response to intubation, reflexes that can potentially cause cardiac or neurologic deterioration in at-risk patients

3. To provide humane conditions for an unpleasant procedure

You are dispatched to the scene of a motor vehicle crash in which a 20-year-old male driver was ejected. You find the patient lying prone on the ground, with snoring respirations. He is unresponsive and bleeding from the nose. His initial blood pressure is 170/90 mm Hg, heart rate is 53 beats/min, respiration rate is 16 breaths/min, and oxygen saturation is 96% on nonrebreather oxygen. The patient is rolled onto and secured to a long spine board with an appropriately sized cervical collar, and a head immobilizer is applied. Your partner establishes an IV line of normal saline while you perform a rapid secondary survey. You estimate the patient's weight to be 190 lb. His left pupil is sluggish and dilated, but the right pupil is normally reactive and 4 mm in diameter. Respirations are adequate with equal breath sounds, the abdomen is mildly distended, and the pelvis is stable.

This patient most likely has a significant closed-head injury, as evidenced by his unresponsiveness and unequal pupils. His relative hypertension and bradycardia may be suggestive of increased intracranial pressure (ICP) and risk for brain herniation. In addition, possible abdominal injuries are a concern given the mild distension. Remember that in every patient who has an altered mental status, a glucose level should be taken at some time during the evaluation (the patient may be a diabetic, and a low glucose level may have caused the accident).

This patient requires endotracheal intubation to protect his airway from aspiration of stomach contents and to prevent hypoxia. Arbabi et al[15] noted an improved outcome when patients with closed-head injury were intubated in the field versus delayed until arrival at an ED. Important considerations in this patient are the potential for increased ICP, the possibility for cervical spine injury, and the potential for internal injuries that could lead to a shock state over time.

This patient is ideally suited for RSI. Barriers to intubation should be recognized by asking yourself the same series of questions:

1. *Can I intubate?*

Be aware of your own skill limitations. Blood may obscure your view, and the need for cervical immobilization imparts a more limited laryngeal view compared with cases in which neck immobilization is not necessary. Applying front-to-back pressure over the thyroid cartilage (Adam's apple) can improve visualization of the laryngeal opening. This maneuver is commonly referred to as a **Sellick maneuver.**

> A modification known as the **BURP maneuver** can provide even better visualization. BURP is a mnemonic for *b*ackward-*u*pward (toward the head), *r*ightward (toward the patient's right), and *p*ressure.

Displacing the jaw anteriorly, as in a jaw or chin thrust airway maneuver, can also improve visualization in these circumstances. This situation is not appropriate for an inexperienced provider to attempt on his or her first RSI.

2. *Can I ventilate?*

Look for anatomic problems that could interfere with your ability to apply a bag-mask device. Such interference can be as simple as a bushy beard that must be quickly trimmed or as complex as massive facial and jaw injuries.

3. *What are my options if I can't intubate or ventilate?*

You must have a rescue airway, such as a dual-lumen device. The esophageal-Combitube (Tyco-Kendall, Mansfield, Mass.) airway is the only specific device listed within the American Society of Anesthesiologists algorithm for difficult airways. Translaryngeal catheter ventilation can temporarily deliver oxygen to a patient who cannot be intubated if you are unable to secure an airway or ventilate conventionally with a bag-mask device.

4. *Is the equipment on hand? Is it assembled?*

After medication administration is not the time to rummage for equipment. Before administration, ensure a functional suction line, a functional laryngoscope, appropriate sizes of endotracheal tubes, a reliable pulse oximeter reading, a bag-mask with a resuscitation bag attached to an ample supply of oxygen, and an end-tidal CO_2 monitor.

5. *Does the patient have any medical contraindications?*

Before you give any drug to any patient for any reason, ask yourself whether any reasons exist why this particular patient should not have a particular medication. As is the case with succinylcholine, certain patients may have lethal reactions. Make a habit of looking for medical identification jewelry on every unconscious patient.

6. *Will this patient die if I do not intubate him or her?*

As with any life-saving maneuver that carries significant risks, you must determine whether the benefits of proceeding outweigh the risks of attempting it. To some extent, the answer depends on your own honest self-assessment of your capabilities. Deferring an airway to the receiving hospital because of a carefully reasoned risk-benefit analysis can be the correct course of action. You may find that the receiving ED team echoes your decision by deferring to the operating room for surgical airway management.

RAPID SEQUENCE INTUBATION PHARMACOLOGY

RSI involves the use of two main classes of drugs, chemical paralytics and sedating agents, in addition to some adjunctive medications.

CHEMICAL PARALYSIS

The first medical use of chemical paralysis dates back to the use of curare in 1932.[16] Most people are familiar with curare's nonmedical use as the poison used on blow darts (as seen in jungle adventure movies). To understand how chemical paralytics work, a review is helpful of how a muscle gets a stimulus for contraction and, in turn, how that stimulus can be blocked.[17]

For voluntary skeletal contracture, such as the muscles in the arms, legs, chest wall, abdominal wall, neck, pharynx, eyes, diaphragm, and larynx, a nerve impulse is generated in the brain cells (neurons), transmitted to a neuron in the spinal canal, and then transmitted to a nerve that directly communicates with the muscle. At each junction between neurons, called **synapses,** the "hand off" occurs by chemicals called **neurotransmitters** being released on one side of the synapse, diffusing across to the other side, and then initiating an electrochemical impulse along the nerve. The final chemical transmission—between nerve and muscle—is crucial to understanding how chemical paralytics work and how to anticipate problems.

The end of the nerve fiber comes into close contact with the portion of the muscle cell that has receptors for the neurotransmitter sent by the nerve cell. This junction between nerve and muscle cell is known as the **neuromuscular junction.** The nerve side is the presynaptic membrane; the muscle side is the postsynaptic membrane, or motor end plate; and the space in between is the **synaptic cleft.** The chemical transmitter used is **acetylcholine.**

As an electrochemical signal reaches the presynaptic membrane of the neuromuscular junction, acetylcholine is released from storage sites at the end of the nerve cell axon and crosses the synaptic cleft to bind to receptors on the postsynaptic (muscle) side. This occurs quite rapidly because the distance across the cleft is only approximately 0.1 micrometer wide (or 1/10,000 of a millimeter). Once the acetylcholine binds to the postsynaptic membrane at special receptor binding sites, specific **acetylcholine receptors** (which act as special cellular gates) are unlocked and opened, resulting in contraction of the muscle fiber.

Muscle cells contracting in synchrony lead to coordinated muscle contraction. Once depolarization and contraction of the muscle fibers occur, the muscle cell membrane must pump out the ions and reestablish its normal electrical potential in preparation for another contraction. This period needed to restore itself is called the **refractory period;** during this time, the muscle cannot contract again.

Once acetylcholine binds to its receptor site on the postsynaptic membrane, ion flow continues until the acetylcholine molecule disengages. However, if it remains in the synaptic cleft, it can simply bind again. That is prevented by a chemical called **acetylcholinesterase,** which rapidly breaks the acetylcholine down and prevents continued binding. This breakdown occurs in approximately one tenth of a second. Nerve gas agents and organophosphate pesticides block the cholinesterase (i.e., act as a cholinesterase inhibitor), resulting in exaggerated cholinergic activity and continuous neuromuscular transmission, which explains the twitching and writhing that accompany their exposure. Anticholinergic medications such as atropine are used to treat nerve gas toxicity. Atropine is also used to prevent some of the adverse consequences of succinylcholine.

PARALYTIC DRUGS

Paralytic drugs are divided into two classes: **depolarizing** and **nondepolarizing paralytics.** The characterization of paralytic drugs into these two groups is key to understanding the complications and contraindications that a particular drug can pose to a particular patient.

Depolarizing Paralytics

Succinylcholine (often referred to as "SUX") is the only depolarizing paralytic. Succinylcholine is chemically similar to acetylcholine; in fact, succinylcholine is effectively two molecules of acetylcholine attached head to head. Because of the structural similarity, succinylcholine binds at the same receptor as acetylcholine. However, it does not let go as easily and is not broken down as readily. The result is that the ion gates remain open and, after initial contraction, the muscle cell cannot reestablish its electrical potential (because the gates are still open for ions to flow in) and therefore cannot generate further contractions. Succinylcholine acts to depolarize the muscle cell membrane and prevent repolarization; thus it is known as a *depolarizing paralytic drug.*

> A baseball pitcher (muscle) is on the mound waiting to receive the ball so that he can throw a pitch. The catcher (nerve) is in a squat, has the ball (acetylcholine) in his glove, and throws it from behind the plate to the pitcher (across the synaptic cleft). The pitcher catches the ball (acetylcholine) in his glove (the receptor binding site), goes into his wind up, and releases the pitch (the contraction).
>
> But wait! If the pitcher's glove is filled with something else, say a football, that stays in the pocket of the glove so that he cannot receive the ball, the pitcher no longer has a baseball to throw. This is what happens with a nondepolarizing paralytic. The receptor site is blocked by a chemical that has a high affinity (attraction) for the binding site but does not initiate a depolarization of the muscle cell (hence a nondepolarizing paralytic) and is not broken down in the synaptic cleft.
>
> If, on the other hand, a baseball is glued to the pitcher's glove, he may make his wind up, but no pitch will be thrown. The glued baseball has a high affinity for the receptor site (it is stuck in the glove) and initiates a wind up (because it is a baseball, not a football), but no pitch (contraction) results until the pitcher removes the glued baseball and cleans his glove. This reflects a depolarizing paralytic—it is similar in size and shape to the neurotransmitter, but it does not disengage from the receptor and results in *continued* depolarization of the muscle membrane, preventing further contractions.

Succinylcholine is the paralytic agent used most often in both ED and out-of-hospital RSI. Its properties that lend itself well to this use include rapid onset of paralysis (approximately 45 seconds IV) and short effective duration (approximately 5 minutes). Unfortunately, it also has detrimental side effects as a consequence of its action to depolarize muscle cell membranes.

The receptors on the postsynaptic motor end plate are relatively few in number. However, when stimulated by acetylcholine in the process of causing muscle cell depolarization, a small amount of potassium is released into the blood. This amount of potassium would be inconsequential in most healthy patients. However, in certain disease states in which the muscle is damaged (e.g., extensive burns) or diseased (e.g., muscular dystrophy) or not receiving nerve stimulation (e.g., neuromuscular disorder), the receptor sites proliferate over the entire muscle cell membrane, not just at the neuromuscular junction. Given the large surface area of the muscle fibers, the increase in the number of receptors is tremendous. Now, instead of an inconsequential release of potassium after succinylcholine-initiated depolarization, a critical and often fatal increase in serum potassium occurs (hyperkalemia), which can lead to sudden cardiac arrest from arrhythmia. Patients who are susceptible to this phenomenon include those with major burns (several days to several months after the burn), neuromuscular disease (e.g., recent stroke, recent cervical spine injury, encephalitis), and myopathic disease (e.g., muscular dystrophy).

> Succinylcholine administration to patients with burns, spinal cord injuries, extensive muscle trauma, renal failure, or muscle disorders can result in life-threatening hyperkalemia.

Also at risk for lethal hyperkalemia are patients who already have a dangerous but unrecognized elevation in serum potassium, for whom a normally inconsequential increase could push their elevated potassium level beyond a dangerous threshold. These patients include those undergoing kidney dialysis or with kidney failure; those with significant crush injury or history of extensive limb entrapment, impairing blood supply for a period; those with certain overdoses such as digoxin or digitalis; and those with overdoses that can cause severe acidosis, such as aspirin, methanol, and ethylene glycol. In the study by Wayne and Friedland,[9] previously mentioned in the context of RSI by paramedics, the only fatality in their series of almost 3000 patients occurred from hyperkalemic arrest in a patient with unknown amyotrophic lateral sclerosis (also called *Lou Gehrig's disease*).

A major concern for the prehospital use of succinylcholine is that the history of many patients is unknown to the prehospital provider. Even in the more controlled setting of elective surgery, deaths have occurred in patients who underwent preoperative screening but who had unrecognized neuromuscular disease, primarily undiagnosed Duchenne muscular dystrophy in children.[18,19] For that reason, succinylcholine is no longer used in routine surgery in children. One subtle sign of Duchenne muscular dystrophy is the presence of significantly enlarged lower leg muscles. What this discussion means for the paramedic is that the question "Does this patient have any contraindications to this medication?" must be carefully considered before succinylcholine is given.

Another potentially fatal side effect of succinylcholine administration is a condition known as **malignant hyperthermia.** This is a genetic abnormality in which a patient has exaggerated and sustained muscle contractions in response to certain inhaled general anesthetics and succinylcholine. The increased muscle activity can lead to fatal hyperthermia. If recognized in family members or previously in the patient, such patients may wear medical identification jewelry indicating that they should not receive inhaled anesthetics or succinylcholine.

Other side effects of succinylcholine, again related to its initial depolarizing effects, include increased intragastric pressure (increased risk of vomiting), increased ocular pressure (risk of extrusion of eye contents if an open eye injury exists), increased ICP (concern in head trauma), and masseter spasm (spasm of cheek and jaw muscles that can delay intubation), Finally, succinylcholine can cause severe bradycardia in children because of their increased sensitivity to vagus nerve effects on the heart and the fact that succinylcholine mimics the action of acetylcholine. For that reason, atropine is recommended before succinylcholine in any child younger than approximately 8 years.

> Succinylcholine administration in children can produce bradycardia. Pretreat children younger than 8 years old with atropine to avoid bradycardia.

Succinylcholine has a short duration of action because it is completely and rapidly metabolized in the blood by an enzyme called **pseudocholinesterase.** Because breakdown by the liver or kidney is not necessary, succinylcholine dosage does not need to be adjusted for patients with kidney or liver disease. Some individuals have a genetically determined pseudocholinesterase deficiency and have a significantly prolonged (hours to days) paralysis. This information may be available on medical identification jewelry.

SUCCINYLCHOLINE (ANECTINE)

Classification: Neuromuscular blocker, depolarizing
Action: Competes with the acetylcholine receptor of the motor end plate on the muscle cell, resulting in muscle paralysis.
Indications: To induce neuromuscular blockade for the facilitation of ET intubation.
Adverse Effects: Anaphylactoid reactions, respiratory depression, apnea, bronchospasm, cardiac arrhythmias, malignant hyperthermia, hypertension, hypotension, muscle fasciculation, postprocedure muscle pain, hypersalivation, rash.
Contraindications: Malignant hyperthermia, burns, trauma. Use with caution in children, cardiac disease, hepatic disease, renal disease, peptic ulcer disease, cholinesterase-inhibitor toxicity, pseudocholinesterase deficiency, digitalis toxicity, glaucoma, hyperkalemia, hypothermia, rhabdomyolysis, myasthenia gravis.

cont'd

SUCCINYLCHOLINE (ANECTINE)—CONT'D

Dosage:
- **Adult:**
  - **IV:** 0.6 mg/kg IV, IO (range 0.3-1.1 mg/kg).
  - **IM:** 3 to 4 mg/kg (max dose: 150 mg).
- **Pediatric:**
  - **IV:**
    - **Adolescents and older children:** 1 mg/kg IV, IO.
    - **Small children and infants:** 2 mg/kg IV, IO.
  - **IM:** 3 to 4 mg/kg (max dose: 150 mg).

Special Considerations:

IV administration results in neuromuscular blockade in 0.5 to 1 minute. IM administration results in neuromuscular blockade in 2 to 3 minutes.

IV administration in infants and children can potentially result in profound bradycardia and, in some cases, asystole. The incidence of bradycardia is greater after the second dose. The occurrence of bradycardia can be reduced with the pretreatment of atropine.

Succinylcholine can have a significantly prolonged effect in the setting of poisoning with nerve gas agents and organophosphate pesticides.

Pregnancy class C

ATROPINE SULFATE

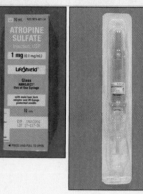

Classification: Anticholinergic (antimuscarinic)

Action: Competes reversibly with acetylcholine at the site of the muscarinic receptor. Receptors affected, in order from the most sensitive to the least sensitive, include salivary, bronchial, sweat glands, eye, heart, and GI tract.

Indications: Symptomatic bradycardia, asystole or PEA, nerve agent exposure, organophosphate poisoning.

Adverse Effects: Decreased secretions resulting in dry mouth and hot skin temperature, intense facial flushing, blurred vision or dilation of the pupils with subsequent photophobia, tachycardia, restlessness. Atropine may cause paradoxical bradycardia if the dose administered is too low or if the drug is administered too slowly.

Contraindications: Acute MI; myasthenia gravis; GI obstruction; closed-angle glaucoma; known sensitivity to atropine, belladonna alkaloids, or sulfites. Will not be effective for infranodal (type II) AV block and new third-degree block with wide QRS complex.

Dosage:

Symptomatic Bradycardia:
- **Adult:** 0.5 mg IV, IO every 3 to 5 minutes to a maximum dose of 3 mg.
- **Adolescent:** 0.02 mg/kg (minimum 0.1 mg/dose; maximum 1 mg/dose) IV, IO up to a total dose of 2 mg.
- **Pediatric:** 0.02 mg/kg (minimum 0.1 mg/dose; maximum 0.5 mg/dose) IV, IO, to a total dose of 1 mg.

Asystole/Pulseless Electrical Activity:
- 1 mg IV, IO every 3 to 5 minutes, to a maximum dose of 3 mg. May be administered via ET tube at 2 to 2.5 mg diluted in 5 to 10 mL of water or normal saline.

Nerve Agent or Organophosphate Poisoning:
- **Adult:** 2 to 4 mg IV, IM; repeat if needed every 20 to 30 minutes until symptoms dissipate. In severe cases, the initial dose can be as large as 2 to 6 mg administered IV. Repeat doses of 2 to 6 mg can be administered IV, IM every 5 to 60 minutes.
- **Pediatric:** 0.05 mg/kg IV, IM every 10 to 30 minutes as needed until symptoms dissipate.
- **Infants <15 lb:** 0.05 mg/kg IV, IM every 5 to 20 minutes as needed until symptoms dissipate.

Special Considerations:

Half-life 2.5 hours

Pregnancy class C; possibly unsafe in lactating mothers.

Nondepolarizing Paralytics

Nondepolarizing muscle relaxants act to bind preferentially to the acetylcholine receptor site, preventing binding of acetylcholine (i.e., blocking the key) and ion flow into the cell, thereby preventing muscle contraction. Because the membrane is not allowed to depolarize, these are known as *nondepolarizing neuromuscular blocking agents*. Curare is a nondepolarizing drug.

Several nondepolarizing muscle relaxants are grouped according to their duration of action: short-, intermediate-, and long-acting agents. Two short-acting agents are mivacurium and rocuronium. Both mivacurium (Mivacron) and rocuronium (Zemuron) have a rapid onset and short duration of action (15 to 30 minutes). Unfortunately, mivacurium (Mivacron) is no longer manufactured and is not available in the United States. Examples of intermediate-acting nondepolarizing agents include vecuronium (Norcuron) and atracurium (Tracrium). Pancuronium (Pavulon) is considered a long-acting agent.

Twelve nondepolarizing agents are currently clinically available for chemical paralysis. They vary in speed of onset, duration of action, mechanism of metabolism, and cost.

> Paralytic agents have no effect on consciousness or reduction of pain. Patients must have adequate sedation and analgesia administered in addition to the paralytic agents.

For prehospital and ED use, vecuronium provides a reliable combination of rapid onset, intermediate duration, and reasonable cost. Vecuronium is an intermediate-acting, nondepolarizing paralytic that induces muscle paralysis by blocking receptors for acetylcholine and preventing muscle contraction. It has no negative effects on cardiovascular function and does not lower blood pressure or affect heart rate. Vecuronium is primarily metabolized by the liver and therefore has an increased duration in patients with liver disease.

Vecuronium has none of the contraindications of succinylcholine and would appear to be an ideal agent. However, the major problem with nondepolarizing agents is that their onset of action is slower than that of succinylcholine, and the duration of action is significantly longer. Whereas succinylcholine results in adequate paralysis for intubation at 45 seconds, vecuronium can require 3 to 5 minutes. Perhaps even more concerning is the fact that vecuronium maintains effective paralysis for 25 to 40 minutes compared with 5 to 8 minutes for succinylcholine.

The onset of action of vecuronium to be effective to create intubating conditions is considered too slow by many for use in RSI. Vecuronium typically is used to maintain neuromuscular paralysis once the patient has been intubated with succinylcholine. Alternatively, vecuronium and other agents can be used to provide paralysis for intubation in conditions in which succinylcholine is contraindicated.

One component of RSI technique is to preoxygenate the patient. This involves applying a tightly fitting nonrebreather mask at 100% oxygen concentration for 5 minutes before the RSI procedure. Alternatively, if the patient is able to cooperate, he or she can take 4 maximal tidal breaths while breathing 100% oxygen. By doing this, the nitrogen that is part of the gas remaining in the alveoli after breathing room air is washed out and replaced by oxygen. This creates a reservoir of oxygen waiting to diffuse from the alveolus into the pulmonary capillaries.

Patients who are properly preoxygenated can sustain up to 6 minutes of complete apnea (as induced by a paralytic) without oxygen saturation dropping below 90%. Note that 6 minutes is ideal; many patients who require intubation require it because of problems with oxygenation in the first place. This illustrates the advantage of succinylcholine over vecuronium. It is conceivably possible, although not assured, to administer succinylcholine, have the patient paralyzed for 6 minutes, and emerge from paralysis without the oxygen saturation level falling below 90%, even if you are unable to intubate or successfully ventilate the patient. This is not possible with vecuronium or any of the other nondepolarizing blockers. Therefore the risk of the vulnerable period of a failed intubation must be weighed against the risk of hyperkalemia and malignant hyperthermia.

However, decreasing the time of onset for vecuronium is possible by using a technique known as *priming* (from the practice of priming a pump). For a muscle to be paralyzed, a nondepolarizing paralytic drug must block 90% of the motor end plate receptors. Muscle weakness does not usually occur until 75% of the receptors are blocked, meaning that blocking fewer than 75% of receptors *should* have no noticeable effect on muscle function. Administering one tenth of the paralyzing dose 2 to 3 minutes before administration of the full dose initiates blockade of some of the receptors, decreasing the time necessary to block the remaining receptors. This can shorten the time of onset to 1 to 1.5 minutes. However, because of individual variability, some patients may have effective paralysis at the priming dose; therefore all equipment should be ready to intubate at that time.

Another method for decreasing the onset time is to increase the paralyzing dose; however, this can also extend the effective paralysis for more than 90 minutes and would significantly increase patient vulnerability if intubation was not successful. A third method for decreasing the *relative* onset of paralysis is a technique called *timing,* in which the sedating agent is withheld until paralysis is about to take effect (generally when hand grip fails) so that the sedating agent takes effect as paralysis ensues and maximal sedation is achieved at the same time as maximal paralysis. The timing approach may be too difficult for use in the prehospital environment.

ROCURONIUM (ZEMURON)

Classification: Neuromuscular blocker, nondepolarizing
Action: Antagonizes acetylcholine at the motor end plate, producing skeletal muscle paralysis.
Indications: To induce neuromuscular blockade for the facilitation of ET intubation.
Adverse Effects: Muscle paralysis, apnea, dyspnea, respiratory depression, sinus tachycardia, urticaria.
Contraindications: Known sensitivity to bromides. Use with caution in heart disease, liver disease.
Dosage:
- **Adult:** 0.6 to 1.2 mg/kg IV, IO.
- **Pediatric (older than 3 months):** 0.6 mg/kg IV, IO.

Special Considerations:
Onset of action is 2 to 8 minutes.
Duration of action is 31 minutes.
Pregnancy class B

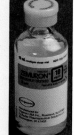

VECURONIUM (NORCURON)

Classification: Neuromuscular blocker, nondepolarizing
Action: Antagonizes acetylcholine at the motor end plate, producing skeletal muscle paralysis.
Indications: To induce neuromuscular blockade for the facilitation of ET intubation.
Adverse Effects: Muscle paralysis, apnea, dyspnea, respiratory depression, sinus tachycardia, urticaria.
Contraindications: Known sensitivity to bromides. Use with caution in heart disease, liver disease.
Dosage:
- **Adult:** 0.08 to 0.1 mg/kg IV, IO.
- **Pediatric:** Dosage is individualized.

Special Considerations:
Pregnancy class C

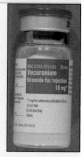

ATRACURIUM (TRACRIUM)

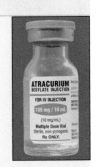

Classification: Nondepolarizing neuromuscular blocker
Action: Antagonizes acetylcholine receptors at the motor end plate, producing muscle paralysis.
Indications: Neuromuscular blockade to facilitate ET intubation.
Adverse Effects: Flushing, edema, urticaria, pruritus, bronchospasm and/or wheezing, alterations in heart rate, decrease in blood pressure.
Contraindications: Cardiac disease, electrolyte abnormalities, dehydration, known sensitivity.
Dosage:
- **Adult:** 0.4 to 0.5 mg/kg IV, IO; repeat with 0.08 to 0.1 mg/kg every 20 to 45 minutes as needed for prolonged paralysis.
- **Pediatric:**
  - **Older than 2 years:** Same as adult dosing.
  - **Younger than 2 years:** 0.3 to 0.4 mg/kg IV, IO.

Special Considerations:
Do not give by IM injection.
Pregnancy class C

PANCURONIUM (PAVULON)

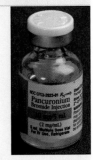

Classification: Nondepolarizing neuromuscular blocker
Action: Antagonizes acetylcholine at the motor end plate, producing skeletal muscle paralysis.
Indications: To induce neuromuscular blockade for the facilitation of ET intubation.
Adverse Effects: Muscle paralysis, apnea, dyspnea, respiratory depression, cutaneous flushing, sinus tachycardia.
Contraindications: Known sensitivity to bromides. Use with caution in heart disease, renal disease.
Dosage:
- **Adult:** 0.04 to 0.1 mg/kg IV, IO; repeat dosing is 0.01 mg/kg every 25 to 60 minutes.
- **Pediatric:** Same as adult dosing.

Special Considerations:
Pregnancy class C

DEEP SEDATION DRUGS

The second major drug component of RSI is the sedating agent. When used with paralytics, sedation improves the intubation success rate.[20] The purposes of sedation are to protect the brain and heart from dangerous fluctuations in blood pressure and heart rate and prevent the patient from being paralyzed while awake. It would be terrifying for patients to be unable to control their breathing, be fully aware of a painful procedure, and be unable to communicate any discomfort. Therefore this situation is absolutely to be avoided. Clinical clues that sedation is insufficient include a significant rise in blood pressure and elevation in heart rate.

Sedation can be provided on a continuum from light sedation (such as the preanesthesia relaxants given before a patient is taken into surgery) to general anesthesia (during which patients are deeply unconscious without the ability to protect their airway). The sedation level at the drug doses that permit RSI approaches and often reaches general anesthesia levels. The following are common sedation agents: midazolam (Versed), etomidate (Amidate), and ketamine (Ketalar).

Midazolam is a benzodiazepine with anticonvulsant properties, sedative properties, and the ability to induce amnesia for events occurring after administration. Midazolam causes a slight decrease in ICP but does not necessarily blunt the rise in pressure that results from laryngoscopy or intubation.[21] Midazolam causes a decrease in vascular resistance from vascular smooth muscle relaxation; in patients who are hypovolemic or in shock, this can result in a sudden drop in blood pressure and/or a compensatory increase in heart rate. Midazolam should therefore be used cautiously in patients with multiple trauma.

Midazolam has no analgesic (pain-killing) effects; do not assume a sedated and paralyzed patient has adequate pain control if only midazolam has been administered. Midazolam can also cause respiratory depression, although this is of clinical concern only if successful intubation is in doubt.

Midazolam has been advocated as a single agent to facilitate prehospital intubation in patients with barriers to intubation, such as clenched jaws or combative behavior, with a success rate of 64% and 85% in two small studies.[22,23] When compared with other sedating agents, midazolam has not always engendered the same success as other agents.[6] One reason may be a tendency to underdose because of concerns for hypotension.[24] Whereas the sedating dose for anxiety is 0.03 mg/kg, the dose recommended for intubation is 10 times that level, or 0.3 mg/kg.[21,24,25] This is more a matter of patient selection than dosing regimen; that is, if potential hypotension is a concern, choose another agent rather than an ineffective dose.

A potential safety feature for midazolam is that its effects can be reversed with flumazenil (Romazicon). Flumazenil is an antagonist to benzodiazepines, just as naloxone (Narcan) is an antagonist to opiates. Flumazenil should be used with caution in people who regularly take benzodiazepine medications because it can produce withdrawal seizures that are difficult to control and complicate airway management efforts.

Etomidate is a unique sedating agent that is not related to narcotics, benzodiazepines, or barbiturates. It was first used in the early 1980s as an alternative to these other classes of medications and has risen rapidly to a preeminent position among the RSI sedation drugs. Etomidate has favorable properties for RSI sedation: it has a very rapid onset (30 seconds), short duration of action (3 to 5 minutes), and minimal effects on the heart and blood vessels. Etomidate lowers ICP and preserves cerebral and heart perfusion; therefore it does not cause hypotension or worsen shock states.[21,25] For these reasons, etomidate is the agent of choice for use in RSI for patients with multiple trauma. In fact, etomidate has emerged as the overall sedation method of choice for RSI in the ED[5,20,26] and is being used with increasing frequency for RSI in the prehospital setting.[27-30]

Because of its favorable hemodynamic profile and the fact that it causes less respiratory depression at comparable levels of deep sedation, etomidate is now being used for sedation in EDs for procedures such as major joint and fracture reductions and cardioversion without intubation. Etomidate has also been used to facilitate removal of patients who are painfully entrapped within motor vehicles.[31]

Note that the effective duration of etomidate of 3 to 5 minutes means that patients can wake up before paralysis wears off. Be prepared to either resedate or administer a longer-acting sedation agent such as midazolam after successful intubation. On the other hand, if the patient has been properly preoxygenated, the short duration is quite advantageous if intubation cannot be accomplished.

> Patients can wake from etomidate before the paralysis wears off. Therefore patients need to be resedated with a longer-acting agent after intubation.

As with midazolam, etomidate has been advocated as a single agent for chemically assisted intubation. However, intubation success rates are not as high as when combined with paralytics.[27-29] Etomidate causes burning pain on injection.

One additional side effect of etomidate is a dose-related suppression of adrenal function. Because adrenal steroid secretion is one of the mechanisms with which the body responds to stress, a suppression of corticosteroid production can have serious effects on recovery from trauma. Some trauma patients who have been maintained on etomidate drips for long-term intensive care unit sedation have died from sepsis because of this effect. Although a decrease in blood corticosteroid levels can be demonstrated after a single dose of etomidate, most experts do not believe that this suppression is clinically important for a single dose.[25]

Ketamine is described as a dissociative anesthetic because patients apparently experience a separation of consciousness from the perception of pain. Ketamine is derived from and has some similar properties to a better-known drug, phencyclidine phosphate, known more commonly as "PCP" or "angel dust." Unfortunately, ketamine has now also emerged as a street drug of abuse, often called "Special K."

Ketamine induces intense sedation, analgesia, and amnesia. Yet protective airway reflexes are generally preserved, even during deep sedation; no significant respiratory depression occurs, and apnea is extremely rare. Ketamine causes a modest increase in blood pressure and heart rate and can increase myocardial oxygen demands. Ketamine should not be used in patients with acute coronary syndromes or myocardial infarction. On the other hand, ketamine does offer some protection against arrhythmias precipitated by epinephrine and other stress responses. Therefore ketamine can work well in patients with hypovolemia. In addition, ketamine has potent bronchodilator properties and is more advantageous than other agents when patients with severe bronchospasm or status asthmaticus are being intubated.[32] Ketamine does cause a rise in ICP and should not be used if a potential for increased ICP exists (closed-head trauma, brain tumor, stroke or intracranial hemorrhage, or status seizures).

> Patients administered ketamine maintain their airway reflexes and do not have significant respiratory depression.

Ketamine has been used extensively for sedation during painful procedures, especially in children, and has an excellent safety record.[33] Ketamine has also been extensively used for RSI in the ED, but few reports of ketamine in the prehospital setting exist.[20,26] This may be caused in part by the potential for diversion and drug abuse with ketamine compared with agents such as etomidate. Ketamine can be a useful addition to the paramedic's drug box, however. Ketamine can provide safer conditions for chemically assisting the extrication of patients entrapped within motor vehicles and from collapsed buildings or structures. It has significant potential in natural and manmade disaster situations, particularly those associated with earthquakes and explosions.[31,34,35]

Because of the low incidence of respiratory depression and the maintenance of protective airway reflexes, the intubation and procedural sedation dosages are the same. Onset of effect is quite rapid, less than 1 minute. Duration of unconsciousness is 15 to 20 minutes, and analgesia continues for an additional 30 minutes. Ketamine can also be effective when administered intramuscularly. Onset can be delayed to 3 to 5 minutes. Duration of effect is also more prolonged when ketamine is given intramuscularly, lasting approximately 1 hour.

Adverse side effects of ketamine include laryngospasm, increased bronchial secretions, and dysphoric (unpleasant) emergence from sedation. To limit bronchial secretions, an anticholinergic agent such as atropine or glycopyrrolate (Robinul) can be administered. Emergence phenomena, such as nightmares and hallucinations, are another adverse effect. In both adults and children the administration of diazepam can reduce the incidence of unpleasant and sometimes psychologically disturbing dreams on awakening from anesthesia.

MIDAZOLAM (VERSED)

Classification: Benzodiazepine, Schedule C-IV
Action: Binds to the benzodiazepine receptor and enhances the effects of the brain chemical (neurotransmitter) GABA. Benzodiazepines act at the level of the limbic, thalamic, and hypothalamic regions of the CNS to produce short-acting CNS depression (including sedation, skeletal muscle relaxation, and anticonvulsant activity).
Indications: Sedation, anxiety, skeletal muscle relaxation.
Adverse Effects: Respiratory depression, respiratory arrest, hypotension, nausea/vomiting, headache, hiccups, cardiac arrest.
Contraindications: Acute-angle glaucoma, pregnant women, known sensitivity.
Dosage:
Sedation:
Note: The dose of midazolam needs to be individualized. Every dose should be administered slowly over a period of 2 minutes. Allow 2 minutes to evaluate the clinical effect of the dose given.

- **Adult:**
  - **Healthy and younger than 60 years:** *Some patients require as little as 1 mg IV, IO. No more than 2.5 mg should be given over a 2-minute interval.* If additional sedation is required, continue to administer small increments over 2-minute periods (max dose: 5 mg). If the patient also has received a narcotic, he or she will typically require 30% less midazolam than the same patient not given the narcotic.
  - **60 years and older and debilitated or chronically ill patients:** This group of patients has a higher risk of hypoventilation, airway obstruction, and apnea. The peak clinical effect can take longer in these patients; therefore dose increments should be smaller, and the rate of injection should be slower. *Some patients require a dose as small as 1 mg IV, IO, and no more than 1.5 mg should be given over a 2-minute period.* If additional sedation is required, additional midazolam should be given at a rate of no more than 1 mg over a 2-minute period (max dose: 3.5 mg). If the patient also has received a narcotic, he or she will typically require 50% less midazolam than the same patient not given the narcotic.
  - **Continuous infusion:** Continuous infusions can be required for prolonged transport of intubated, critically ill, and injured patients. After an initial bolus dose, the adult patient will require a maintenance infusion dose of 0.02 to 0.1 mg/kg/hr (1-7 mg/hr).
- **Pediatric (weight-based):** Pediatric patients typically require higher doses of midazolam than do adults on the basis of weight (in mg/kg). Younger pediatric patients (younger than 6 years) require higher doses (in mg/kg) than older pediatric patients. Midazolam takes approximately 3 minutes to reach peak effect; therefore wait at least 2 minutes to determine effectiveness of drug and need for additional dosing.
  - **12 to 16 years:** Same as adult dosing. Some patients in this age group require a higher dose than that used in adults, but rarely does a patient require more than 10 mg.
  - **6 to 12 years:** 0.025 to 0.05 mg/kg IV, IO up to a total dose of 0.4 mg/kg. Exceeding 10 mg as total dose usually is not necessary.
  - **6 months to 5 years:** 0.05 to 0.1 mg/kg IV, IO up to a total dose of 0.6 mg/kg. Exceeding 6 mg as total dose usually is not necessary.
  - **Younger than 6 months:** Dosing recommendations for this age group is unclear. Because this age group is especially vulnerable to airway obstruction and hypoventilation, use small increments with frequent clinical evaluation. Dose: 0.05 to 0.1 mg/kg IV, IO.

Special Considerations:
Patients receiving midazolam require frequent monitoring of vital signs and pulse oximetry. Be prepared to support patient's airway and ventilation.
Pregnancy class D

FLUMAZENIL (ROMAZICON)

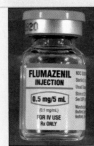

Classification: Benzodiazepine receptor antagonist, antidote
Action: Competes with benzodiazepines for binding at the benzodiazepine receptor, reverses the sedative effects of benzodiazepines.
Indication: Benzodiazepine oversedation
Adverse Effects: Resedation, seizures, dizziness, pain at injection site, nausea/vomiting, diaphoresis, headache, visual impairment.
Contraindications: Cyclic antidepressant overdose; life-threatening conditions that require treatment with benzodiazepines, such as status epilepticus and intracranial hypertension; known sensitivity to flumazenil or benzodiazepines. Use with caution where there is the possibility of unrecognized benzodiazepine dependence and in patients who have a history of substance abuse or who are known substance abusers.
Dosage:
- **Adult:** Initial dose is 0.2 mg IV, IO over a 15-second period. If the desired effect is not observed after 45 seconds, administer a second 0.2-mg dose, again over a 15-second period. Doses can be repeated a total of four times until a total dose of 1 mg has been administered.
- **Pediatric:** Children older than 1 year, 0.01 mg/kg IV, IO given over a 15-second period. May repeat in 45 seconds and then every minute to a maximum cumulative dose of 0.05 mg/kg or 1 mg, whichever is the lower dose.

Special Considerations:
Monitor for signs of hypoventilation and hypoxia for approximately 2 hours.
If the half-life of the benzodiazepine is longer than flumazenil, an additional dose may be needed.
May precipitate withdrawal symptoms in patients dependent on benzodiazepines.
Flumazenil has not been shown to benefit patients who have overdosed on multiple drugs.
Pregnancy class C

ETOMIDATE (AMIDATE)

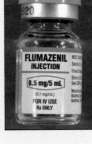

Classification: Hypnotic, anesthesia induction agent
Action: Although the exact mechanism is unknown, etomidate appears to have GABA-like effects.
Indications: Induction for rapid sequence intubation and pharmacologic-assisted intubation, induction of anesthesia.
Adverse Effects: Hypotension, respiratory depression, pain at the site of injection, temporary involuntary muscle movements, frequent nausea/vomiting on emergence, adrenal insufficiency, hyperventilation, hypoventilation, apnea of short duration, hiccups, laryngospasm, snoring, tachypnea, hypertension, cardiac arrhythmias.
Contraindications: Known sensitivity. Use in pregnancy only if the potential benefits justify the potential risk to the fetus. Do not use during labor and avoid in nursing mothers.
Dosage:
- **Adult:** 0.2 to 0.6 mg/kg slow IV, IO (over 30 to 60 seconds). A typical adult intubating dose of etomidate is 20 mg slow IV. Consider less (e.g., 10 mg) in the elderly or patients with cardiac conditions.
- **Pediatric:**
  - **Older than 10 years:** Same as adult dosing.
  - **Younger than 10 years:** Safety has not been established.

Special Considerations:
Etomidate is used to prepare a patient for orotracheal intubation. Both personnel and equipment must be present to manage the patient's airway before administration.
Pregnancy class C

KETAMINE (KETALAR)

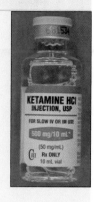

Classification: General anesthetic
Action: Produces a state of anesthesia while maintaining airway reflexes, heart rate, and blood pressure.
Indications: Pain and as anesthesia for procedures of short duration.
Adverse Effects: Emergence phenomena, hypertension and sinus tachycardia, hypotension and sinus bradycardia, other cardiac arrhythmias (rare), respiratory depression, apnea, laryngospasms and other forms of airway obstruction (rare), tonic and clonic movements, vomiting.
Contraindications: Patients in whom a significant elevation in blood pressure would be hazardous (hypertension, stroke, head trauma, increased intracranial mass or bleeding, MI). Use with caution in patients with increased ICP or increased intraocular pressure (glaucoma) and patients with hypovolemia, dehydration, or cardiac disease (especially angina and CHF).
Dosage: Administer slowly over a period of 60 seconds.
IV, IO:

  · **Adult:** 1 to 4.5 mg/kg IV, IO. 1 to 2 mg/kg produces anesthesia usually within 30 seconds that typically lasts 5 to 10 minutes.
  · **Pediatric:** 0.5 to 2 mg IV, IO over a 1-minute period.

IM:

  · **Adult:** 6.5 to 13 mg/kg IM. 10 mg/kg IM is capable of producing anesthesia within 3 to 4 minutes with an effect typically lasting 12 to 25 minutes. In adults, concomitant administration of 5 to 15 mg of diazepam reduces the incidence of emergence phenomena.
  · **Pediatric:** 3 to 7 mg IM.

Special Considerations:
Pregnancy class C

RAPID SEQUENCE INTUBATION

The procedure for RSI can be characterized by following the seven P's (Fig. 20-2):

1. *P*reparations (time $\geq$ t − 5 minutes)

Patient is attached to pulse oximeter, ECG monitor, and end-tidal CO_2 monitor (if available). Medications are chosen after considering underlying patient condition and potential contraindications. Intubation and suction equipment are readied, including rescue devices such as Combitube and manual jet ventilator. Ensure that oxygen is connected and flowing at the maximal rate. Remember personal protective gear because blood and body fluids often erupt from the airways.

2. *P*reoxygenation (time = t − 5 minutes)

Patient is placed on tight-fitting 100% nonrebreather face mask for 5 minutes. Attempt to wash out excess nitrogen from the pulmonary alveoli, providing a reservoir of oxygen to enable tolerance of an apneic period. As much as possible, avoid ventilating the patient with positive pressure unless oxygen saturation falls below 90%. If positive pressure ventilation is required, apply downward pressure over the cricothyroid membrane (Sellick maneuver) to limit passage of air into the stomach, which would otherwise increase the risk of emesis and aspiration. If the patient is alert, coach him or her to take 8 maximal (i.e., as deep as possible) breaths, a technique that also eliminates space-wasting nitrogen.

3. *P*retreatment/priming (time = t − 3 minutes)

If using succinylcholine, administer one tenth of the paralyzing dose. Be sure equipment is ready in the event of premature paralysis. Consider pretreatment with lidocaine. Manipulation of the larynx causes both reflex elevation of ICP and secretion of catecholamines such as epinephrine.[15,25] These can cause decreased blood flow to the brain and put increased stress on cardiac oxygen consumption. Lidocaine has been shown to blunt these effects.[36] Whether any additive protection is applied to deep sedation is unclear, but no downside exists in trying to maximize cerebral and cardiac protection. If a patient does not have a head injury, intracranial process, or cardiac problems, lidocaine can be omitted.

4. **Paralytic/sedation (time = t − 1 minute)**

Administer a sedation agent followed immediately by a paralytic agent. Allow for adequate relaxation before attempting to intubate; the use of a watch is best. Some cases allow you to administer sedation, maintain spontaneous breathing, and assess the ability to visualize the laryngeal opening, following with full paralysis and intubation. Administering sedation before the paralytic is generally better in case IV access is lost.

5. **Protection (Time = t − 1 minute)**

From the point at which sedation and the paralytic are administered until the endotracheal position is confirmed, the Sellick maneuver should be applied.

6. **Pass the tube (Time = 0)**

7. **Prove it! (Time = t+)**

Confirm tube position. Although determining endotracheal position is especially difficult in the prehospital environment, several studies have demonstrated unacceptable rates of undetected endotracheal malposition in field intubations.[37,38] Confirmatory methods must be used, such as end-tidal CO_2 detectors and esophageal detector devices, in addition to clinical assessment of endotracheal tube position.[8,39]

You and your partner respond to a call for a gunshot wound to the face. After the scene is secured by police, you find a 46-year-old man who attempted suicide by placing a shotgun under his chin and firing. He is awake and sitting forward. Although he cannot speak beyond mumbles, he is able to follow commands and communicate. Blood is draining at a moderate rate out of what is left of his mouth. His blood pressure is 150/85 mm Hg, heart rate is 110 beats/min, and respiratory rate is 30 breaths/min and unlabored. Oxygen saturation is 92%. You have concerns about his airway and consider intubating him, using your knowledge of RSI technique.

In this common scenario, the paramedic is faced with several decisions. First, does the patient need immediate intubation (question 6)? As long as he leans forward, he should be able to maintain his airway until he goes into shock. The decision really depends on how much he is bleeding and how far away you are from the destination hospital (or helicopter). If you decide to intubate, maintain him in a position of comfort (sitting up) for as long as possible and consider intubating him while he is sitting up. The patient's risk of cervical spine injury with this mechanism of injury is low. He is at a higher risk for losing his airway.[40]

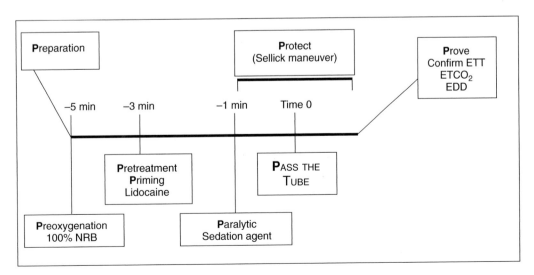

▼ **Fig. 20-2** RSI technique. *EDD*, Esophageal detector device; *ETCO₂*, end-tidal CO_2; *ETT*, endotracheal tube; *NRB*, nonrebreather mask.

If his blood loss, ability to control his airway, and time to the trauma center are too great, a modified intubation plan may be warranted. Following the previously outlined steps, proceed through the seven P's. During preparation, ask yourself the five remaining questions:

1. *Can I intubate?*

Surprisingly, patients who sustain a gunshot wound to their mandible and teeth/tongue are often easy to intubate because of little resistance to laryngoscopy. Bleeding can obscure the view, however, so suction should be optimized. The patient should remain leaning forward throughout the procedure if possible.

2. *Can I ventilate?*

It would not be appropriate to ventilate with a bag-mask.

3. *Do I have other options?*

Plan on an alternate airway. The Combitube has been shown to be a valuable adjunct and may also provide some tamponade of pharyngeal bleeding.[41]

4. *Is the equipment assembled?*

5. *Are any contraindications to medications or technique present?*

The major problem may be visualization. Because the patient is currently breathing, you could choose a technique that maintains his breathing, at least until confirmation that the laryngeal opening can be visualized. Consider using ketamine (if part of approved protocols) or etomidate at a reduced dose (0.15 to 0.2 mg/kg). If you can visualize the laryngeal opening, proceed with full paralysis. If not, defer to the receiving hospital unless the patient deteriorates further. This plan should be established in advance, with alternatives considered at that time, as well.

RSI as a prehospital skill has yet to be fully explored. Currently, paramedics in most systems have only limited opportunity to perform this intervention; data extrapolated from Pittsburgh EMS statistics would project only one RSI per paramedic per decade.[8] Consequently, to remain competent in performing RSI, continual review of the pharmacology of the medications in this chapter is necessary. Equally important, paramedics must fortify airway skills and decision making by participating in continuing education and clinical airway management experiences.

REVIEW QUESTIONS

1. What are six questions to ask yourself when preparing to perform rapid sequence intubation?
2. What is the neurotransmitter used to make muscles contract?
3. What is the chemical that normally breaks down acetylcholine?
4. What are the two classes of paralytics?
5. How quickly does succinylcholine induce paralysis?
6. What electrolyte is released into the bloodstream after administration of succinylcholine?
7. In what medical conditions should a patient *not* be given succinylcholine?
8. What is malignant hyperthermia?
9. In children younger than 8 years, what medication should be administered before succinylcholine? Why?
10. What are the effects of vecuronium on the cardiovascular system?
11. What is the unique relation between the deep sedation medications midazolam and flumazenil?
12. Explain why etomidate is the preferred drug for deep sedation in intubation.
13. List the seven P's of RSI and the timeframe required for each step of the procedure.

REFERENCES

1. Mihic DE, Binkert E, Novoselac M: The first endotracheal intubation, *Anesthesiology* 52:523, 1980.
2. Scott J: Oral endotracheal intubation. In Dailey RH, et al, editors: *The airway: emergency management,* St Louis, 1992, Mosby, pp 73-91.

3. Stept WJ, Safar P: Rapid induction-intubation for prevention of gastric-content aspiration, *Anesth Analg* 49:633, 1970.
4. Rapid-sequence intubation. American College of Emergency Physicians, *Ann Emerg Med* 29:573, 1997.
5. Levitan RM, Rosenblatt B, Meiner EM: Alternating day emergency medicine and anesthesia resident responsibility for management of the trauma airway: a study of laryngoscopy performance and intubation success, *Ann Emerg Med* 43:48, 2004.
6. Sivilotti ML, Ducharme J: Randomized, double-blind study on sedatives and hemodynamics during rapid-sequence intubation in the emergency department: the SHRED study, *Ann Emerg Med* 31:313, 1998.
7. Thompson JD, Fish S, Ruiz E: Succinylcholine for endotracheal intubation, *Ann Emerg Med* 11:526, 1982.
8. Wang HE, Davis DP, Wayne MA: Prehospital rapid-sequence intubation—what does the evidence show? Proceedings from the 2004 National Association of EMS Physicians annual meeting, *Prehosp Emerg Care* 8:366, 2004.
9. Wayne MA, Friedland E: Prehospital use of succinylcholine: a 20-year review, *Prehosp Emerg Care* 3:107, 1999.
10. Davis DP, et al: Paramedic-administered neuromuscular blockade improves prehospital intubation success in severely head-injured patients, *J Trauma* 55:713, 2003.
11. Davis DP, et al: The effect of paramedic rapid sequence intubation on outcome in patients with severe traumatic brain injury, *J Trauma* 54:444, 2003.
12. Ochs M, et al: Paramedic-performed rapid sequence intubation of patients with severe head injuries, *Ann Emerg Med* 40:159, 2002.
13. Davis DP, et al: The impact of hypoxia and hyperventilation on outcome after paramedic rapid sequence intubation of severely head-injured patients, *J Trauma* 57:1, 2004.
14. Davis DP, et al: The use of quantitative end-tidal capnometry to avoid inadvertent severe hyperventilation in patients with head injury after paramedic rapid sequence intubation, *J Trauma* 56:808, 2004.
15. Arbabi S, et al: A comparison of prehospital and hospital data in trauma patients, *J Trauma* 56:1029, 2004.
16. West R: Curare in man, *Proc Roy Soc Med* 25:1107, 1932.
17. Booij LH: Neuromuscular transmission and its pharmacological blockade. Part 1: neuromuscular transmission and general aspects of its blockade, *Pharm World Sci* 19:1-12, 1997.
18. Booij LH: Neuromuscular transmission and its pharmacological blockade. Part 2: pharmacology of neuromuscular blocking agents, *Pharm World Sci* 19:13, 1997.
19. Rosenberg H, Gronert GA: Intractable cardiac arrest in children given succinylcholine, *Anesthesiology* 77:1054, 1992.
20. Sivilotti ML, et al: Does the sedative agent facilitate emergency rapid sequence intubation? *Acad Emerg Med* 10:612, 2003.
21. Simon B: Pharmacologic aids in airway management. In Dailey R, et al, editors: *The airway: emergency management,* St Louis, 1992, Mosby, pp 145-170.
22. Wang HE, et al: The utilization of midazolam as a pharmacologic adjunct to endotracheal intubation by paramedics, *Prehosp Emerg Care* 4:14, 2000.
23. Dickinson ET, Cohen JE, Mechem CC: The effectiveness of midazolam as a single pharmacologic agent to facilitate endotracheal intubation by paramedics, *Prehosp Emerg Care* 3:191, 1999.
24. Sagarin MJ, et al: Underdosing of midazolam in emergency endotracheal intubation, *Acad Emerg Med* 10:329, 2003.
25. Hartmannsgruber MW, et al: The traumatic airway: the anesthesiologist's role in the emergency room, *Int Anesthesiol Clin* 38:87, 2000.
26. Sakles JC, et al: Airway management in the emergency department: a one-year study of 610 tracheal intubations, *Ann Emerg Med* 31:325, 1998.
27. Bozeman WP, Young S: Etomidate as a sole agent for endotracheal intubation in the prehospital air medical setting, *Air Med J* 21:32, 2002.
28. Deitch S, et al: The use of etomidate for prehospital rapid-sequence intubation, *Prehosp Emerg Care* 7:380, 2003.
29. Reed DB, Snyder G, Hogue TD: Regional EMS experience with etomidate for facilitated intubation, *Prehosp Emerg Care* 6:50, 2002.
30. Swanson ER, Fosnocht DE, Jensen SC: Comparison of etomidate and midazolam for prehospital rapid-sequence intubation, *Prehosp Emerg Care* 8:273, 2004.
31. Worf N, White SJ, High K: *Etomidate as a sedative agent to "chemically extricate" motor vehicle crash victims,* Nashville, Tenn, 2005, Vanderbilt University Medical Center.
32. Papiris S, Kotanidou A, Malagari K, et al: Clinical review: severe asthma, *Crit Care* 6:30, 2002.
33. Mace SE, et al: Clinical policy: evidence-based approach to pharmacologic agents used in pediatric sedation and analgesia in the emergency department, *Ann Emerg Med* 44:342, 2004.
34. Bonanno FG: Ketamine in war/tropical surgery (a final tribute to the racemic mixture), *Injury* 33:323, 2002.
35. Porter K: Ketamine in prehospital care, *Emerg Med J* 21:351, 2004.

36. Grover VK, et al: Intracranial pressure changes with different doses of lignocaine under general anaesthesia, *Neurol India* 47:118, 1999.
37. Jemmett ME, et al: Unrecognized misplacement of endotracheal tubes in a mixed urban to rural emergency medical services setting, *Acad Emerg Med* 10:961, 2003.
38. Jones JH, et al: Emergency physician-verified out-of-hospital intubation: miss rates by paramedics, *Acad Emerg Med* 11:707, 2004.
39. White SJ, Slovis CM: Inadvertent esophageal intubation in the field: reliance on a fool's "gold standard," *Acad Emerg Med* 4:89, 1997.
40. Kaups KL, Davis JW: Patients with gunshot wounds to the head do not require cervical spine immobilization and evaluation, *J Trauma* 44:865, 1998.
41. Davis DP, et al: The Combitube as a salvage airway device for paramedic rapid sequence intubation, *Ann Emerg Med* 42:697, 2003.

Medications, Classifications, and Body Systems Affected

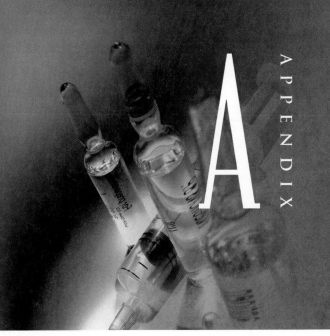

Medication	Classification	Body System Affected	Chapter	Page Number
Abciximab (ReoPro)	GP IIb/IIIa inhibitor	Cardiovascular	6: Acute Coronary Syndromes	124
Activated charcoal	Antidote, adsorbent	Gastrointestinal	13: Poisonings, Overdoses, and Intoxications	214
Adenosine (Adenocard)	Antiarrhythmic	Cardiovascular	9: Cardiac Arrhythmias 19: Special Considerations	165 327
Albumin	Volume expander, colloid	Cardiovascular	5: Intravenous Fluids and Administration	89
Albuterol (Proventil, Ventolin)	Bronchodilator, beta agonist	Respiratory	8: Anaphylaxis 14: Respiratory Emergencies 19: Special Considerations	156 241 313
Albuterol/ipratropium (Combivent)	Combination bronchodilator	Respiratory	14: Respiratory Emergencies	243
Aminophylline	Bronchodilator	Respiratory	14: Respiratory Emergencies	246
Amiodarone (Cordarone)	Antiarrhythmic, class III	Cardiovascular	9: Cardiac Arrhythmias 18: Critical Care Transport 19: Special Considerations	171 294 327
Angiotensin-converting enzyme (ACE) inhibitors: Captopril (Capoten), Enalapril (Vasotec), Lisinopril (Prinivil, Zestril), Ramipril (Altace)	ACE inhibitor	Cardiovascular	6: Acute Coronary Syndromes 10: Congestive Heart Failure	125 183
Aspirin, ASA	Antiplatelet, nonnarcotic analgesic, antipyretic	Cardiovascular, central nervous	6: Acute Coronary Syndromes 7: Analgesia and Sedation 12: Hypertensive Emergencies 13: Poisonings, Overdoses, and Intoxications	115 136 206 225

Medication	Classification	Body System Affected	Chapter	Page Number
Atenolol (Tenormin)	Beta adrenergic antagonist, antianginal, antihypertensive, class II antiarrhythmic	Cardiovascular	1: Principles of Pharmacology 6: Acute Coronary Syndromes 9: Cardiac Arrhythmias	22 121 168
Atracurium (Tracrium)	Nondepolarizing neuromuscular blocker	Musculoskeletal	20: Pharmacology-Assisted Intubation	343
Atropine sulfate	Anticholinergic (antimuscarinic)	Cardiovascular, parasympathetic nervous	1: Principles of Pharmacology 9: Cardiac Arrhythmias 13: Poisonings, Overdoses, and Intoxications 19: Special Considerations 20: Pharmacology-Assisted Intubation	23 162 219 325 340
Butorphanol (Stadol)	Opioid agonist-antagonist; Schedule C-IV controlled substance	Central nervous	7: Analgesia and Sedation	135
Calcium gluconate	Electrolyte solution	Cardiovascular, renal	5: Intravenous Fluids and Administration	91
Carbamazepine (Tegretol)	Anticonvulsant	Central nervous	15: Seizures	254
Clopidogrel (Plavix)	Antiplatelet	Hematologic, cardiovascular	6: Acute Coronary Syndromes	123
Dexamethasone (Decadron)	Corticosteroid	Endocrine, respiratory, immune	18: Critical Care Transport	289
Dextrose (Dextrose 50%, Dextrose 25%, Dextrose 10%)	Antihypoglycemic	Endocrine	5: Intravenous Fluids and Administration 11: Endocrine Emergencies 13: Poisonings, Overdoses, and Intoxications	93 189 228
Diazepam (Valium)	Benzodiazepine; Schedule C-IV	Central nervous	7: Analgesia and Sedation 12: Hypertensive Emergencies 13: Poisonings, Overdoses, and Intoxications 15: Seizures	142 209 218 251
Digoxin (Lanoxin)	Cardiac glycoside	Cardiovascular	10: Congestive Heart Failure	182
Diltiazem (Cardizem)	Calcium channel blocker; class IV antiarrhythmic	Cardiovascular	9: Cardiac Arrhythmias	166
Diphenhydramine hydrochloride (Benadryl)	Antihistamine	Immune system, cardiovascular, respiratory	8: Anaphylaxis 19: Special Considerations	156 312
Dobutamine (Dobutrex)	Adrenergic agent	Cardiovascular	1: Principles of Pharmacology 16: Shock	19 267
Dolasetron (Anzemet)	Antiemetic	Central nervous	7: Analgesia and Sedation	147

Medication	Classification	Body System Affected	Chapter	Page Number
Dopamine (Intropin)	Adrenergic agonist, inotropic, vasopressor	Cardiovascular	1: Principles of Pharmacology 9: Cardiac Arrhythmias 16: Shock	18 163 267
Epinephrine	Adrenergic agent, inotropic	Cardiovascular, respiratory	1: Principles of Pharmacology 8: Anaphylaxis 9: Cardiac Arrhythmias 19: Special Considerations	19 154 162 325
Epinephrine autoinjectors (EpiPen, EpiPen Jr)	Adrenergic agonist inotropic	Cardiovascular, respiratory	8: Anaphylaxis	154
Eptifibatide (Integrilin)	GP IIb/IIIa inhibitor	Hematologic, cardiovascular	6: Acute Coronary Syndromes 18: Critical Care Transport	124 294
Esmolol (Brevibloc)	Beta adrenergic antagonist, class II antiarrhythmic	Cardiovascular	6: Acute Coronary Syndromes 9: Cardiac Arrhythmias 11: Endocrine Emergencies 12: Hypertensive Emergencies	121 169 196 202
Etomidate (Amidate)	Hypnotic, anesthesia induction agent	Central nervous	7: Analgesia and Sedation 20: Pharmacology-Assisted Intubation	140 347
Felbamate (Felbatol)	Anticonvulsant	Central nervous	15: Seizures	253
Fentanyl citrate (Sublimaze)	Narcotic analgesic; Schedule C-II	Central nervous	7: Analgesia and Sedation 18: Critical Care Transport	134 299
Fibrinolytics: Tissue Plasminogen Activator (tPA), Streptokinase (Streptase, Kabikinase), Reteplase (Retavase), Tenecteplase (TNKase)	Thrombolytic agent	Hematologic, cardiovascular	6: Acute Coronary Syndromes	128
Flumazenil (Romazicon)	Benzodiazepine receptor antagonist, antidote	Central nervous	7: Analgesia and Sedation 20: Pharmacology-Assisted Intubation	145 347
Fosphenytoin (Cerebyx)	Anticonvulsant	Central nervous	15: Seizures	254
Furosemide (Lasix)	Loop diuretic	Renal	10: Congestive Heart Failure 12: Hypertensive Emergencies	180 203
Gabapentin (Neurontin)	Anticonvulsant	Central nervous	15: Seizures	255
Glucagon	Hormone	Endocrine	11: Endocrine Emergencies 13: Poisonings, Overdoses, and Intoxications	190 220

Medication	Classification	Body System Affected	Chapter	Page Number
Haloperidol (Haldol)	Antipsychotic agent	Central nervous	13: Poisonings, Overdoses, and Intoxications	223
Heparin (unfractionated heparin)	Anticoagulant	Hematologic, cardiovascular	6: Acute Coronary Syndromes	123
Hetastarch (Hespan)	Volume expander, colloid	Cardiovascular	5: Intravenous Fluids and Administration	89
HMG Coenzyme A Statins: Atorvastatin (Lipitor), Fluvastatin (Lescol), Lovastatin (Mevacor), Pravastatin (Pravachol), Rosuvastatin (Crestor), Simvastatin (Zocor)	HMG coenzyme A statins	Cardiovascular	6: Acute Coronary Syndromes	126
Hydralazine (Apresoline)	Antihypertensive agent, vasodilator	Cardiovascular	12: Hypertensive Emergencies 18: Critical Care Transport 19: Special Considerations	208 291 318
Hydrocortisone sodium succinate (Cortef, Solu-Cortef)	Corticosteroid	Endocrine, respiratory, immune	8: Anaphylaxis 11: Endocrine Emergencies 14: Respiratory Emergencies 19: Special Considerations	157 195 245 316
Hypertonic saline (3% saline)	Volume expander, electrolyte solution	Central nervous, cardiovascular	5: Intravenous Fluids and Administration 17: Traumatic Brain Injury and Spinal Cord Injury	90 277
Ibuprofen	NSAID	Cadiovascular, central nervous	7: Analgesia and Sedation	137
Insulin, regular (Humulin R, Novolin R)	Hormone	Endocrine, renal	5: Intravenous Fluids and Administration 11: Endocrine Emergencies 18: Critical Care Transport 19: Special Considerations	92 193 297 320
Ipratropium bromide (Atrovent)	Bronchodilator, anticholinergic	Respiratory	14: Respiratory Emergencies 19: Special Considerations	243 314
Ketamine (Ketalar)	General anesthetic	Central nervous	7: Analgesia and Sedation 20: Pharmacology-Assisted Intubation	140 348
Ketorolac (Toradol)	NSAID	Central nervous, peripheral tissue	7: Analgesia and Sedation	137
Labetalol (Normodyne, Trandate)	Beta adrenergic antagonist, antianginal, antihypertensive	Cardiovascular	1: Principles of Pharmacology 6: Acute Coronary Syndromes 11: Endocrine Emergencies 12: Hypertensive Emergencies 18: Critical Care Transport 19: Special Considerations	21 122 197 204 291 318

Medication	Classification	Body System Affected	Chapter	Page Number
Lamotrigine (Lamictal)	Anticonvulsant, antimanic agent	Central nervous	15: Seizures	256
Levalbuterol (Xopenex)	Beta agonist	Respiratory	14: Respiratory Emergencies	242
Lidocaine (Xylocaine)	Antiarrhythmic, class IB	Cardiovascular	9: Cardiac Arrhythmias 19: Special Considerations	172 328
Lorazepam (Ativan)	Benzodiazepine; Schedule C-IV	Central nervous	7: Analgesia and Sedation 13: Poisonings, Overdoses, and Intoxications 15: Seizures	144 222 252
Magnesium sulfate	Electrolyte, tocolytic, mineral	Cardiovascular	9: Cardiac Arrhythmias 12: Hypertensive Emergencies 13: Poisonings, Overdoses, and Intoxications 14: Respiratory Emergencies 18: Critical Care Transport 19: Special Considerations	173 208 216 246 290 319
Mannitol (Osmitrol)	Osmotic diuretic	Central nervous, cardiovascular, renal	17: Traumatic Brain Injury and Spinal Cord Injury 18: Critical Care Transport	276 300
Meperidine (Demerol)	Narcotic analgesic, Schedule C-II	Central nervous	7: Analgesia and Sedation	135
Methylprednisolone sodium succinate (Solu-Medrol)	Corticosteroid	Central nervous, endocrine, respiratory, immune	8: Anaphylaxis 14: Respiratory Emergencies 17: Traumatic Brain Injury and Spinal Cord Injury 19: Special Considerations	157 245 277 315
Metoprolol (Lopressor, Toprol XL)	Beta adrenergic antagonist, antianginal, antihypertensive, class II antiarrhythmic	Cardiovascular	1: Principles of Pharmacology 6: Acute Coronary Syndromes 9: Cardiac Arrhythmias 10: Congestive Heart Failure 11: Endocrine Emergencies	22 120 168 183 197
Midazolam (Versed)	Benzodiazepine, Schedule C-IV	Central nervous	7: Analgesia and Sedation 13: Poisonings, Overdoses, and Intoxications 18: Critical Care Transport 20: Pharmacology-Assisted Intubation	143 221 293 346
Milrinone (Primacor)	Inotropic	Cardiovascular	16: Shock	268
Morphine sulfate	Opiate agonist, Schedule C-II	Cardiovascular, central nervous	6: Acute Coronary Syndromes 7: Analgesia and Sedation 10: Congestive Heart Failure 13: Poisonings, Overdoses, and Intoxications	119 134 180 226
Nalbuphine (Nubain)	Synthetic opioid agonist-antagonist	Central nervous	7: Analgesia and Sedation	135

Medication	Classification	Body System Affected	Chapter	Page Number
Naloxone (Narcan)	Opioid antagonist	Central nervous	7: Analgesia and Sedation 13: Poisonings, Overdoses, and Intoxications	146 228
Nicardipine (Cardene)	Calcium channel blocker	Cardiovascular	12: Hypertensive Emergencies	203
Nitroglycerin (Nitrolingual, NitroQuick, Nitro-Dur)	Antianginal agent	Cardiovascular	6: Acute Coronary Syndromes 10: Congestive Heart Failure 12: Hypertensive Emergencies 13: Poisonings, Overdoses, and Intoxications	118 181 206 224
Nitrous oxide	Inorganic gas, inhaled anesthetic	Central nervous	7: Analgesia and Sedation	139
Norepinephrine (Levophed)	Adrenergic agonist, inotropic, vasopressor	Cardiovascular	1: Principles of Pharmacology 13: Poisonings, Overdoses, and Intoxications 16: Shock	18 217 268
Oxygen	Elemental gas	Respiratory, cardiovascular	6: Acute Coronary Syndromes 14: Respiratory Emergencies	115 236
Pancuronium (Pavulon)	Nondepolarizing neuromuscular blocker	Musculoskeletal	20: Pharmacology-Assisted Intubation	343
Phenobarbital (Luminal)	Anticonvulsant, barbiturate, Schedule C-IV	Central nervous	15: Seizures	255
Phentolamine (Regitine)	Alpha antagonist, antihypertensive	Cardiovascular	12: Hypertensive Emergencies 13: Poisonings, Overdoses, and Intoxications	210 226
Phenylephrine (Neo-Synephrine)	Adrenergic agonist	Cardiovascular	1: Principles of Pharmacology 13: Poisonings, Overdoses, and Intoxications 16: Shock	19 216 270
Phenytoin (Dilantin)	Anticonvulsant	Central nervous	13: Poisonings, Overdoses, and Intoxications 15: Seizures 18: Critical Care Transport	218 254 290
Potassium chloride	Electrolyte replacement	Cardiovascular, central nervous, renal	5: Intravenous Fluids and Administration	94
Pralidoxime (2-PAM, Protopam)	Cholinergic agonist, antidote	Parasympathetic nervous	13: Poisonings, Overdoses, and Intoxications	230
Prednisone	Corticosteroid	Endocrine, respiratory, immune	19: Special Considerations	315
Procainamide (Pronestyl)	Antiarrhythmic, class IA	Cardiovascular	9: Cardiac Arrhythmias 19: Special Considerations	172 328

Medication	Classification	Body System Affected	Chapter	Page Number
Promethazine (Phenergan)	Antiemetic, antihistamine	Central nervous	7: Analgesia and Sedation	147
Propofol (Diprivan)	Anesthetic	Central nervous	7: Analgesia and Sedation 18: Critical Care Transport	141 298
Propranolol (Inderal)	Beta adrenergic antagonist, antianginal, antihypertensive, antiarrhythmic class II	Cardiovascular	1: Principles of Pharmacology 6: Acute Coronary Syndromes 9: Cardiac Arrhythmias	21 121 168
Racemic epinephrine/ racepinephrine (microNefrin, S_2)	Bronchodilator, adrenergic agent	Respiratory	14: Respiratory Emergencies	247
Rocuronium (Zemuron)	Neuromuscular blocker, nondepolarizing	Musculoskeletal	20: Pharmacology-Assisted Intubation	342
Scopolamine (Transderm Scop)	Neurologic antivertigo, antimuscarinic	Cardiovascular, parasympathetic nervous	1: Principles of Pharmacology	24
Sodium bicarbonate	Electrolyte replacement	Cardiovascular, pulmonary, renal	5: Intravenous Fluids and Administration 13: Poisonings, Overdoses, and Intoxications	92 215
Sodium nitroprusside (Nipride, Nitropress)	Antihypertensive agent	Cardiovascular	12: Hypertensive Emergencies	204
Succinylcholine (Anectine)	Neuromuscular blocker, depolarizing	Musculoskeletal	20: Pharmacology-Assisted Intubation	339
Terbutaline (Brethine)	Adrenergic agonist	Respiratory	19: Special Considerations	313
Thiamine (Vitamin B_1)	Vitamin B_1	Central nervous	11: Endocrine Emergencies 13: Poisonings, Overdoses, and Intoxications	190 227
Tirofiban (Aggrastat)	GP IIb/IIIa inhibitor	Cardiovascular	6: Acute Coronary Syndromes	125
Valproic acid (Depakote)	Anticonvulsant, antimanic	Central nervous	15: Seizures	255
Vasopressin	Nonadrenergic vasopressor	Cardiovascular	9: Cardiac Arrhythmias	175
Vecuronium (Norcuron)	Neuromuscular blocker, nondepolarizing	Musculoskeletal	18: Critical Care Transport 20: Pharmacology-Assisted Intubation	294 342
Verapamil (Isoptin)	Calcium channel blocker; class IV antiarrhythmic	Cardiovascular	9: Cardiac Arrhythmias	166

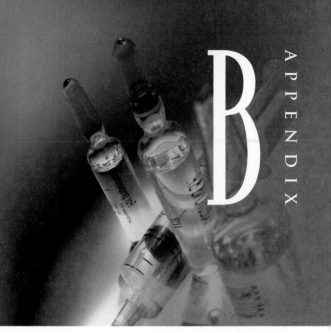

Compilation of Drug Profiles

ABCIXIMAB (REOPRO)

Classification: GP IIb/IIIa inhibitor
Action: Prevents the aggregation of platelets by inhibiting the integrin GP IIb/IIIa receptor.
Indications: UA/NSTEMI patients undergoing planned or emergent percutaneous coronary intervention.
Adverse Effects: Bleeding from the GI tract, internal bleeding, intracranial hemorrhage, hypotension, stroke, anaphylactic shock.
Contraindications: Bleeding from any source, severe uncontrolled hypertension, surgery or trauma within the previous 6 weeks, stroke within the previous 30 days, renal failure, thrombocytopenia, intracranial mass.
Dosage:
UA/NSTEMI with Planned PCI within 24 Hours:
· 0.25 mg/kg IV, IO (10 to 60 minutes prior to procedure), then 0.125 mcg/kg/min IV, IO infusion for 12 to 24 hours.
Percutaneous Coronary Intervention Only:
· 0.25 mg/kg IV, IO, then 10 mcg/min IV, IO infusion.
Special Considerations:
Pregnancy class C

ACTIVATED CHARCOAL

Classification: Antidote, adsorbent
Action: When certain chemicals and toxins are in proximity to the activated charcoal, the chemical will attach to the surface of the charcoal and become trapped.
Indications: Toxic ingestion
Adverse Effects: Nausea/vomiting, constipation, or diarrhea. If aspirated into the lungs, charcoal can induce a potentially fatal form of pneumonitis.
Contraindications: Ingestion of acids, alkalis, ethanol, methanol, cyanide, ferrous sulfate or other iron salts, lithium; coma; GI obstruction.
Dosage:
· **Adult:** 50 to 100 g/dose.
· **Pediatric:** 1 to 2 g/kg.
Special Considerations:
Pregnancy class C

ADENOSINE (ADENOCARD)

Classification: Antiarrhythmic
Action: Slows the conduction of electrical impulses at the AV node.
Indications: Stable reentry SVT. Does not convert AF, atrial flutter, or VT.
Adverse Effects: Common adverse reactions are generally mild and short-lived: sense of impending doom, complaints of flushing, chest pressure, throat tightness, numbness. Patients will have a brief episode of asystole after administration.
Contraindications: Sick sinus syndrome, second- or third-degree heart block, poison-/drug-induced tachycardia.
Dosage: Note: Adenosine should be delivered only by rapid IV bolus with a peripheral IV or directly into a vein, in a location as close to the heart as possible, preferably in the antecubital fossa. Administration of adenosine must be immediately followed by a saline flush, and then the extremity should be elevated.

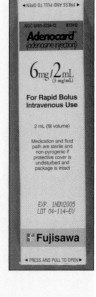

- **Adult:** Initial dose 6 mg rapid IV, IO (over a 1- to 3-second period) immediately followed by a 20-mL rapid saline flush. If the first dose does not eliminate the rhythm in 1 to 2 minutes, 12 mg rapid IV, IO, repeat a second time if required.
- **Pediatric:**
  - **Children >50 kg:** Same as adult dosing.
  - **Children <50 kg:** Initial dose 0.1 mg/kg IV, IO (max dose: 6 mg) immediately followed by a ≥5-mL rapid saline flush; may repeat at 0.2 mg/kg (max dose: 12 mg).

Special Considerations:
Use with caution in patients with preexisting bronchospasm and those with a history of AF.
Elderly patients with no history of PSVT should be carefully evaluated for dehydration and rapid sinus tachycardia requiring volume fluid replacement rather than simply treated with adenosine.
Pregnancy class C

ALBUMIN

Classification: Volume expander, colloid
Action: Increases oncotic pressure in intravascular space.
Indications: Expand intravascular volume.
Adverse Effects: Allergic reaction in some patients; an excessive volume of fluid can result in CHF and pulmonary edema in susceptible patients.
Contraindications: Severe anemia or cardiac failure in the presence of normal or increased intravascular volume, solution appears turbid or after 4 hours since opening the container, known sensitivity.
Dosage: Two preparations: 500 mL of a 5% solution and 100 mL of a 25% solution.

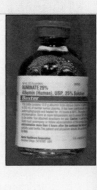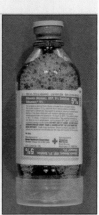

- **Adult:**
  - **5% albumin:** 500 to 1000 mL IV, IO.
  - **25% albumin:** 50 to 200 mL IV, IO.
- **Pediatric:**
  - **5% albumin:** 12 to 20 mL/kg IV; the initial dose may be repeated in 15 to 30 minutes if the clinical response is inadequate.
  - **25% albumin:** 2.5 to 5 mL/kg IV, IO.
  - Alternatively, one may administer based on grams of albumin at 0.5 to 1 g/kg/dose IV, IO. May repeat as needed (max dose: 6 g/kg/day).

Special Considerations:
Patients with a history of CHF, cardiac disease, hypertension, and pulmonary edema should be given 5% albumin, or the 25% albumin should be diluted. Because 25% of albumin increases intravascular volume greater than the volume administered, slowly administer 25% albumin in normovolemic patients to prevent complications such as pulmonary edema.
Pregnancy class C

ALBUTEROL (PROVENTIL, VENTOLIN)

Classification: Bronchodilator, beta agonist
Action: Binds and stimulates beta$_2$ receptors, resulting in relaxation of bronchial smooth muscle.
Indications: Asthma, bronchitis with bronchospasm, and COPD.
Adverse Effects: Hyperglycemia, hypokalemia, palpitations, sinus tachycardia, anxiety, tremor, nausea/vomiting, throat irritation, dry mouth, hypertension, dyspepsia, insomnia, headache, epistaxis, paradoxical bronchospasm.
Contraindications: Angioedema, sensitivity to albuterol or levalbuterol. Use with caution in lactating patients, cardiovascular disorders, cardiac arrhythmias.

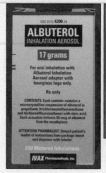
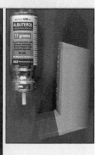

Dosage:
Acute Bronchospasm:
- **Adult:**
  - **MDI:** 4 to 8 puffs every 1 to 4 hours may be required.
  - **Nebulizer:** 2.5 to 5 mg every 20 minutes for a maximum of three doses. After the initial three doses, escalate the dose or start a continuous nebulization at 10 to 15 mg/hr.
- **Pediatric:**
  - **MDI:**
    - **4 years and older:** 2 inhalations every 4 to 6 hours; however, in some patients, 1 inhalation every 4 hours is sufficient. More frequent administration or more inhalations are not recommended.
    - **Younger than 4 years:** Administer by nebulization.
  - **Nebulizer:**
    - **Older than 12 years:** The dose for a continuous nebulization is 0.5 mg/kg/hr.
    - **Younger than 12 years:** 0.15 mg/kg every 20 minutes for a maximum of three doses. Alternatively, continuous nebulization at 0.5 mg/kg/hr can be delivered to children younger than 12 years.

Asthma in Pregnancy:
- **MDI:** Two inhalations every 4 hours. In acute exacerbation, start with 2 to 4 puffs every 20 minutes.
- **Nebulizer:** 2.5 mg (0.5 mL) by 0.5% nebulization solution. Place 0.5 mL of the albuterol solution in 2.5 mL of sterile normal saline. Flow is regulated to deliver the therapy over a 5- to 20-minute period. In refractory cases, some physicians order 10 mg nebulized over a 60-minute period.

Special Considerations:
Pregnancy class C

ALBUTEROL/IPRATROPIUM (COMBIVENT)

Classification: Combination bronchodilator
Action: Binds and stimulates beta$_2$ receptors, resulting in relaxation of bronchial smooth muscle, and antagonizes the acetylcholine receptor, producing bronchodilation.
Indications: Second-line treatment (if bronchodilator is ineffective) in COPD or severe acute asthma exacerbations during medical transport.
Adverse Effects: Headache, cough, nausea, arrhythmias, paradoxical acute bronchospasm.
Contraindications: Allergy to soybeans or peanuts; known sensitivity to atropine, albuterol, or their respective derivatives. Used with caution in patients with asthma, hypertension, angina, cardiac arrhythmias, tachycardia, cardiovascular disease, congenital long QT syndrome, closed-angle glaucoma.

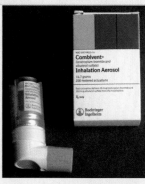

Dosage:
- **Adult:** 2 puffs inhaled every 6 hours by MDI, with a maximum daily dose of 12 puffs/day.
- **Pediatric:** Not recommended for pediatric patients.

Special Considerations:
Pregnancy class C

AMINOPHYLLINE

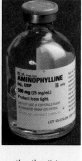

Classification: Bronchodilator
Action: Relaxes the smooth muscle of the bronchial airways and pulmonary blood vessels. May also have antiinflammatory properties.
Indications: Bronchospasm
Adverse Effects: Seizures, cardiac arrest, arrhythmias, nausea/vomiting, abdominal pain or cramping, headache, tachycardia, palpitations, anxiety, ventricular arrhythmias.
Contraindications: Known sensitivity. Use with caution in liver disease, kidney disease, seizures, cardiac arrhythmias.
Dosage: A loading dose is first administered, followed by an infusion.
- **Adult:** Load with 5 mg/kg IV, IO slowly over a 20- to 30-minute period, followed by an infusion. An infusion rate of 0.4 mg/kg/hr is effective for a nonsmoker, but a patient who smokes can require a high infusion rate at 0.8 mg/kg/hr IV, IO. When treating patients with CHF, reduce the dose to 0.2 mg/kg/hr.
- **Pediatric:** Load with 5 mg/kg slow IV, IO over a 20-minute period.
  - **Older than 12 years:** 0.4 mg/kg/hr IV, IO.
  - **10 to 12 years:** 0.7 mg/kg/hr IV, IO.
  - **1 to 9 years:** 0.8 to 1 mg/kg/hr IV, IO.
  - **6 months to 1 year:** 0.6 to 0.7 mg/kg/hr IV, IO.
  - **6 to 24 weeks:** 0.5 mg/kg/hr IV, IO.

Special Considerations:
Pregnancy class C

AMIODARONE (CORDARONE)

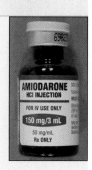

Classification: Antiarrhythmic, class III
Action: Acts directly on the myocardium to delay repolarization and increase the duration of the action potential.
Indications: Ventricular arrhythmias; second-line agent for atrial arrhythmias.
Adverse Effects: Burning at the IV site, hypotension, bradycardia.
Contraindications: Sick sinus syndrome, second- and third-degree heart block, cardiogenic shock, when episodes of bradycardia have caused syncope, sensitivity to benzyl alcohol and iodine.
Dosage:
Ventricular Fibrillation and Pulseless Ventricular Tachycardia:
- **Adult:** 300 mg IV, IO. May be followed by one dose of 150 mg in 3 to 5 minutes.
- **Pediatric:** 5 mg/kg (max dose: 300 mg); may repeat 5 mg/kg IV, IO up to 15 mg/kg.

Relatively Stable Patients with Arrhythmias such as Premature Ventricular Contractions or Wide-Complex Tachycardias with a Strong Pulse:
- **Adult:** 150 mg in 100 mL D5W IV, IO over a 10-minute period; may repeat in 10 minutes up to a maximum dose of 2.2 g over 24 hours.
- **Pediatric:** 5 mg/kg very slow IV, IO (over 20 to 60 minutes); may repeat in 5-mg/kg doses up to 15 mg/kg (max dose: 300 mg).

Special Considerations:
Pregnancy class D

ANGIOTENSIN-CONVERTING ENZYME (ACE) INHIBITORS: CAPTOPRIL (CAPOTEN), ENALAPRIL (VASOTEC), LISINOPRIL (PRINIVIL, ZESTRIL), RAMIPRIL (ALTACE)

Classification: ACE inhibitor

Action: Blocks the enzyme responsible for the production of angiotensin II, resulting in a decrease in blood pressure.

Indications: Congestive heart failure, hypertension, post–myocardial infarction.

Adverse Effects: Headache, dizziness, fatigue, depression, chest pain, hypotension, palpitations, cough, dyspnea, upper respiratory infection, nausea/vomiting, rash, pruritus, angioedema, renal failure.

Contraindications: Angioedema related to previous treatment with an ACE inhibitor, known sensitivity. Use with caution in aortic stenosis, bilateral renal artery stenosis, hypertrophic obstructive cardiomyopathy, pericardial tamponade, elevated serum potassium levels, acute kidney failure.

Dosage:
- **Adult:** Medication is administered orally. Dosage is individualized.
- **Pediatric:** Medication is administered orally. Dosage is individualized.

Special Considerations:
Pregnancy class D

ASPIRIN, ASA

Classification: Antiplatelet, nonnarcotic analgesic, antipyretic

Action: Prevents the formation of a chemical known as thromboxane A_2, which causes platelets to clump together, or aggregate, and form plugs that cause obstruction or constriction of small coronary arteries.

Indications: Fever, inflammation, angina, acute MI, and patients complaining of pain, pressure, squeezing, or crushing in the chest that may be cardiac in origin.

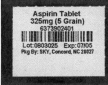

Adverse Effects: Anaphylaxis, angioedema, bronchospasm, bleeding, stomach irritation, nausea/vomiting.

Contraindications: GI bleeding, active ulcer disease, hemorrhagic stroke, bleeding disorders, children with chickenpox or flulike symptoms, known sensitivity.

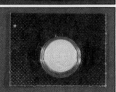

Dosage: Note: "Baby aspirin" 81 mg, standard adult aspirin dose 325 mg.

Myocardial Infarction:
- **Adult:** 160 to 325 mg PO (alternatively, four 81-mg baby aspirin are often given), 300-mg rectal suppository.
- **Pediatric:** 3 to 5 mg/kg/day to 5 to 10 mg/kg/day given as a single dose.

Pain or Fever:
- **Adult:** 325 to 650 mg PO (1 to 2 adult tablets) every 4 to 6 hours.
- **Pediatric:** 60 to 90 mg/kg/day in divided doses every 4 to 6 hours.

Special Considerations:
Pregnancy class C except the last 3 months of pregnancy, when aspirin is considered pregnancy class D.

ATENOLOL (TENORMIN)

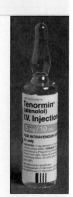

Classification: Beta adrenergic antagonist, antianginal, antihypertensive, class II antiarrhythmic
Action: Inhibits the strength of the heart's contractions and heart rate, resulting in a decrease in cardiac oxygen consumption. Also saturates the beta receptors and inhibits dilation of bronchial smooth muscle ($beta_2$ receptor).
Indications: ACS, hypertension, SVT, atrial flutter, AF.
Adverse Effects: Bradycardia, bronchospasm, hypotension.
Contraindications: Cardiogenic shock, AV block, bradycardia, known sensitivity. Use with caution in hypotension, chronic lung disease (asthma and COPD).
Dosage: ACS:
- **Adult:** 5 mg IV, IO over a 5-minute period; repeat in 5 minutes.
- **Pediatric:** Not recommended for pediatric patients.

Special Considerations:
Pregnancy class D

ATRACURIUM (TRACRIUM)

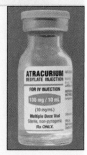

Classification: Nondepolarizing neuromuscular blocker
Action: Antagonizes acetylcholine receptors at the motor end plate, producing muscle paralysis.
Indications: Neuromuscular blockade to facilitate ET intubation.
Adverse Effects: Flushing, edema, urticaria, pruritus, bronchospasm and/or wheezing, alterations in heart rate, decrease in blood pressure.
Contraindications: Cardiac disease, electrolyte abnormalities, dehydration, known sensitivity.
Dosage:
- **Adult:** 0.4 to 0.5 mg/kg IV, IO; repeat with 0.08 to 0.1 mg/kg every 20 to 45 minutes as needed for prolonged paralysis.
- **Pediatric:**
  - **Older than 2 years:** Same as adult dosing.
  - **Younger than 2 years:** 0.3 to 0.4 mg/kg IV, IO.

Special Considerations:
Do not give by IM injection.
Pregnancy class C

ATROPINE SULFATE

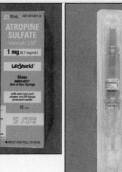
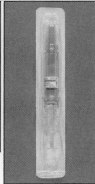

Classification: Anticholinergic (antimuscarinic)
Action: Competes reversibly with acetylcholine at the site of the muscarinic receptor. Receptors affected, in order from the most sensitive to the least sensitive, include salivary, bronchial, sweat glands, eye, heart, and GI tract.
Indications: Symptomatic bradycardia, asystole or PEA, nerve agent exposure, organophosphate poisoning.
Adverse Effects: Decreased secretions resulting in dry mouth and hot skin temperature, intense facial flushing, blurred vision or dilation of the pupils with subsequent photophobia, tachycardia, restlessness. Atropine may cause paradoxical bradycardia if the dose administered is too low or if the drug is administered too slowly.
Contraindications: Acute MI; myasthenia gravis; GI obstruction; closed-angle glaucoma; known sensitivity to atropine, belladonna alkaloids, or sulfites. Will not be effective for infranodal (type II) AV block and new third-degree block with wide QRS complex.

cont'd

ATROPINE SULFATE—CONT'D

Dosage:
Symptomatic Bradycardia:
- **Adult:** 0.5 mg IV, IO every 3 to 5 minutes to a maximum dose of 3 mg.
- **Adolescent:** 0.02 mg/kg (minimum 0.1 mg/dose; maximum 1 mg/dose) IV, IO up to a total dose of 2 mg.
- **Pediatric:** 0.02 mg/kg (minimum 0.1 mg/dose; maximum 0.5 mg/dose) IV, IO, to a total dose of 1 mg.

Asystole/Pulseless Electrical Activity:
- 1 mg IV, IO every 3 to 5 minutes, to a maximum dose of 3 mg. May be administered via ET tube at 2 to 2.5 mg diluted in 5 to 10 mL of water or normal saline.

Nerve Agent or Organophosphate Poisoning:
- **Adult:** 2 to 4 mg IV, IM; repeat if needed every 20 to 30 minutes until symptoms dissipate. In severe cases, the initial dose can be as large as 2 to 6 mg administered IV. Repeat doses of 2 to 6 mg can be administered IV, IM every 5 to 60 minutes.
- **Pediatric:** 0.05 mg/kg IV, IM every 10 to 30 minutes as needed until symptoms dissipate.
- **Infants <15 lb:** 0.05 mg/kg IV, IM every 5 to 20 minutes as needed until symptoms dissipate.

Special Considerations:
Half-life 2.5 hours
Pregnancy class C; possibly unsafe in lactating mothers.

BUTORPHANOL (STADOL)

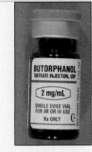

Classification: Opioid agonist-antagonist; Schedule C-IV controlled substance
Action: Produces analgesia by binding to the opioid receptor.
Indications: Moderate to severe pain.
Adverse Effects: Drowsiness, dizziness, confusion, respiratory depression, nausea/vomiting, bradycardia, hypotension.
Contraindications: Patients with active substance abuse, sensitivity to opiate agonists. Use with caution in kidney, liver, or pulmonary problems.
Dosage:
- **Adult:** 0.5 to 2 mg IV, IO every 3 to 4 hours.
- **Pediatric:** Not recommended for pediatric patients.

Special Considerations:
Pregnancy class C

CALCIUM GLUCONATE

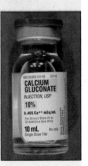

Classification: Electrolyte solution
Action: Counteracts the toxicity of hyperkalemia by stabilizing the membranes of the cardiac cells, reducing the likelihood of fibrillation.
Indications: Hyperkalemia, hypocalcemia, hypermagnesemia.
Adverse Effects: Soft tissue necrosis, hypotension, bradycardia (if administered too rapidly).
Contraindications: VF, digitalis toxicity, hypercalcemia.
Dosage: Supplied as 10% solution; therefore each milliliter contains 100 mg of calcium gluconate.
- **Adult:** 500 to 1000 mg IV, IO administered slowly at a rate of approximately 1 to 1.5 mL/min; maximum dose 3 g IV, IO.
- **Pediatric:** 60 to 100 mg/kg IV, IO slowly over a 5- to 10-minute period; maximum dose 3 g IV, IO.

Special Considerations:
Do not administer by IM or Sub-Q routes, which causes significant tissue necrosis.
Pregnancy class C

CARBAMAZEPINE (TEGRETOL)

Classification: Anticonvulsant
Action: Decreases the spread of the seizure.
Indications: Partial and generalized tonic-clonic seizures.
Adverse Effects: Dizziness, drowsiness, ataxia, nausea/vomiting, blurred vision, confusion, headache, transient diplopia, visual hallucinations, life-threatening rashes.
Contraindications: AV block, bundle branch block, agranulocytosis, bone marrow suppression, MAOI therapy, hypersensitivity to carbamazepine or tricyclic antidepressants. Use with caution in petit mal, atonic, or myoclonic seizures; liver disease; patients with blood dyscrasia caused by drug therapies or blood disorders; patients with a history of cardiac disease; or patients with a history of alcoholism.
Dosage:
- **Adult:** 200 mg PO every 12 hours.
- **Pediatric:**
  - **6 to 11 years:** 100 mg PO twice daily.
  - **Younger than 6 years:** 10 to 20 mg/kg/day PO 2 or 3 times per day.

Special Considerations:
Pregnancy class D

CLOPIDOGREL (PLAVIX)

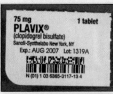
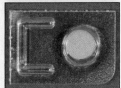

Classification: Antiplatelet
Action: Blocks platelet aggregation by antagonizing the GP IIb/IIIa receptors.
Indications: ACS, chronic coronary and vascular disease, ischemic stroke.
Adverse Effects: Nausea, abdominal pain, and hemorrhage.
Contraindications: History of intracranial hemorrhage, GI bleed or trauma, known sensitivity.
Dosage:
Unstable Angina Pectoris or Non–Q-Wave Acute Myocardial Infarction:
- **Adult:** Single loading dose of 300 mg PO followed by a daily dose of 75 mg PO.
- **Pediatric:** Not recommended for pediatric patients.

Special Considerations:
Pregnancy class B

DEXAMETHASONE (DECADRON)

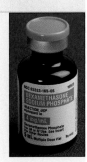

Classification: Corticosteroid
Action: Reduces inflammation and immune responses.
Indications: Various inflammatory conditions, adrenal insufficiency, nonresponsive forms of shock.
Adverse Effects: Nausea/vomiting, edema, hypertension, hyperglycemia, immunosuppression.
Contraindications: Fungal infections, known sensitivity.
Dosage:
- **Adult:** 1 to 6 mg/kg IV to a maximum dose of 40 mg.
- **Pediatric:** 0.03 to 0.3 mg/kg IV, IO divided into doses every 6 hours.

Special Considerations:
Pregnancy class C

DEXTROSE (DEXTROSE 50%, DEXTROSE 25%, DEXTROSE 10%)

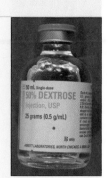

Classification: Antihypoglycemic
Action: Increases blood glucose concentrations.
Indications: Hypoglycemia
Adverse Effects: Hyperglycemia, warmth, burning from IV infusion. Concentrated solutions may cause pain and thrombosis of the peripheral veins.
Contraindications: Intracranial and intraspinal hemorrhage, delirium tremens, solution is not clear, seals are not intact.
Dosage:
Hyperkalemia:
- **Adult:** 25 g of dextrose 50% IV, IO.
- **Pediatric:** 0.5 to 1 g/kg IV, IO.
Hypoglycemia:
- **Adult:** 10 to 25 g of dextrose 50% IV (20 to 50 mL of dextrose solution).
- **Pediatric:**
  - **Older than 2 years:** 2 mL/kg of dextrose 50%.
  - **Younger than 2 years:** 2 to 4 mL/kg of dextrose 10%.
Special Considerations:
Pregnancy class C

DIAZEPAM (VALIUM)

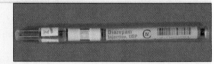

Classification: Benzodiazepine; Schedule C-IV
Action: Binds to the benzodiazepine receptor and enhances the effects of GABA. Benzodiazepines act at the level of the limbic, thalamic, and hypothalamic regions of the CNS and can produce any level of CNS depression required (including sedation, skeletal muscle relaxation, and anticonvulsant activity).
Indications: Anxiety, skeletal muscle relaxation, alcohol withdrawal, seizures.
Adverse Effects: Respiratory depression, drowsiness, fatigue, headache, pain at the injection site, confusion, nausea, hypotension, oversedation.
Contraindications: Children younger than 6 months, acute-angle glaucoma, CNS depression, alcohol intoxication, known sensitivity.
Dosage:
Anxiety:
- **Adult:**
  - **Moderate:** 2 to 5 mg slow IV, IM.
  - **Severe:** 5 to 10 mg slow IV, IM (administer no faster than 5 mg/min).
  - **Low:** Low dosages are often required for elderly or debilitated patients.
- **Pediatric:** 0.04 to 0.3 mg/kg/dose IV, IM every 4 hours to a maximum dose of 0.6 mg/kg.
Delirium Tremens from Acute Alcohol Withdrawal:
- **Adult:** 10 mg IV
Seizure:
- **Adult:** 5 to 10 mg slow IV, IO every 10 to 15 minutes; maximum total dose 30 mg.
- **Pediatric:**
- **IV, IO:**
  - **5 years and older:** 1 mg over a 3-minute period every 2 to 5 minutes to a maximum total dose of 10 mg.
  - **Older than 30 days to younger than 5 years:** 0.2 to 0.5 mg over a 3-minute period; may repeat every 2 to 5 minutes to a maximum total dose of 5 mg.
  - **Neonate:** 0.1 to 0.3 mg/kg/dose given over a 3- to 5-minute period; may repeat every 15 to 30 minutes to a maximum total dose of 2 mg. (Not a first-line agent due to sodium benzoic acid in the injection.)

cont'd

DIAZEPAM (VALIUM)—CONT'D

- **Rectal administration:** If vascular access is not obtained, diazepam may be administered rectally to children.
  - **12 years and older:** 0.2 mg/kg.
  - **6 to 11 years:** 0.3 mg/kg.
  - **2 to 5 years:** 0.5 mg/kg.
  - **Younger than 2 years:** Not recommended.

Special Considerations:
Make sure that IV, IO lines are well secured. Extravasation of diazepam causes tissue necrosis.
Diazepam is insoluble in water and must be dissolved in propylene glycol. This produces a viscous solution; give slowly to prevent pain on injection.
Pregnancy class D

DIGOXIN (LANOXIN)

Classification: Cardiac glycoside
Action: Inhibits sodium-potassium-adenosine triphosphatase membrane pump, resulting in an increase in calcium inside the heart muscle cell, which causes an increase in the force of contraction of the heart.
Indications: CHF, to control the ventricular rate in chronic AF and atrial flutter, narrow-complex PSVT.
Adverse Effects: Headache, weakness, GI disturbances, arrhythmias, nausea/vomiting, diarrhea, vision disturbances.
Contraindications: Digitalis allergy, VT and VF, heart block, sick sinus syndrome, tachycardia without heart failure, pulse lower than 50 to 60 beats/min, MI, ischemic heart disease, patients with preexcitation AF or atrial flutter (i.e., a delta wave, characteristic of Wolff-Parkinson-White syndrome, visible during normal sinus rhythm).
Dosage: Dosage is individualized.

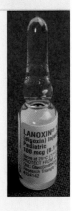

Special Considerations:
Low levels of serum potassium can lead to digoxin toxicity and bradycardia. Conditions such as administration of steroids or diuretics or vomiting and diarrhea can produce low levels of potassium and subsequent digoxin toxicity.
Pregnancy class C

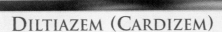

DILTIAZEM (CARDIZEM)

Classification: Calcium channel blocker, class IV antiarrhythmic
Action: Blocks calcium from moving into the heart muscle cell, which prolongs the conduction of electrical impulses through the AV node.
Indications: Ventricular rate control in rapid AF.
Adverse Effects: Flushing; headache; bradycardia; hypotension; heart block; myocardial depression; severe AV block; and, at high doses, cardiac arrest.
Contraindications: Hypotension, heart block, heart failure.
Dosage:

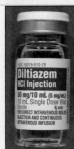

- **Adult:** Optimum dose is 0.25 mg/kg IV, IO over a 2-minute period to control rapid AF; 20 mg is a reasonable dose for the average adult patient. A second, higher dose of 0.35 mg/kg IV, IO (25 mg is a typical second dose) may be administered over a 2-minute period if rate control is not obtained with the lower dose. For continued reduction in heart rate, a continuous infusion can be started at a dose range of 5 to 15 mg/hr.
- **Pediatric:** Not recommended for pediatric patients.

Special Considerations:
Use with extreme caution in patients who are taking beta blockers because these two drug classes potentiate each other's effects and toxicities.
Patients with a history of heart failure and heart block are at a higher risk for toxicity.
Pregnancy class C

DIPHENHYDRAMINE HYDROCHLORIDE (BENADRYL)

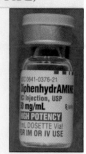

Classification: Antihistamine
Action: Binds and blocks H_1 histamine receptors.
Indications: Anaphylactic reactions
Adverse Effects: Drowsiness, dizziness, headache, excitable state (children), wheezing, thickening of bronchial secretions, chest tightness, palpitations, hypotension, blurred vision, dry mouth, nausea/vomiting, diarrhea.
Contraindications: Acute asthma, which thickens secretions; patients with cardiac histories; known sensitivity.
Dosage:
- **Adult:** 25 to 50 mg IV, IO, IM.
- **Pediatric: 2 to 12 years:** 1 to 1.25 mg/kg IV, IO, IM.

Special Considerations:
Pregnancy class B

DOBUTAMINE (DOBUTREX)

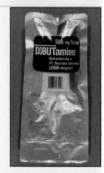

Classification: Adrenergic agent
Action: Acts primarily as an agonist at $beta_1$ adrenergic receptors with minor $beta_2$ and $alpha_1$ effects. Consequently, dobutamine increases myocardial contractility and stroke volume with minor chronotropic effects, resulting in increased cardiac output.
Indications: CHF, cardiogenic shock.
Adverse Effects: Tachycardia, PVCs, hypertension, hypotension, palpitations, arrhythmias.
Contraindications: Suspected or known poisoning/drug-induced shock, systolic blood pressure <100 mm Hg with signs of shock, idiopathic hypertrophic subaortic stenosis, known sensitivity (including sulfites). Use with caution in hypertension, recent MI, arrhythmias, hypovolemia.
Dosage:
- **Adult:** 2 to 20 mcg/kg/min IV, IO. At doses >20 mcg/kg/min, increases of heart rate of >10% may induce or exacerbate myocardial ischemia.
- **Pediatric:** Same as adult dosing.

Special Considerations:
Half-life 2 minutes
Pregnancy class C

DOLASETRON (ANZEMET)

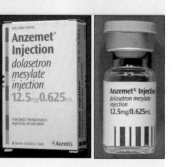

Classification: Antiemetic
Action: Prevents/reduces nausea/vomiting by binding and blocking a receptor for the brain chemical serotonin.
Indications: Prevent and treat nausea/vomiting.
Adverse Effects: Headache, fatigue, diarrhea, dizziness, abdominal pain, hypotension, hypertension, ECG changes (prolonged PR and QT intervals, widened QRS), bradycardia, tachycardia, syncope.
Contraindications: Known sensitivity. Use with caution in hypokalemia, hypomagnesemia, cardiac arrhythmias.
Dosage:
- **Adult:** 12.5 mg IV, IO.
- **Pediatric: 2 to 16 years:** 0.35 mg/kg IV, IO (max dose: 12.5 mg).

Special Considerations:
Pregnancy class B

DOPAMINE (INTROPIN)

Classification: Adrenergic agonist, inotropic, vasopressor
Action: Stimulates alpha and beta adrenergic receptors. At moderate doses (2-10 mcg/kg/min), dopamine stimulates beta$_1$ receptors, resulting in inotropy and increased cardiac output while maintaining dopaminergic-induced vasodilatory effects. At high doses (>10 mcg/kg/min), alpha adrenergic agonism predominates, and increased peripheral vascular resistance and vasoconstriction result.
Indications: Hypotension and decreased cardiac output associated with cardiogenic shock and septic shock, hypotension after return of spontaneous circulation following cardiac arrest, symptomatic bradycardia unresponsive to atropine.
Adverse Effects: Tachycardia, arrhythmias, skin and soft tissue necrosis, severe hypertension from excessive vasoconstriction, angina, dyspnea, headache, nausea/vomiting.
Contraindications: Pheochromocytoma, VF, VT, or other ventricular arrhythmias, known sensitivity (including sulfites). Correct any hypovolemia with volume fluid replacement before administering dopamine.
Dosage:
- **Adult:** 2 to 20 mcg/kg/min IV, IO infusion. Starting dose 5 mcg/kg/min; may gradually increase the infusion by 5 to 10 mcg/kg/min to desired effect. Cardiac dose is usually 5 to 10 mcg/kg/min; vasopressor dose is usually 10 to 20 mcg/kg/min. Little benefit is gained beyond 20 mcg/kg/min.
- **Pediatric:** Same as adult dosing.

Special Considerations:
Half-life 2 minutes
Pregnancy class C

EPINEPHRINE

Classification: Adrenergic agent, inotropic
Action: Binds strongly with both alpha and beta receptors, producing increased blood pressure, increased heart rate, bronchodilation.
Indications: Bronchospasm, allergic and anaphylactic reactions, restoration of cardiac activity in cardiac arrest.
Adverse Effects: Anxiety, headache, cardiac arrhythmias, hypertension, nervousness, tremors, chest pain, nausea/vomiting.
Contraindications: Arrhythmias other than VF, asystole, PEA; cardiovascular disease; hypertension; cerebrovascular disease; shock secondary to causes other than anaphylactic shock; closed-angle glaucoma; diabetes; pregnant women in active labor; known sensitivity to epinephrine or sulfites.

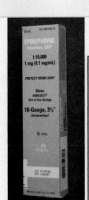
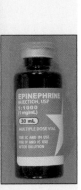

Dosage:
Cardiac Arrest:
- **Adult:** 1 mg (1:10,000 solution) IV, IO; may repeat every 3 to 5 minutes.
- **Pediatric:** 0.01 mg/kg (1:10,000 solution) IV, IO; repeat every 3 to 5 minutes as needed (max dose: 1 mg).

Symptomatic Bradycardia:
- **Adult:** 1 mcg/min (1:10,000 solution) as a continuous IV infusion; usual dosage range: 2 to 10 mcg/min IV; titrate to effect.
- **Pediatric:** 0.01 mg/kg (1:10,000 solution) IV, IO; may repeat every 3 to 5 minutes (max dose: 1 mg). If giving epinephrine by ET tube, administer 0.1 mg/kg.

Asthma Attacks and Certain Allergic Reactions:
- **Adult:** 0.3 to 0.5 mg (1:1000 solution) IM or Sub-Q; may repeat every 10 to 15 minutes (max dose: 1 mg).
- **Pediatric:** 0.01 mg/kg (1:1000 solution) IM or Sub-Q (max dose: 0.5 mg).

cont'd

EPINEPHRINE—CONT'D

Anaphylactic Shock:
- **Adult:** 0.1 mg (1:10,000 solution) IV slowly over 5 minutes, or IV infusion of 1 to 4 mcg/min, titrated to effect.
- **Pediatric:** Continuous IV infusion rate of 0.1 to 1 mcg/kg/min (1:10,000 solution); titrate to response.

Special Considerations:
Half-life 1 minute
Pregnancy class C

EPINEPHRINE AUTOINJECTORS (EPIPEN, EPIPEN JR)

Classification: Adrenergic agonist, inotropic
Action: Binds strongly with both alpha and beta receptors, producing increased blood pressure, increased heart rate, bronchodilation.
Indications: Anaphylactic shock, certain allergic reactions, asthma attacks.
Adverse Effects: Headaches, nervousness, tremors, arrhythmias, hypertension, chest pain, nausea/vomiting.
Contraindications: Arrhythmias other than VF, asystole, PEA; cardiovascular disease; hypertension; cerebrovascular disease; shock secondary to causes other than anaphylactic shock; closed-angle glaucoma; diabetes; pregnant women in active labor; known sensitivity to epinephrine or sulfites.
Dosage:
- **Adult:** An EpiPen contains 0.3 mg epinephrine to be administered IM into the anterolateral thigh area.
- **Pediatric:** For children weighing <30 kg, an EpiPen Jr delivers 0.15 mg IM.

Special Considerations:
Half-life 1 minute
Pregnancy class C

EPTIFIBATIDE (INTEGRILIN)

Classification: GP IIb/IIIa inhibitor
Action: Prevents the aggregation of platelets by binding to the GP IIb/IIIa receptor.
Indications: UA/NSTEMI—to manage medically and for those undergoing percutaneous coronary intervention.
Adverse Effects: Bleeding from the GI tract, internal bleeding, intracranial hemorrhage, hypotension, stroke, anaphylactic shock.
Contraindications: Bleeding from any source, severe uncontrolled hypertension, surgery or trauma within the previous 6 weeks, stroke within the previous 30 days, renal failure, thrombocytopenia.
Dosage:

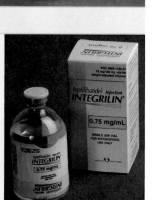

- **Adult:** Loading dose: 180 mcg/kg IV, IO (max dose: 22.6 mg) over 1 to 2 minutes, then 2 mcg/kg/min IV, IO infusion (max dose: 15 mg/hr).
- **Pediatric:** No current dosing recommendations exist for pediatric patients.

Special Considerations:
Half-life approximately 90 to 120 minutes
Pregnancy class B

ESMOLOL (BREVIBLOC)

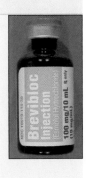

Classification: Beta adrenergic antagonist, class II antiarrhythmic

Action: Inhibits the strength of the heart's contractions, as well as heart rate, resulting in a decrease in cardiac oxygen consumption.

Indications: ACS, MI, acute hypertension, supraventricular tachyarrhythmias, thyrotoxicosis.

Adverse Effects: Hypotension, sinus bradycardia, AV block, cardiac arrest, nausea/vomiting, hypoglycemia, injection site reaction.

Contraindications: Acute bronchospasm, COPD, second- or third-degree heart block, bradycardia, cardiogenic shock, pulmonary edema, sick sinus syndrome, known sensitivity. Use with caution in patients with pheochromocytoma, Prinzmetal's angina, cerebrovascular disease, stroke, poorly controlled diabetes mellitus, hyperthyroidism, thyrotoxicosis, renal disease.

Dosage:
- **Adult:** 500 mcg/kg (0.5 mg/kg) IV, IO over a 1-minute period, followed by a 50-mcg/kg/min (0.05 mg/kg) infusion over a 4-minute period (maximum total: 200 mcg/kg). If patient response is inadequate, administer a second bolus 500 mcg/kg (0.5 mg/kg) over a 1-minute period, and then increase infusion to 100 mcg/kg/min. Maximum infusion rate: 300 mcg/kg/min.
- **Pediatric:** 500 mcg/kg (0.5 mg/kg) IV, IO over a 1-minute period, followed by an infusion at 25 to 200 mcg/kg/min.

Special Considerations:

Half-life 5 to 9 minutes

Any adverse effects caused by administration of esmolol are brief because of the drug's short half-life.

Resolution of effects usually within 10 to 20 minutes.

Pregnancy class C

ETOMIDATE (AMIDATE)

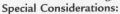

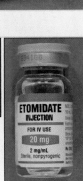

Classification: Hypnotic, anesthesia induction agent

Action: Although the exact mechanism is unknown, etomidate appears to have GABA-like effects.

Indications: Induction for rapid sequence intubation and pharmacologic-assisted intubation, induction of anesthesia.

Adverse Effects: Hypotension, respiratory depression, pain at the site of injection, temporary involuntary muscle movements, frequent nausea/vomiting on emergence, adrenal insufficiency, hyperventilation, hypoventilation, apnea of short duration, hiccups, laryngospasm, snoring, tachypnea, hypertension, cardiac arrhythmias.

Contraindications: Known sensitivity. Use in pregnancy only if the potential benefits justify the potential risk to the fetus. Do not use during labor and avoid in nursing mothers.

Dosage:
- **Adult:** 0.2 to 0.6 mg/kg slow IV, IO (over 30 to 60 seconds). A typical adult intubating dose of etomidate is 20 mg slow IV. Consider less (e.g., 10 mg) in the elderly or patients with cardiac conditions.
- **Pediatric:**
  - **Older than 10 years:** Same as adult dosing.
  - **Younger than 10 years:** Safety has not been established.

Special Considerations:

Etomidate is used to prepare a patient for orotracheal intubation. Both personnel and equipment must be present to manage the patient's airway before administration.

Pregnancy class C

FELBAMATE (FELBATOL)

Classification: Anticonvulsant
Action: Although the mechanism of action is not known, it is believed that felbamate antagonizes the effects of glycine, increases the seizure threshold in absence seizures, and prevents the spread of generalized tonic-clonic and partial seizures.
Indications: Partial seizures with and without generalization in epileptic adults; partial and generalized seizures associated with Lennox-Gastaut syndrome in children.
Adverse Effects: Nausea/vomiting, suicidal ideation and behavior, depression, insomnia, dyspepsia, upper respiratory tract infection, fatigue, headache, constipation, diarrhea, rhinitis, anxiety, aplastic anemia, photosensitivity.
Contraindications: Blood dyscrasias, hepatic disease, known sensitivity to carbomates.
Dosage: Should be individualized based on condition.
Special Considerations:
Pregnancy class C

FENTANYL CITRATE (SUBLIMAZE)

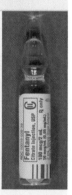

Classification: Narcotic analgesic; Schedule C-II
Action: Binds to opiate receptors, producing analgesia and euphoria.
Indications: Pain
Adverse Effects: Respiratory depression, apnea, hypotension, nausea/vomiting, dizziness, sedation, euphoria, sinus bradycardia, sinus tachycardia, palpitations, hypertension, diaphoresis, syncope, pain at injection site.
Contraindications: Known sensitivity. Use with caution in traumatic brain injury, respiratory depression.
Dosage: Note: Dosage should be individualized.
· **Adult:** 50 to 100 mcg/dose (0.05 to 0.1 mg) IM or slow IV, IO (administered over 1 to 2 minutes).
· **Pediatric:** 1 to 2 mcg/kg IM or slow IV, IO (administered over 1 to 2 minutes).
Special Considerations:
Pregnancy class B

FIBRINOLYTICS: TISSUE PLASMINOGEN ACTIVATOR (tPA), STREPTOKINASE (STREPTASE, KABIKINASE), RETEPLASE (RETAVASE), TENECTEPLASE (TNKASE)

Classification: Thrombolytic agent
Action: Dissolves thrombi plugs in the coronary arteries and reestablishes blood flow.
Indications: ST-segment elevation (≥ 1 mm in two or more contiguous leads), new or presumed-new left bundle branch block.
Adverse Effects: Bleeding, intracranial hemorrhage, stroke, cardiac arrhythmias, hypotension, bruising.
Contraindications: ST-segment depression, cardiogenic shock, recent (within 10 days) major surgery, cerebrovascular disease, recent (within 10 days) GI bleeding, recent trauma, hypertension (systolic blood pressure ≥ 180 mm Hg or diastolic blood pressure ≥ 110 mm Hg), high likelihood of left heart thrombus, acute pericarditis, subacute bacterial endocarditis, severe renal or liver failure with bleeding complications, significant liver dysfunction, diabetic hemorrhagic retinopathy, septic thrombophlebitis, advanced age (older than 75 years), patients taking warfarin (Coumadin).
Dosage: Dosing per medical direction.
Special Considerations:
Pregnancy class C

FLUMAZENIL (ROMAZICON)

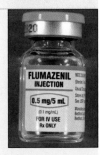

Classification: Benzodiazepine receptor antagonist, antidote

Action: Competes with benzodiazepines for binding at the benzodiazepine receptor, reverses the sedative effects of benzodiazepines.

Indication: Benzodiazepine oversedation

Adverse Effects: Resedation, seizures, dizziness, pain at injection site, nausea/vomiting, diaphoresis, headache, visual impairment.

Contraindications: Cyclic antidepressant overdose; life-threatening conditions that require treatment with benzodiazepines, such as status epilepticus and intracranial hypertension; known sensitivity to flumazenil or benzodiazepines. Use with caution where there is the possibility of unrecognized benzodiazepine dependence and in patients who have a history of substance abuse or who are known substance abusers.

Dosage:
- **Adult:** Initial dose is 0.2 mg IV, IO over a 15-second period. If the desired effect is not observed after 45 seconds, administer a second 0.2-mg dose, again over a 15-second period. Doses can be repeated a total of four times until a total dose of 1 mg has been administered.
- **Pediatric:** Children older than 1 year, 0.01 mg/kg IV, IO given over a 15-second period. May repeat in 45 seconds and then every minute to a maximum cumulative dose of 0.05 mg/kg or 1 mg, whichever is the lower dose.

Special Considerations:

Monitor for signs of hypoventilation and hypoxia for approximately 2 hours.

If the half-life of the benzodiazepine is longer than flumazenil, an additional dose may be needed.

May precipitate withdrawal symptoms in patients dependent on benzodiazepines.

Flumazenil has not been shown to benefit patients who have overdosed on multiple drugs.

Pregnancy class C

FOSPHENYTOIN (CEREBYX)

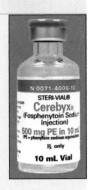

Classification: Anticonvulsant

Action: Alters the movement of sodium and calcium into nervous tissue and prevents the spread of seizure activity.

Indications: Partial and generalized seizures, status epilepticus, seizure prophylaxis.

Adverse Effects: Phenytoin can cause several adverse effects often related to drug dose, including sedation, nystagmus, tremors, ataxia, dysarthria, gingival hypertrophy, hirsutism, and facial coarsening. Too-rapid administration can cause hypotension.

Contraindications:

Bradycardia, bundle branch blocks, agranulocytosis, Adams-Stokes syndrome, hydantoin hypersensitivity.

Dosage: The dose and concentration of fosphenytoin is expressed in PE to simplify the conversion between phenytoin and fosphenytoin.
- **Adult:** The usual loading dose of fosphenytoin is 15 to 20 mg PE/kg IV, not to exceed 150 mg PE/min IV rate.
- **Pediatric:** The usual loading dose of fosphenytoin is 15 to 20 mg PE/kg IV, not to exceed 3 mg PE/kg/min (max dose: 150 mg PE/min) IV rate.

Special Considerations:

Pregnancy class D

Compatible with breast-feeding

FUROSEMIDE (LASIX)

Classification: Loop diuretic
Action: Inhibits the absorption of the sodium and chloride ions and water in the loop of Henle, as well as the convoluted tubule of the nephron. This results in decreased absorption of water and increased production of urine.
Indications: Pulmonary edema, CHF, hypertensive emergency.
Adverse Effects: Vertigo, dizziness, weakness, orthostatic hypotension, hypokalemia, thrombophlebitis. Patients with anuria, severe renal failure, untreated hepatic coma, increasing azotemia, and electrolyte depletion can develop life-threatening consequences.
Contraindications: Known sensitivity to sulfonamides or furosemide.
Dosage:
Congestive Heart Failure and Pulmonary Edema:
- **Adult:** 40 mg IV, IO administered slowly over a 1- to 2-minute period. If a satisfactory response is not achieved within 1 hour, an additional dose of 80 mg can be given. A maximum single IV dose is 160 to 200 mg.
- **Pediatric:** 1 mg/kg IV, IO or IM. If the response is not satisfactory, an additional dose of 2 mg/kg may be administered no sooner than 2 hours after the first dose.
Hypertensive Emergency:
- **Adult:** 40 to 80 mg IV, IO.
- **Pediatric:** 1 mg/kg IV or IM.
Special Considerations:
Onset of action for IV, IO administration occurs within 5 minutes and will peak within 30 minutes.
Furosemide is a diuretic, so the patient will likely have urinary urgency. Be prepared to help the patient void.
Pregnancy class C

GABAPENTIN (NEURONTIN)

Classification: Anticonvulsant
Action: The exact mechanism of action has not been determined.
Indications: Seizures, neuropathic pain syndromes.
Adverse Effects: Dizziness, ataxia, sleepiness, gait disturbances, upset stomach.
Contraindications: Known sensitivity. Use with caution in elderly patients, renal impairment.
Dosage:
- **Adult:** 300 to 1800 mg PO daily.
- **Pediatric:**
  - **5 to 12 years:** 25 to 35 mg/kg/day PO divided in three divided doses daily.
  - **3 to 4 years:** 40 mg/kg/day PO divided in three divided doses daily.
Special Considerations:
Pregnancy class C

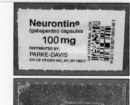
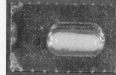

GLUCAGON

Classification: Hormone
Action: Converts glycogen to glucose.
Indications: Hypoglycemia, beta blocker overdose.
Adverse Effects: Nausea/vomiting, rebound hyperglycemia, hypotension, sinus tachycardia.
Contraindications: Pheochromocytoma, insulinoma, known sensitivity.

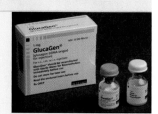

cont'd

GLUCAGON—CONT'D

Dosage:
Hypoglycemia:
- **Adult:** 1 mg IM, IV, IO, or Sub-Q.
- **Pediatric (<20 kg):** 0.5 mg IM, IV, IO, or Sub-Q.

Beta blocker overdose:
- **Adult:** 2 to 5 mg IV, IO over a 1-minute period, followed by a second dose of 10 mg IV if the symptoms of bradycardia and hypotension recur. (Note that this dose is much higher than the dose required to treat hypoglycemia.)
- **Pediatric:** For patients weighing <20 kg, the dose is 0.5 mg.

Special Considerations:
Pregnancy class B

HALOPERIDOL (HALDOL)

Classification: Antipsychotic agent
Action: Selectively blocks postsynaptic dopamine receptors.
Indications: Psychotic disorders, agitation.
Adverse Effects: Extrapyramidal symptoms, drowsiness, tardive dyskinesia, hypotension, hypertension, VT, sinus tachycardia, QT prolongation, torsades de pointes.
Contraindications: Depressed mental status, Parkinson's disease.
Dosage:
- **Adult:**
  - **Mild agitation:** 0.5 to 2 mg PO or IM.
  - **Moderate agitation:** 5 to 10 mg PO or IM.
  - **Severe agitation:** 10 mg PO or IM.
- **Pediatric:** Not recommended for pediatric patients.

Special Considerations:
Pregnancy class C

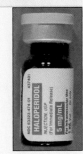

HEPARIN (UNFRACTIONATED HEPARIN)

Classification: Anticoagulant
Action: Acts on antithrombin III to reduce the ability of the blood to form clots, thus preventing clot deposition in the coronary arteries.
Indications: ACS, acute pulmonary embolism, deep venous thrombosis.
Adverse Effects: Bleeding, thrombocytopenia, allergic reactions.
Contraindications: Predisposition to bleeding, aortic aneurysm, peptic ulceration; known sensitivity or history of heparin-induced thrombocytopenia, severe thrombocytopenia, sulfite sensitivity.
Dosage:
Cardiac Indications:
- **Adult:** 60 U/kg IV (max 4000 units), followed by 12 U/kg/hr (max 1000 units). Once in the hospital, additional dosing is determined based on laboratory blood tests.
- **Pediatric:** 75 U/kg followed by 20 U/kg/hr.

Pulmonary Embolism and Deep Vein Thrombosis:
- **Adult:** 80 U/kg IV, followed by 18 U/kg/hr.
- **Pediatric:** 75 U/kg IV followed by 20 U/kg/hr.

Special Considerations:
Half-life approximately 90 minutes
Pregnancy class C

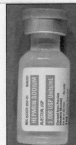

HETASTARCH (HESPAN)

Classification: Volume expander, colloid
Action: Causes water to move from interstitial spaces, thereby increasing the oncotic pressure within the intravascular space.
Indications: Hypovolemia when volume must be increased only in the intravascular compartment.
Adverse Effects: Anaphylactic reactions, CHF, pulmonary edema, cardiac arrhythmias, cardiac arrest, severe hypotension, pruritus, edema, platelet dysfunction, bleeding complications, dilution of the serum proteins responsible for the formation of blood clots, nausea/vomiting.
Contraindications: Bleeding disorders, intracranial bleeding, CHF, pulmonary edema, renal failure, thrombocytopenia or other coagulopathy (e.g., hemophilia), known sensitivity to hetastarch or corn.
Dosage: Note: The dosage of hetastarch required is determined by the clinical situation and the severity of the hypovolemia.
- **Adult:** 500 to 1000 mL IV, IO; more than 1500 mL of hetastarch typically is not administered because of concerns that larger doses can interfere with platelet function and promote bleeding.
- **Pediatric:** 10 mL/kg per dose IV; the total daily dosage should not exceed 20 mL/kg.
Special Considerations:
Pregnancy class C

HMG COENZYME A STATINS: ATORVASTATIN (LIPITOR), FLUVASTATIN (LESCOL), LOVASTATIN (MEVACOR), PRAVASTATIN (PRAVACHOL), ROSUVASTATIN (CRESTOR), SIMVASTATIN (ZOCOR)

Classification: HMG coenzyme A statins
Action: Reduces the level of circulating total cholesterol, LDL cholestrol, and serum triglycerides; reduces the incidence of reinfarction, recurrent angina, rehospitalization, and stroke when initiated within a few days after onset of ACS.
Indications: Acute coronary syndromes/acute myocardial infarction prophylaxis, hypercholesterolemia, hyperlipoproteinemia, hypertriglyceridemia, stroke prophylaxis.
Adverse Effects: Constipation, flatulence, dyspepsia, abdominal pain, infection, headache, flu-like symptoms, back pain, allergic reaction, asthenia, diarrhea, sinusitis, pharyngitis, rash, arthralgia, nausea/vomiting, myopathy, myasthenia, renal failure, rhabdomyolysis, chest pain, bronchitis, rhinitis, insomnia.
Contraindications: Active hepatic disease, pregnancy, breast-feeding, rhabdomyolysis.
Dosage:
- **Adult:** Medication is administered orally. Dosage is individualized.
- **Pediatric:** Safe use has not been established.
Special Considerations:
Pregnancy class X

HYDRALAZINE (APRESOLINE)

Classification: Antihypertensive agent, vasodilator
Action: Directly dilates the peripheral blood vessels.
Indications: Hypertension associated with preeclampsia and eclampsia, hypertensive crisis.
Adverse Effects: Headache, angina, flushing, palpitations, reflex tachycardia, anorexia, nausea/vomiting, diarrhea, hypotension, syncope, peripheral vasodilation, peripheral edema, fluid retention, paresthesias.
Contraindications: Patients taking diazoxide or MAOIs, coronary artery disease, stroke, angina, dissecting aortic aneurysm, mitral valve and rheumatic heart diseases.

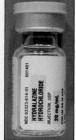

cont'd

HYDRALAZINE (APRESOLINE)—CONT'D

Dosage:
Preeclampsia and Eclampsia:
- **Adult:** 5 to 10 mg IV, IO. Repeat every 20 to 30 minutes until systolic blood pressure of 90 to 105 mm Hg is attained.

Acute Hypertension Not Associated with Preeclampsia:
- **Adult:** 10 to 20 mg IV, IO, or IM.
- **Pediatric:**
  - **1 month to 12 years:** 0.1 to 0.6 mg/kg IV, IO, or IM (max: 20 mg/dose).

Special Considerations:
Pregnancy class C

HYDROCORTISONE SODIUM SUCCINATE (CORTEF, SOLU-CORTEF)

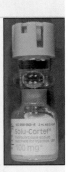

Classification: Corticosteroid
Action: Reduces inflammation by multiple mechanisms. As a steroid, it replaces the steroids that are lacking in adrenal insufficiency.
Indications: Adrenal insufficiency, allergic reactions, anaphylaxis, asthma, COPD.
Adverse Effects: Leukocytosis, hyperglycemia, increased infection, decreased wound healing, increased rate of death from sepsis.
Contraindications: Cushing's syndrome, known sensitivity to benzyl alcohol. Use with caution in diabetes, hypertension, CHF, known systemic fungal infection, renal disease, idiopathic thrombocytopenia, psychosis, seizure disorder, GI disease, glaucoma, known sensitivity.
Dosage:
Anaphylactic Shock:
- **Adult:** 100 to 500 mg IV, IO, or IM.
- **Pediatric:** 2 to 4 mg/kg/day IV, IO, or IM (max: 500 mg).

Adrenal Insufficiency:
- **Adult:** 100 to 500 mg IV, IO, or IM.
- **Pediatric:** 1 to 2 mg/kg IV, IO, or IM.

Asthma and Chronic Obstructive Pulmonary Disease:
- **Adult:** 100 to 500 mg IV, IO, IM.
- **Pediatric:** 1 mg/kg IV, IO. The dose may be reduced for infants and children, but it is governed more by the severity of the condition and response of the patient than by age or body weight. Dose should not be less than 25 mg daily.

Special Considerations:
Pregnancy class C

HYPERTONIC SALINE (3% SALINE)

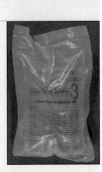

Classification: Volume expander, electrolyte solution
Action: The hypertonic nature of this fluid pulls extravascular fluid into the vascular space. Hypertonic saline may therefore be used as a volume expander in cases of hypovolemia or to reduce the edema of the swollen brain. Three percent saline has an electrolyte concentration of 514 mEq/L sodium.
Indications: Reduction of increased intracranial pressure resulting from traumatic brain injury, hypovolemic shock.
Adverse Effects: Increased rate of bleeding, alteration of blood clotting ability, osmotic demyelination syndrome.
Contraindications: Pulmonary congestion, pulmonary edema, known sensitivity. Hypertonic saline should not be administered by the IO route.
Dosage: Note: Hypertonic saline is available in several concentrations from 3% to 5%.
- **Adult:** 250-mL bag of hypertonic saline infused IV slowly over a 1-hour period.
- **Pediatric:** 6.5 to 10 mL/kg infused slowly IV over a 2-hour period.

Special Considerations:
Hypertonic saline can cause damage to the vein in which it is administered.
Pregnancy class C

IBUPROFEN

Classification: NSAID

Action: Inhibits prostaglandin synthesis by inhibiting cyclooxygenase (COX) isoenzymes, resulting in analgesic, antipyretic, and antiinflammatory effects.

Indications: Mild to moderate pain, fever, osteoarthritis, rheumatoid arthritis.

Adverse Effects: Anorexia, nausea/vomiting, epigastric/abdominal pain, dyspepsia, constipation, diarrhea, gastritis, melena, flatulence, headache, dizziness.

Contraindications: Sensitivity to NSAID or salicylate. Use with caution in asthma, hepatic disease, renal disease, congestive heart failure, hypertension, cardiac disease, cardiomyopathy, cardiac arrhythmias, significant coronary artery disease, peripheral vascular disease, cerebrovascular disease, fluid retention, or edema.

Dosage:

Mild to Moderate Pain:

- **Adult:** 400 mg PO every 4 hours as needed, not to exceed 1200 mg per day.
- **Pediatric: 6 months to 12 yrs:** 5 to 10 mg/kg PO every 6 to 8 hours as needed, not to exceed 40 mg/kg/day.

Fever:

- **Adult:** 200 to 400 mg PO every 4 to 6 hours as needed, not to exceed 1200 mg per day.
- **Pediatric: 6 months to 12 years:** 5 mg/kg PO if baseline temperature is less than 102.5° F, or 10 mg/kg PO if baseline temperature is greater than 102.5° F (max dose: 40 mg/kg/day).

Osteoarthritis or Rheumatoid Arthritis:

- **Adult:** 400 to 800 mg PO 3 to 4 times per day, not to exceed 3200 mg/day.
- **Pediatric: 1 to 12 years:** 30 to 40 mg/kg/day PO in 3 to 4 divided doses, not to exceed 50 mg/kg/day.

Special Considerations:

Pregnancy class B

INSULIN, REGULAR (HUMULIN R, NOVOLIN R)

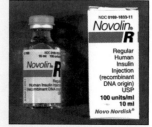

Classification: Hormone

Action: Binds to a receptor on the membrane of cells and facilitates the transport of glucose into cells.

Indications: Hyperglycemia, insulin-dependent diabetes mellitus, hyperkalemia.

Adverse Effects: Hypoglycemia, tachycardia, palpitations, diaphoresis, anxiety, confusion, blurred vision, weakness, depression, seizures, coma, insulin shock, hypokalemia.

Contraindications: Hypoglycemia, known sensitivity.

Dosage:

Diabetic Ketoacidosis:

- **Adult:** 0.1 U/kg IV, IO, or Sub-Q. Because of poor perfusion of the peripheral tissues, Sub-Q administration is much less effective than the IV, IO route. IV, IO insulin has a very short half-life; therefore IV, IO insulin without an infusion is not that effective. The rate for an insulin infusion is 0.05 to 0.1 U/kg/hr IV, IO. When dosing insulin, use a U-100 insulin syringe to measure and deliver the insulin. The time from administration to action, as well as the duration of action, varies greatly among different individuals, as well as at different times in the same individual.

Hyperkalemia:

- **Adult:** 10 U IV, IO of regular insulin (Insulin R), coadministered with 50 mL of $D_{50}W$ over 5 minutes.
- **Pediatric:** 0.1 U/kg Insulin R IV, IO.

Special Considerations:

Only regular insulin can be given IV, IO.

Pregnancy class B

IPRATROPIUM BROMIDE (ATROVENT)

Classification: Bronchodilator, anticholinergic
Action: Antagonizes the acetylcholine receptor on bronchial smooth muscle, producing bronchodilation.
Indications: Asthma, bronchospasm associated with COPD.
Adverse Effects: Paradoxical acute bronchospasm, cough, throat irritation, headache, dizziness, dry mouth, palpitations.
Contraindications: Closed-angle glaucoma, bladder neck obstruction, prostatic hypertrophy, known sensitivity including peanuts or soybeans and atropine or atropine derivatives.

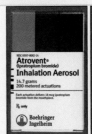
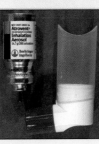

Dosage:
MDI:
- **Adult:** 4 inhalations every 10 minutes, with no more than 24 inhalations per day or closer than 4 hours apart.
- **Pediatric:**
  - **Older than 12 years:** 2 to 3 puffs inhaled every 6 to 8 hours. Maximum of 12 puffs/day.
  - **5 to 12 years:** 1 to 2 puffs inhaled every 6 to 8 hours. Maximum of 8 puffs/day.

Nebulization:
- **Adult:** 0.5 mg every 6 to 8 hours.
- **Pediatric: 5 to 14 years:** 0.25 to 0.5 mg every 20 minutes for 3 doses as needed.

Special Considerations:
Ipratropium bromide is not typically used as a sole medication in the treatment of acute exacerbation of asthma. Ipratropium bromide is commonly administered after a beta agonist.
Care should be taken to not allow the aerosol spray (especially in the MDI) to come into contact with the eyes. This can cause temporary blurring of vision that resolves without intervention within 4 hours.
Pregnancy class B

KETAMINE (KETALAR)

Classification: General anesthetic
Action: Produces a state of anesthesia while maintaining airway reflexes, heart rate, and blood pressure.
Indications: Pain and as anesthesia for procedures of short duration.
Adverse Effects: Emergence phenomena, hypertension and sinus tachycardia, hypotension and sinus bradycardia, other cardiac arrhythmias (rare), respiratory depression, apnea, laryngospasms and other forms of airway obstruction (rare), tonic and clonic movements, vomiting.
Contraindications: Patients in whom a significant elevation in blood pressure would be hazardous (hypertension, stroke, head trauma, increased intracranial mass or bleeding, MI). Use with caution in patients with increased ICP or increased intraocular pressure (glaucoma) and patients with hypovolemia, dehydration, or cardiac disease (especially angina and CHF).

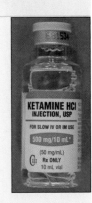

Dosage: Administer slowly over a period of 60 seconds.
IV, IO:
- **Adult:** 1 to 4.5 mg/kg IV, IO. 1 to 2 mg/kg produces anesthesia usually within 30 seconds that typically lasts 5 to 10 minutes.
- **Pediatric:** 0.5 to 2 mg IV, IO over a 1-minute period.

IM:
- **Adult:** 6.5 to 13 mg/kg IM. 10 mg/kg IM is capable of producing anesthesia within 3 to 4 minutes with an effect typically lasting 12 to 25 minutes. In adults, concomitant administration of 5 to 15 mg of diazepam reduces the incidence of emergence phenomena.
- **Pediatric:** 3 to 7 mg IM.

Special Considerations:
Pregnancy class C

KETOROLAC (TORADOL)

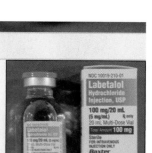

Classification: NSAID
Action: Inhibits the production of prostaglandins in inflamed tissue, which decreases the responsiveness of pain receptors.
Indications: Moderately severe acute pain.
Adverse Effects: Headache, drowsiness, dizziness, abdominal pain, dyspepsia, nausea/vomiting, diarrhea.
Contraindications: Patients with a history of peptic ulcer disease or GI bleed, patients with renal insufficiency, hypovolemic patients, pregnancy (third trimester), nursing mothers, allergy to aspirin or other NSAIDs, stroke or suspected stroke or head trauma, need for major surgery in the immediate or near future (i.e., within 7 days).
Dosage: Note: The following dosage regimen applies to single-dose administration only. IV, IO administration should occur over a period of at least 15 seconds.
  · **Adult:**
    · **Younger than 65 years:** 30 mg IV, IO or 60 mg IM.
    · **Older than 65 years:** 15 mg IV, IO or 30 mg IM.
  · **Pediatric:** 0.5 mg/kg IV, IO to a maximum dose of 15 mg, or 1 mg/kg IM to a maximum dose of 30 mg.
Special Considerations:
Pregnancy class C; class D in third trimester

LABETALOL (NORMODYNE, TRANDATE)

Classification: Beta adrenergic antagonist, antianginal, antihypertensive
Action: Binds with both the beta$_1$ and beta$_2$ receptors and alpha$_1$ receptors in vascular smooth muscle. Inhibits the strength of the heart's contractions, as well as heart rate. This results in a decrease in cardiac oxygen consumption.
Indications: ACS, SVT, severe hypertension.
Adverse Effects: Usually mild and transient; hypotensive symptoms, nausea/vomiting, bronchospasm, arrhythmia, bradycardia, AV block.
Contraindications: Hypotension, cardiogenic shock, acute pulmonary edema, heart failure, severe bradycardia, sick sinus syndrome, second- or third-degree heart block, asthma or acute bronchospasm, cocaine-induced ACS, known sensitivity. Use caution in pheochromocytoma, cerebrovascular disease or stroke, poorly controlled diabetes, with hepatic disease. Use with caution at lowest effective dose in chronic lung disease.
Dosage:
Cardiac Indications: Note: Monitor blood pressure and heart rate closely during administration.
  · **Adult:** 10 mg IV, IO over a 1- to 2-minute period. May repeat every 10 minutes to a maximum dose of 150 mg or give initial bolus and then follow with infusion at 2 to 8 mg/min.
  · **Pediatric:** 0.4 to 1 mg/kg/hr to a maximum dosage of 3 mg/kg/hr.
Severe Hypertension:
  · **Adult:** Initial dose is 20 mg IV, IO slow infusion over a 2-minute period. After the initial dose, blood pressure should be checked every 5 minutes. Repeat doses can be given at 10-minute intervals. The second dose should be 40 mg IV, IO, and subsequent doses should be 80 mg IV, IO, to a maximum total dose of 300 mg. The effect on blood pressure typically will occur within 5 minutes from the time of administration. Alternatively, may be administered via IV infusion at 2 mg/min to a total maximum dose of 300 mg.
  · **Pediatric:** 0.4 to 1 mg/kg/hr IV, IO infusion with a maximum dose of 3 mg/kg/hr.
Special Considerations:
Pregnancy class C

LAMOTRIGINE (LAMICTAL)

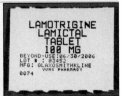
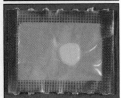

Classification: Anticonvulsant, antimanic agent
Action: The exact mechanism of action has not been determined. Studies suggest lamotrigine stabilizes neuronal membranes by acting at voltage-sensitive sodium channels, thereby decreasing presynaptic release of glutamate and aspartate, resulting in decreased seizure activity.
Indications: Seizures, bipolar disorders.
Adverse Effects: Headache, dizziness, nausea/vomiting, ataxia, diplopia.
Contraindications: Known sensitivity.
Dosage:
 · **Adult:** Medication is administered orally. Dosage is individualized.
 · **Pediatric:** Medication is administered orally. Dosage is individualized.
Special Considerations:
Pregnancy class C

LEVALBUTEROL (XOPENEX)

Classification: Beta agonist
Action: Stimulates beta$_2$ receptors, resulting in relaxation of the smooth muscle in the lungs, uterus, and vasculature that supply skeletal muscle.
Indications: Acute bronchospasm or bronchospasm prophylaxis in patient with asthma.
Adverse Effects: Hyperglycemia, hypokalemia, palpitations, sinus tachycardia, anxiety, tremor, nausea/vomiting, throat irritation, hypertension, dyspepsia, insomnia, headache.
Contraindications: Angioedema, sensitivity to albuterol or levalbuterol. Use with caution in lactating patients, cardiovascular disorders, cardiac arrhythmias. Do not use in patients taking phenothiazines because this may cause prolonged QT interval and cardiac arrhythmias. Also avoid use in patients getting sotalol because they may decrease bronchodilating effects and cause bronchospasm, prolonged QT interval, and cardiac arrhythmias.
Dosage:
MDI:
 · **Adult:** 2 inhalations every 4 to 6 hours. In some patients, 1 inhalation may be sufficient. For acute exacerbations, 4 to 8 inhalations every 20 minutes up to 4 hours, then every 1 to 4 hours as needed.
 · **Pediatric:**
  · **4 to 12 years:** 2 inhalations every 4 to 6 hours. In some patients, 1 inhalation may be sufficient. For acute exacerbations, 2 to 4 inhalations every 20 minutes for 3 doses, then 2 to 4 inhalations every 1 to 4 hours as needed.
  · **Younger than 4 years:** Safe and effective use has not been established. For acute exacerbations, 2 to 4 inhalations holding a valved holding chamber and face mask every 20 minutes for 3 doses, then 2 to 4 inhalations every 1 to 4 hours as needed.
Nebulizer:
 · **Adult:** Usually, 0.63 mg 3 times/day. For acute exacerbations, 1.25 to 2.5 mg every 20 minutes for 3 doses, then 1.25 to 5 mg every 1 to 4 hours as needed.
 · **Pediatric:**
  · **6 to 11 years:** Usually, 0.31 mg 3 times/day. For acute exacerbations, 0.075 mg/kg (1.25 mg minimum) every 20 minutes for 3 doses, then 0.075 to 0.15 mg/kg (5 mg maximum) every 1 to 4 hours as needed.
  · **Younger than 6 years:** Safe and effective use has not been established. For acute exacerbations, 1.25 to 2.5 mg every 20 minutes for 3 doses, then 1.25 to 5 mg every 1 to 4 hours as needed.
Special Considerations:
Pregnancy class C

LIDOCAINE (XYLOCAINE)

Classification: Antiarrhythmic, class IB
Action: Blocks sodium channels, increasing the recovery period after repolarization; suppresses automaticity in the His-Purkinje system and depolarization in the ventricles.
Indications: Ventricular arrhythmias, when amiodarone is not available: cardiac arrest from VF/VT, stable monomorphic VT with preserved ventricular function, stable polymorphic VT with normal baseline QT interval and preserved left ventricular function (when ischemia and electrolyte imbalance are treated), stable polymorphic VT with baseline QT prolongation suggestive of torsades de pointes.
Adverse Effects: Toxicity (signs may include anxiety, apprehension, euphoria, nervousness, disorientation, dizziness, blurred vision, facial paresthesias, tremors, hearing disturbances, slurred speech, seizures, sinus bradycardia), seizures without warning, cardiac arrhythmias, hypotension, cardiac arrest, pain at injection site.
Contraindications: AV block; bleeding; thrombocytopenia; known sensitivity to lidocaine, sulfite, or paraben. Use with caution in bradycardia, hypovolemia, cardiogenic shock, Adams-Stokes syndrome, Wolff-Parkinson-White syndrome.
Dosage:
Pulseless Ventricular Tachycardia and Ventricular Fibrillation:
- **Adult IV, IO:** 1 to 1.5 mg/kg IV, IO; may repeat at half the original dose (0.5-0.75 mg/kg) every 5 to 10 minutes to a maximum dose of 3 mg/kg. If a maintenance infusion is warranted, the rate is 1 to 4 mg/min.
- **Adult ET tube:** 2 to 10 mg/kg ET tube, diluted in 10 mL normal saline or sterile distilled water.
- **Pediatric IV, IO:** 1 mg/kg IV, IO (maximum: 100 mg). If a maintenance infusion is warranted, the rate is 20 to 50 mcg/kg/min.
- **Pediatric ET tube:** 2 to 3 mg/kg ET tube, followed by a 5-mL flush of normal saline.
Perfusing Ventricular Rhythms:
- **Adult:** 0.5 to 0.75 mg/kg IV, IO (up to 1-1.5 mg/kg may be used). Repeat 0.5 to 0.75 mg/kg every 5 to 10 minutes to a maximum total dose of 3 mg/kg. A maintenance infusion of 1 to 4 mg/min (30-50 mcg/kg/min) is acceptable.
- **Pediatric:** 1 mg/kg IV, IO. May repeat every 5 to 10 minutes to a maximum dose of 3 mg/kg. Maintenance infusion rate is 20 to 50 mcg/kg/min.
Special Considerations:
Half-life approximately 90 minutes
Pregnancy class B

LORAZEPAM (ATIVAN)

Classification: Benzodiazepine; Schedule C-IV
Action: Binds to the benzodiazepine receptor and enhances the effects of the brain chemical GABA, an inhibitory transmitter, and may result in a state of sedation, hypnosis, skeletal muscle relaxation, anticonvulsant activity, coma.
Indications: Preprocedure sedation induction, anxiety, status epilepticus.
Adverse Effects: Headache, drowsiness, ataxia, dizziness, amnesia, depression, dysarthria, euphoria, syncope, fatigue, tremor, vertigo, respiratory depression, paradoxical CNS stimulation.
Contraindications: Known sensitivity to lorazepam, benzodiazepines, polyethylene glycol, propylene glycol, or benzyl alcohol; COPD; sleep apnea (except while being mechanically ventilated); shock; coma; acute closed-angle glaucoma.
Dosage: Note: IV, IO lorazepam needs to be administered slowly.
Analgesia and Sedation:
- **Adult:** 2 mg or 0.44 mg/kg IV, IO, whichever is smaller. This dosage will provide adequate sedation in most patients and should not be exceeded in patients older than 50 years.
- **Pediatric:** 0.05 mg/kg IV, IO. Each dose should not exceed 2 mg IV, IO.

cont'd

LORAZEPAM (ATIVAN)—CONT'D

Seizures:
- **Adult:** 4 mg IV, IO given over 2 to 5 minutes; may repeat in 10 to 15 minutes (max total dose: 8 mg in a 12-hour period).
- **Pediatric:**
  - **Adolescents:** 0.07 mg/kg slow IV, IO given over 2 to 5 minutes (max single dose: 4 mg). May repeat in 10 to 15 minutes (max dose: 8 mg in a 12-hour period).
  - **Children and infants:** 0.1 mg/kg slow IV, IO given over 2 to 5 minutes (max single dose: 4 mg). May repeat at half the original dose in 10 to 15 minutes if seizure activity resumes.
  - **Neonates:** 0.05 mg/kg slow IV, IO given over 2 to 5 minutes. May repeat in 10 to 15 minutes.

Special Considerations:
Be prepared to support the patient's airway and ventilation.
Pregnancy class D

MAGNESIUM SULFATE

Classification: Electrolyte, tocolytic, mineral
Action: Required for normal physiologic functioning. Magnesium is a cofactor in neurochemical transmission and muscular excitability. Magnesium sulfate controls seizures by blocking peripheral neuromuscular transmission. Magnesium is also a peripheral vasodilator and an inhibitor of platelet function.
Indications: Torsades de pointes, cardiac arrhythmias associated with hypomagnesemia, eclampsia and seizure prophylaxis in preeclampsia, status asthmaticus.

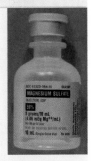

Adverse Effects: Magnesium toxicity (signs include flushing, diaphoresis, hypotension, muscle paralysis, weakness, hypothermia, and cardiac, CNS, or respiratory depression).
Contraindications: AV block, GI obstruction. Use with caution in renal impairment.
Dosage:
Pulseless Ventricular Fibrillation/Ventricular Tachycardia with Torsades de Pointes or Hypomagnesemia:
- **Adult:** 1 to 2 g in 10 mL D₅W IV, IO administered over 5 to 10 minutes.
- **Pediatric:** 25 to 50 mg/kg IV, IO over 10 to 20 minutes; may administer faster for torsades de pointes (max single dose: 2 g).

Torsades de Pointes with a Pulse or Cardiac Arrhythmias with Hypomagnesemia:
- **Adult:** 1 to 2 g in 50 to 100 mL D₅W IV, IO administered over 5 to 60 minutes. Follow with 0.5 to 1 g/hr IV, IO titrated to control torsades de pointes.
- **Pediatric:** 25 to 50 mg/kg IV, IO over 10 to 20 minutes (max single dose: 2 g).

Eclampsia and Seizure Prophylaxis in Preeclampsia:
- **Adult:** 4 to 6 g IV, IO over 20 to 30 minutes, followed by an infusion of 1 to 2 g/hr.

Status Asthmaticus:
- **Adult:** 1.2 to 2 g slow IV, IO (over 20 minutes).
- **Pediatric:** 25 to 50 mg/kg (diluted in D₅W) slow IV, IO (over 10 to 20 minutes).

Special Considerations:
Pregnancy class A

MANNITOL (OSMITROL)

Classification: Osmotic diuretic
Action: Facilitates the flow of fluid out of tissues (including the brain) and into interstitial fluid and blood, thereby dehydrating the brain and reducing swelling. Reabsorption by the kidney is minimal, consequently increasing urine output.
Indications: Increased ICP.
Adverse Effects: Pulmonary edema, headache, blurred vision, dizziness, seizures, hypovolemia, nausea/vomiting, diarrhea, electrolyte imbalances, hypotension, hypertension, sinus tachycardia, PVCs, angina, phlebitis.
Contraindications: Active intracranial bleeding, CHF, pulmonary edema, severe dehydration. Use with caution in hypovolemia, renal failure.
Dosage:
· **Adult:** 0.5 to 2 g/kg IV, IO followed by 0.25 to 1 g/kg administered every 4 hours.
· **Pediatric:** 0.25 to 1 g/kg IV, IO followed by 0.25 to 0.5 g/kg every 4 hours.
Special Considerations:
Mannitol should not be given in the same IV, IO line as blood.
Pregnancy class C

MEPERIDINE (DEMEROL)

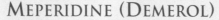

Classification: Narcotic analgesic, Schedule C-II
Action: Binds to opiate receptors, producing analgesia and euphoria.
Indications: Moderate to severe pain.
Adverse Effects: Respiratory depression, nausea/vomiting, sinus bradycardia, sinus tachycardia, palpitations, hypertension, hypotension, orthostatic hypotension, diaphoresis, syncope, shock, cardiac arrest.
Contraindications: Patients who have taken a MAOI in the past 2 weeks, patients who are using other CNS depressants or alcohol, known sensitivity. Use with caution in patients with chronic respiratory conditions (asthma or COPD), pregnant or nursing women, atrial flutter.
Dosage: If given IV, IO, administer slowly.
· **Adult:** 50 to 150 mg IV, IO, IM, or Sub-Q. Elderly: 50 mg IV, IO, IM, or Sub-Q.
· **Pediatric:** 1 to 2 mg/kg IV, IO, IM, or Sub-Q.
Special Considerations:
In adults, half-life approximately 4 hours, but its active metabolites may last 30 hours.
Pregnancy class C; class D near term.

METHYLPREDNISOLONE SODIUM SUCCINATE (SOLU-MEDROL)

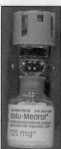

Classification: Corticosteroid
Action: Reduces inflammation by multiple mechanisms.
Indications: Anaphylaxis, asthma, COPD.
Adverse Effects: Depression, euphoria, headache, restlessness, hypertension, bradycardia, nausea/vomiting, swelling, diarrhea, weakness, fluid retention, paresthesias.
Contraindications: Cushing's syndrome, fungal infection, measles, varicella, known sensitivity (including sulfites). Use with caution in active infections, renal disease, penetrating spinal cord injury, hypertension, seizures, CHF.
Dosage:
Asthma and Chronic Obstructive Pulmonary Disease:
· **Adult:** 40 to 80 mg IV.
· **Pediatric:** 1 mg/kg (up to 60 mg) IV, IO per day in two divided doses.

cont'd

METHYLPREDNISOLONE SODIUM SUCCINATE (SOLU-MEDROL)—CONT'D

Anaphylactic Shock:
- **Adult:** 1 to 2 mg/kg/dose, then 0.5 to 1 mg/kg every 6 hours.
- **Pediatric:** Same as adult dosing.

Blunt Spinal Cord Injury:
- **Adult:** 30 mg/kg IV, IO over a period of 1 hour, then as an infusion to run for the remaining 23 hours at a dose of 5.4 mg/kg/hr.
- **Pediatric:** Same as adult dosing.

Special Considerations:
May mask signs and symptoms of infection.
Pregnancy class C

METOPROLOL (LOPRESSOR, TOPROL XL)

Classification: Beta adrenergic antagonist, antianginal, antihypertensive, class II antiarrhythmic

Action: Inhibits the strength of the heart's contractions, as well as heart rate. This results in a decrease in cardiac oxygen consumption. Also saturates the beta receptors and inhibits dilation of bronchial smooth muscle (beta$_2$ receptor).

Indications: ACS, hypertension, SVT, atrial flutter, AF, thyrotoxicosis.

Adverse Effects: Tiredness, dizziness, diarrhea, heart block, bradycardia, bronchospasm, drop in blood pressure.

Contraindications: Cardiogenic shock, AV block, bradycardia, known sensitivity. Use with caution in hypotension, chronic lung disease (asthma and COPD).

Dosage:

Cardiac Indications:
- **Adult:** 5 mg slow IV, IO over a 5-minute period; repeat at 5-minute intervals up to a total of three infusions totaling 15 mg IV, IO.
- **Pediatric:** Not recommended for pediatric patients; no studies available.

Special Considerations:
Blood pressure, heart rate, and ECG should be monitored carefully.
Use with caution in patients with asthma.
Pregnancy class C

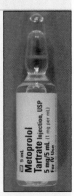

MIDAZOLAM (VERSED)

Classification: Benzodiazepine, Schedule C-IV

Action: Binds to the benzodiazepine receptor and enhances the effects of the brain chemical (neurotransmitter) GABA. Benzodiazepines act at the level of the limbic, thalamic, and hypothalamic regions of the CNS to produce short-acting CNS depression (including sedation, skeletal muscle relaxation, and anticonvulsant activity).

Indications: Sedation, anxiety, skeletal muscle relaxation.

Adverse Effects: Respiratory depression, respiratory arrest, hypotension, nausea/vomiting, headache, hiccups, cardiac arrest.

Contraindications: Acute-angle glaucoma, pregnant women, known sensitivity.

Dosage:

Sedation:
Note: The dose of midazolam needs to be individualized. Every dose should be administered slowly over a period of 2 minutes. Allow 2 minutes to evaluate the clinical effect of the dose given.

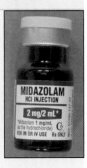

cont'd

MIDAZOLAM (VERSED)—CONT'D

- **Adult:**
  - **Healthy and younger than 60 years:** *Some patients require as little as 1 mg IV, IO. No more than 2.5 mg should be given over a 2-minute interval.* If additional sedation is required, continue to administer small increments over 2-minute periods (max dose: 5 mg). If the patient also has received a narcotic, he or she will typically require 30% less midazolam than the same patient not given the narcotic.
  - **60 years and older and debilitated or chronically ill patients:** This group of patients has a higher risk of hypoventilation, airway obstruction, and apnea. The peak clinical effect can take longer in these patients; therefore dose increments should be smaller, and the rate of injection should be slower. *Some patients require a dose as small as 1 mg IV, IO, and no more than 1.5 mg should be given over a 2-minute period.* If additional sedation is required, additional midazolam should be given at a rate of no more than 1 mg over a 2-minute period (max dose: 3.5 mg). If the patient also has received a narcotic, he or she will typically require 50% less midazolam than the same patient not given the narcotic.
  - **Continuous infusion:** Continuous infusions can be required for prolonged transport of intubated, critically ill, and injured patients. After an initial bolus dose, the adult patient will require a maintenance infusion dose of 0.02 to 0.1 mg/kg/hr (1-7 mg/hr).
- **Pediatric (weight-based):** Pediatric patients typically require higher doses of midazolam than do adults on the basis of weight (in mg/kg). Younger pediatric patients (younger than 6 years) require higher doses (in mg/kg) than older pediatric patients. Midazolam takes approximately 3 minutes to reach peak effect; therefore wait at least 2 minutes to determine effectiveness of drug and need for additional dosing.
  - **12 to 16 years:** Same as adult dosing. Some patients in this age group require a higher dose than that used in adults, but rarely does a patient require more than 10 mg.
  - **6 to 12 years:** 0.025 to 0.05 mg/kg IV, IO up to a total dose of 0.4 mg/kg. Exceeding 10 mg as total dose usually is not necessary.
  - **6 months to 5 years:** 0.05 to 0.1 mg/kg IV, IO up to a total dose of 0.6 mg/kg. Exceeding 6 mg as total dose usually is not necessary.
  - **Younger than 6 months:** Dosing recommendations for this age group is unclear. Because this age group is especially vulnerable to airway obstruction and hypoventilation, use small increments with frequent clinical evaluation. Dose: 0.05 to 0.1 mg/kg IV, IO.

Special Considerations:
Patients receiving midazolam require frequent monitoring of vital signs and pulse oximetry. Be prepared to support patient's airway and ventilation.
Pregnancy class D

MILRINONE (PRIMACOR)

Classification: Inotropic
Action: Milrinone is a positive inotropic drug and vasodilator with minimal chronotropic effect. Milrinone inhibits an enzyme, cAMP phosphodiesterase, which results in an increase in the concentration of calcium inside the cardiac cell. The result is improvement in diastolic function and myocardial contractility.
Indications: Cardiogenic shock, CHF.
Adverse Effects: Cardiac arrhythmias, nausea/vomiting, hypotension.
Contraindications: Valvular heart disease, known sensitivity.
Dosage:

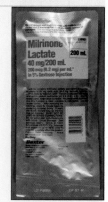

- **Adult:** 50 mcg/kg IV, IO over a period of 10 minutes, followed by an infusion of 0.375 to 0.5 mcg/kg/min (max dose: 0.75 mcg/kg/min).
- **Pediatric:** Same as adult dosing.

Special Considerations:
Pregnancy class C

MORPHINE SULFATE

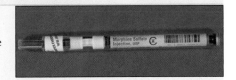

Classification: Opiate agonist, Schedule C-II
Action: Binds with opioid receptors. Morphine is capable of inducing hypotension by depression of the vasomotor centers of the brain, as well as release of the chemical histamine. In the management of angina, morphine reduces stimulation of the sympathic nervous system caused by pain and anxiety. Reduction of sympathetic stimulation reduces heart rate, cardiac work, and myocardial oxygen consumption.
Indications: Moderate to severe pain, including chest pain associated with ACS, CHF, pulmonary edema.
Adverse Effects: Respiratory depression, hypotension, nausea/vomiting, dizziness, lightheadedness, sedation, diaphoresis, euphoria, dysphoria, worsening of bradycardia and heart block in some patients with acute inferior wall MI, seizures, cardiac arrest, anaphylactoid reactions.
Contraindications: Respiratory depression, shock, known sensitivity. Use with caution in hypotension, acute bronchial asthma, respiratory insufficiency, head trauma.
Dosage:
Pain:
- **Adult:** 2.5 to 15 mg IV, IO, IM, or Sub-Q administered slowly over a period of several minutes. The dose is the same whether administered IV, IO, IM, or Sub-Q.
- **Pediatric:**
  - **6 months to 12 years:** 0.05 to 0.2 mg/kg IV, IO, IM, or Sub-Q.
  - **Younger than 6 months:** 0.03 to 0.05 mg/kg IV, IO, IM, or Sub-Q.

Chest Pain Associated with Acute Coronary Syndromes, Congestive Heart Failure, and Pulmonary Edema:
Administer small doses and reevaluate the patient. Large doses may lead to respiratory depression and worsen the patient's hypoxia.
- **Adult:** 2 to 4 mg slow IV, IO over a 1- to 5-minute period with increments of 2 to 8 mg repeated every 5 to 15 minutes until patient relieved of chest pain.
- **Pediatric:** 0.1 to 0.2 mg/kg/dose IV, IO.

Special Considerations:
Monitor vital signs and pulse oximetry closely. Be prepared to support patient's airway and ventilations.
Overdose should be treated with naloxone.
Pregnancy class C

NALBUPHINE (NUBAIN)

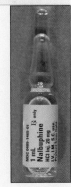

Classification: Synthetic opioid agonist-antagonist
Action: Produces analgesia by binding to the opioid receptor.
Indications: Moderate to severe pain.
Adverse Effects: Drowsiness, diaphoresis, headache, nausea/vomiting, dry mouth, respiratory depression, hypotension, bradycardia.
Contraindications: Known sensitivity.
Dosage:
- **Adult:** 10 mg IV, IO, IM, or Sub-Q.
- **Pediatric:** Not recommended for pediatric patients.
Special Considerations:
Pregnancy class B

NALOXONE (NARCAN)

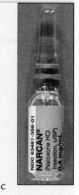

Classification: Opioid antagonist
Action: Binds the opioid receptor and blocks the effect of narcotics.
Indications: Narcotic overdoses, reversal of narcotics used for procedure-related anesthesia.
Adverse Effects: Nausea/vomiting, restlessness, diaphoresis, tachycardia, hypertension, tremulousness, seizures, cardiac arrest, narcotic withdrawal. Patients who have gone from a state of somnolence from a narcotic overdose to wide awake may become combative.
Contraindications: Known sensitivity to naloxone, nalmefene, or naltrexone. Use with caution in patients with supraventricular arrhythmias or other cardiac disease, head trauma, brain tumor.
Dosage:
- **Adult:** 0.4 to 2 mg IV, IO, ET, IM, or Sub-Q. Alternatively, administer 2 mg intranasally. Higher doses (10-20 mg) may be required for overdoses of synthetic narcotics. A repeat dose of one third to two thirds the original dose is often necessary.
- **Pediatric:**
  - **5 years or older or weight >20 kg:** 2 mg IV, IO, ET, IM, or Sub-Q.
  - **Younger than 5 years or weight <20 kg:** 0.1 mg/kg IV, IO, ET, IM, or Sub-Q; may repeat every 2 to 3 minutes.

Special Considerations:
Pregnancy class C

NICARDIPINE (CARDENE)

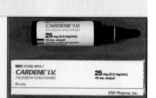

Classification: Calcium channel blocker
Action: Blocks calcium movement into the smooth muscle of the blood vessel walls, causing vasodilation.
Indications: Hypertension
Adverse Effects: Edema, headaches, flushing, sinus tachycardia, hypotension.
Contraindications: Aortic stenosis, hypotension, known sensitivity.
Use with caution in heart failure, cardiac conduction abnormalities, cerebrovascular disease, depressed AV node conduction.
Dosage:
- **Adult:** 5 mg/hr IV, IO; may increase by 2.5 mg/hr every 5 to 15 minutes (max dose: 15 mg/hr). Once the patient has achieved the desired blood pressure, decrease infusion to a maintenance dose of 3 mg/hr.
- **Pediatric:** 0.5 to 1 mcg/kg/min IV, IO infusion.

Special Considerations:
Pregnancy class C

NITROGLYCERIN (NITROLINGUAL, NITROQUICK, NITRO-DUR)

Classification: Antianginal agent

Action: Relaxes vascular smooth muscle, thereby dilating peripheral arteries and veins. This causes pooling of venous blood and decreased venous return to the heart, which decreases preload. Nitroglycerin also reduces left ventricular systolic wall tension, which decreases afterload.

Indications: Angina, ongoing ischemic chest discomfort, hypertension, myocardial ischemia associated with cocaine intoxication.

Adverse Effects: Headache, hypotension, bradycardia, lightheadedness, flushing, cardiovascular collapse, methemoglobinemia.

Contraindications: Hypotension, severe bradycardia or tachycardia, increased ICP, intracranial bleeding, patients taking any medications for erectile dysfunction (such as sildenafil [Viagra], tadalafil [Cialis], or vardenafil [Levitra]), known sensitivity to nitrates. Use with caution in anemia, closed-angle glaucoma, hypotension, postural hypotension, uncorrected hypovolemia.

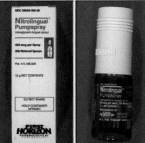
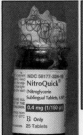
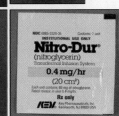

Dosage:
- **Adult:**
  - **Sublingual tablets:** 1 tablet (0.3-0.4 mg) at 5-minute intervals to a maximum of 3 doses.
  - **Translingual spray:** 1 (0.4 mg) spray at 5-minute intervals to a maximum of 3 sprays.
  - **Ointment:** 2% topical (Nitro-Bid ointment): Apply 1 to 2 inches of paste over the chest wall, cover with transparent wrap, and secure with tape.
  - **IV:**
    - **Bolus:** 12.5 to 25 mcg
    - **Infusion:** 5 mcg/min; may increase rate by 5 to 10 mcg/min every 5 to 10 minutes as needed. End points of dose titration for nitroglycerin include a drop in the blood pressure of 10%, relief of chest pain, and return of ST segment to normal on a 12-lead ECG.
  - **Pediatric IV infusion:** The initial pediatric infusion is 0.25 to 0.5 mcg/kg/min IV, IO titrated by 0.5 to 1 mcg/kg/min. Usual required dose is 1 to 3 mcg/kg/min to a maximum dose of 5 mcg/kg/min.

Special Considerations:
Administration of nitroglycerin to a patient with right ventricular MI can result in hypotension.
Pregnancy class C

NITROUS OXIDE

Classification: Inorganic gas, inhaled anesthetic

Action: Exact mechanism is not known.

Indications: Mild to severe pain.

Adverse Effects: Delirium, hypoxia, respiratory depression, nausea/vomiting.

Contraindications: Use with caution in head trauma, increased ICP, pneumothorax, bowel obstruction, patients with COPD who require a hypoxic respiratory drive.

Dosage: Inhaled: 20% to 50% concentration mixed with oxygen.

Special Considerations:
Ensure the safety of healthcare professionals. Use only with a scavenger gas system to ensure that unused gas is collected, or scavenged, and that providers are not exposed to significant levels of the agent.
Pregnancy class not noted

NOREPINEPHRINE (LEVOPHED)

Classification: Adrenergic agonist, inotropic, vasopressor
Action: Norepinephrine is an $alpha_1$, $alpha_2$, and $beta_1$ agonist. Alpha-mediated peripheral vasoconstriction is the predominant clinical result of administration, resulting in increasing blood pressure and coronary blood flow. Beta adrenergic action produces inotropic stimulation of the heart and dilates the coronary arteries.
Indications: Cardiogenic shock, septic shock, severe hypotension.
Adverse Effects: Dizziness, anxiety, cardiac arrhythmias, dyspnea, exacerbation of asthma.
Contraindications: Patients taking MAOIs, known sensitivity. Use with caution in hypovolemia.
Dosage:
- **Adult:** Add 4 mg to 250 mL of D_5W or D_5NS, but not normal saline alone. 0.5 to 1 mcg/min as IV, IO, titrated to maintain systolic blood pressure >80 mm Hg. Refractory shock may require doses as high as 30 mcg/min.
- **Pediatric:** 0.05 to 2 mcg/kg/min IV, IO infusion, to a maximum dose of 2 mcg/kg/min.

Special Considerations:
Do not administer in same IV line as alkaline solutions.
Half-life 1 minute
Pregnancy class C

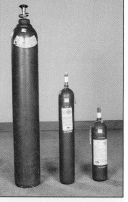

OXYGEN

Classification: Elemental gas
Action: Facilitates cellular energy metabolism.
Indications: Hypoxia, ischemic chest pain, respiratory distress, suspected carbon monoxide poisoning, traumatic injuries, shock.
Adverse Effects: High concentrations can cause decreased level of consciousness and respiratory depression in patients with chronic carbon dioxide retention or chronic lung disease.
Contraindications: Known paraquat poisoning.
Dosage:
Low-Concentration Oxygen:
- A dose of 1 to 4 L/min by a nasal cannula is appropriate.

High-Concentration Oxygen:
- A dose of 10 to 15 L/min via nonrebreather mask is appropriate.

Special Considerations:
Pregnancy class A

PANCURONIUM (PAVULON)

Classification: Nondepolarizing neuromuscular blocker
Action: Antagonizes acetylcholine at the motor end plate, producing skeletal muscle paralysis.
Indications: To induce neuromuscular blockade for the facilitation of ET intubation.
Adverse Effects: Muscle paralysis, apnea, dyspnea, respiratory depression, cutaneous flushing, sinus tachycardia.
Contraindications: Known sensitivity to bromides. Use with caution in heart disease, renal disease.
Dosage:
- **Adult:** 0.04 to 0.1 mg/kg IV, IO; repeat dosing is 0.01 mg/kg every 25 to 60 minutes.
- **Pediatric:** Same as adult dosing.

Special Considerations:
Pregnancy class C

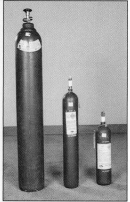

PHENOBARBITAL (LUMINAL)

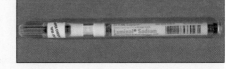

Classification: Anticonvulsant, barbiturate, Schedule C-IV

Action: Depresses seizure activity in the cortex, thalamus, and limbic system; increases threshold for electrical stimulation of motor cortex; produces state of sedation.

Indications: Seizures

Adverse Effects: Depression, agitation, respiratory depression, accelerated metabolism of several other medications.

Contraindications: Liver dysfunction, porphyria, agranulocytosis, known sensitivity to barbiturates. Use with caution with respiratory dysfunction.

Dosage:
- **Adult:** 15 to 18 mg/kg IV, IO; infuse at a rate not faster than 60 mg/min.
- **Pediatric:** 15 to 20 mg/kg IV, IO; infuse at a rate not faster than 2 mg/kg/min.

Special Considerations:
Be prepared to manage the patient's airway.
Pregnancy class D

PHENTOLAMINE (REGITINE)

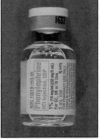

Classification: Alpha antagonist, antihypertensive

Action: Blocks alpha adrenergic receptors, causing vasodilation.

Indications: Hypertensive emergencies and hypertension caused by pheochromocytoma, cocaine-induced vasospasm of the coronary arteries.

Adverse Effects: Sinus tachycardia, angina, dizziness, orthostatic hypotension, prolonged hypotensive episodes, nausea/vomiting, diarrhea, weakness, flushing, nasal congestion.

Contraindications: Known sensitivity. Use with caution in acute MI, angina, coronary insufficiency, evidence suggestive of coronary artery disease, peptic ulcer disease.

Dosage:
Hypertensive Crisis:
- **Adult:** 5 to 15 mg IV, IO or IM.
- **Pediatric:** Not recommended for pediatric patients.

Cocaine-Induced Vasospasm:
- **Adult:** 5 mg IV, IO or IM.
- **Pediatric:** Not recommended for pediatric patients.

Special Considerations:
Pregnancy class C

PHENYLEPHRINE (NEO-SYNEPHRINE)

Classification: Adrenergic agonist

Action: Stimulates the alpha receptors, causing vasoconstriction, which results in increased blood pressure.

Indications: Neurogenic shock, spinal shock, cases of shock in which the patient's heart rate does not need to be increased, drug-induced hypotension.

Adverse Effects: Hypertension, VT, headache, excitability, tremor, MI, exacerbation of asthma, cardiac arrhythmias, reflex bradycardia, soft tissue necrosis.

Contraindications: Acute MI, angina, cardiac arrhythmias, severe hypertension, coronary artery disease, pheochromocytoma, narrow-angle glaucoma, cardiomyopathy, MAOI therapy, known sensitivity to phenylephrine or sulfites.

cont'd

PHENYLEPHRINE (NEO-SYNEPHRINE)—CONT'D

Dosage:
- **Adult:** 100 to 180 mcg/min IV, IO. Once the blood pressure has been stabilized, the dose can be reduced to 40 to 60 mcg/min.
- **Pediatric (2 to 12 years):** 5 to 20 mcg/kg IV, IO followed by 0.1 to 0.5 mcg/kg/min IV, IO (max dose: 3 mcg/kg/min IV, IO).

Special Considerations:
Pregnancy class C

PHENYTOIN (DILANTIN)

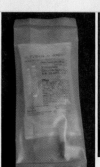

Classification: Anticonvulsant
Action: Depresses seizures by affecting the movement of sodium and calcium into neural tissue.
Indications: Generalized tonic-clonic seizures.
Adverse Effects: Nausea/vomiting, depression of cardiac conduction, sedation, nystagmus, tremors, ataxia, dysarthria, gingival hypertrophy, hirsutism, facial coarsening, hypotension.
Contraindications: Sinus bradycardia, sinoatrial block, second- and third-degree heart block, Adams-Stokes syndrome, known sensitivity to hydantoins.
Dosage:
- **Adult:** 15 to 20 mg/kg IV, IO should be administered slowly at a rate not exceeding 50 mg/min. (This requires approximately 20 minutes in a 70-kg patient.)
- **Pediatric:** 15 to 20 mg/kg IV, IO, administered at a rate of 1 to 3 mg/kg/min.

Special Considerations:
Continuously monitor the ECG and blood pressure during administration.
Pregnancy class D

POTASSIUM CHLORIDE

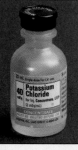

Classification: Electrolyte replacement
Action: Replaces potassium. Slight alterations in extracellular potassium levels can cause serious alterations in both cardiac and nervous function.
Indications: Hypokalemia
Adverse Effects: Hyperkalemia; AV block; cardiac arrest; GI bleeding, obstruction, or perforation; tissue necrosis if the infusion infiltrates into the soft tissues.
Contraindications: Use with caution in patients with cardiac arrhythmias, renal failure, muscle cramps, severe tissue trauma.
Dosage:
- **Adult:** Dosage must be individualized according to patient serum potassium concentration.
- **Pediatric:** Dosage must be individualized according to patient serum potassium concentration.

Special Considerations:
Pregnancy class C

PRALIDOXIME (2-PAM, PROTOPAM)

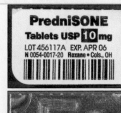

Classification: Cholinergic agonist, antidote
Action: Reactivates cholinesterase.
Indications: Toxicity from nerve agents (organophosphates) having cholinesterase activity.
Adverse Effects: Dizziness, blurred vision, hypertension, diplopia, hyperventilation, laryngospasm, nausea/vomiting, sinus tachycardia.
Contraindications: Myasthenia gravis, renal failure, inability to control the airway.
Dosage:
- **Adult:** 1 to 2 g (dilute in 100 mL normal saline) over a 15- to 30-minute period. If this is not practical or if pulmonary edema is present, the dose should be given slowly (≥5 min) by IV as a 5% solution in water.
- **Autoinjector:** Pralidoxime is also available as an autoinjector that delivers 600 mg IM. Repeat doses can be given every 15 minutes to a total of three doses (1800 mg). Pralidoxime autoinjector is not recommended for pediatric patients.
- **Pediatric:** 20 to 50 mg/kg IV, IO over a 10-minute period.

Special Considerations:
Pregnancy class C

PREDNISONE

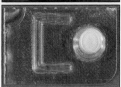

Classification: Corticosteroid
Action: Reduces inflammation
Indications: Inflammatory conditions, such as asthma with bronchospasm.
Adverse Effects: Many adverse effects of steroid use are not related to short-term use but typically are seen with long-term use and during withdrawal.
Contraindications: Cushing's syndrome, fungal infections, measles, varicella, known sensitivity.
Dosage:
- **Adult:** Dosage must be individualized.
- **Pediatric:** Dosage must be individualized.

Special Considerations:
Pregnancy class C

PROCAINAMIDE (PRONESTYL)

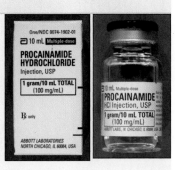

Classification: Antiarrhythmic, class IA
Action: Blocks influx of sodium through membrane pores, consequently suppresses atrial and ventricular arrhythmias by slowing conduction in myocardial tissue.
Indications: Alternative to amiodarone for stable monomorphic VT with normal QT interval and preserved ventricular function, reentry SVT if uncontrolled by adenosine and vagal maneuvers if blood pressure stable, AF with rapid rate in Wolff-Parkinson-White syndrome.
Adverse Effects: Asystole, VF, flushing, hypotension, PR prolongation, QRS widening, QT prolongation.
Contraindications: AV block, QT prolongation, torsades de pointes. Use with caution in hypotension, heart failure.
Dosage:
- **Adult:** 20 mg/min slow IV, IO (max total dose: 17 mg/kg until one of the following occurs: arrhythmia resolves, hypotension, QRS widens by >50% of original width).

cont'd

PROCAINAMIDE (PRONESTYL)—CONT'D

- **Maintenance:** Infusion (after resuscitation from cardiac arrest): mix 1 g in 250 mL solution (4 mg/mL), infuse at 1 to 4 mg/min.
- **Pediatric:** 15 mg/kg slow IV, IO over 30 to 60 minutes.

Special Considerations:
Pregnancy class C

PROMETHAZINE (PHENERGAN)

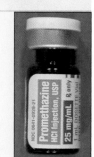

Classification: Antiemetic, antihistamine
Action: Decreases nausea and vomiting by antagonizing H_1 receptors.
Indications: Nausea/vomiting
Adverse Effects: Paradoxic excitation in children and elderly patients.
Contraindications: Altered level of consciousness, jaundice, bone marrow suppression, known sensitivity. Use with caution in seizure disorder.
Dosage:
- **Adult:** 12.5 to 25 mg IV, IO or IM.
- **Pediatric:**
  - **2 years and older:** 0.25 to 1 mg/kg IV, IO, IM (maximum rate of IV, IO administration is 25 mg/min).

Special Considerations:
Pregnancy class C

PROPOFOL (DIPRIVAN)

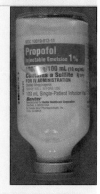

Classification: Anesthetic

Action: Produces rapid and brief state of general anesthesia.

Indications: Anesthesia induction.

Adverse Effects: Apnea, cardiac arrhythmias, asystole, hypotension, hypertension, pain at injection site.

Contraindications: Hypovolemia, known sensitivity (including soybean oil, eggs).

Dosage: A general induction dose used to produce a state of unconsciousness rapidly is 1.5 to 3 mg/kg IV, IO.

Patient Group	Dosage	Rate of Administration (10 mg/mL)
Healthy adults younger than 55 years	2 to 2.5 mg/kg IV, IO	40 mg every 10 seconds
Elderly or debilitated patients	1 to 1.5 mg/kg IV, IO	20 mg every 10 seconds
Cardiac patients	0.5 to 1.5 mg/kg IV, IO	20 mg every 10 seconds
Patients with head injuries	1 to 2 mg/kg IV, IO	20 mg every 10 seconds
Pediatric (3 to 16 years)	2.5 to 3.5 mg/kg IV, IO	20 mg every 10 seconds

After the induction bolus, the patient must be given intermittent boluses or a maintenance infusion. For an average adult, an intermittent dose is 20 to 50 mg as needed. Alternatively, a propofol infusion may be ordered. Maintenance of anesthesia with a propofol infusion can be achieved by following the following protocols:
- **Adult patients:** 25 to 75 mcg/kg/min IV, IO.
- **Elderly, debilitated, or head-injured patients:** Use approximately 80% of the normal adult dose.
- **Pediatric:** 125 to 300 mcg/kg/min IV, IO.

cont'd

PROPOFOL (DIPRIVAN)—CONT'D

Special Considerations:
Propofol should be administered only by personnel trained and equipped to manage the patient's airway and provide mechanical ventilation. In elderly and debilitated patients, avoid rapid administration to prevent hypotension, apnea, airway obstruction, and/or oxygen desaturation. Continue to monitor the patient's oxygenation and vital signs and try to limit use of propofol to patients who are intubated. Propofol should not be administered through the same IV catheter as blood or plasma. Pain can occur at the site of injection, which can be minimized by use of larger veins, slower rates of administration, and administration of 1 mL 1% lidocaine before propofol administration.
Propofol is listed as a pregnancy class B; however, propofol should be avoided in pregnant women because it crosses the placenta and can cause neonatal depression.

PROPRANOLOL (INDERAL)

Classification: Beta adrenergic antagonist, antianginal, antihypertensive, antiarrhythmic class II
Action: Nonselective beta antagonist that binds with both the beta$_1$ and beta$_2$ receptors. Propranolol inhibits the strength of the heart's contractions, as well as heart rate. This results in a decrease in cardiac oxygen consumption.
Indications: Angina; narrow-complex tachycardias that originate from either a *reentry mechanism* (reentry SVT) or an *automatic focus* (junctional, ectopic, or multifocal tachycardia) uncontrolled by vagal maneuvers and adenosine in patients with preserved ventricular function; AF and atrial flutter in patients with preserved ventricular function; hypertension; migraine headaches.
Adverse Effects: Bradycardia, AV block, bronchospasm, hypotension.
Contraindications: Cardiogenic shock, heart failure, AV block, bradycardia, pulmonary edema, sick sinus syndrome, known sensitivity. Use with caution in chronic lung disease (asthma and COPD).
Dosage:
· **Adult:** 1 to 3 mg IV, IO at a rate of 1 mg/min; may repeat the dose 2 minutes later.
· **Pediatric:** 0.01 to 0.1 mg/kg slow IV, IO over a 10-minute period.
Special Considerations:
Monitor blood pressure and heart rate closely during administration.
Pregnancy class C

RACEMIC EPINEPHRINE/RACEPINEPHRINE (MICRONEFRIN, S$_2$)

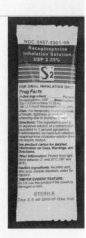

Classification: Bronchodilator, adrenergic agent
Action: Stimulates both alpha and beta receptors, causing vasoconstriction, reduced mucosal edema, and bronchodilation.
Indications: Bronchial asthma, croup.
Adverse Effects: Anxiety, dizziness, headache, tremor, palpitations, tachycardia, cardiac arrhythmias, hypertension, nausea/vomiting.
Contraindications: Glaucoma, elderly, cardiac disease, hypertension, thyroid disease, diabetes, known sensitivity to sulfites.
Dosage:
· **Adult:** Add 0.5 mL to nebulizer; for hand-bulb nebulizer, administer 1 to 3 inhalations; for jet nebulizer, add 3 mL of diluent, swirl the nebulizer and administer for 15 minutes.
· **Pediatric:**
· **Older than 4 years:** Same as adult dosing.
· **Younger than 4 years:** Safe and effective use has not been demonstrated.
Special Considerations:
Monitor blood pressure, heart rate, and cardiac rhythm for changes.
Onset of action is 1 to 5 minutes.
Pregnancy class C

ROCURONIUM (ZEMURON)

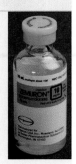

Classification: Neuromuscular blocker, nondepolarizing
Action: Antagonizes acetylcholine at the motor end plate, producing skeletal muscle paralysis.
Indications: To induce neuromuscular blockade for the facilitation of ET intubation.
Adverse Effects: Muscle paralysis, apnea, dyspnea, respiratory depression, sinus tachycardia, urticaria.
Contraindications: Known sensitivity to bromides. Use with caution in heart disease, liver disease.
Dosage:
- **Adult:** 0.6 to 1.2 mg/kg IV, IO.
- **Pediatric (older than 3 months):** 0.6 mg/kg IV, IO.

Special Considerations:
Onset of action is 2 to 8 minutes.
Duration of action is 31 minutes.
Pregnancy class B

SCOPOLAMINE (TRANSDERM SCOP)

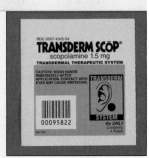

Classification: Neurologic antivertigo, antimuscarinic
Action: Antagonizes acetylcholine at muscarinic receptors.
Indications: Motion sickness
Adverse Effects: Dry mouth, drowsiness, dilated pupils and blurred vision, hallucinations, confusion.
Contraindications: Glaucoma, cardiac arrhythmias, coronary artery disease, known sensitivity.
Dosage:
- **Adult and children older than 12 years:** 1 disc applied to skin behind ear.

Special Considerations:
Half-life 8 hours
Pregnancy class C

SODIUM BICARBONATE

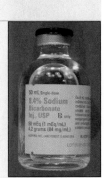

Classification: Electrolyte replacement
Action: Counteracts existing acidosis.
Indications: Acidosis, drug intoxications (e.g., barbiturates, salicylates, methyl alcohol).
Adverse Effects: Metabolic alkalosis, hypernatremia, injection site reaction, sodium and fluid retention, peripheral edema.
Contraindications: Metabolic alkalosis.
Dosage:
Metabolic Acidosis during Cardiac Arrest:
- **Adult:** 1 mEq/kg slow IV, IO; may repeat at 0.5 mEq/kg in 10 minutes.
- **Pediatric:** Same as adult dosing.

Metabolic Acidosis Not Associated with Cardiac Arrest:
- **Adult:** Dosage should be individualized.
- **Pediatric:** Dosage should be individualized.

Special Considerations:
Do not administer into an IV, IO line in which another medication is being given.
Because of the high concentration of sodium within each ampule of sodium bicarbonate, use with caution in patients with CHF and renal disease.
Pregnancy class C

SODIUM NITROPRUSSIDE (NIPRIDE, NITROPRESS)

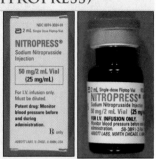

Classification: Antihypertensive agent
Action: Causes direct relaxation of both arteries and veins.
Indications: Hypertensive emergencies.
Adverse Effects: Cyanide or thiocyanate toxicity, nausea/vomiting, dizziness, headache, restlessness, abdominal pain, methemoglobinemia.
Contraindications: Hypotension, increased ICP, cerebrovascular disease, coronary artery disease, hepatic disease, renal disease, pulmonary disease.
Dosage:
  · **Adult:** 0.3 to 10 mcg/kg/min IV, IO. Titrate to desired blood pressure.
  · **Pediatric:** Same as adult dosing.
Special Considerations:
Nitroprusside will break down when exposed to ultraviolet light. Therefore the infusion should be shielded from light by wrapping the bag with aluminum foil.
Pregnancy class C

SUCCINYLCHOLINE (ANECTINE)

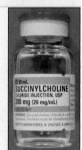

Classification: Neuromuscular blocker, depolarizing
Action: Competes with the acetylcholine receptor of the motor end plate on the muscle cell, resulting in muscle paralysis.
Indications: To induce neuromuscular blockade for the facilitation of ET intubation.
Adverse Effects: Anaphylactoid reactions, respiratory depression, apnea, bronchospasm, cardiac arrhythmias, malignant hyperthermia, hypertension, hypotension, muscle fasciculation, postprocedure muscle pain, hypersalivation, rash.
Contraindications: Malignant hyperthermia, burns, trauma. Use with caution in children, cardiac disease, hepatic disease, renal disease, peptic ulcer disease, cholinesterase-inhibitor toxicity, pseudocholinesterase deficiency, digitalis toxicity, glaucoma, hyperkalemia, hypothermia, rhabdomyolysis, myasthenia gravis.
Dosage:
  · **Adult:**
    · **IV:** 0.6 mg/kg IV, IO (range 0.3-1.1 mg/kg).
    · **IM:** 3 to 4 mg/kg (max dose: 150 mg).
  · **Pediatric:**
    · **IV:**
      · **Adolescents and older children:** 1 mg/kg IV, IO.
      · **Small children and infants:** 2 mg/kg IV, IO.
    · **IM:** 3 to 4 mg/kg (max dose: 150 mg).
Special Considerations:
IV administration results in neuromuscular blockade in 0.5 to 1 minute. IM administration results in neuromuscular blockade in 2 to 3 minutes.
IV administration in infants and children can potentially result in profound bradycardia and, in some cases, asystole. The incidence of bradycardia is greater after the second dose. The occurrence of bradycardia can be reduced with the pretreatment of atropine.
Succinylcholine can have a significantly prolonged effect in the setting of poisoning with nerve gas agents and organophosphate pesticides.
Pregnancy class C

TERBUTALINE (BRETHINE)

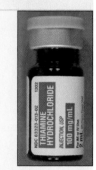

Classification: Adrenergic agonist

Action: Stimulates the beta$_2$ receptor, producing relaxation of bronchial smooth muscle and bronchodilation.

Indications: Prevention and reversal of bronchospasm.

Adverse Effects: Cardiac arrhythmias, arrhythmia exacerbation, angina, anxiety, headache, tremor, palpitations, dizziness.

Contraindications: Known sensitivity to sympathomimetics. Use with caution in hypertension, cardiac disease, cardiac arrhythmias, diabetes, elderly, MAOI therapy, pheochromocytoma, thyrotoxicosis, seizure disorder.

Dosage:
- **Adult:** 0.25 mg Sub-Q every 20 minutes for 3 doses. The usual site for the Sub-Q injection is the lateral deltoid.
- **Pediatric:** 0.01 mg/kg Sub-Q every 20 minutes for 3 doses.

Special Considerations:
Pregnancy class B

THIAMINE (VITAMIN B$_1$)

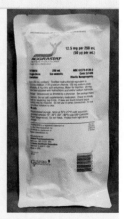

Classification: Vitamin B$_1$

Action: Thiamine combines with adenosine triphosphate to produce thiamine diphosphate, which acts as a coenzyme in carbohydrate metabolism.

Indications: Wernicke-Korsakoff syndrome, beriberi, nutritional supplementation.

Adverse Effects: Itching, rash, pain at injection site.

Contraindications: Known sensitivity.

Dosage:
Wernicke-Korsakoff Syndrome:
- **Adult:** 100 mg IV, IO.
- **Pediatric:** Not recommended for pediatric patients.

Special Considerations:
Pregnancy class A

TIROFIBAN (AGGRASTAT)

Classification: GP IIb/IIIa inhibitor

Action: Prevents the aggregation of platelets by binding to the GP IIb/IIIa receptor.

Indications: UA/NSTEMI—to manage medically and for those undergoing percutaneous coronary intervention.

Adverse Effects: Bleeding from the GI tract, internal bleeding, intracranial hemorrhage, hypotension, stroke, anaphylactic shock.

Contraindications: Bleeding from any source, severe uncontrolled hypertension, surgery or trauma within the previous 6 weeks, stroke within the previous 30 days, renal failure, thrombocytopenia.

Dosage: 0.4 mcg/kg/min IV, IO for 30 minutes, then 0.1 mcg/kg/min IV, IO infusion for 48 to 96 hours.

Special Considerations:
Half-life approximately 2 hours
Pregnancy class B

VALPROIC ACID (DEPAKOTE)

Classification: Anticonvulsant, antimanic
Action: Although the exact mechanism of action is unknown, it is suggested that valproic acid increases brain concentrations of GABA.
Indications: Seizures, mood disorders.
Adverse Effects: Tremor, transient hair loss, weight gain, weight loss.
Contraindications: Liver disease.
Dosage: Dosing is individualized.
Special Considerations:
Although generally well tolerated, valproic acid does require regular monitoring of blood levels to ensure maintenance of therapeutic levels while minimizing adverse drug reactions.
Pregnancy class D

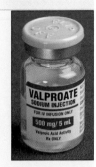

VASOPRESSIN

Classification: Nonadrenergic vasoconstrictor
Action: Vasopressin causes vasoconstriction independent of adrenergic receptors or neural innervation.
Indications: Adult shock-refractory VF or pulseless VT, asystole, PEA, vasodilatory shock.
Adverse Effects: Cardiac ischemia, angina.
Contraindications: Responsive patients with cardiac disease.
Dosage:
  · **Adult:** 40 U IV, IO may replace either the first or second dose of epinephrine.
  · May be given ET but the optimal dose is not known.
Special Considerations:
Pregnancy class C

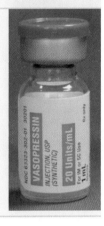

VECURONIUM (NORCURON)

Classification: Neuromuscular blocker, nondepolarizing
Action: Antagonizes acetylcholine at the motor end plate, producing skeletal muscle paralysis.
Indications: To induce neuromuscular blockade for the facilitation of ET intubation.
Adverse Effects: Muscle paralysis, apnea, dyspnea, respiratory depression, sinus tachycardia, urticaria.
Contraindications: Known sensitivity to bromides. Use with caution in heart disease, liver disease.
Dosage:
  · **Adult:** 0.08 to 0.1 mg/kg IV, IO.
  · **Pediatric:** Dosage is individualized.
Special Considerations:
Pregnancy class C

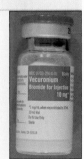

VERAPAMIL (ISOPTIN)

Classification: Calcium channel blocker; class IV antiarrhythmic

Action: Blocks calcium from moving into the heart muscle cell, which prolongs the conduction of electrical impulses through the AV node. Also dilates arteries.

Indications: Atrial fibrillation, hypertension, PSVT, PSVT prophylaxis.

Adverse Effects: Sinus bradycardia; first-, second-, or third-degree AV block; congestive heart failure; reflex sinus tachycardia; transient asystole; AV block; hypotension.

Contraindications: Second- or third- degree AV block (except in patients with a functioning artificial pacemaker); hypotension (systolic pressure <90 mm Hg) or cardiogenic shock; sick sinus syndrome (except in patients with a functioning artificial pacemaker); Wolff-Parkinson-White syndrome; Lown-Ganong-Levine syndrome; severe left ventricular dysfunction; known sensitivity to verapamil or any component of the formulation; atrial flutter or fibrillation and an accessory bypass tract (WPW, Lown-Ganong-Levine syndrome); in infants <1 yr.

Dosage:
- **Adult:** 2.5 to 5 mg IV, IO over 2 minutes (3 minutes in elderly patients). May repeat at 5 to 10 mg every 15 to 30 minutes to a maximum dose of 30 mg.
- **Pediatric:**
  - **Children 1 to 16 years:** 0.1 mg/kg IV, IO (maximum 5 mg/dose) over 2 minutes. May repeat in 30 minutes to a maximum dose of 10 mg.
  - **Infants <1 year:** Not recommended.

Special Considerations:

Pregnancy class C

Commonly Prescribed and Over-the-Counter Medications

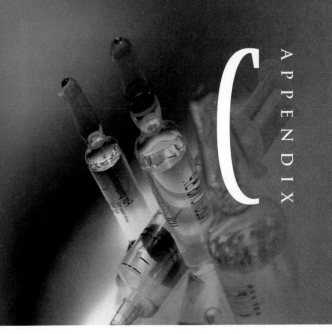

Generic Name	Trade Names	Classifications	Indications
acetaminophen	Tylenol	Analgesic/antipyretic	Pain, fever
acyclovir	Acyclo-V, Zovirax, others	Antiviral	Herpes
adapalene	Differin	Dermatologic	Acne
albuterol	Proventil, Proventil HFA, Ventolin, others	Bronchodilator/adrenergic agonist	Asthma, bronchospasm
alendronate	Fosamax, others	Bisphosphonate	Osteoporosis, Paget disease
allopurinol	Zyloprim	Antigout	Gout
alprazolam	Xanax, others	Anxiolytic/benzodiazepine/ sedative-hypnotic	Anxiety, panic disorder
amitriptyline HCl	Elavil, others	Tricyclic antidepressant	Depression
amlodipine besylate	Norvasc	Calcium channel blocker	Angina, hypertension
amlodipine besylate/ benazepril HCl	Lotrel	ACE inhibitor/calcium channel blocker	Hypertension
amoxicillin	Amoxil, Trimox	Antibiotic, penicillin	Infection
amoxicillin/clavulanate	Augmentin, Augmentin ES-600	Antibiotic, penicillin	Infection
amphetamine mixed salts	Adderall and Adderall XR	Adrenergic agent/amphetamine/ central nervous system stimulant	ADHD, narcolepsy
aspirin	Zorprin, others	Analgesic/antipyretic/ salicylate	Arthritis, pain
atenolol	Tenormin, others	Antiadrenergic/beta blocker	Angina, hypertension, myocardial infarction

Generic Name	Trade Names	Classifications	Indications
atomoxetine	Strattera	Norepinephrine reuptake inhibitor	ADHD
atorvastatin	Lipitor	Antihyperlipidemic	High cholesterol
azelastine	Astelin	Antihistamine	Allergy
azithromycin	Zithromax	Antibiotic	Infection
benazepril HCl	Lotensin	ACE inhibitor	Hypertension
benazepril HCl/ hydrochlorothiazide	Lotensin HCT	ACE inhibitor/diuretic	Hypertension
benzonatate	Tessalon Perles	Antitussive	Cough
benzoyl peroxide/ clindamycin	BenzaClin	Antibiotic/dermatologic	Acne
benztropine mesylate	Cogentin, others	Anticholinergic (antiparkinson)	Parkinson disease, extrapyramidal disorder
bimatoprost	Lumigan	Ophthalmologic	Glaucoma
bisoprolol/HCTZ	Ziac	Beta blocker/diuretic	Hypertension
brimonidine	Alphagan P	Adrenergic agonist; ophthalmologic	Glaucoma
budesonide	Pulmicort, Rhinocort, others	Inhaled corticosteroid	Asthma, Crohn disease, inflammatory bowel disease, rhinitis
budesonide	Rhinocort Aqua	Corticosteroid	Rhinitis
bupropion HCl	Wellbutrin, Zyban	Antidepressant	Depression, smoking cessation
buspirone HCl	BuSpar	Anxiolytic	Anxiety
butalbital/APAP/ caffeine	Fioricet with codeine	Analgesic/barbiturate/xanthine	Pain
calcitonin	Miacalcin	Hormone	High calcium levels, Paget disease
candesartan	Atacand	Angiotensin II receptor antagonist	Hypertension
captopril	Capoten	ACE inhibitor	Congestive heart failure, hypertension, myocardial infarction, diabetic neuropathy
carisoprodol	Soma, others	Skeletal muscle relaxant	Musculoskeletal pain
carvedilol	Coreg	Antiadrenergic/beta blocker	Hypertension, myocardial infarction
cefdinir	Omnicef	Antibiotic/cephalosporin	Infection
cefprozil	Cefzil	Antibiotic	Infection

Generic Name	Trade Names	Classifications	Indications
cefuroxime axetil	Ceftin	Antibiotic	Infection
celecoxib	Celebrex	Analgesic/NSAID	Arthritis
cephalexin	Keflex	Antibiotic/cephalosporin	Infection
cetirizine HCl	Zyrtec	Antihistamine	Allergy
cetirizine/ pseudoephedrine	Zyrtec-D	Antihistamine/ decongestant	Allergy
cimetidine HCl	Tagamet, others	Antihistamine, H_2/gastrointestinal	Gastroesophageal reflux disease, ulcer
ciprofloxacin HCl	Ciloxan, Cipro, others	Antibiotic	Infection (e.g., bone, respiratory, urinary), anthrax
citalopram hydrobromide	Celexa	SSRI antidepressant	Depression
clarithromycin	Biaxin	Antibiotic	Infection
clindamycin HCl	Cleocin	Antibiotic	Infection
clonazepam	Klonopin	Anxiolytic/benzodiazepine	Epilepsy
clonidine HCl	Catapres, Catapres-TTS, others	Antiadrenergic (central)	Pain, hypertension
clopidogrel bisulfate	Plavix	Platelet inhibitor	Myocardial infarction and stroke prevention
clotrimazole	Lotrimin	Antifungal	Fungal infection
clotrimazole/ betamethasone	Lotrisone	Antifungal	Fungal infection
codeine phosphate	Codeine Phosphate	Narcotic analgesic	Pain
conjugated estrogens	Premarin	Hormone (estrogen)	Cancer, menopause
conjugated estrogens/ medroxyprogesterone	Prempro	Hormone	Menopause
cyclobenzaprine HCl	Flexeril	Skeletal muscle relaxant	Muscle spasm
desloratadine	Clarinex	Antihistamine	Allergy
desogestrel/ethinyl estradiol	Apri, Desogen, Kariva, Mircette	Contraceptive	Contraception
dexamethasone/ tobramycin	TobraDex	Antiinfective/corticosteroid; ophthalmologic	Eye injury, infection
diazepam	Valium	Anxiolytic/benzodiazepine/muscle relaxant	Ethyl alcohol withdrawal, epilepsy, muscle spasm

Generic Name	Trade Names	Classifications	Indications
diclofenac	Voltaren	Analgesic/NSAID	Pain, arthritis
digoxin	Digitek, Lanoxin	Antiarrhythmic/cardiac glycoside/ inotropic	Atrial fibrillation, congestive heart failure
diltiazem	Tiazac	Calcium channel blocker	Angina, hypertension, atrial fibrillation or flutter, paroxysmal supraventricular tachycardia
diltiazem HCl	Cardizem, Cardizem CD, Cartia XT, others	Calcium channel blocker	Angina, hypertension, atrial fibrillation or flutter, paroxysmal supraventricular tachycardia
diphenhydramine	Benadryl	Antihistamine	Allergic reaction
divalproex	Depakote	Anticonvulsant	Epilepsy
docetaxel	Taxotere	Antineoplastic	Breast cancer
donepezil HCl	Aricept	Cholinesterase inhibitor	Dementia, Alzheimer's disease
dorzolamide HCl/ timolol maleate	Cosopt	Antiadrenergic/beta blocker/ ophthalmologic	Glaucoma
doxazosin mesylate	Cardura	Alpha$_1$ blocker	Benign prostatic hypertrophy, hypertension
doxepin HCl	Sinequan	Tricyclic antidepressant	Anxiety, depression
doxycycline	Vibramycin, others	Antibiotic/tetracycline	Infection
drosperinone/ethinyl estradiol	Yasmin 28	Contraceptive	Contraception
enalapril maleate	Vasotec	ACE inhibitor	Congestive heart failure, hypertension, left ventricular dysfunction
epoetin alfa	Epogen, Procrit	Hematopoietic/hormone	Anemia
erythromycin	Ilotycin	Antibiotic	Infection
escitalopram	Lexapro	SSRI antidepressant	Depression
esomeprazole	Nexium	Gastrointestinal/PPI	Ulcer, gastroesophageal reflux disease, esophagitis
estradiol	Climara, Estraderm, Vivelle-DOT, others	Estrogen hormone	Menopause, cancer, vaginal atrophy
estradiol/ norethindrone acetate	Activella	Hormone	Menopause

Generic Name	Trade Names	Classifications	Indications
ethinyl estradiol/ norethindrone	Ovcon-35	Contraceptive	Contraception
ethinyl estradiol/ ethynodiol diacetate	Zovia 1/35	Contraceptive	Contraception
ethinyl estradiol/ ferrous fumarate/ norethindrone acetate	Estrostep Fe	Contraceptive/ hormone	Contraception
ethinyl estradiol/ levonorgestrel	Levora, Triphasil, Trivora-28	Contraceptive	Contraception
ethinyl estradiol/ norethindrone	Necon	Contraceptive	Contraception
ethinyl estradiol/ norgestimate	Ortho-Cyclen, Ortho Tri-Cyclen	Contraceptive	Contraception
ethinyl estradiol/ norgestromin	Ortho Evra	Contraceptive	Contraception
famotidine	Pepcid	Antihistamine, H_2 blocker/ gastrointestinal	Adenoma, gastroesophageal reflux disease, ulcer
felodipine	Plendil	Calcium channel blocker	Hypertension
fenofibrate	Lipidil, TriCor	Antihyperlipidemic	High triglyceride level
fentanyl citrate	Duragesic	Narcotic analgesic	Pain
fexofenadine HCl	Allegra	Antihistamine	Rhinitis, seasonal allergy
fexofenadine HCl/ pseudoephedrine HCl	Allegra-D	Antihistamine/decongestant	Rhinitis, seasonal allergy
finasteride	Proscar	Antiandrogen/hormone	Hair loss, benign prostatic hypertrophy
fluconazole	Diflucan	Antifungal	Candidiasis, meningitis, bone marrow transplant adjunct
fluoxetine HCl	Prozac	SSRI antidepressant	Depression, bulimia, obsessive-compulsive disorder
fluticasone propionate	Flonase, Flovent	Inhaled corticosteroid	Allergic rhinitis, dermatosis
fluticasone propionate, salmeterol xinafoate	Advair Diskus	Adrenergic agonist/bronchodilator/ inhaled corticosteroid	Asthma
fluvastatin	Lescol XL	Antihyperlipidemic	High cholesterol
folic acid	Folvite	Hematinic/vitamin	Anemia
fosinopril	Monopril	ACE inhibitor	Hypertension, congestive heart failure

Generic Name	Trade Names	Classifications	Indications
flunisolide inhaled	AeroBid	Inhaled corticosteroid	Asthma prophylaxis
furosemide	Lasix	Loop diuretic	Edema, pulmonary conditions, congestive heart failure, hypertension
gabapentin	Neurontin	Anticonvulsant	Epilepsy
gatifloxacin	Tequin	Antibiotic	Infection
gemfibrozil	Lopid	Antihyperlipidemic	High cholesterol
glimepiride	Amaryl	Antidiabetic agent	Diabetes mellitus
glipizide	Glucotrol, Glucotrol XL	Antidiabetic agent	Diabetes mellitus
glyburide	DiaBeta, others	Antidiabetic agent	Diabetes mellitus
glyburide/metformin	Glucovance	Antidiabetic agent	Diabetes mellitus
human insulin 70/30	Humulin 70/30	Antidiabetic agent/insulin	Diabetes mellitus
human insulin NPH	Humulin N	Antidiabetic agent/insulin	Diabetes mellitus
hydrochlorothiazide	Esidrix	Diuretic	Edema, hypertension
hydrochlorothiazide/ losartan	Hyzaar	Angiotensin II receptor antagonist/ diuretic	Hypertension
hydrocodone/ ibuprofen	Vicoprofen	Narcotic analgesic/NSAID	Pain
hydroxyzine	Atarax	Antiemetic/antihistamine/anxiolytic/ sedative	Ethyl alcohol withdrawal, anxiety, nausea and vomiting
hyoscyamine sulfate	Levsin, others	Anticholinergic/gastrointestinal	Bladder, bowel, pancreatic problems; Parkinson disease
ibuprofen	Advil, Motrin, others	Analgesic/antiinflammatory/antipyretic/ NSAID	Rheumatoid arthritis and osteoarthritis, mild to moderate pain, primary dysmenorrhea, fever, pain
infliximab	Remicade	Antirheumatic/gastrointestinal/ immunomodulator	Rheumatoid arthritis, Crohn disease
insulin glargine	Lantus	Antidiabetic agent/insulin	Diabetes mellitus
insulin lispro	Humalog	Antidiabetic agent/insulin	Diabetes mellitus
ipratropium	Atrovent	Anticholinergic bronchodilator	Bronchospasm associated with chronic obstructive pulmonary disease
ipratropium/albuterol	Combivent	Adrenergic agonist/anticholinergic/ bronchodilator	Bronchitis, chronic obstructive pulmonary disease

Generic Name	Trade Names	Classifications	Indications
irbesartan	Avapro	Angiotensin II receptor antagonist	Hypertension
irbesartan/HCTZ	Avalide	Angiotensin II receptor antagonist/ diuretic	Hypertension
isosorbide mononitrate	Isomer, others	Nitrate/vasodilator	Angina
isotretinoin	Accutane	Acne	Acne
ketoconazole	Nizoral shampoo	Antifungal	Skin infection
lamivudine/zidovudine	Combivir	Antiviral	HIV
lamotrigine	Lamictal	Anticonvulsant	Epilepsy
lansoprazole	Prevacid	Gastrointestinal/PPI	Esophagitis, gastroesophageal reflux disease, ulcer
latanoprost	Xalatan	Ophthalmologic	Glaucoma
leuprolide acetate	Lupron Depot	Antineoplastic/hormone	Cancer, endometriosis
levalbuterol HCl	Xopenex	Adrenergic agonist/ bronchodilator	Asthma
levofloxacin	Levaquin	Antibiotic	Infection
levonorgestrel/ethinyl estradiol	Alesse, Aviane	Contraceptive/ hormone	Contraception
levothyroxine	Levothroid, Levoxyl, Synthroid, others	Hormone (thyroid)	Goiter, hypothyroidism
lisinopril	Prinivil, Zestril, others	ACE inhibitor	Congestive heart failure, hypertension
lisinopril/HCTZ	Zestoretic	ACE inhibitor/diuretic	Congestive heart failure, hypertension
loratadine	Claritin	Antihistamine	Allergy
losartan	Cozaar	Angiotensin II receptor antagonist	Hypertension
lovastatin/niacin	Advicor	Cholesterol lowering	Elevated cholesterol
meclizine	Antivert, others	Antiemetic/antivertigo	Motion sickness, vertigo
medroxyprogesterone acetate	Depo-Provera	Hormone/antineoplastic/ contraceptive	Amenorrhea, cancer, contraception, uterine bleeding
mesalamine	Asacol, Rowasa, others	Gastrointestinal/salicylate	Colitis, proctitis
metaxalone	Skelaxin	Musculoskeletal relaxant	Pain
metformin HCl	Glucophage	Antidiabetic	Diabetes mellitus

Generic Name	Trade Names	Classifications	Indications
methotrexate	Folex, Rheumatrex, others	Antineoplastic/antirheumatic	Arthritis, cancer
methylphenidate XR	Concerta	Central nervous system stimulant	ADHD
methylprednisolone	Medrol	Corticosteroid	Adrenocortical insufficiency, anemia, arthritis, allergy, gastrointestinal conditions, inflammatory conditions
metoclopramide	Reglan	Antiemetic/gastrointestinal stimulant	Gastrointestinal conditions
metolazone	Zaroxolyn	Diuretic	Edema, hypertension
metoprolol succinate	Toprol XL	Antiadrenergic/beta blocker	Angina, hypertension, myocardial infarction, congestive heart failure
metoprolol tartrate	Lopressor	Antiadrenergic/beta blocker	Angina, hypertension, myocardial infarction, congestive heart failure
metronidazole	Flagyl	Antibiotic	Infection
minocycline HCl	Minocin	Antibiotic/tetracycline	Infection
mirtazapine	Remeron, others	Tricyclic antidepressant	Depression
mometasone	Elocon, Nasonex	Inhaled corticosteroid	Dermatosis, rhinitis
montelukast	Singulair	Leukotriene blocker/inhibitor	Asthma
mupirocin	Bactroban	Antiinfective/dermatologic	Skin infection
nabumetone	Relafen	Analgesic/NSAID	Arthritis
naproxen	Naprosyn	Analgesic/NSAID	Arthritis, pain
nefazodone HCl	Serzone	Antidepressant	Depression
niacin	Niaspan	Antihyperlipidemic/vitamin	High cholesterol, high triglyceride level
Nifedipine	Adalat, Nifediac CC, NIFEdipine ER, Procardia XL	Calcium channel blocker	Angina, hypertension
nitrofurantoin	Macrobid	Antibiotic	Urinary tract infection
nitroglycerin	NitroQuick, Transderm, others	Vasodilator	Angina, congestive heart failure, hypertension
norethindrone/ethinyl estradiol	Microgestin Fe, Ortho-Novum, Ortho-Novum 7/7/7, Loestrin Fe 1/20, Lo-Ovral, Low-Ogestrel	Hormone/contraceptive	Contraception
nortriptyline HCl	Pamelor	Tricyclic antidepressant	Depression

Generic Name	Trade Names	Classifications	Indications
ofloxacin	Floxin, Ocuflox	Antibiotic/antifungal	Infection
olanzapine	Zyprexa	Antipsychotic	Schizophrenia, bipolar disorder
olmesartan medoxomil	Benicar	Angiotensin II receptor blocker	Hypertension
olopatadine HCl	Patanol	Antihistamine	Conjunctivitis
omeprazole	Prilosec, others	Gastrointestinal/PPI	Esophagitis, gastroesophageal reflux disease, ulcer
oseltamivir	Tamiflu	Antiviral	Influenza
oxybutynin	Ditropan XL	Anticholinergic	Incontinence, bladder dysfunction
oxycodone HCl	OxyContin	Narcotic analgesic	Pain
oxycodone/ acetaminophen	Percocet, Roxicet, Endocet	Narcotic analgesic	Pain
pantoprazole	Protonix	Gastrointestinal/PPI	gastroesophageal reflux disease
paroxetine HCl	Paxil	SSRI antidepressant	Anxiety, panic disorder, depression, obsessive-compulsive disorder
penicillin VK	Penicillin VK, Veetids	Antibiotic	Infection
phenazopyridine HCl	Pyridium	Analgesic	Dysuria
phenobarbital	Luminal, Phenobarbital, others	Anticonvulsant/barbiturate/sedative	Epilepsy, insomnia
phenytoin	Dilantin	Anticonvulsant	Epilepsy
pimecrolimus	Elidel	Dermatologic	Dermatitis
pioglitazone	Actos	Antidiabetic	Diabetes mellitus
potassium chloride	K-Dur, Klor-Con, Klor-Con M20	Electrolyte	Hypokalemia
pravastatin	Pravachol	Antihyperlipidemic	High cholesterol
prednisone	Deltasone	Corticosteroid	Adrenal insufficiency, inflammatory conditions
progesterone	Prometrium, Progestasert, others	Antiemetic/antihistamine/ phenothiazine	Amenorrhea, uterine bleeding
promethazine HCl	Phenergan, Promethegan, others	Antiemetic/antihistamine/ phenothiazine	Allergy, motion sickness

Generic Name	Trade Names	Classifications	Indications
propoxyphene napsylate	Darvon	Narcotic analgesic	Pain
propranolol	Inderal, Inderal LA, others	Antiadrenergic/beta blocker/ antiarrhythmic	Angina, atrial arrhythmia, migraine, hypertension, myocardial infarction
quetiapine fumarate	Seroquel	Antipsychotic	Schizophrenia
quinapril	Accupril	ACE inhibitor	Congestive heart failure, hypertension
rabeprazole	Aciphex	PPI	Gastroesophageal reflux disease, ulcers
raloxifene HCl	Evista	Hormone (estrogen)	Osteoporosis
ramipril	Altace	ACE inhibitor	Myocardial infarction and stroke prevention, congestive heart failure, hypertension
ranitidine HCl	Zantac	Antihistamine, H_2/gastrointestinal	Esophagitis, gastroesophageal reflux disease, ulcer
risedronate	Actonel	Bisphosphonate	Paget disease
risperidone	Risperdal	Antipsychotic	Psychosis, schizophrenia
rivastigmine tartrate	Exelon	Cholinesterase inhibitor	Dementia, Alzheimer's disease
salmeterol	Serevent	Adrenergic agonist/ bronchodilator	Asthma, bronchospasm
sertraline HCl	Zoloft	SSRI antidepressant	Depression, obsessive-compulsive disorder, panic disorder, premenstrual syndrome, posttraumatic stress disorder
sildenafil citrate	Viagra	Impotence agent	Erectile dysfunction
simvastatin	Zocor	Antihyperlipidemic	Congestive heart failure and myocardial infarction prevention, high cholesterol
spironolactone	Aldactone	Diuretic	Adenoma, edema, hypertension
sulfamethoxazole/ trimethoprim	Bactrim, Cotrim, SMX-TMP, others	Antibiotic/sulfonamide	Infection
sumatriptan	Imitrex	Serotonin receptor agonist	Migraine headache
tadalafil	Cialis	Impotence agent	Erectile dysfunction
tamoxifen citrate	Nolvadex	Antineoplastic/hormone	Breast cancer
tamsulosin	Flomax	Antiadrenergic/alpha blocker	Benign prostatic hypertrophy

Generic Name	Trade Names	Classifications	Indications
temazepam	Restoril	Benzodiazepine/sedative	Insomnia
terazosin HCl	Hytrin	Alpha$_1$ blocker	Benign prostatic hypertrophy
terbinafine HCl	Lamisil Oral	Antifungal	Fungal infection
theophylline	Theophylline SR	Methylxanthine bronchodilator	Asthma, bronchospasm
timolol	Timoptic	Beta blocker, ophthalmologic	Glaucoma
tolterodine tartrate	Detrol, Detrol LA	Anticholinergic/urinary tract relaxant	Incontinence
topiramate	Topamax	Anticonvulsant	Epilepsy
tramadol HCl	Ultram	Narcotic-like analgesic	Pain
tramadol/ acetaminophen	Ultracet	Narcotic-like analgesic	Pain
trandolapril	Mavik	ACE inhibitor	Hypertension, congestive heart failure
trazodone HCl	Desyrel	Antidepressant	Depression
triamcinolone	Aristocort	Corticosteroid	Anemia, inflammatory conditions
triamcinolone acetonide	Nasacort AQ	Corticosteroid	Anemia, inflammatory conditions
triamterene	Dyrenium	Diuretic	Edema, congestive heart failure
valacyclovir	Valtrex	Antiviral	Herpes
valdecoxib	Bextra	Analgesic/NSAID	Arthritis, dysmenorrhea
valsartan	Diovan	Angiotensin II receptor blocker	Hypertension, congestive heart failure
valsartan/HCTZ	Diovan HCT	Angiotensin II antagonist/diuretic	Hypotension, congestive heart failure
vardenafil HCl	Levitra	Impotence agent	Erectile dysfunction
venlafaxine HCl	Effexor, Effexor XR	Antidepressant	Depression, anxiety
verapamil	Calan	Calcium channel blocker	Angina, arrhythmia, hypertension
warfarin	Coumadin	Anticoagulant	Arrhythmia, pulmonary embolism, deep vein thrombosis
zolpidem tartrate	Ambien	Sedative-hypnotic	Insomnia

ACE, Angiotensin-converting enzyme; *ADHD,* attention deficit–hyperactivity disorder; *APAP,* acetaminophen; *HCl,* hydrochloride; *HCTZ,* hydrochlorothiazide; *NSAID,* nonsteroidal antiinflammatory drug; *PPI,* proton pump inhibitor; *SSRI,* selective serotonin reuptake inhibitor.

Common Herbal Supplements

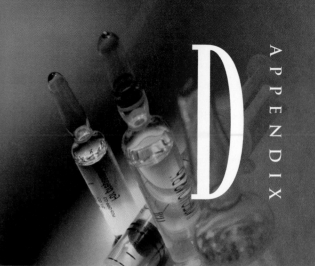

Data from Skidmore-Roth L: *Mosby's handbook of herbs and natural supplements*, ed 3, St Louis, 2006, Mosby.

Herbal Product	Uses	Important Facts
Alfalfa	Digestive disorders, arthritis, to increase blood clotting, as a diuretic, cystitis	Should not be used during pregnancy or in patients with lupus erythematosus; seeds should not be eaten; may increase prothrombin time and prolong bleeding when taken with anticoagulants; may potentiate hypoglycemic action; avoid concurrent use with estrogen and oral contraceptives; may cause hypotension, photosensitivity
Aloe	Minor burns, sunburns, cuts, abrasions, bed sores, diabetic ulcers, acne, stomatitis	Should not be used internally during pregnancy; should not be given to children younger than 12 years; should not be used by persons with kidney disease, cardiac disease, or bowel obstruction; should not be used topically by persons hypersensitive to aloe, garlic, onions, or tulips; may cause gastrointestinal spasms, intestinal mucosa damage, hemorrhagic diarrhea, red-colored urine, nephrotoxicity, contact dermatitis, delayed healing of deep wounds, hypokalemia, uterine contractions causing spontaneous abortion, premature labor; aloe products taken internally may increase the effects of antiarrhythmics, cardiac glycosides, antidiabetics, loop diuretics, potassium-wasting drugs, systemic steroids, and thiazides; if taken internally, avoid concurrent use with licorice, which may cause hypokalemia; aloe may lower serum potassium levels with long-term use
Arginine	Congestive heart failure, erectile dysfunction, peripheral vascular disease, angina, interstitial cystitis, chronic renal failure	Safety in pregnancy and children not established; should not be used by persons with severe hepatic disease; may cause nausea, vomiting, anorexia, increased blood urea nitrogen level, hyperkalemia; angiotensin-converting enzyme inhibitors taken with arginine IV may lead to fatal hypokalemia; concurrent use of alcohol, NSAIDs, platelet inhibitors, and salicylates may cause gastric irritation
Astragalus	Bronchitis, chronic obstructive pulmonary disease, colds, flu, gastrointestinal conditions, weakness, fatigue, chronic hepatitis, ulcers, hypertension, viral myocarditis	Should not be used during pregnancy and lactation; should not be used by persons with acute infections, in the presence of fever, or inflammation; may cause allergic reactions; may decrease or increase action of antihypertensives, avoid concurrent use

Herbal Product	Uses	Important Facts
Belladonna	Irritable bowel syndrome, nervous system disorders, headache, menopausal symptoms, premenstrual syndrome, radiation burns, muscle and bone aches	Should not be used during pregnancy and lactation; should not be used in children; may cause dilated pupils, flushed skin, dry mouth, tachycardia, confusion, nervousness, hallucinations, allergic rashes; should not be used in persons sensitive to anticholinergic drugs or who are allergic to members of the nightshade family such as bell peppers, potatoes, and eggplant; atropine is an ingredient in belladonna, therefore drugs that interact with atropine will interact with belladonna
Betel nut	Central nervous system stimulation, schizophrenia, anemia	Should not be used during pregnancy and lactation; should not be used in children; may cause skin color changes, dilated pupils, blurred vision, difficulty breathing, increased salivation, incontinence, diaphoresis, fever, confusion, psychosis, amnesia, feeling of euphoria; may cause tremors, stiffness in persons also taking antipsychotic medications; chewing betel nuts may cause nausea, vomiting, stomach cramps, diarrhea, chest pain, arrhythmias; do not use concurrently with alcohol, antiglaucoma agents, beta blockers, calcium channel blockers, cardiac glycosides, monoamine oxidase inhibitors, neuroleptics
Bilberry	To improve night vision; prevent cataracts, macular degeneration, and glaucoma; treat varicose veins and hemorrhoids; prevent hemorrhage after surgery; prevent and treat diabetic retinopathy and myopia; decrease diarrhea and dyspepsia; control insulin levels	Safety in pregnancy not established; may cause constipation; use caution if taking concurrently with anticoagulants, antiplatelets, aspirin, insulin, iron (avoid concurrent use), NSAIDs, oral antidiabetics
Black cohosh	Menopausal symptoms, arthritis	Use during pregnancy may cause uterine stimulation; should not be used during lactation; should be given to children only under supervision of a qualified herbalist; should not be used in patients with a history of estrogen receptor–positive breast cancer; may cause hypotension, bradycardia, uterine stimulation, spontaneous abortion, nausea, vomiting, anorexia; avoid concurrent use with antihypertensives, oral contraceptives, sedatives/hypnotics; use cautiously with hormone replacement therapy
Blessed thistle	Anorexia; gastrointestinal discomfort; memory improvement; for liver disorders such as jaundice, hepatitis, and dyspepsia	Should not be used during pregnancy; may cause nausea, vomiting, anorexia, contact dermatitis
Burdock	Arthritis, diabetes, some skin disorders (e.g., psoriasis, eczema, poison ivy)	May cause hypotension, hypoglycemia; use with caution in persons with diabetes or cardiac disorders; avoid concurrent use with antidiabetics, antihypertensives, calcium channel blockers
Chondroitin	Joint conditions (in combination with glucosamine), coronary artery disease, interstitial cystitis, hyperlipidemia	Safety in pregnancy and children not established; should not be used in persons with bleeding disorders or renal failure; may cause headache, restlessness, euphoria, nausea, vomiting, anorexia, bleeding; do not use concurrently with anticoagulants, NSAIDs, or salicylates

Herbal Product	Uses	Important Facts
Coenzyme Q10	Ischemic heart disease, congestive heart failure, angina pectoris, hypertension, arrhythmias, diabetes mellitus, breast cancer, deafness, Bell's palsy, decreased immunity, mitral valve prolapse, periodontal disease, infertility	Should not be used at excessive levels during pregnancy and lactation; safety in children not established; may cause nausea, vomiting, anorexia, diarrhea, epigastric pain; avoid concurrent use with anticoagulants, beta blockers, HMG-CoA reductase inhibitors, oral antidiabetics, phenothiazines, tricyclic antidepressants
Cranberry	Urinary tract disorders, susceptibility to kidney stones	Should not be used by persons with oliguria, anuria; may cause diarrhea (large doses), hypersensitivity reactions
Creatine	Enhanced athletic performance	Safety in pregnancy and children not established; may cause nausea, vomiting, anorexia, bloating, weight gain, diarrhea, dehydration, cramping (high doses)
Dandelion	As a laxative, antihypertensive, diuretic	Should not be used during pregnancy and lactation; safety in children not established; should be used with caution in persons with diabetes mellitus or fluid and electrolyte imbalances; avoid use in persons with irritable bowel syndrome, digestive diseases, bile duct obstruction, intestinal obstruction, latex allergy; may cause nausea, vomiting, anorexia, cholelithiasis, gallbladder inflammation, contact dermatitis; avoid concurrent use with antihypertensives, diuretics, insulin, lithium, oral antidiabetics
Devil's claw	Anorexia, joint pain and inflammation, allergies, headache, heartburn, dysmenorrhea, gastrointestinal upset, malaria, gout, nicotine poisoning	Should not be used during pregnancy and lactation; should not be given to children; avoid use in persons with peptic or duodenal ulcer disease, cholecystitis; may cause nausea, vomiting, anorexia; use cautiously with antiarrhythmics
DHEA	Atherosclerosis, hyperglycemia, cancer, to improve memory and cognitive functioning	Safety in pregnancy and children not established; avoid use in persons with estrogen-sensitive tumors, prostate cancer, or benign prostatic hypertrophy; may cause arrhythmias (high doses), insomnia, restlessness, irritability, anxiety, increased mood, aggressiveness, acne; avoid concurrent use with hormone replacement therapy
Dong quai	Menopausal symptoms, menstrual irregularities (e.g., dysmenorrhea, premenstrual syndrome, menorrhagia), headache, neuralgia, herpes infections, malaria	Safety in pregnancy and children not established; avoid use in persons with bleeding disorders, excessive menstrual flow, or acute illness; may cause nausea, vomiting, diarrhea, anorexia, increased menstrual flow, hypersensitivity reactions, photosensitivity, fever, bleeding; use cautiously with antiplatelets, oral anticoagulants, chamomile, dandelion, horse chestnut, red clover, St. John's Wort
Echinacea	Prevention and treatment of infection (especially a cold or the flu); impaired immune status	Should not be used during pregnancy and lactation; should not be given to children younger than 2 years; avoid use in persons with autoimmune diseases; may cause hepatotoxicity, hypersensitivity reactions, acute asthma attack, angioedema

Herbal Product	Uses	Important Facts
Ephedra	Asthma, bronchitis, headache, pulmonary congestion, joint pain and inflammation, to promote weight loss	**Note: On February 6, 2004, the Food and Drug Administration issued a final rule prohibiting the sale of dietary supplements containing ephedra.** May cause palpitations, tachycardia, hypertension, chest pain, arrhythmias, stroke, myocardial infarction, cardiac arrest, anxiety, nervousness, insomnia, hallucinations, headache, dizziness, poor concentration, tremors, confusion, seizures, psychosis, nausea, vomiting, anorexia, constipation or diarrhea, hepatotoxicity, dysuria, urinary retention, hypersensitivity reactions, exfoliative dermatitis, uterine contractions, dyspnea; should not be used during pregnancy and lactation; should not be given to children; should not be used by persons with hypersensitivity to sympathomimetics, narrow-angle glaucoma, seizure disorders, hyperthyroidism, diabetes mellitus, prostatic hypertrophy, arrhythmias, heart block, hypertension, psychosis, tachycardia, angina pectoris; avoid concurrent use with anesthetics, antidiabetics, beta blockers, monoamine oxidase inhibitors, oxytocics, phenothiazines, sympathomimetics, tricyclics, xanthines
Evening primrose oil	Premenstrual syndrome, hot flashes, inflammatory disorders, migraine headache	May cause uterine contraction in pregnant women; may lower seizure threshold in seizure disorders or individuals taking phenothiazines; do not use concurrently with phenothiazines
Garlic	Improve circulation, lower blood lipid levels, hypertension, inflammatory/menstrual disorders, earaches, diarrhea, cold and flu symptoms	May increase bleeding time; should not be used before or immediately after surgery or with drugs or herbs that affect clotting; should not be used medicinally during pregnancy and lactation, may stimulate labor and cause colic in infants; should not be used by persons with hypothyroidism, stomach inflammation, gastritis; may cause dizziness, headache, irritability, nausea, vomiting, anorexia, hypothyroidism, hypersensitivity reactions, contact dermatitis, diaphoresis, garlic odor, irritation of the oral cavities, decreased red blood cells; do not use concurrently with anticoagulants
Ginger	Nausea, indigestion, sore throat, motion and morning sickness, inflammation, migraine headaches	Safety in pregnancy not established; should not be used by persons with cholelithiasis; may cause nausea, vomiting, anorexia, hypersensitivity reactions; may increase the risk of bleeding when used concurrently with anticoagulants or antiplatelets
Ginkgo	Decrease disturbances of cerebral functioning and peripheral vascular insufficiency in persons with Alzheimer's disease or other types of age-related dementia, as an antioxidant, to improve peripheral artery disease, enhance circulation throughout the body, depressive mood disorders, sexual dysfunction, asthma, glaucoma, menopausal symptoms, multiple sclerosis, headaches, tinnitus, dizziness, arthritis, altitude sickness, intermittent claudication	Safety in pregnancy and children not established; should not be used in persons with coagulation or platelet disorders, hemophilia; may cause transient headache, anxiety, restlessness, nausea, vomiting, anorexia, diarrhea, hypersensitivity reactions, rash; avoid concurrent use with anticonvulsants, anticoagulants, monoamine oxidase inhibitors, platelet inhibitors
Ginseng	Physical/mental exhaustion, stress, viral infection, diabetes, headache	Safety in pregnancy and children not established; should not be used by persons with hypertension, cardiac disorders; may cause decreased diastolic blood pressure, increased QT interval, hypertension, chest pain, palpitations, edema, insomnia, hypertonia, anxiety, insomnia, restlessness (high doses), headache, nausea, vomiting, anorexia, diarrhea (high doses), hypersensitivity reactions, rash; avoid concurrent use with immunosuppressants, insulin, monoamine oxidase inhibitors, oral antidiabetics, stimulants

Herbal Product	Uses	Important Facts
Glucosamine	Joint conditions (in combination with chondroitin)	Should not be used during pregnancy and lactation, should not be given to children; may cause drowsiness, headache, nausea, vomiting, anorexia, constipation or diarrhea, heartburn, epigastric pain, cramps, indigestion, hypersensitivity reactions, rash (rare); may increase the effects of antidiabetics
Goldenseal	Gastritis, gastrointestinal ulceration, peptic ulcer disease, mouth ulcer, bladder infection, sore throat, postpartum hemorrhage, skin disorders (e.g., pruritus, boils, hemorrhoids, anal fissures, eczema), cancer, tuberculosis, may promote wound healing and reduce inflammation	Uterine stimulant—should not be used during pregnancy; safety during lactation and in children not established; should not be used by persons with cardiovascular conditions such as heart block, arrhythmias, hypertension; should not be used locally by persons with purulent ear discharge or by those with ruptured eardrum; may cause bradycardia, asystole, heart block, central nervous system depression, seizures, paralysis (increased doses), paresthesia, dyspnea (prolonged use), restlessness, nervousness, irritability, cardiovascular collapse, coma, death, hallucinations, delirium (prolonged use), nausea, vomiting, anorexia, diarrhea or constipation, abdominal cramping, mouth ulcers, hypersensitivity reactions, rash, contact dermatitis, phototoxicity (topical); do not use concurrently with alcohol, antiarrhythmics, anticoagulants, antihypertensives, azole antifungals, benzodiazepines, beta blockers, calcium channel blockers, cardiac glycosides, central nervous system depressants, statins, vitamin B
Gotu kola	**Internally:** Hypertension, cancer, hepatic disorders, leprosy, varicose veins, chronic interstitial cystitis, cellulite, periodontal disease, to increase fertility **Externally:** To promote wound healing, treat skin disorders (e.g., psoriasis, eczema, keloids)	Safety in pregnancy and children not established; may cause sedation, hypersensitivity reactions (e.g., burning [topical use], contact dermatitis, rash, pruritus), increased blood glucose, increased cholesterol levels; do not use concurrently with antidiabetics, antilipidemics
Grapeseed	Antioxidant, disease prevention, leg cramps, inflammation, vision problems	Safety in pregnancy and children not established; may cause dizziness, nausea, anorexia, hepatotoxicity, rash
Green tea	Used as a general antioxidant, anticancer agent, diuretic, antibacterial, antilipidemic, antiatherosclerotic	Should not be used by persons with kidney inflammation, gastrointestinal ulcers, insomnia, cardiovascular disease, increased intraocular pressure; contains caffeine; may cause hypertension, palpitations, arrhythmia (high doses), anxiety, nervousness, insomnia (high doses), nausea, heartburn, increased stomach acid (high doses), hypersensitivity reactions; antacids may decrease the therapeutic effects of green tea; large amounts may increase the action of xanthines and some bronchodilators; do not use concurrently with monoamine oxidase inhibitors
Hawthorn	Cardiovascular disorders (e.g., hypertension, arrhythmias, arteriosclerosis, congestive heart disease, Buerger disease, stable angina pectoris)	Safety in pregnancy and children not established; may cause hypotension, arrhythmias, fatigue, sedation, nausea, vomiting, anorexia, hypersensitivity reactions; avoid concurrent use with antihypertensives, central nervous system depressants; carefully monitor concurrent use with cardiac glycosides

Herbal Product	Uses	Important Facts
Horse chestnut	Fever, phlebitis, hemorrhoids, prostate enlargement, edema, inflammation, diarrhea, varicose veins	Safety in pregnancy and children not established; may cause nephropathy, nephrotoxicity, hepatotoxicity, severe bleeding, shock, nausea, vomiting, anorexia, pruritus, hypersensitivity, rash, urticaria, muscle spasms; do not use concurrently with anticoagulants, aspirin, and other salicylates; may increase the hypoglycemic effects of diabetic medications
Horsetail	**Internally:** Oral diuretic for treatment of edema, osteoporosis **Externally:** To promote wound healing	Safety in pregnancy and children not established; may cause weakness, dizziness, fever, weight loss, cold feeling in extremities (very large quantities), nausea, vomiting, anorexia, hypersensitivity reactions, thiamine deficiency; avoid use in persons with edema, cardiac disease, kidney disease, nicotine sensitivity; contains nicotine and should not be used for prolonged periods; the active chemicals in this herb are absorbed through the skin and can cause death; avoid concurrent use with cardiac glycosides, cerebral stimulants, diuretics, lithium, xanthines
Kava	Anxiety, depression, insomnia, stress, to promote wound healing	Safety in pregnancy not established; should not be used in children younger than 12 years; should not be used by persons with major depressive disorder or Parkinson disease; most side effects and adverse reactions occur when high doses are taken for a long period; may include pulmonary hypertension, liver damage, increased reflexes, blurred vision, red eyes, nausea, vomiting, anorexia, weight loss, hematuria; decreased platelets, lymphocytes, bilirubin, protein, and albumin; increased red blood cell volume, hypersensitivity reactions, skin yellowing and scaling (high doses), dyspnea; do not use concurrently with antiparkinsonian, benzodiazepines, central nervous system depressants; antipsychotics taken with kava may result in neuroleptic movement disorders; concurrent use with barbiturates may result in increased sedation
Lavender	Anxiety, insomnia	Safety in pregnancy and children not established; may cause central nervous system depression, headache, drowsiness, dizziness, euphoria, nausea, vomiting, increased appetite, constipation, hypersensitivity reactions, contact dermatitis; avoid concurrent use with alcohol, antihistamines, opioids, sedatives/hypnotics
Licorice	Constipation, asthma, malaria, hepatitis, abdominal pain, gastrointestinal disorders, infections, eczema, chronic fatigue syndrome, insomnia	Safety in pregnancy and children not established; should not be used by persons with liver disease, renal disease, hypokalemia, hypertension, arrhythmias, congestive heart failure; may cause cardiac arrest, hypokalemia, hypertension, edema, headache, weakness, nausea, vomiting, anorexia, hypersensitivity reactions; do not use concurrently with antiarrhythmics, antihypertensives, azole antifungals, cardiac glycosides, corticosteroids, diuretics
Lycopene	Cancer prevention	Safety of lycopene supplements in pregnancy and children not established; may cause nausea, anorexia
Marshmallow	Cough, sore throat, gastric disorders (e.g., irritable bowel syndrome, gastritis, constipation), minor skin disorders	Safety in pregnancy and children not established; may cause nausea, vomiting, anorexia, hypersensitivity reactions; may reduce the absorption of oral medications, do not use concurrently
Melatonin	Insomnia, to inhibit cataract formation, increase longevity, treat jet lag, prevent weight loss in cancer patients	Safety in pregnancy and children not established; may cause tachycardia, headache, change in sleep patterns, confusion, hypothermia, sedation; nausea, vomiting, anorexia; hypersensitivity reactions (rash, pruritus); decreased progesterone, estradiol, luteinizing hormone levels; use cautiously with benzodiazepines; avoid concurrent use with cerebral stimulants, DHEA, magnesium, succinylcholine, zinc

Herbal Product	Uses	Important Facts
Milk thistle	Hepatotoxicity caused by poisonous mushrooms, cirrhosis of the liver, chronic candidiasis, hepatitis C, exposure to toxic chemicals, liver transplantation	Safety in pregnancy and children not established; may cause nausea, vomiting, anorexia, diarrhea, menstrual changes, hypersensitivity reactions; should not be used with drugs metabolized by the cytochrome P-450 enzyme
Passion flower	Anxiety, sleep disorders, neuralgia, nervous tachycardia, restlessness, opiate withdrawal	Safety in pregnancy and children not established; may cause central nervous system depression (high doses), severe nausea, vomiting, drowsiness, prolonged QT interval, nonsustained ventricular tachycardia, liver toxicity, hypersensitivity reactions, anorexia; avoid concurrent use with central nervous system depressants and monoamine oxidase inhibitors
Propolis	Inflammation, to promote wound healing	Safety in pregnancy and children not established; may cause nausea, anorexia, oral mucositis, stomatitis, hypersensitivity reactions, dermatitis, eczema
Pycnogenol	Hypoxia in cardiac or cerebral infarction, inflammation, also used as an antioxidant and an antitumor	Safety in pregnancy and children not established; may cause reduced blood platelet aggregation
Pygeum	Urinary tract infections, benign prostatic hypertrophy, to increase prostatic secretions that may cause sterility	Safety in pregnancy and children not established; may cause nausea, vomiting, anorexia, gastrointestinal irritation; avoid concurrent use with anticoagulants, antiplatelets, hormones, immunostimulants, NSAIDs
Saw palmetto	Benign prostatic hypertrophy; urinary problems; chronic and subacute cystitis; to increase breast size, sperm count, and sexual potency	Should not be used during pregnancy; safety during lactation and in children not established; may cause headache, nausea, vomiting, anorexia, constipation or diarrhea, abdominal pain and cramping, dysuria, urine retention, impotence, hypersensitivity reactions, back pain
Slippery elm	Cough, gastrointestinal conditions; topically, for smoothing skin and as a poultice to treat skin inflammation, wounds, burns	May cause spontaneous abortion if used during pregnancy; safety during lactation and in children not established; may cause nausea, vomiting, anorexia
Soy	To lower cholesterol, treat hyperactivity, fever, headache, anorexia, chronic hepatitis, menopausal symptoms, osteoporosis, various cancers	No absolute contraindications are known; may cause hypersensitivity reactions, nausea, bloating, diarrhea, abdominal pain; avoid concurrent use with thyroid agents
Spirulina	Malnutrition, promote weight loss, decrease cholesterol, treat fibromyalgia	Safety in pregnancy and children not established; may cause nausea, vomiting, anorexia, hypersensitivity reactions; avoid concurrent use with thyroid hormones

Herbal Product	Uses	Important Facts
St. John's Wort	Anxiety, depression, sleep disorders, viral infection, hemorrhoids, vitiligo, burns	Safety in pregnancy and children not established; may cause dizziness, insomnia, restlessness, fatigue, constipation, abdominal cramps, photosensitivity, rash, hypersensitivity reactions; avoid concurrent use with angiotensin-converting enzyme inhibitors, loop diuretics, thiazide diuretics, alcohol (inconclusive research), immunosuppressants, monoamine oxidase inhibitors (inconclusive research), NSAIDs, oral contraceptives, selective serotonin reuptake inhibitors, sulfonamides, sulfonylureas, tetracyclines; concurrent use of amphetamines, antidepressants, trazodone may cause serotonin syndrome; taken orally in combination with indinavir may decrease the antiretroviral action of this drug
Valerian root	Anxiety, stress, depression, insomnia	Safety in pregnancy and children not established; may cause insomnia, headache, restlessness, nausea, vomiting, anorexia, hepatotoxicity (overdose), hypersensitivity reactions, vision changes, palpitations; may enhance effects of alcohol or sedating substances; avoid if taking antidepressants, pain medications, tranquilizers, antihistamines, anticholinergic drugs, or kava; may increase effects of anesthetic; avoid before surgery; avoid concurrent use with central nervous system depressants, monoamine oxidase inhibitors, phenytoin, warfarin

NSAIDs, Nonsteroidal antiinflammatory drugs.

Answers to Chapter Review Questions

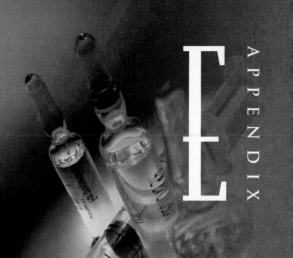

PART I

CHAPTER 1

1. The generic name is usually an abbreviated form of the drug's chemical name. These names often describe the chemical structure or properties of the drug molecule. Generic names are often long and difficult to remember and are registered with the U.S. Food and Drug Administration. Generic drug names are written in lower case. Trade names are names created by the drug companies, often created to help providers remember the action or properties of the drug. Trade names always begin with a capital letter.

2. The properties of medications include mechanism of action, absorption, distribution, metabolism, elimination, and toxicity.

3. Typically, the higher the dosage, the higher the concentration of the medication at the site of action. The greater the amount of drug at the site of action, the greater the physiologic effect. Typically, as the dosage of a medication is increased, the physiologic effect manifested by the drug is increased. This effect continues with increasing doses of the medication up to a point at which increasing the medication no longer produces an increase in the desired physiologic effect.

4. A patient having an asthmatic attack requires a medication that has nearly immediate delivery and action. Once swallowed, the oral medication needs to be absorbed and delivered to the site of action, which may take more than half an hour. Additionally, a patient having difficulty breathing may not be able to swallow an oral medication or any water to help swallow the pill.

5. Medications absorbed through the gastrointestinal tract must first pass through the liver before being distributed throughout the body. While passing through the liver, the drug is often partially metabolized, reducing the amount of medication available for distribution to the body.

6. Factors include age of the patient, route of drug administration, dosage of the medication, genetic predisposition of the patient, diet or starvation, and preexisting disease.

7. Both active transport and carrier-mediated diffusion require a macromolecule to assist in transport. Both processes require specific binding of the drug molecule to the macromolecule, and both are capable of reaching a point of saturation.

8. A half-life is the period of time required to eliminate half of an administered medication from the body.

9. The two factors required to calculate the therapeutic index are the effective dose 50 (ED50) and lethal dose 50 (LD50). The lethal dose is fatal in 50% of the laboratory animals tested. The ED50 produces a therapeutic effect in 50% of the animals tested. Once these two values are determined, the therapeutic index is calculated as LD50/ED50. The closer the therapeutic index is to 1, the more dangerous the drug. In contrast, the closer this number is to 0, the safer the drug.

10. An agonist is a drug that produces the desired physiologic effect upon binding with a drug receptor. Agonists turn things on. In contrast, an antagonist is a drug that either diminishes or eradicates the physiologic effect of the agonist. Antagonists turn things off.

11. A drug interaction occurs when the actions of one drug modify or interfere with the actions of a second drug.

12. The two types of drug interactions alter the plasma level of a medication or alter the effects of a medication.

13. Epinephrine binds to both the alpha and beta receptors. This results in an increase in blood pressure, heart rate, and cardiac contractility. Epinephrine is quite arrhythmogenic; that is, it is prone to causing cardiac arrhythmias.

14. Stimulation of beta$_1$ receptors increases the heart rate (chronotropism) and the force of cardiac contraction (inotropism).

15. Stimulation of beta$_2$ receptors causes relaxation of bronchial smooth muscle.

16. In a dose smaller than recommended, atropine causes a paradoxic slowing of the heart rate.

CHAPTER 2

1. Ordinary negligence is failure to exercise the degree of care that another reasonable person would exercise in the same or a similar situation in which harm to another person results.

2. The basic principle of Good Samaritan laws is to encourage others to assist an ill or injured person to the best of their ability without the fear of a lawsuit for potential mistakes they may make.

3. To prove that a paramedic was negligent after a medication error, it must be proven that the paramedic breached his or her duty to the patient and the paramedic deviated from the standard of care. Under these conditions, proving negligence is difficult.

4. Standing orders and protocols are advance orders from a medical director and are to be followed in the event that certain medical conditions are determined by the paramedic. When protocols and standing orders are used, online medical direction is not necessary. They tend to be rigid and do not allow for unique patient conditions or situations. Standing orders are usually part of a larger treatment protocol.

5. Schedule I drugs are the most dangerous and have the highest abuse potential. Drugs in this class have no recognized medical use and include agents such as heroin, LSD, and methaqualone.

6. Shelf life is the period that a medication may be stored and remain suitable for administration to patients. Drugs that have exceeded the expiration date have expired. Expired medications may not produce the intended beneficial effects when administered to patients.

7. The Ryan White Law provides safeguards for EMS personnel in the event of a needlestick. If a patient tests positive for HIV, EMS personnel will be advised of the necessary precautions and other steps to take.

8. The EMS system medical director ultimately approves which medications will be used by a local EMS system.

9. The paramedic must ensure that the patient is competent to make that refusal. All refusals of care must be carefully documented to prevent the risk of a claim of abandonment or negligence. Failure to assess the patient's ability to give consent properly and improper documentation of a refusal of care are significant areas of liability risk.

10. A partial refusal occurs when a patient agrees to some, but not all, of the treatment offered. If a patient refuses a portion of treatment, such as the administration of a specific medication, the paramedic can still provide other treatment that the patient does consent to receive. A complete refusal occurs in situations in which the patient refuses all aspects of treatment.

11. Minors are usually permitted by most state laws to be able to consent to treatment, but they usually are not considered legally competent to refuse treatment.

12. Under advanced directives, the healthcare provider is allowed to treat the patient with palliative or comfort measures and restrict the use of resuscitative measures such as cardiopulmonary resuscitation, endotracheal intubation, and medication administration.

13. (1) Do not scribble or write illegibly. (2) Do not misspell words or medication names. (3) Do not forget to check the patient's response to the medication. (4) Do not create abbreviations or use inappropriate acronyms in documentation. Use only approved abbreviations. (5) Do not assume that other crew members will take care of your documentation. (6) Do not prepare your report late if you can avoid it.

14. Once an incident report is completed, submit it to your immediate supervisor. In many cases, attaching the incident report to the patient care record is not wise because anything attached to it can become part of the medical record.

CHAPTER 3

1. Standing orders are instructions for treatment that are usually specific to a particular patient presentation and may or may not require consultation with medical control. Standing orders are most appropriate for life-threatening conditions that require immediate intervention.

2. As-needed orders can be obtained from medical control to treat a condition if it develops.

3. The six patient rights of drug administration are right patient, right drug, right dose, right route, right time, and right documentation.

4. Parenteral drug administration is a more effective route for drug administration in the prehospital environment because medications given intravenously produce blood levels that are reliable and almost immediately available. Enteral medications enter the bloodstream by absorption through the gastrointestinal tract.

5. Oral medications have several disadvantages for use in emergencies. A patient with an altered or depressed level of consciousness will not be able to take an oral medication safely. Oral medication must be transported through the gastrointestinal tract and then absorbed into the bloodstream, which delays transport and absorption. Thus a medication that is administered orally is not rapidly available for treatment of a potentially life-threatening condition.

6. A provider should never attempt to recap or bend a needle. Immediately after using a needle or sharp, place it in an approved, puncture-resistant, leak-proof needle box.

7. Some medications used in IM injections are irritating to the soft tissues and can result in permanent staining of the skin. The Z-track technique allows delivery of medications deep into muscle tissue and prevents the medication from leaking into the surrounding soft tissue and skin.

8. Medications that can be delivered by endotracheal tube include lidocaine, epinephrine, atropine, and naloxone. These medications can be remembered by the mnemonic LEAN.

9. When administering a medication by endotracheal tube, the paramedic needs to give 2 to 2.5 times the standard IV dose. In addition to this increased dose, the medication should be diluted in 10 mL of normal saline. This exposes the medication to the large surface area of the lung and facilitates greater absorption.

CHAPTER 4

Answers to Practical Application Problems

1. 10 mL
2. 2 mL
3. 6 mL
4. 3 mL

5. 250 gtt/min
6. 4 gtt/sec
7. 5 mL
8. 2 tablets
9. 50 kg; 200 mcg/min
10. 1600 mcg/mL
11. 7 to 8 gtt/min
12. 1 gtt/7 to 8 sec
13. 4 mcg/mL
14. 30 gtt/min
15. 1 gtt/sec
16. 4 mL
17. 0.5 mL
18. 75 mL
19. 5 mL
20. 2 mL

CHAPTER 5

1. Intracellular fluid is found inside the cells. Intracellular fluid composes two thirds of the total body water.
2. Extracellular fluid is composed of the fluid between the cells (the interstitial fluid) and the fluid inside the blood vessels.
3. Osmosis is the movement of water across a semipermeable membrane.
4. 83 mL
5. 250 mL
6. Crystalloid solutions are IV fluids in which sodium is the primary particle that controls volume distribution. The most common types of crystalloid fluids used by prehospital providers are Ringer's lactate and normal saline. Colloid solutions use complex molecules such as proteins and complex sugars to provide osmotic pressure. Crystalloid solutions use electrolytes for osmotic pressure. Isotonic fluids contain sodium and other electrolyte concentrations that closely mimic the concentration of the extracellular fluid.
7. Hyperkalemia may be caused by kidney failure, burns, crush injuries, diabetic ketoacidosis, and severe infections.
8. A fluid bolus in a pediatric patient is 10 to 20 mL/kg.
9. Drop factor is the number of drops into the chamber required to administer 1 mL.
10. Microdrip chambers have 60 gtt/mL.
11. 60 mL/hr
12. Factors affecting the drip rate include the height of the IV bag, position of the extremity with the IV, caliber of the IV catheter, and coiling of the IV tubing.
13. The size of the IV catheter is the principal determinant of the maximal rate of fluid administration.
14. Infiltration occurs when the tip of the catheter dislodges from the lumen of the vein and the fluid or medication is delivered to soft tissues around the vein.
15. The paramedic should suspect IV infiltration when the IV no longer drips freely and when a patient has pain or swelling at the IV site.
16. The way to prevent catheter shear is to never try to resheath an angiocatheter back over the needle while the needle is still inside the patient.

PART II

CHAPTER 6

1. The American Heart Association has identified the following risk factors for the development of acute myocardial ischemia: cigarette smoking, high blood pressure, high blood cholesterol, lack of exercise, obesity, and heart disease.

2. Stable angina pectoris occurs when the oxygen demands of the heart exceed the body's ability to deliver oxygen to the heart muscle. Providing the patient with oxygen increases oxygen delivery to the heart.

3. Erectile dysfunction. Administration of nitroglycerin to a patient taking a medication for erectile dysfunction, such as sildenafil (Viagra), tadalafil (Cialis), and vardenafil (Levitra), can result in profound hypotension.

4. Morphine helps relieve the pain from myocardial ischemia and causes vasodilation, which increases blood flow to the heart.

5. Beta blockers are widely prescribed to patients with heart disease. Beta blockers decrease the heart rate, which decreases the amount of oxygen consumed by the heart. Also, blood flows through the heart during the diastolic portion of the cardiac cycle; therefore slowing the heart rate increases the blood through the coronary arteries.

6. Contraindications for the use of beta blockers include current cocaine use, signs of heart failure, evidence of low output state, cardiogenic shock or increased risk for cardiogenic shock, PR interval greater than 0.24 second, second- or third-degree heart block, and active asthma or reactive airway disease.

7. Drugs that block or antagonize the glycoprotein IIb/IIIa receptors prevent platelet aggregation and reduce platelet plugs within the coronary arteries.

8. Contraindications to administration of fibrinolytic drugs include age greater than 75 years, ST-segment depression, cardiogenic shock, surgery within the previous 10 days, cerebrovascular disease, gastrointestinal bleeding within the previous 10 days, recent trauma, systolic blood pressure greater than 180 mm Hg or diastolic blood pressure greater than 110 mm Hg, recent trauma, high likelihood of left heart thrombus, acute pericarditis, subacute bacterial endocarditis, severe kidney or liver failure with bleeding complications, diabetic hemorrhagic retinopathy, septic thrombophlebitis, and warfarin (Coumadin) administration.

CHAPTER 7

1. Pain

2. Patients in pain may not be given narcotics because of concerns of respiratory depression and hypotension. Other concerns that prevent narcotic use include the masking of symptoms in patients with head injuries or acute abdominal pain.

3. Morphine can produce hypotension by the release of histamine, which produces vasodilation and subsequently hypotension. This hypotension can be especially profound in patients who are hypovolemic.

4. Fentanyl administration does not release histamine and is less likely to cause hypotension after administration.

5. Administration of narcotics to a patient with abdominal pain can mask the progression of an intraabdominal disease process (e.g., appendicitis), which typically manifests as an increase in the intensity of pain. The patient can subjectively feel better, but in reality the condition is worsening.

6. Ketorolac (Toradol) is a powerful nonsteroidal antiinflammatory analgesic that can be given parenterally.

7. Nitrous oxide is self-administered, and once the patient has received an adequate dose the mask falls away from the patient's face. Nitrous oxide provides mild analgesia while allowing the patient to maintain and protect the airway.

8. Benzodiazepines

9. Antegrade amnesia is the inability to remember events from a point in time forward. Antegrade amnesia is an effect of benzodiazepine administration. Therefore, before an unpleasant procedure or situation, administer a benzodiazepine and the patient will be unable to recall the event.

10. Nausea and vomiting are common adverse effects of narcotic administration.

CHAPTER 8

1. The symptoms of anaphylactic shock are shortness of breath, syncope, itching, swelling of the throat, and a sudden fall in blood pressure.

2. The antigen triggers the body's allergic response. An antigen provokes the body to produce an allergic response, which in turn stimulates cells within the body to release the chemicals histamine, serotonin, bradykinin, and slow-reacting substance of anaphylaxis. These chemicals, when released, cause vasodilation, increased capillary permeability, and smooth muscle spasm.

3. Histamine is the chemical released by the body that is responsible for many of the symptoms associated with anaphylaxis.

4. The most common cause of death in patients with anaphylaxis is airway obstruction.

5. Allergy to shellfish is a common food allergy, and the patient reports a history of such reactions to seafood in the past.

6. Epinephrine is the first-line drug therapy for patients having an anaphylactic reaction. The concentration and dose of epinephrine depend on the route of administration.

7. Epinephrine causes the relaxation of bronchial smooth muscle and constriction of blood vessels.

8. EpiPen and EpiPen Jr.

CHAPTER 9

1. Electrical defibrillation is the single best method of treatment for the patient with VF. The likelihood that a patient will survive an arrest from VF will significantly diminish the longer this rhythm is not converted using electrical therapy. When defibrillation is applied within 1 minute of the development of VF, the survival rate is greater than 70%. This rate of successful defibrillation drops by 10% for each minute defibrillation is delayed.

2. Atropine is used to treat sinus bradycardia because it inhibits the effects of the vagus nerve. The vagus nerve, when stimulated, causes slowing of the heart rate, much like applying the brakes when driving a vehicle. Therefore a drug that inhibits the vagus nerve will increase the heart rate, as if you took your foot off the brake pedal in the vehicle.

3. The half-life of adenosine is 5 to 20 seconds.

4. Class I antiarrhythmics are sodium channel blockers. These agents are further divided into subclasses based on what effect they have on the sodium channel. Class IA agents block the fast sodium channels and depress depolarization. Class IB sodium channel blockers shorten the action potential duration. Class IC sodium channel blockers depress depolarization and conductivity. This subclass is the most potent sodium channel blocker. Class II agents are beta blockers. Class III agents block potassium channels. Class IV agents block calcium channels.

5. Calcium channel blockers are class IV agents. The overall effect is that the rapid electrical impulses traveling down from the atria to the ventricles through the atrioventricular (AV) node are slowed, and the ventricular rate is slowed.

6. Beta blockers exert their pharmacologic effects on both $beta_1$ and $beta_2$ receptors. $Beta_1$ receptors are located in the heart and act as the main mediator of rate and contractility. Beta blockers are negative inotropic drugs that decrease the force and velocity of myocardial contractility, thus lowering blood pressure and oxygen consumption. The negative chronotropic effects of beta blockers result in a lower heart rate, automaticity, and conduction. Thus beta blockers can dramatically decrease cardiac output.

7. The drug of choice for ventricular arrhythmias is amiodarone.

8. Magnesium sulfate should be used for the treatment of torsades de pointes.

9. Pulseless electrical activity is characterized by detectable electrical activity on the monitor but no mechanical cardiac activity as detected by the presence of a pulse or audible heart tones. In asystole, the patient has neither electrical nor mechanical cardiac activity.

CHAPTER 10

1. Heart failure may be the result of ischemic heart disease, diabetes mellitus, hypertension, or disease of the heart valves. The onset of heart failure may be rather acute after a myocardial infarction or may take years to develop in conditions such as valvular heart disease, hypertension, or diabetes mellitus.

2. Diuretics increase urine output and decrease the intravascular volume. Diuretics are commonly used in the treatment of congestive heart failure in patients with pulmonary edema. The decrease in the intravascular volume offloads the weakened and failing heart and reduces the congestion, or the backing up, of fluids in the lung.

3. In the treatment of congestive heart failure, morphine is beneficial by causing venodilation, which reduces patient anxiety and lowers myocardial oxygen demand.

4. Diastole is the portion of the cardiac cycle at which the heart is relaxed and blood is flowing through the coronary arteries. Systole is the portion of the cardiac cycle when the heart squeezes and ejects blood out of the ventricles. During systole, when the heart is contracting, blood cannot flow through the coronary arteries. With an elevated heart rate, the time in systole remains constant, but the diastolic time decreases. Because blood flows through the coronary arteries during diastole, an elevated heart rate causes decrease coronary blood flow and decreased myocardial oxygen delivery. Therefore decreasing heart rate improves oxygen delivery to the diseased heart.

5. Digoxin is used in patients with congestive heart failure to increase myocardial contractility and often to slow the heart rate. Digoxin helps the heart beat stronger and more slowly.

6. Angiotensin-converting enzyme (ACE) inhibitors inhibit the production of the most powerful vasoconstrictor in the body (angiotensinogen). As a result, the patient has a decrease in blood pressure and mild diuresis. ACE inhibitors also reduce cardiac ischemic events, mortality rate, and hospital admissions for individuals with congestive heart failure.

7. After a beta blocker is administered, the blood pressure, heart rate, and ECG should be carefully monitored.

CHAPTER 11

1. Patients with type 1 diabetes do not produce insulin. In type 2 diabetes, patients are capable of making insulin; however, the insulin is not used properly by the body, a condition known as *insulin resistance.* Most people with diabetes have type 2.

2. The use of beta blockers in patients with diabetes can render the patient unaware of low blood sugar and create a condition known as *hypoglycemic unawareness.* Beta blockers mask the common symptoms of hypoglycemia: increased heart rate, hypertension, sweating, and a sense of anxiety.

3. After glucagon is administered, the patient may have nausea and vomiting.

4. Too-aggressive fluid resuscitation can lead to cerebral edema. A patient with diabetic ketoacidosis will be dehydrated; note that the dehydration developed over a protracted period. Therefore do not replace all the patient's fluid losses in the first hour or two of treatment.

5. Diabetic ketoacidosis can be treated by prehospital providers without insulin. Patients with this condition have blood sugar levels that are alarming, but correcting the blood sugar levels too rapidly can be more harmful than no immediate treatment at all. Often the initiation of IV fluids is sufficient initial therapy for treatment of the hyperglycemia and metabolic acidosis until the patient can be treated at the hospital.

6. In times of stress, cortisol prepares the body by increasing the blood pressure, heart rate, and blood sugar level.

7. Patients with thyrotoxicosis commonly have tachycardia, tremor, diaphoresis, weight loss, and intolerance for warm rooms and environments.

CHAPTER 12

1. Specific hypertensive emergencies include hypertensive encephalopathy, hypertensive intracranial hemorrhage, pulmonary edema with hypertension, myocardial ischemia with hypertension, and preeclampsia and eclampsia (hypertension with proteinuria in pregnancy).
2. When treating a patient with a hypertensive emergency, do not reduce the diastolic blood pressure by more than 10% to 15%. Overzealous reduction of blood pressure can result in cerebral ischemia.
3. Contraindications to the use of nitroprusside include coronary ischemia or infarction, pregnancy, and conditions associated with elevated intracranial pressure.
4. Nitroprusside should be protected from light by wrapping the IV bag with aluminum foil. Nitroprusside will break down when exposed to ultraviolet light.
5. Labetalol decreases blood pressure by blocking beta-mediated contraction of vascular smooth muscle.
6. Labetalol should not be used in patients who are hypertensive as a result of cocaine intoxication. A patient whose blood pressure is elevated as a result of cocaine intoxication will have an increase in blood pressure after administration of labetalol.
7. Nitroglycerin is the drug of choice for treating elevated blood pressure in a patient having a myocardial infarction.
8. Magnesium sulfate
9. Administration of hydralazine will cause a drop in blood pressure but a reflexive increase in heart rate.
10. Contraindications to the use of beta blockers include asthma, heart failure, pheochromocytoma, cocaine toxicity, and heart block.

CHAPTER 13

1. Administration of activated charcoal commonly induces vomiting; if aspirated into the lungs, the charcoal can induce a sometimes fatal pneumonitis.
2. Do not give activated charcoal to someone who has overdosed on acetaminophen (Tylenol) because activated charcoal interferes with the absorption of medications that are administered at the hospital to treat the poisoning.
3. If the patient is having wide-complex QRS rhythms, treatment with sodium bicarbonate is appropriate.
4. Too-rapid administration results in hypotension.
5. Glucagon
6. Methamphetamines increase the body's levels of norepinephrine and epinephrine, resulting in tachycardia, hypertension, hyperthermia, agitation, and mydriasis.
7. Neither gastric lavage nor activated charcoal has a role in methamphetamine intoxication because the majority of the drug has been absorbed by the time the patient is seen by a prehospital provider.
8. The initial treatment for cocaine-related agitation is diazepam (Valium).
9. Thiamine, dextrose, and naloxone
10. The most dangerous clinical manifestations of organophosphate poisoning are excessive respiratory secretions (bronchorrhea), bronchospasm, and respiratory insufficiency.
11. Succinylcholine should not be used because it cannot be broken down, resulting in prolonged paralysis of the patient.

CHAPTER 14

1. Increasing the concentration of inspired oxygen increases the content of oxygen in the blood and subsequently the amount of oxygen delivered to the heart and peripheral tissues.
2. Rebreather face masks, or partial rebreathing face masks, have a face mask and a reservoir bag. Oxygen accumulates in the reservoir bag. During inhalation, the

patient inhales the oxygen in the reservoir, as well as some room air through the side ports. When the patient exhales, some of the exhaled breath goes back into the reservoir bag, where it is then rebreathed. Partial rebreather masks are capable of delivering 60% oxygen. Nonrebreather face masks are similar to rebreather masks in appearance and function, with the exception of having one-way exhalation valves on the sides of the mask and on the reservoir bag. The valves on the sides of the mask prevent inhalation of room air during inhalation. The valve on the reservoir prevents any of the exhaled breath from entering the oxygen-rich reservoir. Nonrebreather face masks require a higher flow rate of 12 to 15 L/min and are capable of delivering oxygen concentrations close to 100%.

3. The class of drugs commonly used to treat bronchospasm are beta$_2$-specific agonists. These drugs cause dilation of bronchial smooth muscle by stimulating the beta$_2$ receptor.

4. The two methods of delivering medications directly to the bronchioles are the pneumatically powered nebulizer and metered-dose inhaler.

5. The objective of delivering inhaled medications is to deliver the medications to the lung. Particles that are too large will not make it to their intended site of action, the lung. Particles that are too small will be inhaled and then exhaled without binding to their receptors inside the lung.

6. The purpose of using the spacer is to slow the velocity of the medication particles so that they do not collide with the soft tissues of the oropharynx and the medication particles can reach their intended site in the lung.

7. The principal goal in the management of the asthmatic patient is reversal of the acute bronchospasm.

8. In a drug with a narrow therapeutic index, the margin between the drug being effective and being toxic is quite thin. Therefore, to avoid the complications of toxicity, the paramedic must carefully dose the patient.

9. Patients with a long-standing history of chronic obstructive pulmonary disease require a mild degree of hypoxia to continue breathing. This need for mild hypoxia to continue a respiratory drive is known as *hypoxic respiratory drive*. If the patient is given too much oxygen, the hypoxic respiratory drive is removed, as well as the patient's stimulus for spontaneous respirations.

CHAPTER 15

1. Status epilepticus is defined as continuous seizure activity for more than 30 minutes or a series of seizures without full recovery of consciousness between seizures.

2. Rectal medication administration may be required in a patient who is actively having a seizure and in whom IV access is not obtainable.

3. The most common class of agents used in the initial management of seizure activity, particularly in the prehospital setting, are the benzodiazepines.

4. Acute-angle glaucoma is a contraindication to benzodiazepine administration because the drug relaxes the ciliary muscle of the pupil and can cause an acute increase in intraocular pressure.

5. A prodrug is a medication administered in an inactive form and then converted to the active form after administration. Fosphenytoin (Cerebyx) is an example of a prodrug.

CHAPTER 16

1. The early clinical signs of shock in patients include delayed capillary refill, cold and clammy skin, and an increased respiratory rate.

2. The five types of shock are hypovolemic, cardiogenic, neurogenic, septic, and anaphylactic shock.

3. A common therapy for any patient in shock is expansion of the intravascular volume with IV fluids.

4. An initial therapy for the treatment of hypovolemic shock is to stop the bleeding. This may be difficult for someone in shock from a gastrointestinal bleed. Control

of hemorrhage from traumatic blood loss can be achieved by direct pressure or tourniquets.

5. The preferred IV fluid for use in trauma is normal saline. The principal reason for this choice is that saline is compatible with the administration of blood products in the same IV line.

6. Patients who demonstrate improved perfusion, heart rate, or blood pressure with crystalloid infusion can be categorized as rapid responders, transient responders, or nonresponders. Rapid responders do not need further aggressive resuscitation. They have no ongoing hemorrhage; the source of bleeding has been controlled with pressure or the patient's normal hemostatic mechanisms. Transient responders improve as their intravascular volume is replenished. However, with ongoing manifestations of poor perfusion return, transient responders require blood transfusion and control of hemorrhage. Nonresponders have uncontrolled hemorrhage and require blood transfusion and control of bleeding.

7. Standard blood banking practices involve separating donated whole blood into components. Red blood cells, platelets, and plasma are all separated. In this manner, a single unit of blood can provide therapy for many patients.

8. Rh⁻ patients who receive Rh⁺ blood develop antibodies against the Rh factor in approximately 80% of cases. The seroconversion that occurs can complicate a subsequent pregnancy if the Rh⁻ mother becomes pregnant with an Rh⁺ fetus. The fetus can have chronic hemolytic disease of the newborn.

9. Milrinone, a drug classified as a phosphodiesterase inhibitor, is a good drug to use in a patient in cardiogenic shock but not responding to an adrenergic agonist such as dobutamine. Milrinone works by a different mechanism than dobutamine.

10. Fluid infusion to improve preload is the initial therapy for neurogenic shock. Neurogenic shock mainly involves managing a bigger vascular container, and fluid administration simply refills that vascular container. Fluids, not vasopressors, are the initial treatment for neurogenic shock.

11. In septic shock, the patient has a source of infection that initiates a complex sequence of events in the body known as a *systemic inflammatory response.* The inflammatory reaction produces toxins within the body that result in dilation of the blood vessels. Another effect of the produced toxins is that the blood vessels become "leaky," and the patient can become hypovolemic as he or she loses intravascular fluid to the extravascular space. Therefore these patients have vasodilation such as that seen in neurogenic shock and decreased intravascular volume as seen in hypovolemic shock.

CHAPTER 17

1. Two types of trauma can occur to the brain: primary brain injury occurs directly to the brain from mechanical forces at the time of the initial insult. Secondary brain injury occurs hours after the time of the injury. In a significant number of patients, secondary brain injury leads to delayed death and disability in head-injured patients.

2. Hypotension and hypoxia result in a significant increase in mortality rate from traumatic brain injury. Therefore the paramedic should strive to prevent or treat these conditions rapidly.

3. The treatment of severe traumatic brain injury has two goals: to identify an intracranial injury that may require surgery rapidly and to prevent conditions that result in secondary brain injury (hypoxia and hypotension).

4. Mannitol is an osmotic diuretic that decreases brain swelling by dehydrating the brain.

5. Hypertonic saline must be administered slowly to avoid an increase in the rate of bleeding and an alteration of the ability to clot blood. Too-rapid infusion can result in osmotic demyelination syndrome.

6. Methylprednisolone (Solu-Medrol)

PART III

CHAPTER 18

1. Types of infusion sets include macrodrip infusion sets, microdrip infusion sets, blood tubing sets, volume-control chamber sets, vented and nonvented infusion sets, and multiple-drip infusion sets.

2. The drip rate is 30 gtt/min.

3. Historically in the treatment of HELLP, dexamethasone at a dosage of 10 mg IV every 12 hours has been shown to improve blood pressure, urine output, platelet count, and liver function tests. On the other hand, studies have suggested that high-dose steroids decrease the acuity of the syndrome and concurrently reduce the need for additional treatments.

4. The treatment for magnesium toxicity includes the administration of IV calcium gluconate.

5. Amiodarone prevents the patient from experiencing additional arrhythmias.

6. Blood glucose level should not be decreased at a rate faster than 10% per hour. Dextrose in the form of D_5 should be added to the IV fluids once the blood glucose is less than 250 mg/dL.

7. Cerebral perfusion pressure is calculated from the mean arterial pressure and intracranial pressure. A goal for the cerebral perfusion pressure of 70 mm Hg is needed to ensure adequate cerebral perfusion. Therefore increases in intracranial pressure and decreases in mean arterial pressure can result in an insufficient blood flow to the brain.

8. Fluid replacement is essential in preventing hypovolemia in critically ill burn patients. Major fluid shifts and losses occur during the first 24 hours of a burn injury. Large amounts of fluids leak from the vascular space to the extravascular space. Additionally, with large areas of burned skin, the body also loses large amounts of fluids from evaporation from the burns. Large amounts of crystalloid must be administered to replace the intravascular fluid loss that results from shifts to the interstitial space.

9. The rule of nines divides the patient's body surface area into units that are divisible by nine. This calculation is accurate for use in adult patients but is not adequate for calculating total body surface area of children because of the disproportion of their body surface area.

10. If a transfusion reaction is suspected, stop the transfusion and flush the line with saline.

CHAPTER 19

1. Pregnant women have a delay in gastric emptying that results in a delay from the time a patient takes an oral medication to the time the drug is delivered to the intestine, where oral medications are absorbed. Pregnant women have higher minute ventilation than nonpregnant women, so inhaled medications result in more rapid systemic effects than in nonpregnant women. Pregnancy increases the percentage of body fat, which creates a larger volume of distribution for fat-soluble drugs. Pregnancy also induces a decrease in liver function and an increase in renal function. As a result, the breakdown of a drug by the liver can be slowed, but the excretion of that drug's by-products can be increased by an improvement in kidney function.

2. Teratogenic drugs are medications that result in a characteristic set of malformations in the fetus.

3. Drugs are categorized as A, B, C, D, or X. A is the safest, with B, C, and D progressively more dangerous. Category X drugs are the most dangerous to use in pregnancy and should be avoided. The Pregnancy Safety Category system is limited in its usefulness because most research studies conducted to determine the safety of drugs have used animals.

4. Peanut or soy allergy is a contraindication to ipratropium bromide.

5. When the initial peak expiratory flow rate is less than 50% of predicted, corticosteroids should be administered after ipratropium bromide. Corticosteroids should also be considered when the peak expiratory flow rate does not improve by at least 10% after bronchodilator therapy or is less than 70% after 1 hour of therapy.

6. Chronic hypertension occurs when the pregnant woman has a history of hypertension that precedes the pregnancy. Gestational hypertension is elevated blood pressure that first occurs during pregnancy but does not meet the diagnostic criteria of eclampsia.

7. The threshold for treatment that has been suggested is a diastolic blood pressure greater than 105 mm Hg or a systolic blood pressure in excess of 160 mm Hg.

8. Diabetic ketoacidosis is a state of insulin deficiency that produces a condition of hyperglycemia, dehydration, and metabolic acidosis. Diabetic ketoacidosis in pregnancy can be fatal for the fetus, with fetal mortality rates approaching 50%.

9. A decrease in blood pressure is a late sign of shock in both adults and children. Tachycardia is a more reliable sign than hypotension.

10. Stroke volume is the amount of blood ejected by the heart with each heartbeat. An adult has some variability of stroke volume; however, the stroke volume is held relatively stable in children.

11. Complications of intraosseous infusions include osteomyelitis, cellulitis, infiltration of fluid, anterior compartment syndrome, tibial fractures, and fat embolus.

12. Information on pediatric drug dosing is usually given based on age, weight, or body surface area. In most cases, drugs recommended for pediatric use usually propose a particular dose in milligrams per kilogram or pound. For many drugs, the recommended weight-based dose (or weight-normalized dose) is presented for children of different ages or weight groups. For many drugs, the weight-normalized dose increases as the weight of the child decreases. These changes in weight-based doses are attributable to changes in the child's body composition and metabolism. The percentage of total body water of an infant is approximately 80%, and this proportion decreases to approximately 60% by adulthood. In the first year of life the percentage of fat nearly doubles in infants. Infants have a much smaller percentage of muscle mass than do adults, but they have much larger brains and livers in relation to their total body weight. Infants and children also have large volumes of distribution and rapid metabolic rates. Because of differences in a child's metabolism during the various stages of development, a simple linear reduction of an adult drug dose is not appropriate.

13. Hypoxia

14. Adenosine administration can cause transient atrioventricular block, which can appear to be asystole for the first 10 seconds.

15. Too-aggressive fluid administration in a child with diabetic ketoacidosis can result in cerebral edema.

16. Polypharmacy occurs when an individual patient is taking multiple medications for the treatment of several medical disorders. The danger of polypharmacy is the increased likelihood of an adverse effect or serious drug interaction.

17. With increasing age comes a normal decrease in renal function. By the age of 70 years, a normal individual has 50% of the renal function of a younger adult.

18. The causes of renal failure include trauma, pregnancy, hemorrhage, and complications of drug therapy.

19. Hypertension and diabetes mellitus

20. Medications that have the potential of becoming toxic in kidney disease include digoxin, antibiotics, antihypertensives, and antiarrhythmics.

21. Hemodialysis is the removal of toxic substances from the bloodstream by filtering the patient's blood through a machine and then passing the blood back to the patient.

CHAPTER 20

1. If I give these drugs and if/when this patient stops breathing, will I be able to intubate? If I am unable to intubate the patient, will I be able to ventilate? If I am unable

to either intubate or ventilate this patient, do I have other options? Do I have the right equipment on hand? Is the equipment assembled? Does the patient have any medical problems or conditions for which these drugs and techniques are contra-indicated? If I do not act, will this patient die or have permanent brain damage?

2. Acetylcholine
3. Acetylcholinesterase
4. Depolarizing and nondepolarizing
5. Succinylcholine is able to induce paralysis in approximately 45 seconds.
6. Potassium
7. Patients who should not be given succinylcholine are those with major burns, neuromuscular conditions, myopathic diseases, or hyperkalemia. Succinylcholine should be used with caution in patients with renal failure because these patients often have elevated potassium levels.
8. Malignant hyperthermia is a genetic abnormality in which a patient has exaggerated, sustained muscle contractions in response to certain inhaled general anesthetics and succinylcholine. The increased muscle activity can lead to fatal hyperthermia.
9. To avoid bradycardia after administration of succinylcholine, the paramedic should administer atropine to children younger than 8 years.
10. Vecuronium has no negative effects on cardiovascular function and does not lower blood pressure or raise or lower heart rate. For these reasons it is a safe drug to use in a potentially hypovolemic patient.
11. Flumazenil can completely reverse the effects of midazolam.
12. Etomidate has favorable properties for rapid sequence intubation sedation; it has a rapid onset (30 seconds), short duration of action (3 to 5 minutes), and minimal effects on the heart and blood vessels.
13. (1) Preparations (Time = t − 5 minutes or greater); (2) preoxygenation (Time = t − 5 minutes); (3) pretreatment/priming (Time = t − 3 minutes); (4) paralytic/sedation (Time = t − 1 minute); (5) protection (Time = t − 1 minute); (6) pass the tube (Time = 0); (7) prove it! (Time = t +).

Glossary

5-HT₃ receptor antagonist receptor for the neurotransmitter and peripheral signal mediator serotonin, also known as *5-hydroxytryptamine* or *5-HT*. 5-HT receptors are located on the cell membrane of nerve cells and other cell types, including smooth muscle in animals, and mediate the effects of serotonin as the endogenous ligand and of a broad range of pharmaceutical and hallucinogenic drugs. 5-HT receptors affect the release and activity of other neurotransmitters such as glutamate, dopamine, and GABA. 5-HT₂ₐ receptors increase the activity of glutamate in many areas of the brain, whereas some other serotonin receptors have the effect of suppressing glutamate.

A

A³E³P³ ("A three, E three, P three") refusal guidelines a method of remembering and documenting the critical considerations when a patient refuses treatment. A³E³P³ stands for *a*ssess, *a*dvise, *a*void; *e*nsure, *e*xplain; *p*ersist, *p*rotocols, *p*rotect.

absorption the incorporation of matter by other matter through chemical, molecular, or physical action, such as the dissolving of a gas in a liquid or the taking up of a liquid by a porous solid.

acetylcholine a direct-acting cholinergic neurotransmitter agent widely distributed in body tissues, with a primary function of mediating synaptic activity of the nervous system and skeletal muscles.

acetylcholine receptor a receptor that specifically binds the neurotransmitter acetylcholine and results in contraction of a muscle fiber.

acetylcholinesterase an enzyme present at endings of voluntary nerves, parasympathetic involuntary nerves, and autonomic nerve ganglia. It inactivates and prevents accumulation of the neurotransmitter acetylcholine released during nerve impulse transmission by hydrolyzing the substance to choline and acetate.

activated charcoal a general-purpose emergency antidote and a powerful pharmaceutical adsorbent prescribed in the treatment of acute poisoning.

active transport the movement of materials across the membranes and epithelial layers of a cell by chemical activity that allows the cell to admit otherwise impermeable molecules against a concentration gradient.

acute adrenal insufficiency a life-threatening emergency caused by inadequate amounts of cortisol and stress hormones at times of stress, such as injury and illness.

acute coronary syndrome (ACS) a classification encompassing clinical presentations ranging from unstable angina through myocardial infarction not characterized by alterations in Q waves. The classification sometimes also includes myocardial infarction characterized by altered Q waves.

adrenal medulla the inner portion of the adrenal gland. Adrenal medulla cells secrete epinephrine and norepinephrine when stimulated by the sympathetic division of the autonomic nervous system.

adrenergic agonist medication that acts on the adrenergic receptor to stimulate the sympathetic nervous system.

adrenergic receptor a site in a sympathetic effector cell that reacts to adrenergic stimulation. Two types of adrenergic receptors are recognized: alpha adrenergic, which act in response to sympathomimetic stimuli, and beta adrenergic, which block sympathomimetic activity.

adrenocorticotropin (ACTH) the adrenocorticotropic hormone secreted by the anterior pituitary gland that stimulates secretion of corticosteroid hormones by the adrenal cortex.

advance directive an advance declaration by a person of treatment preferences if he or she is unable to communicate his or her wishes.

adverse effect an undesirable or harmful effect from a medication.

affinity the measure of the binding strength of the antibody-antigen reaction.

agonist a drug that produces a desired physiologic effect on binding with the receptor. Agonists turn things on.

albumin a water-soluble, heat-coagulable protein containing carbon, hydrogen, oxygen, nitrogen, and sulfur.

allergen an environmental substance that can produce a hypersensitive allergic reaction in the body but may not be intrinsically harmful. Common allergens include pollen, animal dander, house dust, feathers, and various foods.

allergic response an exaggerated hypersensitivity reaction to a previously encountered antigen; a potentially life-threatening series of events that affects multiple body systems. Also called an *anaphylactic response*.

alpha₁ receptor receptor in the sympathetic nervous system located on the peripheral blood vessels that, when stimulated with an alpha agonist, typically produces constriction of blood vessels and an increase in blood pressure.

alpha₂ receptor receptor located on nerve endings that provides negative feedback to nerves in the sympathetic nervous system.

alveolus a small outpouching of walls of alveolar space through which gas exchange between alveolar air and pulmonary capillary blood takes place. The term is often used interchangeably with *acinus*.

ampule a small, sterile glass or plastic container that usually contains a single dose of a solution.

analgesic a drug that relieves pain. The opioid analgesics act on the central nervous system and alter the patient's perception; they are more often used for severe pain.

anaphylactic reaction acute allergic response involving immunoglobulin E–mediated, antigen-stimulated mast cell activation resulting in histamine release. Exposure to the antigen may result in dyspnea, airway obstruction, shock, urticaria and, in some cases, death.

anaphylactic shock a severe and sometimes fatal systemic allergic reaction to a sensitizing substance, such as a drug, vaccine, specific food, serum, allergen extract, insect venom, or chemical.

anaphylaxis an exaggerated, life-threatening hypersensitivity reaction to a previously encountered antigen.

anemia a decrease in hemoglobin in the blood to levels below the normal range of 12 to 16 g/dL for women and 13.5 to 18 g/dL for men. Anemia may be caused by a decrease in red cell production, an increase in red cell destruction, or a loss of blood.

angina pectoris a paroxysmal thoracic pain most often caused by myocardial anoxia as a result of atherosclerosis or spasm of the coronary arteries.

angioedema swelling of the mucous membranes of the airway.

angiotensin-converting enzyme (ACE) inhibitor protease inhibitor found in serum that promotes vasodilation by blocking the formation of angiotensin II and slowing the degradation of bradykinin and other kinins. It decreases sodium retention, water retention, blood pressure, and heart size and increases cardiac output.

angiotensin II a potent vasoconstrictor that also acts to stimulate the secretion of antidiuretic hormone.

angiotensinogen a serum glycoprotein produced in the liver that is the precursor of angiotensin.

antagonist a drug that diminishes or eradicates the physiologic effect of an agonist. Antagonists turn things off.

anterograde amnesia the inability to recall events that occur after the onset of amnesia.

antibody an immunoglobulin produced by lymphocytes in response to bacteria, viruses, or other antigenic substances. An antibody is specific to an antigen. Each class of antibody is named for its action.

anticonvulsant a substance or procedure that prevents or reduces the severity of epileptic or other convulsive seizures.

antigen a substance, usually a protein, that the body recognizes as foreign and that can evoke an immune response.

antiplatelet any agent that destroys platelets or inhibits their function.

antisialagogue a substance or medication that reduces or prevents the production of saliva or secretions.

apothecary system an obsolete unit of measure used in pharmaceutical preparations. The basic unit of weight is the grain (gr), and the basic unit of volume is the minim (m).

arrhythmia any deviation from the normal pattern of the heartbeat.

arterial line an arterial blood monitoring system consisting of a catheter inserted into an artery and connected to pressure tubing, a transducer, and a monitor. The device permits continuous direct blood pressure readings, as well as access to the arterial blood supply when samples are needed for analysis.

as-needed order order that applies as necessary for a certain and specified condition; often referred to as a **prn order** (prn is an abbreviation for the Latin phrase *pro re nata,* which means "as the situation demands").

assisted medication administration the act of assisting a patient in self-administering medications previously prescribed by a personal physician for preexisting or chronic medical conditions.

asthma a respiratory disorder characterized by recurring episodes of paroxysmal dyspnea, wheezing on expiration, and/or inspiration caused by constriction of the bronchi, coughing, and viscous mucoid bronchial secretions.

atrial fibrillation (AF) a cardiac arrhythmia characterized by disorganized electrical activity in the atria accompanied by an irregular ventricular response that is usually rapid.

atrial flutter a type of atrial tachycardia characterized by contraction rates between 230 and 380 per minute. Two kinds, typical and atypical, have been identified and are distinguished from each other by their rates and ECG patterns.

atrioventricular (AV) node an area of specialized cardiac muscle that receives the cardiac impulse from the sinoatrial (SA) node and conducts it to the AV bundle and then to the Purkinje fibers and walls of the ventricles. The AV node is located in the septal wall between the left and right atria.

autonomic nervous system the part of the nervous system that regulates involuntary body functions, including the activity of the cardiac muscle, smooth muscles, and glands. It has two divisions, the sympathetic nervous system and the parasympathetic nervous system.

autoresuscitate the shift of fluid from extravascular fluid spaces (intracellular and interstitial spaces) to the intravascular space in an attempt to compensate for a state of hypovolemia.

B

baroreceptor one of the pressure-sensitive nerve endings in the walls of the atria of the heart, the aortic arch, and the carotid sinuses. Baroreceptors stimulate central reflex mechanisms that allow physiologic adjustment and adaptation to changes in blood pressure by changes in heart rate, vasodilation, or vasoconstriction.

barrel the portion of the syringe that contains the medication.

belladonna alkaloids a group of anticholinergic alkaloids occurring in belladonna (*Atropa belladonna*).

benzodiazepine a class of medications that reduces anxiety (anxiolysis), relaxes muscles, and treats seizures. Benzodiazepines induce a state of anterograde amnesia.

beta agonist medication that exerts a positive effect by binding to the beta receptor. Beta agonists increase heart rate, increase the cardiac force of contraction, and produce bronchodilation.

beta blocker a popular term for beta agonist, a medication that binds and blocks the receptor. Beta blockers mediate a negative effect on the beta receptor. Such medications bind the beta receptor and have the potential to decrease heart rate, decrease force of contraction, and even produce bronchospasm.

beta$_1$ receptor a type of beta receptor found on the heart and blood vessels. When stimulated with an agonist, beta$_1$ receptors increase heart rate, increase the force of cardiac contraction, and produce vasodilation.

beta$_2$ receptor a type of beta receptor found on bronchial smooth muscle. When stimulated with an agonist, beta$_2$ receptors produce bronchodilation.

bevel the angled tip of a hypodermic needle.

bioavailability the degree of activity or amount of an administered drug or other substance that becomes available for activity in the target tissue.

biotransformation the chemical changes a substance undergoes in the body, such as by the action of enzymes.

blood tubing set tubing specific for the administration of blood and blood products.

bradykinin a peptide containing nine amino acid residues produced from alpha$_2$-globulin by the enzyme kallikrein. Bradykinin is a potent vasodilator.

breach of duty to act failure to provide a level of care dictated by the local EMS policies or protocols.

bronchodilator a substance, especially a drug, that relaxes contractions of the smooth muscle of the bronchioles to improve ventilation to the lungs. Pharmacologic bronchodilators are prescribed to improve aeration in asthma, bronchiectasis, bronchitis, and emphysema.

bronchospasm an excessive and prolonged contraction of the smooth muscle of the bronchi and bronchioles, resulting in an acute narrowing and obstruction of the respiratory airway.

buccal administration (of medication) oral administration of a drug, usually in the form of a tablet, by placing it between the cheek and the teeth or gum until it dissolves.

buccal area the vestibule of the mouth, specifically the area lying between the teeth and cheeks.

BURP maneuver a mnemonic for a series of manual techniques to improve visualization during endotracheal intubation. BURP stands for *b*ackward-*u*pward (toward the head), *r*ightward (toward the patient's right), and *p*ressure.

butterfly needle a short needle attached to plastic stabilizers at 90 degrees. It is used for IV access of small veins of adults and children. Usual gauge is 22 to 25.

C

calcium channel blocker a drug that inhibits the flow of calcium ions across the membranes of smooth muscle cells. By reduction of the calcium flow, smooth muscle tone is relaxed and the risk of muscle spasms is diminished.

cardiac output (CO) the volume of blood expelled by the ventricles of the heart with each beat (the stroke volume) multiplied by the heart rate.

cardiogenic shock an abnormal condition often characterized by a low cardiac output associated with acute myocardial infarction and congestive heart failure.

cardioselective beta blocker the common name for a beta$_1$ antagonist.

carrier-mediated facilitated diffusion transportation of a drug into a particular cell by using a second molecule to carry the drug molecule.

catheter shear the cutting, separating, and perhaps embolization of an IV catheter by the reinsertion of a needle while the catheter is still in the patient.

causation the existence of a reasonable connection between the misfeasance, malfeasance, or nonfeasance of the defendant and the injury or damage suffered by the plaintiff.

centi combining form meaning "one hundred" or "one hundredth."

central nervous system (CNS) one of the two main divisions of the nervous system, consisting of the brain and the spinal cord.

central venous catheter a catheter that is threaded through the internal jugular, antecubital, or subclavian vein, usually with the tip resting in the superior vena cava or the right atrium of the heart. It is used to administer fluids or medications for hemodynamic monitoring and to measure central venous pressure.

cholinergic agonist a class of drugs that act on the parasympathetic nervous system by binding and stimulating cholinergic receptors.

cholinergic receptor a specialized sensory nerve ending that responds to the stimulation of acetylcholine.

chronic hypertension a long-standing condition of elevated blood pressure.

chronic obstructive pulmonary disease (COPD) a progressive and irreversible condition characterized by diminished inspiratory and expiratory capacity of the lungs.

chronotropic drug a medication that increases heart rate.

chronotropism the act or process of affecting the regularity of a periodic function, especially interference with the rate of heartbeat.

colloid solution a solution in which small particles, such as large polymeric molecules, are homogenously dispersed through a liquid medium.

coma cocktail a combination of medications used to treat a patient with an altered mental status and no history of trauma.

competitive antagonist a substance that interferes with usual metabolic activity by competing for binding sites on a substrate (the substance on which an enzyme acts in a chemical reaction) or on an enzyme that ordinarily attacks the substrate. The antagonist is usually an analog of the substrate.

complete refusal the right of a patient to refuse treatment after the provider has informed the patient of the diagnosis, prognosis, available alternative interventions, risks and benefits of those options, and risks and probable outcomes of no intervention.

congenital adrenal hyperplasia (CAH) a group of disorders that have in common an enzyme defect resulting in low levels of cortisol and increased secretion of adrenocorticotrophic hormone. The net effects are adrenal gland hyperplasia and increased production of cortisol precursors and androgens.

congestive heart failure (CHF) an abnormal condition that reflects impaired cardiac pumping. Its causes include myocardial infarction, ischemic heart disease, and cardiomyopathy.

consent to give approval, assent, or permission.

cortisol a steroid hormone produced naturally by the adrenal gland, identical to chemically synthesized hydrocortisone.

crystalloid a substance in a solution that can diffuse through a semipermeable membrane.

cyclic adenosine monophosphate (cAMP) a cyclic nucleotide formed from adenosine triphosphate by the action of adenylyl cyclase. This cyclic compound, known as the "second messenger," participates in the action of catecholamines, vasopressin, adrenocorticotropic hormone, and many other hormones.

cytochrome P-450 a protein involved with extramitochondrial electron transport in the liver and during drug detoxification.

D

decompensated shock loss of physiologic adaptation to a condition that predisposes and eventually leads to a shock condition characterized by tachycardia, hypotension, and tachypnea.

dehydration excessive loss of water from body tissues. Dehydration is accompanied by a disturbance in the balance of essential electrolytes, particularly sodium, potassium, and chloride. It may follow prolonged fever, diarrhea, vomiting, acidosis, and any condition in which rapid depletion of body fluids occurs.

deltoid muscle a large, thick, triangular muscle that covers the shoulder joint.

depolarization the reduction of a membrane potential caused by the influx of cations, such as sodium and calcium, through ion channels in the membrane.

diabetic ketoacidosis (DKA) diabetic coma, an acute, life-threatening complication of uncontrolled diabetes mellitus. In this condition, urinary loss of water, potassium, ammonium, and sodium results in hypovo-lemia, electrolyte imbalance, extremely high blood glucose levels, and breakdown of free fatty acids, causing acidosis, often with coma.

distribution the location of medications in various organs and tissues after administration.

diuresis increased formation and secretion of urine.

diuretic a drug or other substance that tends to promote the formation and excretion of urine.

dorsogluteal injection injection of a medication into a region of the upper outer quadrant of the buttocks where intramuscular injections can safely be administered.

dosage the regimen governing the size, amount, frequency, and number of doses of a therapeutic agent to be administered to a patient.

dose the amount of a drug or other substance to be administered at one time.

dose-response curve a range of doses over which response occurs. Doses lower than the threshold produce no response, whereas those in excess of the threshold exert no additional response.

dose-response relationship a mathematic relationship between the dose of a drug or radiation and the body's reaction to it.

drip chamber the compartment immediately below the IV bag where the IV fluid drips at a predetermined volume.

drop factor the number of drops into the chamber required to administer 1 mL of fluid.

drug interaction an occurrence in which the effects of one drug are modified by or interfere with the effects of a second drug administered concurrently.

DUMBBELS a mnemonic used to remember the effects of muscarinic receptor blockage. The abbreviation stands for *D*iarrhea, *U*rination, *M*iosis (contraction of pupils), *B*radycardia, *B*ronchospasm and bronchorrhea, *E*mesis, *L*acrimation, *S*alivation, secretion, and sweating.

duration of action the period from which the drug initially exhibits its desired action to the point in time when the effect is no longer perceptible. Duration of action is different than biologic half-life.

duty to act a duty to respond to the patient and provide the level of care that reasonable paramedics are expected to provide.

E

eclampsia the gravest form of pregnancy-induced hypertension. It is characterized by grand mal seizure, coma, hypertension, proteinuria, and edema.

ectopy a condition in which an organ or substance is not in its natural or proper place, such as an ectopic pregnancy that develops outside the uterus or an ectopic heartbeat.

effective dose 50 (ED50) the dose needed to cause the desired response in 50% of the people to whom it is given.

efficacy (of a drug or treatment) the ability of a drug or treatment to produce a specific result, regardless of dosage.

electrical cardioversion the restoration of the heart's normal sinus rhythm through an electrical shock delivered by a defibrillator. Application of the shock is synchronized to the QRS complex.

electrocardiogram (ECG) a graphic record produced by an electrocardiograph, a device for recording electrical conduction through the heart.

emergence phenomena a condition often experienced by patients awakening from ketamine-induced anesthesia; characterized by frightening and vivid nightmares.

endocytosis uptake by a cell of material from the environment by invagination of its plasma membrane, which may be either phagocytosis or pinocytosis.

endotracheal (ET) tube a large-bore catheter inserted through the mouth or nose and into the trachea to a point above the bifurcation of the trachea. It is used for delivering oxygen under pressure when ventilation must be totally controlled and in general anesthetic procedures.

end-stage renal disease (ESRD) a point at which the kidney is so badly damaged or scarred that dialysis or transplantation is required for patient survival.

enteral administration (of medication) the provision of nutrients through the gastrointestinal tract when the patient cannot ingest, chew, or swallow food but can digest and absorb nutrients.

enzyme a complex produced by living cells that catalyzes chemical reactions in organic matter.

epidural hematoma accumulation of blood in the epidural space, caused by damage to and leakage of blood from the middle meningeal artery, producing compression of the dura mater and thus of the brain.

erythropoietin a glycoprotein hormone synthesized mainly in the kidneys and released into the bloodstream in response to anoxia. The hormone acts to stimulate and regulate the production of erythrocytes and thus increases the oxygen-carrying capacity of the blood.

essential hypertension an elevated systemic arterial pressure for which no cause can be found.

excretion the process of eliminating, shedding, or getting rid of substances by body organs or tissues as part of a natural metabolic activity. Excretion usually begins at the cellular level, where water, carbon dioxide, and other waste products of cellular life are emptied into the capillaries.

exponential kinetics of absorption another name for *first-order kinetics of absorption*. A constant fraction of the medication is absorbed into the bloodstream over a defined period.

extracellular fluid (ECF) the portion of the body fluid composing the interstitial fluid and blood plasma.

extrinsic pertaining to anything external or originating outside a structure or organism, including parts of an organ that are not wholly contained within it, such as an extrinsic muscle.

F

fight-or-flight response the reaction of the body to stress in which the sympathetic nervous system and the adrenal medulla act to increase the cardiac output; dilate the pupils of the eyes; increase the rate of the heartbeat; constrict the blood vessels of the skin; increase the levels of glucose and fatty acids in the circulation; and induce an alert, aroused mental state.

first-order kinetics a chemical reaction in which the rate of decrease in the number of molecules of a substrate is proportional to the concentration of substrate molecules remaining.

first-pass metabolism medications absorbed through the gastrointestinal tract pass through the liver and are partially metabolized before distribution to the rest of the body. This metabolism reduces the amount of medication available for distribution.

flow controller a device used to regulate the flow of an IV fluid or medication though IV tubing.

fluid bolus the rapid administration of a volume of IV fluid.

fluid warmer an instrument that warms administered IV fluids or blood to a safe temperature and helps prevent hypothermia.

fraction of inspired oxygen (FiO₂) the proportion of oxygen in the air that is inspired.

G

gamma-aminobutyric acid (GABA) an amino acid that functions as an inhibitory neurotransmitter in the brain and spinal cord. It is also found in the heart, lungs, and kidneys.

gastrointestinal (GI) pertaining to the organs of the gastrointestinal tract, from mouth to anus.

generic name the official established nonproprietary name assigned to a drug.

gestational hypertension elevated blood pressure that first occurs during pregnancy but does not meet the diagnostic criteria of eclampsia.

glucagon a polypeptide hormone, produced by alpha cells in the islets of Langerhans, that stimulates the conversion of glycogen to glucose in the liver.

glucocorticoid an adrenocortical steroid hormone that increases gluconeogenesis, exerts an antiinflammatory effect, and influences many body functions.

glycogen a polysaccharide that is the major carbohydrate stored in animal cells. It is formed from repeating units of glucose and stored chiefly in the liver and, to a lesser extent, in muscle cells.

glycoprotein (GP) any of the large group of conjugated proteins in which the nonprotein substance is a carbohydrate. These include the mucins, the mucoids, and the chondroproteins.

Good Samaritan legislation laws enacted in some states to protect health professionals from liability in rendering emergency medical or dental aid, unless willful wrong or gross negligence is proven.

gram (g) a unit of mass in the metric system equal to 1/1000 kilogram.

gross negligence the commission of an act that a prudent person would not have done or the omission of a duty that a prudent person would have fulfilled, resulting in injury or harm to another person.

H

half-life the time required for a radioactive substance to lose 50% of its activity through decay. Each radionuclide has a unique half-life.

harm to the patient physical or emotional injury that causes damage to the patient as a result of negligence by the provider.

HELLP syndrome mnemonic for a form of severe preeclampsia, a hypertensive complication of late pregnancy. The abbreviation stands for *h*emolysis, *e*levated *l*iver function, and *l*ow *p*latelet level.

hemodialysis a procedure in which impurities or wastes are removed from the blood. It is used in treating patients with renal failure and various toxic conditions.

heparin a naturally occurring substance that prevents intravascular clotting. The substance is produced by basophils and mast cells, which are found in large numbers in the connective tissue surrounding capillaries, particularly in the lungs and liver.

histamine a compound found in all cells that is produced by the breakdown of histidine. It is released in allergic inflammatory reactions and causes dilation of capillaries, a decrease in blood pressure, an increase in the secretion of gastric juice, and constriction of smooth muscles of the bronchi and uterus.

hub the part of a syringe where the needle attaches.

Huber needle a special needle used to access implantable medical ports. The Huber needle has a hole on the side rather than on the tip. This design slices through the membrane of the implantable medication port and does not core out a segment of the membrane. This reduces the chance of leaking through the opening of the port.

hyperkalemia greater than normal amounts of potassium in the blood.

hypersensitivity reaction an inappropriate and excessive response of the immune system to a sensitizing antigen called an **allergen.**

hypertension a common disorder that is a known cardiovascular disease risk factor. Hypertension is characterized by elevated blood pressure over the normal values of 120/80 mm Hg in an adult older than 18 years.

hypertensive emergency a severe elevation in blood pressure complicated by evidence of end-organ damage. End-organ damage can occur in the kidneys (kidney failure), heart (heart failure), and brain (intracranial bleed or altered level of consciousness). Also known as **malignant hypertension.**

hypertensive urgency a severe elevation of blood pressure without evidence of end-organ damage.

hypertonic pertaining to a solution that causes cells to shrink. Hypertonic solution increases the degree of osmotic pressure on a semipermeable membrane.

hypertonic saline solution a saline solution that contains 1% to 23.4% sodium chloride (compared with normal saline solution at 0.9%).

hypoglycemia a less than normal amount of glucose in the blood, usually caused by administration of too much insulin, exces-

sive secretion of insulin by the islet cells of the pancreas, or dietary deficiency.

hypoglycemic unawareness the inability to recognize impending hypoglycemic episodes; often considered an adverse effect of beta blockers.

hypokalemia a condition in which an inadequate amount of potassium, the major intracellular cation, is found in the circulating bloodstream.

hypotension an abnormal condition in which the blood pressure is not adequate for normal perfusion and oxygenation of the tissues.

hypotensive resuscitation a resuscitation strategy to provide fluids to a trauma patient in which the goal is not to return the vital signs to normal, but to maintain physiologic functioning until the source of hemorrhage can be controlled.

hypotonic a solution having a lower concentration of solute than another solution and thus exerting less osmotic pressure than that solution.

hypovolemic shock a state of physical collapse and prostration caused by massive blood loss, approximately one fifth or more of total blood volume.

hypoxia inadequate oxygen tension at the cellular level.

hypoxic respiratory drive a condition in which patients require a mild degree of hypoxia to continue breathing as a result of chronic respiratory disease.

I

idiosyncratic response a rare and unpredicted response to a drug that is unique to the patient experiencing the response. Such a response is not allergic in nature.

immunities exemption from a duty or an obligation generally required by law, such as an exemption from taxation or penalty for wrongdoing, or protection against liability.

infiltration the process in which a fluid passes into the tissues, such as when a local anesthetic is administered or an IV infusion infiltrates.

infusion pump an apparatus designed to deliver measured amounts of a drug or IV solution through injection over time.

infusion set another term to describe IV administration sets, or setups. Includes a bag of IV fluids, drip chamber, roller clamp, administration port, and IV catheter.

inhalation administration (of medication) the administration of a drug by inspiration of the vapor released from a fragile ampule packed in a fine mesh that is crushed for immediate administration.

inhaled medication medication that can be administered parenterally to bronchi and lungs by having the patient breathe or inhale the medication. In the prehospital setting, inhaled medications can be administered in two basic ways: the metered-dose inhaler and the pneumatically powered nebulizer.

inhaler a device for administering medications to be inhaled, such as vapors, fine powders, or volatile substances.

injectable medication parenteral delivery of a medication by using either IV, intramuscular, or subcutaneous routes of administration.

injection port area placed along the IV tubing where the provider can inject the contents of a syringe into the IV line.

inotropic drug a drug or substance that increase the force of cardiac contractions.

insulin a naturally occurring polypeptide hormone secreted by the beta cells of the islets of Langerhans in the pancreas in response to increased levels of glucose in the blood, as well as the parasympathetic nervous system and other stimuli.

insulin syringe a specially designed and labeled syringe in which the barrel is calibrated and labeled with the units of insulin and not volume, as most syringes are labeled. Most insulin syringes are calibrated and labeled for use with U-100 insulin.

interstitial fluid an extracellular fluid that fills the spaces between most of the cells of the body and provides a substantial portion of the liquid environment of the body.

intracellular fluid (ICF) an extracellular fluid that fills the spaces between most of the cells of the body and provides a substantial portion of the liquid environment of the body.

intracranial pressure (ICP) following injury to the brain, the brain will swell within the confines of the rigid skull, increasing the pressure within the skull and on the brain.

intramedullary space the highly vascular, central cavity of the bone in which an intraosseous needle can be placed to allow the administration of IV fluids, blood, and medications.

intramuscular (IM) the introduction of a hypodermic needle into a muscle to administer a medication.

intraosseous (IO) infusion the injection of blood, medications, or fluids into bone marrow rather than into a vein.

intraparenchymal hematoma typically refers to bleeding within the brain caused by trauma or hemorrhagic stroke. Also can be used to refer to bleeding within the substance of other organs such as the liver or spleen.

intravascular space pertaining to the inside of a blood vessel.

intravenous (IV) pertaining to the inside of a vein, or a route of administration of a injection, infusion, or catheter.

intravenous infusion a solution administered into a vein through an infusion set that includes a plastic or glass vacuum bottle or bag containing the solution and tubing connecting the bottle to a catheter or a needle in the patient's vein.

intravenous pump a pump designed to regulate the rate of flow of a fluid administered through an IV catheter.

intrinsic originating from or situated within an organ or tissue.

intubation the insertion of a breathing tube through the mouth or nose into the trachea to ensure a patent airway for the delivery of anesthetic gases, oxygen, or both.

irreversible binding a condition in which a drug permanently binds to a receptor.

ischemia a decreased supply of oxygenated blood to a body part.

ischemic heart disease a pathologic condition caused by lack of oxygen in cells of the myocardium.

isotonic fluids pertaining to a solution that causes no change in cell volume.

IV piggyback (IVPB) a special coupling in the primary tubing that allows a supplementary, or piggyback, solution to run into the IV system.

IV push (IVP) a rapid form of a bolus typically used in life-threatening conditions in which a syringe containing a medication is connected to the injection port of IV tubing and then injected slowly into the IV line.

K

ketoacidosis acidosis accompanied by an accumulation of ketones in the body, resulting from extensive breakdown of fats because of faulty carbohydrate metabolism.

ketone bodies products of lipid pyruvate metabolism, beta-hydroxybutyric acid, and aminoacetic acid, from which acetone may spontaneously arise. Excessive production leads to their excretion in urine, such as in diabetes mellitus.

ketonemia the presence of ketones, mainly acetone, in the blood. It is characterized by the fruity breath odor of ketoacidosis.

kilo combining form meaning "one thousand."

KVO a common abbreviation meaning "keep vein open."

L

lactic acidosis a disorder characterized by an accumulation of lactic acid in the blood, resulting in a lowered pH in muscle and serum.

latent period the interval between the time of exposure to an injurious dose of radiation and the adverse response. The term is also used to refer to the interval from administration of a drug to the desired effect. When speaking of medications, another name for latent period is "onset of action."

lethal dose (LD50) the amount of toxin that produces death in all members of a species population within a specified period of time.

lipophilic a drug or substance that dissolves in lipids (fat). Medications that are lipophilic are able to be dissolved in body fat and easily cross the membranes that separate the various body compartments.

lipophobic a drug or substance that does not dissolve in lipids (fat). Medications that are lipophobic are not able to dissolve in body fat and cannot cross the membranes that separate the various body compartments.

loading dose a rapidly administered and often larger dose of a medication used to elevate serum drug concentration to a therapeutic concentration.

loop of Henle the U-shaped part of a renal tubule, consisting of a thin descending limb and a thick ascending limb.

low-molecular-weight heparin a class of drugs used to prevent potentially fatal blood clots in patients undergoing surgery or other patients at risk for blood clots.

Luer-lock syringes a syringe fitted with a threaded tip, allowing a needle to be screwed into the tip. The Luer-lock allows the needle to be attached to the barrel with greater security. This type of syringe is required for use in needleless IV systems.

M

macrodrip chamber the drip compartment immediately below the IV bag where the IV fluid drips at a predetermined volume. Macrodrip chambers drip at 10, 12, 15, and 20 drops/mL.

macrodrip infusion set an IV tubing set that contains a macrodrip chamber.

malignant hypertension the most lethal form of hypertension, characterized by severely elevated blood pressure that commonly damages the intima of small vessels, the brain, the retina, the heart, and the kidneys.

malignant hyperthermia a rare genetic hypermetabolic condition characterized by severe hyperthermia and rigidity of the skeletal muscles occurring in affected people exposed to inhalation anesthetics and succinylcholine, a nondepolarizing muscle relaxant.

mechanism of action the chemical or physiologic method of how a medication affects the target tissue.

medical direction the process by which physicians direct and monitor the care given in the prehospital environment within an EMS system.

metabolism the aggregate of all chemical processes that take place in living organisms, resulting in growth, generation of energy, elimination of wastes, and other body functions as they relate to the distribution of nutrients in the blood after digestion.

metered-dose inhaler (MDI) a device designed to deliver a measured dose of an inhaled drug.

methemoglobin A poisonous form of hemoglobin that does not release oxygen as well as normal hemoglobin.

metric system a decimal system of measurement based on the meter (39.37 inches) as the unit of length, on the gram (15.432 grains) as the unit of weight or mass, and—as a derived unit—on the liter (0.908 U.S. dry quart or 1.0567 U.S. liquid quart) as the unit of volume.

micro prefix meaning "one millionth."

microdrip chamber the compartment immediately below the IV bag where the IV fluid drips at a predetermined volume. Microdrip chambers administer 60 gtt/mL. The number of drops per minute equals the rate of infusion in milliliters per hour. Therefore if 30 drops occur per minute, the infusion rate is 30 mL/hr.

microdrip infusion set an apparatus for delivering relatively small amounts of IV solution at specific flow rates. The size of the drop is controlled by the fixed diameter of the plastic delivery tube. With a microdrip set, 60 drops delivers 1 mL of solution. Microdrip sets deliver small amounts of solution over time, such as when it is necessary to keep a vein open.

microgram (mcg) a unit of measurement of mass equal to one millionth of a gram.

milli combining form meaning "one thousandth."

milligram (mg) a metric unit of weight equal to one thousandth of a gram.

milliliter (mL) a metric unit of volume that is one thousandth (10^{-3}) of a liter, or 1 cm.

mineralocorticoid a hormone secreted by the adrenal cortex that maintains normal blood volume, promotes sodium and water retention, and increases urinary excretion of potassium and hydrogen ions.

monoamine oxidase inhibitor (MAOI) any of a chemically heterogeneous group of drugs used primarily in the treatment of depression.

motor end plate a large special synaptic contact between motor axons and each skeletal muscle fiber. Each muscle fiber forms one end plate.

MTWHF a mnemonic for remembering the effects of nicotinic receptor blockage. The abbreviation stands for *M*ydriasis (dilation of pupils), *T*achycardia, *W*eakness, *H*ypertension and hyperglycemia, and *F*asciculations (involuntary contractions, twitching).

multidrip infusion set an infusion set that allows the paramedic to alternate among a 10-, 15-, and 60-drop set in one system.

muscarinic receptor a type of cholinergic receptor in the parasympathetic nervous system. Muscarinic receptors are found in the cardiac and smooth muscle, exocrine glands, and brain.

myocardial infarction (MI) necrosis of a portion of cardiac muscle caused by an obstruction in a coronary artery from atherosclerosis, a thrombus, or a spasm.

N

narcotic a drug that acts by binding to opiate receptors in the central nervous system and alters perception of pain; induces euphoria, mood changes, mental clouding, and deep sleep; depresses respirations and the cough reflex; constricts the pupils; and causes smooth muscle spasm, decreased peristalsis, emesis, and nausea.

narcotic antagonist a drug that binds to the opiate or narcotic receptor to prevent the opiate from exerting its effects of altered mental status, hypotension, and respiratory depression. Also known as *opiate antagonist.*

nasal cannula a device for delivering oxygen by way of two small tubes inserted into the nares.

nasogastric (NG) pertaining to the nose and stomach, as in (nasogastric) aspiration of the stomach's contents.

nebulization a method of administering a drug by spraying it into the respiratory passages of the patient.

nebulize to vaporize or disperse a liquid in a fine spray.

nebulizer a device for producing a fine spray of medication.

nephrolithiasis a disorder characterized by the presence of calculi in the kidney.

neurogenic shock a form of shock that results from peripheral vascular dilation due to loss of neural input maintaining vascular tone.

neuromuscular junction the area of contact between the ends of a large myelinated nerve fiber and a fiber of skeletal muscle.

Neurotransmitters communicate with the muscle tissue in this area.

neurotransmitter any one of numerous chemicals that modify or result in the transmission of nerve impulses between synapses.

nicotinic receptor a type of cholinergic receptor in the parasympathetic nervous system. Nicotinic receptors are found in the central nervous system, autonomic ganglia, and striated muscle.

noncompetitive antagonist an antagonist that irreversibly binds to a receptor. Regardless of how much of the agonist is given, the effect of the noncompetitive antagonists on the receptor cannot be overcome.

nondepolarizing muscle relaxant medication that produces relaxation of skeletal muscles by preferentially binding to the acetylcholine receptor site, preventing binding of acetylcholine and thereby preventing muscle contraction.

nondepolarizing paralytic another name for a nondepolarizing muscle relaxant.

non–Luer-lock syringe a syringe in which the needle fits tightly on the tip, which is not threaded.

nonrebreather face mask oxygen face mask with one-way exhalation valves on the sides of the mask and the reservoir bag. Nonrebreather face masks require a higher flow rate of 12 to 15 L/min and are capable of delivering oxygen concentrations close to 100%.

nonselective beta blocker beta blockers that bind at both the beta$_1$ and the beta$_2$ receptor.

nonsteroidal antiinflammatory drug (NSAID) any of a group of drugs having antipyretic, analgesic, and antiinflamatory effects.

nonvented infusion set infusion sets that do not have a port for air to flow into the closed fluid container. Nonvented sets are used for fluids not packaged in glass containers, such as crystalloid solutions.

O

offline medical direction medical control in which the physician is not available for real-time interactions.

one-time order when a prehospital provider consults medical direction and receives an order for immediate drug intervention.

online medical direction medical direction in which the prehospital provider is able to consult and obtain direction and orders in real time by radio or telephone communication.

onset of action the time required after administration of a drug for a response to be observed.

opiate an opioid drug that contains opium, derivatives of opium, or any of several semisynthetic or synthetic drugs with opiumlike activity. A substance that causes sleep or relief of pain.

opiate receptor transmembrane protein that binds to endogenous opioid neuropeptides and exogenous morphine and similar natural or synthetic compounds.

ordinary negligence the failure to exercise the degree of care that another reasonable person would exercise in the same or similar situation in which harm to another person results. Also known as *basic negligence.*

organophosphate a class of anticholinesterase chemicals used in certain pesticides and war gases. They act by causing irreversible inhibition of cholinesterase.

osmosis the movement of a pure solvent, such as water, through a differentially permeable membrane, from a solution that has a lower solute concentration to one that has a higher solute concentration.

osmotic demyelination syndrome (ODS) a neurologic condition associated with the too-rapid correction of hyponatremia. Symptoms include headache, alterations in behavior, obtundation, coma, and death.

osmotic diuretic a medication that when excreted by the kidneys cannot be reabsorbed by the kidneys and prevents the reabsorption of excreted water. This produces the rate of urine production.

P

packed red blood cells (PRBCs) a preparation of blood cells separated from liquid plasma, often administered in severe anemia to restore adequate levels of hemoglobin and red cells without overloading the vascular system with excess fluids.

parasympathetic nervous system the division of the autonomic nervous system that slows heart rate, increases intestinal peristalsis and gland activity, and relaxes sphincters.

parenteral administration route that bypasses the GI tract.

parenteral route pertaining to a medication administered by a route other than the gastrointestinal tract, such as a drug given by injection.

paroxysmal supraventricular tachycardia (PSVT) an ectopic heart rhythm with a rate of 170 to 250 beats/min. It begins abruptly with a premature atrial or ventricular beat and is supported by an atrioventricular nodal reentry mechanism or by an atrioventricular reentry mechanism involving an accessory pathway.

partial rebreather face mask see **rebreather face mask.**

partial refusal when a patient agrees to some, but not all, of the treatment offered.

passive diffusion when medications penetrate cells by diffusion through the cell membrane.

passive transport the movement of small molecules across the membrane of a cell by diffusion. Passive transport occurs when the chemicals outside a cell become concentrated and start moving into the cell, changing the intracellular equilibrium.

peak expiratory flow rate (PEFR) the greatest rate of airflow that can be achieved during forced expiration beginning with the lungs fully inflated.

percutaneous coronary intervention (PCI) the management of coronary artery occlusion by any of various catheter-based techniques, such as percutaneous transluminal coronary angioplasty, atherectomy, angioplasty using the excimer laser, and implementation of coronary stents and related devices.

percutaneous transluminal coronary angioplasty (PTCA) a technique in the treatment of atherosclerotic coronary heart disease and angina pectoris in which some plaques in the arteries of the heart are flattened against the arterial walls, resulting in improved circulation.

pericardial tamponade compression of the heart produced by the accumulation of blood or other fluid in the pericardial sac.

peripheral line a term that applies to an IV catheter inserted in a peripheral vein.

peripherally inserted central catheter (PICC line) a long catheter introduced through a vein in the arm, then through the subclavian vein into the superior vena cava or right atrium to administer parenteral fluids or medications or to measure central venous pressure.

peritoneal dialysis a dialysis procedure performed to correct an imbalance of fluid or electrolytes in the blood or to remove toxins, drugs, or other wastes normally excreted by the kidney. The peritoneum is used as a diffusible membrane.

pharmacodynamics the study of how a drug acts on a living organism, including the pharmacologic response and the duration and magnitude of response observed relative to the concentration of the drug at an active site in the organism.

pharmacokinetics the study of the action of drugs within the body, including studies of the mechanisms of drug absorption, distribution, metabolism, and excretion; onset of action; duration of effect; biotransformation; and effects and routes of excretion of the metabolites of the drug.

pharmacologic antagonism occurs when a drug binds to a receptor and prevents the biologic effect of that receptor.

pharmacology the study of the preparation, properties, uses, and actions of drugs.

phenytoin equivalent (PE) to avoid the need to perform dose conversions between phenytoin and fosphenytoin, the dosage for fosphenytoin is prescribed in phenytoin equivalents (PE).

pheochromocytoma a vascular tumor of chromaffin tissue of the adrenal medulla or sympathetic paraganglia, characterized by hypersecretion of epinephrine and norepinephrine, causing persistent or intermittent hypertension.

phlebitis inflammation of a vein accompanied by the formation of a clot.

phosphodiesterase inhibitor a class of drugs that increase inotropism by increasing the concentration of calcium inside the cardiac cell.

photophobia abnormal sensitivity to light, especially by the eyes. The condition is prevalent in albinism and various diseases of the conjunctiva and cornea and may be a symptom of such disorders as measles, psittacosis, encephalitis, Rocky Mountain spotted fever, and Reiter's syndrome.

piggyback infusion see **IV piggyback**

placenta a highly vascular fetal organ that exchanges with the maternal circulation, mainly by diffusion of oxygen, carbon dioxide, and other substances.

plunger the inner portion of the syringe that pushes the liquid medication to the tip of the syringe and out the needle.

pneumothorax the presence of air or gas in the pleural space, causing a lung or collapse. Pneumothorax may be the result of an open chest wound that permits the entrance of air, the rupture of an emphysematous vesicle on the surface of the lung, or without apparent cause.

Poiseuille's law the law of physics that governs the movement of an incompressible fluid through a circular tube.

polypharmacy the use of a number of different drugs, possibly prescribed by different doctors and filled in different pharmacies, by a patient who may have one or several health problems.

potency a term used to compare the different doses of two medications in producing the same effect.

potentiation when a drug lacking a particular effect of its own increases the effect of a second drug.

precursor a prognostic characteristic or feature of a patient's health data, such as a radiographic or laboratory finding, that is associated with a higher or lower risk of death than average.

preeclampsia an abnormal condition of pregnancy characterized by the onset of acute hypertension after the twenty-fourth week of gestation.

prefilled tube a medication-filled cylinder to assist in medication administration.

preloaded syringe a two-piece kit with a medication-filled cylinder that rapidly screws to an included syringe to allow rapid drug administration.

premature ventricular complex (PVC) a ventricular depolarization that occurs earlier than expected.

pressure bag a sleeve placed around a bag of IV fluids to increase the pressure of the IV fluids and increase the flow rate of the IV fluid. Pressure bags may be applied to arterial lines to prevent backflow of blood into the tubing.

primary brain injury injury that occurs directly to the brain from mechanical forces at the time of the initial insult.

Prinzmetal's angina chest pain caused by reversible, severe coronary artery spasm. It is associated with ST-segment elevation that reverts to normal within minutes. The ST-segment elevation indicates total occlusion of the epicardial coronary artery.

prn order abbreviation for *pro re nata*, a Latin phrase meaning "as needed," referring to administration times that are determined by the patient's needs.

prodrug an inactive or partially active drug that is metabolically changed in the body to an active drug.

protocol a written plan specifying the procedures to be followed in giving a particular examination, conducting research, or providing care for a particular condition.

proximate cause a legal concept of cause-and-effect relations in determining, for example, whether an injury would have resulted from a particular cause.

pseudocholinesterase an enzyme that acts as a catalyst in the hydrolysis of acetylcholine to choline and acetate; provides the "off" mechanism during cholinergic neurotransmission.

pulmonary edema the accumulation of extravascular fluid in lung tissues and alveoli, caused most commonly by congestive heart failure.

pulseless electrical activity (PEA) continued electrical rhythmicity of the heart in the absence of effective mechanical function.

pulseless ventricular tachycardia a rapid heart rate that originates in the ventricles and is not associated with a pulse.

Q

qualified immunity immunity that has qualification; the caregiver may not act in a reckless, wanton manner in total disregard to the patient.

R

rapid sequence induction a series of techniques to start general anesthesia with a lower risk of aspiration.

rapid sequence intubation adoption of the techniques of **rapid sequence induction** for the use of emergency intubation.

rebreather face mask breathing device with a face mask and a reservoir bag. Oxygen accumulates in the reservoir bag. During inhalation, the patient inhales oxygen in the reservoir, as well as some room air through the side ports. When the patient exhales, some of the exhaled breath goes back into the reservoir bag, where it is then rebreathed.

receptor a chemical structure, usually of protein/carbohydrate, on the surface of a cell that combines with an antigen to produce a discrete immunologic component.

rectal administration (of a medication) the instillation of a medicated suppository, cream, or gel into the rectum.

refractory period a period during the action potential in which the nerve or muscle tissue will not produce a response if stimulated.

reperfusion therapy administration of a medication that dissolves clots within an artery and reestablishes blood flow.

reversible binding a condition in which a drug is able to separate from the cell's receptor, as in removing a key from a lock. When the drug is removed from the receptor, the effect of the drug stops.

Reye's syndrome a combination of acute encephalopathy and fatty infiltration of the internal organs that may follow acute viral infections. The cause is unknown; however, the administration of aspirin seems to be an association.

roller clamp a device, usually made of plastic, equipped with a small roller that may be rolled counterclockwise to close off primary IV tubing or clockwise to open it.

S

sarin a nerve agent used in chemical warfare.

saturable process when referring to movement of drugs across membranes, a process in which the external concentrations of the drug can reach a point at which increasing the concentration does not result in an increase in the rate of transportation into the cell.

Schedule I a category of drugs not considered legitimate for medical use. Special licensing procedures must be followed to use these substances.

Schedule II a category of drugs considered to have a strong potential for abuse or addiction but that have legitimate medical use.

Schedule III a category of drugs that have less potential for abuse or addiction than Schedule II or I drugs.

Schedule IV a category of drugs that have less potential for abuse or addiction than those of Schedules I to III.

Schedule V a category of drugs that have a small potential for abuse or addiction. The specific drugs in Schedule V vary greatly from state to state.

scope of practice the legally approved skills or practices that may be performed by a provider and the medications authorized to administer as defined in state law.

secondary brain injury a delayed injury to the brain that occurs from swelling of the brain within the rigid confines of the skull, resulting in a decrease in blood flow and oxygen delivery.

sedative an agent that decreases functional activity, diminishes irritability, and allays excitement. Some sedatives have a general effect on all organs; others principally affect the activities of the heart, stomach, intestines, nerve trunks, respiratory system, or vasomotor system.

selective beta blocker a beta blocker that binds with either the beta$_1$ or the beta$_2$ receptor but not both.

Sellick maneuver a technique to reduce the risk of aspiration of stomach contents during induction of general anesthesia; applied before intubation, immediately after injection of anesthetic drugs, and as a part of rapid sequence intubation.

septic shock a form of shock that occurs in septicemia when endotoxins or exotoxins are released from certain bacteria in the bloodstream.

serotonin a naturally occurring derivative of tryptophan found in platelets and cells of the brain and the intestine. Serotonin is released from platelets when damage occurs to the blood vessel walls.

shaft the long portion of the needle that attaches to the hub.

shelf life the period of time a medication can be stored and remain suitable for use.

side effect any reaction to or consequence of a medication or therapy, usually undesirable.

single dose administration of one dose of a medication without the need for repeat administration to be therapeutic.

sinus rhythm a cardiac rhythm stimulated by the sinus node. A rate of 60 to 100 beats/min is normal.

six patient rights of drug administration a checklist that should be performed before administering a medication to a patient to improve patient safety in drug administration. The six patient rights are right patient, right drug, right dose, right route, right time, and right administration.

slow-reacting substance of anaphylaxis (SRS-A) a group of active substances, including histamine and leukotrienes, that are released during an anaphylactic reaction. They cause the smooth muscle contraction and vascular dilation that result in the signs and symptoms of anaphylaxis.

somatic nervous system the division of the nervous system that controls skeletal muscles and movement.

spacer device on a metered-dose inhaler, a chamber between the inhaler canister and the patient's mouth where droplets of medication can slow and evaporate so that there is less direct impact on the oropharynx.

stable angina pectoris transient episode of chest pain resulting from myocardial ischemia that predictably occurs with exercise, exertion, and stressful situations.

standard of care a written statement describing the rules, actions, or conditions that direct patient care. Standards of care guide practice and can be used to evaluate performance.

standing orders instructions for treatment that are usually specific to a particular patient presentation and may or may not require consultation with medical direction. Standing orders are most appropriate for life-threatening conditions that require immediate intervention.

status epilepticus a medical emergency characterized by continuous seizures occurring without interruptions and lasting more than 30 minutes.

sternum the elongated flattened bone forming the middle part of the thorax.

steroid hormones any of the ductless gland secretions that contain the basic steroid nucleus in their chemical formulas. The natural steroid hormones include the androgens, estrogens, and adrenal cortex secretions.

stroke volume the amount of blood ejected by a ventricle during contraction.

subcutaneous (Sub-Q) the introduction of a hypodermic needle into the subcutaneous tissue beneath the skin, usually on the upper arm, thigh, or abdomen.

subcutaneous (Sub-Q) space a continuous layer of connective tissue over the entire body between the skin and the deep fascial investment of the specialized structures of the body, such as the muscles.

subdural hematoma an accumulation of blood in the subdural space, usually caused by an injury.

sublingual (SL) administration (of a medication) the administration of a drug, usually in tablet form, by placing it beneath the tongue until the tablet dissolves.

substrate a chemical acted on and changed by an enzyme in a chemical reaction.

summation the concentration of a neurotransmitter at a synapse, either by increasing the frequency of nerve impulses in each fiber or by increasing the number of fibers stimulated, so that the threshold of the postsynaptic neuron is overcome and an impulse is transmitted.

suppurative thrombophlebitis an infection of a vein that can be complicated by septic thrombosis, bacteremia, metastatic abscesses, and even death.

supraventricular tachycardia (SVT) any cardiac rhythm with a rate exceeding 100 beats/min that originates above the branching part of the atrioventricular bundle.

sympathetic nervous system the division of the autonomic nervous system that accelerates heart rate, constricts blood vessels, and raises blood pressure.

sympathomimetic drug a pharmacologic agent that mimics the effects of stimulation of organs and structures by the sympathetic nervous system. It functions by occupying adrenergic receptor sites and acting as an agonist or by increasing the release of the neurotransmitter norepinephrine at postganglionic nerve endings.

synapse the region surrounding the point of contact between two neurons or between a neuron and an effector organ, across which nerve impulses are transmitted through the action of a neurotransmitter.

synaptic cleft the microscopic extracellular space at the synapse that separates the membrane of the terminal nerve endings of a presynaptic neuron and the membrane of a postsynaptic cell.

synergism the observed effect of two medications, when given at the same time, being greater than the effects of the medications when given individually.

syringe a device for withdrawing, injecting, or instilling fluids. A syringe for the injection of medication usually consists of a calibrated glass or plastic cylindric barrel that has a close-fitting plunger at one end and a small opening at the other to which the head of a hollow-bore needle is fitted.

syrup of ipecac an emetic preparation of ipecac fluid extract, glycerin, and syrup used to treat certain types of poisonings and drug overdoses.

T

tardive dyskinesia an abnormal condition characterized by involuntary repetitious movements of the muscles of the face, limbs, and trunk. This disorder most commonly affects older people who have been treated for extended periods with phenothiazine.

teratogenic any substance, agent, or process that interferes with normal prenatal development, causing the formation of one or more developmental abnormalities in the fetus.

therapeutic index (TI) the difference between the minimal therapeutic and minimal toxic concentrations of a drug.

thionamide agent oral antithyroid medications commonly used for long-term management of hyperthyroidism.

thrombolytic a drug or other agent that dissolves thrombi.

thrombophlebitis inflammation of a vein accompanied by the formation of a clot.

thyrotoxicosis a multisystemic autoimmune disorder characterized by pronounced hyperthyroidism, usually associated with an enlarged thyroid gland and exophthalmos (abnormal protrusion of the eyeball).

tibial tuberosity a characteristic elevation on the anterior and proximal portion of the tibia that can be palpated as a small bony bump on the lower leg immediately below the knee.

tip the portion of a syringe where the needle attaches.

TKO an abbreviation for "to keep open,"

referring to a minimal IV infusion rate to keep the catheter from clotting.

tonic-clonic seizure an epileptic seizure characterized by a generalized involuntary muscular contraction and cessation of respiration followed by tonic and clonic spasms of the muscles.

torsades de pointes a type of ventricular tachycardia with a spiral-like appearance ("twisting of the points") and complexes that at first appear to be positive and then negative on an electrocardiogram.

total body water (TBW) all the water within the body, including intracellular and extracellular water plus the water in the gastrointestinal and urinary tracts.

trade name a name for a drug created by pharmaceutical companies; also known as a *proprietary* or *brand name.* Trade names always begin with a capital letter.

transdermal/topical administration (of a medication) a method of applying a drug to unbroken skin. The drug is continuously absorbed through the skin and enters the systemic system.

traumatic brain injury a broad term applied to mechanical injury to the brain, including such injuries as concussion, subarachnoid hemorrhage, subdural hematoma, and epidural hematoma.

triple-lumen catheter (TLC) any catheter with three separate passages.

type 1 diabetes an autoimmune disease characterized by inability to metabolize fuels, carbohydrates, protein, and fat because of absolute insulin deficiency; can occur at any age, but its incidence is more common in children.

type 2 diabetes a type of diabetes mellitus characterized by insulin resistance in appropriate hepatic glucose production and impaired insulin secretion; onset is usually after 40 years of age but can occur at any age, including during childhood and adolescence.

U

United States Pharmacopeia-National Formulary (USP-NF) a compendium recognized officially by the Federal Food, Drug, and Cosmetic Act that contains descriptions, uses, strengths, and standards of purity for selected drugs and for all their forms of dosage.

unstable angina pectoris (UA) angina pectoris, commonly known as angina, is chest pain due to ischemia (a lack of blood and hence oxygen supply) of the heart muscle, generally due to obstruction or spasm of the coronary arteries (the heart's blood vessels). Coronary artery disease, the main cause of angina, is due to atherosclerosis of the cardiac arteries. The term derives from the Greek *ankhon* (strangling) and the Latin *pectus* (chest), and can therefore be translated as "a strangling feeling in the chest."

V

variant angina see **Prinzmetal's angina**

vastus lateralis the largest of the four muscles of the quadriceps femoris group, situated on the lateral side of the thigh.

vented infusion set infusion sets necessary for the administration of fluids. Vented sets have a side port at the drip chamber that can be opened to allow air to flow into the closed fluid container.

ventricular fibrillation (VF) a cardiac arrhythmia marked by rapid depolarizations of the ventricular myocardium.

ventricular tachycardia (VT) tachycardia of at least three consecutive ventricular complexes with a rate greater than 100 per minute. It originates in a focus within the ventricle.

ventrogluteal injection a region of the hip where injections can be safely administered in children.

Venturi mask a respiratory therapy face mask designed to allow inspired air to mix with oxygen, which is supplied through a jet at a fixed concentration.

vial a glass container with a metal-enclosed rubber seal.

volume the amount of space occupied by a body, expressed in cubic units.

volume-control chamber any one of several types of transparent plastic reservoirs with graduated volumetric markings used to regulate the flow of IV solutions. These devices are components of IV volume control sets and accommodate the injection and mixing of medications by special built-in ports.

volume of distribution a measure of how rapidly and to what extent a drug can move throughout the body. A drug with a high volume of distribution is fat soluble and can easily pass through membranes and into the various body compartments.

VX A thin, amber-colored, odorless liquid that resembles motor oil and may be used as a nerve agent.

W

Wernicke-Korsakoff syndrome the coexistence of Wernicke's encephalopathy and Korsakoff's syndrome.

Wolff-Parkinson-White (WPW) syndrome a disorder of atrioventricular conduction involving an accessory pathway; often identified by a characteristic delta wave seen on an electrocardiogram at the beginning of the QRS complex.

Z

Z-track technique a technique for injecting irritating preparations into muscle without tracking residual medication through sensitive tissues.

zero-order kinetics a state at which the rate of an enzyme reaction is independent of the concentration of the substrate.

Index

Page numbers followed by *f* indicate figures; *t*, tables; *b*, boxes.